Coronary Heart Disease: Diagnosis and Assessment

Coronary Heart Disease: Diagnosis and Assessment

Edited by Janice Hunter

hayle medical
New York

Hayle Medical,
750 Third Avenue, 9th Floor,
New York, NY 10017, USA

Visit us on the World Wide Web at:
www.haylemedical.com

ISBN: 978-1-63241-487-8

The publisher's policy is to use permanent paper from mills that operate a sustainable forestry policy. Furthermore, the publisher ensures that the text paper and cover boards used have met acceptable environmental accreditation standards.

Printed in China.

Cataloging-in-Publication Data

Coronary heart disease : diagnosis and assessment / edited by Janice Hunter
p. cm.
Includes bibliographical references and index.
ISBN 978-1-63241-487-8
1. Coronary heart disease. 2. Coronary heart disease--Diagnosis.
I. Hunter, Janice.

RC685.C6 C67 2018
616.123--dc23

Table of Contents

Preface

Coronary heart disease is a group of diseases that include stable angina, unstable angina, myocardial infraction, sudden cardiac death, etc. Unhealthy food habits, smoking and alcoholism are some of the main causes of this group of diseases. Interventions that can stop progressive development of heart disease include peripheral and valvular surgery, implantable devices and heart transplantation. The extensive contents of this book provide the readers with a thorough understanding of the subject. For all those who are interested in coronary heart disease, this book can prove to be an essential guide.

Various studies have approached the subject by analyzing it with a single perspective, but the present book provides diverse methodologies and techniques to address this field. This book contains theories and applications needed for understanding the subject from different perspectives. The aim is to keep the readers informed about the progresses in the field; therefore, the contributions were carefully examined to compile novel researches by specialists from across the globe.

Indeed, the job of the editor is the most crucial and challenging in compiling all chapters into a single book. In the end, I would extend my sincere thanks to the chapter authors for their profound work. I am also thankful for the support provided by my family and colleagues during the compilation of this book.

Editor

Chronic Total Occlusions in Sweden – A Report from the Swedish Coronary Angiography and Angioplasty Registry (SCAAR)

Truls Råmunddal[1]*, Loes Hoebers[2], Jose P. S. Henriques[2], Christian Dworeck[1], Oskar Angerås[1], Jacob Odenstedt[1], Dan Ioanes[1], Göran Olivecrona[3], Jan Harnek[3], Ulf Jensen[4], Mikael Aasa[4], Risto Jussila[4], Stefan James[5], Bo Lagerqvist[5], Göran Matejka[1], Per Albertsson[1], Elmir Omerovic[1]

1 Department of Cardiology, Sahlgrenska University Hospital, Gothenburg, Sweden, **2** Department of Cardiology, Academic Medical Center, Amsterdam, The Netherlands, **3** Department of Coronary Heart Disease, Skåne University Hospital, Scania, Sweden, **4** Department of Cardiology, Stockholm South General Hospital, Stockholm, Sweden, **5** Department of Medical Sciences, Uppsala University, Uppsala, Sweden

Abstract

Introduction: Evidence for the current guidelines for the treatment of patients with chronic total occlusions (CTO) in coronary arteries is limited. In this study we identified all CTO patients registered in the Swedish Coronary Angiography and Angioplasty Registry (SCAAR) and studied the prevalence, patient characteristics and treatment decisions for CTO in Sweden.

Methods and Results: Between January 2005 and January 2012, 276,931 procedures (coronary angiography or percutaneous coronary intervention) were performed in 215,836 patients registered in SCAAR. We identified all patients who had 100% luminal diameter stenosis known or assumed to be ≥3 months old. After exclusion of patients with previous coronary artery bypass graft (CABG) surgery or coronary occlusions due to acute coronary syndrome, we identified 16,818 CTO patients. A CTO was present in 10.9% of all coronary angiographies and in 16.0% of patients with coronary artery disease. The majority of CTO patients were treated conservatively and PCI of CTO accounted for only 5.8% of all PCI procedures. CTO patients with diabetes and multivessel disease were more likely to be referred to CABG.

Conclusion: CTO is a common finding in Swedish patients undergoing coronary angiography but the number of CTO procedures in Sweden is low. Patients with CTO are a high-risk subgroup of patients with coronary artery disease. SCAAR has the largest register of CTO patients and therefore may be valuable for studies of clinical importance of CTO and optimal treatment for CTO patients.

Editor: Ingo Ahrens, University Hospital Medical Centre, Germany

Funding: The SCAAR registry is sponsored by the Swedish Health Authorities only and is independent of commercial funding. No current funding sources for this study. The funders had no role in study design, data collection and analysis, decision to publish, or preparation of the manuscript.

Competing Interests: Dr Stefan James has during the last 3 years received institutional research grants from Medtronic, Terumo Inc,Vascular Solutions and served as an advisory board member for Medtronic. Dr Jose P.S. Henriques has received unrestricted research grant from Abbott Vascular. Dr Elmir Omerovic serves as an advisory board member for Astra Zeneca and has received lecturing fees from Medtronic and Astra Zeneca. All other co-authors have no disclosures or potential conflicts of interest.

* Email: truls@wlab.gu.se

These authors contributed equally to this work.

Introduction

Chronic total occlusions (CTO) are difficult to treat with percutaneous coronary intervention (PCI) [1]. Revascularization of CTO demands expert skills, longer procedural time and is associated with higher procedural risks such as coronary perforation, contrast nephropathy, radiation exposure, and loss of collateral circulation [1,2]. According to the European and American guidelines, PCI of CTO has class-IIa recommendation (weight of evidence in favour of the treatments usefulness/efficacy) [3,4] but this recommendation is based on small retrospective studies and on expert consensus.

The true prevalence of a CTO in the general population is unknown and few studies have addressed this question. In observational studies, a CTO was found in approximately one third of the patients referred for coronary angiography [5–7]. However, these studies were based on low number of patients and participating hospitals, and may therefore be prone to selection bias. To date, no epidemiological study has investigated the prevalence and clinical characteristics of CTO patients at the nationwide level.

The Swedish Coronary Angiography and Angioplasty Registry (SCAAR) is a prospective national registry that collects data about all patient undergoing coronary angiography and PCI in Sweden [8]. Therefore, we identified all CTO patients registered in SCAAR and studied prevalence, patient characteristics and treatment decision for CTO in Sweden.

Methods

Swedish Coronary Angiography and Angioplasty Registry (SCAAR)

The SCAAR registry was established in 1999 after the unification of Swedish Coronary Angiography registry (Acta Coronaria) and the Swedish Coronary Angioplasty registry (SCAP). SCAAR, which is a part of the national SWEDEHEART registry, holds data on all consecutive patients from all centres that perform coronary angiography and PCI in Sweden. The registry is independent of commercial funding and is sponsored by the Swedish Health Authorities only. The technology has been developed and administered by the Uppsala Clinical Research Center. Since 2001, SCAAR has been Internet-based, with recording of data online through an Internet interface in the catheterization laboratory; data are transferred in an encrypted format to a central server at the Uppsala Clinical Research Center.

In total, there are 30 hospitals with cardiac catheterization facilities in Sweden of which 9 are university hospitals. In SCAAR, a coronary angiography procedure is described by approximately 50 variables while a PCI procedure allows for is described by approximately 200 variables. The information about clinical characteristics and procedural details is entered into the registry immediately after the procedure by the PCI physician after the review of clinical information.

Ethics statement

The study was approved by the regional ethical review board of Gothenburg University, Gothenburg,Sweden. The regional ethical review board waived the need for written informed consent from the participants according to Swedish legislation and because data were de-identified and anonymized before analysis.

Definitions

We defined CTO as 100% luminal diameter stenosis and the absence of antegrade flow known or assumed to be ≥3 months duration [6,9,10]. Coronary artery disease was defined as a luminal narrowing ≥50% on angiography. Procedural success after PCI treatment of the coronary lesion is defined as residual stenosis <50%, decreased grade of stenosis after intervention by at least 20%, normal blood flow and no serious complications.

Study cohort

We used two different methods to identify CTO patients in SCAAR between January 2005 and January 2012.

The first method is based on the information about %-luminal stenosis at the level of coronary segments that was introduced in 2005. From this date onwards, the information derived from a diagnostic coronary angiogram can also be used to determine if a coronary segment was totally occluded. In order to differentiate between acute and chronic occlusions, we excluded patients who underwent a procedure for acute coronary syndrome in whom the occlusion was located in the same coronary artery as the culprit vessel. Furthermore, we excluded patients who underwent a procedure in the same vessel within the previous 3 months. The CTO patients identified by this method constitute the *coronary segment subcohort*.

The second method is based on the separate variable by which PCI operators classify a treated occlusion either as a chronic occlusion ≥3 months duration or as an acute/subacute occlusion ≤3 months duration.

The patients with previous coronary artery bypass graft (CABG) surgery were excluded from analysis as the patency of the graft could not be determined. The study was scrutinised and approved by the ethics board according to the Swedish law and regulations.

Total CTO cohort

The total CTO cohort contains all CTO patients identified by either of the two methods (**Figure 1**). Patients and procedures in which the same CTO lesion was registered through both methods or at multiple occasions were identified and duplicate observations were excluded from the analysis. For each patient, the procedure where the CTO was observed first was selected.

Coronary segment subcohort

We also present data from the subcohort of patients who were identified according to whether they had a 100% luminal stenosis and considered to be a CTO based on the above mentioned inclusion criteria. We compared patient characteristics and treatment decisions between patients with significant coronary artery disease in whom a CTO was observed or not. Prevalence of a CTO was calculated only from the coronary segment subcohort and in relation to three different denominators: the number of unique procedures, the number of unique patients and the number of unique patients with significant coronary artery disease.

Validation of CTO

Validation of the CTO definition was performed in a subgroup of 955 patients from one university hospital (Sahlgrenska University Hospital) and from three county hospitals (Norra Älvsborgs Hospital, Borås Hospital, Skövde Hospital). This subgroup represents 5.7% of all identified CTO patients in SCAAR in the study period. The patients were randomly selected by means of random number generator using Stata software (Version 12.1, StataCorp, College Station, Texas, USA). The validation procedure was conducted by a panel consisting of five experienced interventional cardiologists. The panellists examined individual coronary angiograms according to a monitoring plan defined in advance. Each angiogram was evaluated in regard to whether the patient had previous CABG, whether the treated occlusion was ≥3 months old and whether 100% segmental stenosis on angiogram was an occlusion ≥3 months old. The results from the validation procedure were then compared to the data entered in SCAAR.

Statistical analysis

Differences in baseline characteristics between the groups were tested by the χ^2 test for categorical variables while Mann–Whitney U test and Kruskal-Wallis test were used for comparison of continuous non-normally distributed variables. We used Shapiro-Wilks test to test for normal distribution. Tests for trends were made using linear contrasts of means in a one-way analysis of variance model for numerical data and the Armitage-Cohrane trend test for categorical data. We used logistic regression with test for linear trend to evaluate whether annual incidence of CTO and success rate for PCI of CTO changed during the study period. Statistical significance was defined as a P-value<0.05. All analyses were performed using Stata software (Version 13.1, StataCorp, College Station, Texas, USA).

Results

Prevalence of CTO in Sweden

As of January 2012, 497,572 procedures (coronary angiographies and PCIs) performed in 348,863 patients were registered in SCAAR. The numbers of PCIs and coronary angiographies

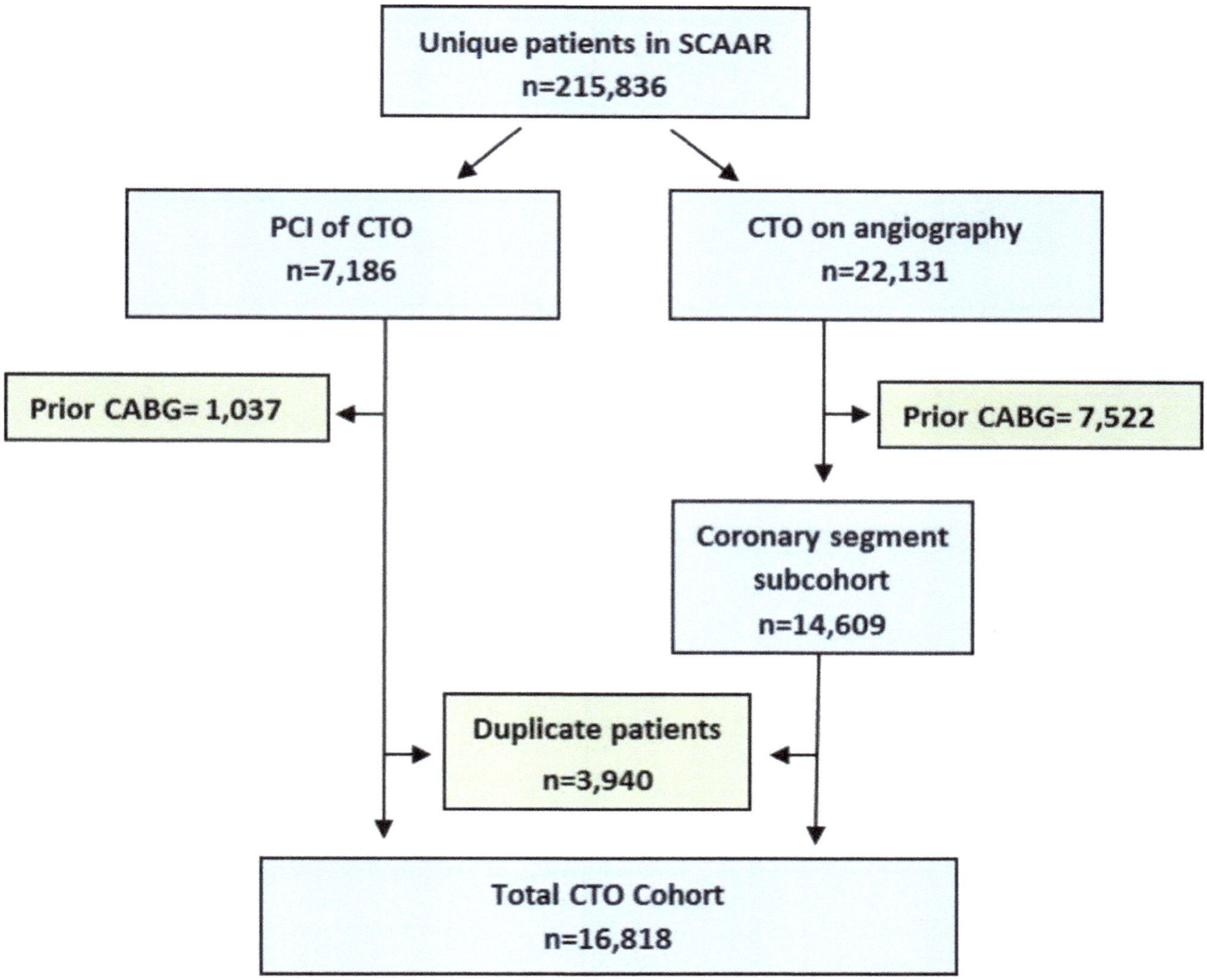

Figure 1. Flow chart for identification and selection of CTO patients in SCAAR. Based on the selection methods we have defined two CTO groups. The first group - *the total CTO cohort*- contains all CTO patients recognized by one or both methods during the period. The second group is the subcohort that contains the patients in whom a CTO was identified through the %-luminal stenosis on the coronary segments – *the coronary segment subcohort.*

increased since 1999 (**Figure 2**). The annual rate of PCIs for CTO remained low (~1200 in 2011).

Between January 2005 and January 2012, Swedish interventionalists completed 276,931 procedures in 215,836 patients. The total number of CTO patients without previous CABG during the same period was 16,818 and these patients constitute the total CTO cohort (**Figure 1**).

Information about age of the treated CTO was missing in 0.8% (n = 1077) of all procedures. Of the 134,087 reported PCIs, 7,816 (5.8%) involved the treatment of a CTO. These procedures were performed in 29 different hospitals on 7,186 unique patients of whom 6,149 without prior CABG. Almost half (43%) of all CTO procedures were performed at university hospitals. Data on procedural success was missing in 12 procedures (0.2%). The overall success rate was 53.1%. The annual success rate did not change significantly during the study period with 54.4% in 2005 and 56.6% in 2012 (OR 1.02, 95% CI 0.99–1.06; P = 0.15 test for linear trend).

Complete information about luminal %-stenosis was available in 160,159 (57.8%) angiographies of which 144,744 were from in patients without previous CABG. A CTO was observed in 10.6% of angiographies from 126,745 patients. Of these patients, 14,609 had at least one CTO resulting in a prevalence of 11.5%. Coronary artery disease was diagnosed in 91,154 patients of which 16.0% had a CTO. In patients who underwent multiple procedures, the CTO was diagnosed on the first diagnostic angiogram in 90% of the cases. The annual number of diagnosed CTO in patients undergoing coronary angiography decreased gradually by 25% from 11.5% in 2005 to 8.6% in 2012 (OR 0.97; 95% CI 0.96–0.98; P<0.001 test for linear trend). In patients with significant coronary artery disease, CTO decreased by 12% from 17.2 in 2005 to 15.1 in 2012 (OR 0.95; 95% CI 0.94–0.96; P< 0.001 test for linear trend).

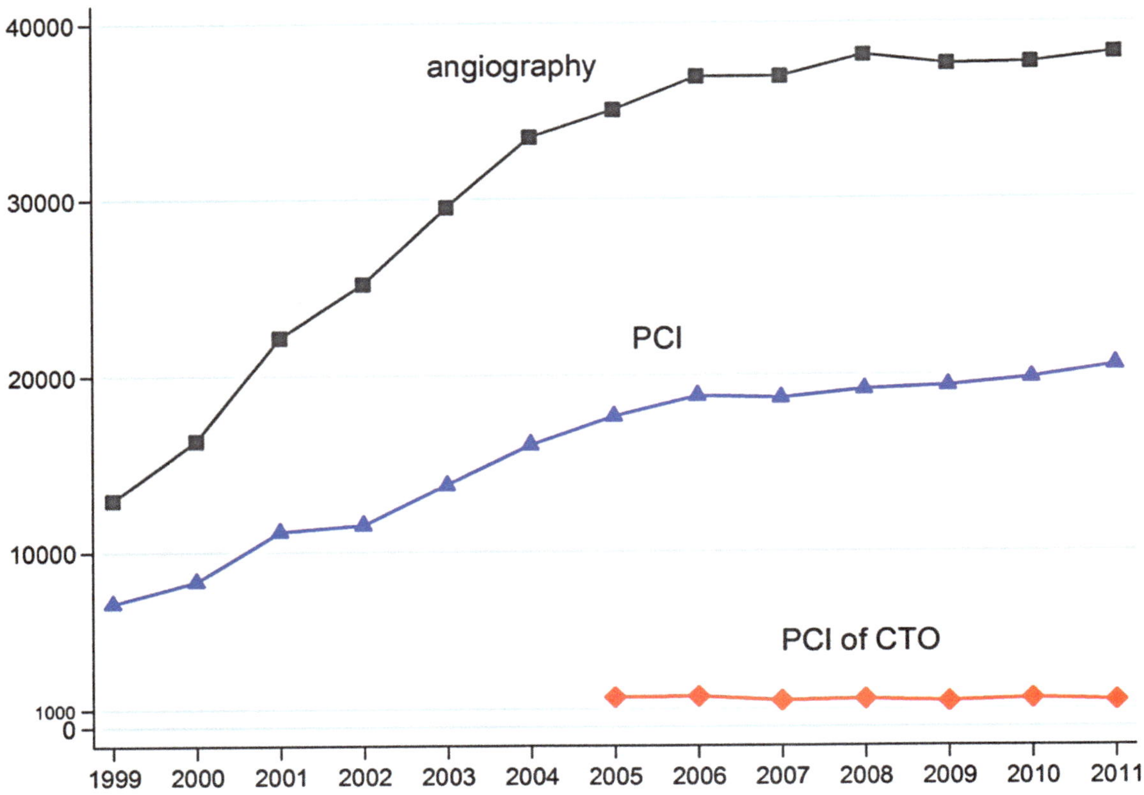

Figure 2. Annual number of coronary angiographies, PCI's, and PCI's performed in CTO patients in Sweden reported in SCAAR since 1999.

Patient characteristics

The clinical characteristics of all CTO patients - the total CTO cohort - registered in SCAAR since 2005 are summarized in **Table 1**. The majority of CTO patients were male. The high occurrence of previous MI (37%) and the presence of traditional cardiovascular risk factors make CTO patients a high-risk population.

Table 2 shows the baseline demographic and angiographic characteristics of patients with coronary artery disease stratified for the presence of a CTO on angiography (coronary segment subcohort). CTO patients were more often males and were more likely to have risk factors including previous MI. In addition, the extent of coronary artery disease was more severe in CTO patients with more multivessel and left main disease. Although CTO was diagnosed in the majority of cases during a coronary angiography for stable angina, a substantial proportion was diagnosed in patients with acute coronary syndrome. Furthermore, patients with a CTO more often presented in cardiogenic shock at presentation for STEMI compared to patients without a CTO. The CTO was more frequently located in the right coronary artery (RCA) followed by the left anterior descending artery (LAD) and left circumflex artery (LCx) (**Figure 3**). In approximately 14%, CTOs were observed in more than one vessel of which only 0.1% included the left main.

Treatment of CTO patients

Table 3 shows the differences in baseline demographic and angiographic characteristics of CTO patients identified through the coronary segment stenosis, according to the received treatment at baseline. After diagnosis, the majority of the CTO patients (56%) received medical treatment only. The CTO patients who received invasive treatment were evenly distributed between PCI (22.3%) and referral for CABG (21.7%). CTO patients, who received medical treatment only, had more often previous MI, presented more often with STEMI, had a lower creatinine clearance and had less severe angina symptoms in comparison to the patients who were treated invasively for a CTO. Patients who were referred for CABG were more often male with a higher prevalence of cardiovascular risk factors including diabetes, had less often previous MI or PCI, presented more often with stable angina and suffered more frequently from extensive coronary artery disease than CTO patients treated with PCI. CTO patients treated for stable angina received medical treatment in 41.6%, PCI in 20.6% and CABG in 37.8%. CTO patients who were treated for acute coronary syndrome received medical treatment in 28.6%, PCI in 71.2%, and were referred to CABG in 0.2%. Procedure-related complications were reported in 5.4% CTO patients treated with PCI. The following complications were reported: death (0%), major bleeding (1.3%), stroke (0.3%), pericardial tamponade (0.4%) renal insufficiency (0.7%), emergency PCI (0.1%), emergency CABG (0%), procedure-related MI (1.1%), anaphylactic reaction (0.1%), other (1.4%)

Validation of CTO

The validation analysis revealed 36 (3.8%) erroneously classified patients. Of these, 18 patients did not have a 100% occluded coronary artery on the coronary angiogram. Another 5 patients

Table 1. Baseline characteristics of the total CTO cohort in SCAAR at the time of diagnosis based on data collected during the period 2005–2012.

	All CTO patients (n = 16,818)	Missing %
Male (%)	77.5	0.0
Age (median, IQR)	68 (60–76)	0.2
Diabetes (%)	23.9	1.0
Hypertension (%)	61.9	2.5
Hyperlipidemia (%)	62.7	2.9
Smoking status (%)		6.2
Current smoker	19.9	
Previous smoker	40.2	
Previous MI (%)	37.2	3.8
Previous PCI (%)	18.4	0.1
Cardiogenic shock (%)*	10.2	1.2
Creatinine Clearance (ml/min)	81 (61–104)	28.2
CCS class (%)**		7.0
I	9.0	
II	52.2	
III	37.4	
IV	1.4	
Indication (%)		0.0
Stable CAD	45.5	
Unstable CAD/NSTEMI	27.5	
STEMI	14.3	
Other	12.7	
Extent of CAD (%)		1.1
1 vessel	20.4	
2 vessel	35.1	
3 vessel	36.1	
Left main disease***	8.4	

CAD: coronary artery disease, CCS: Canadian cardiovascular society, CTO: chronic total occlusion, IQR: inter quartile range, MI: myocardial infarction, (N)STEMI: (non-)ST-elevation myocardial infarction, PCI: percutaneous coronary intervention.
* Cardiogenic shock only displayed for the indication STEMI.
**CCS class only displayed for the indication stable CAD.
*** Left main (LM) disease includes: LM+1 vessel, LM+2 vessel and LM+3 vessel.

had prior CABG and 13 patients had acute or subacute coronary occlusions.

Discussion

In this study, we identified and studied 16,818 CTO patients in SCAAR. We found CTO in every tenth patient undergoing coronary angiography, and that the prevalence of CTO in Sweden decreased by one quarter in these patients between January 2005 and January 2012.

The true prevalence of a CTO in the general population is unknown and not well studied. In a few older studies based on small populations, CTO prevalence was 35% [7] and 52% [5] in patients with significant coronary artery disease. In a recent study from Canada based on 1697 patients, CTO prevalence was 14.7% in all patients undergoing angiography [6]. However, our study shows that the prevalence of CTO was 11.5% in Sweden. The reason for the difference in CTO prevalence between Sweden and other countries may be due to selection bias. While all previous studies were based on selected and relatively small populations, SCAAR holds information from all hospitals that perform coronary angiography and PCI in Sweden which reduces selection bias. Another explanation may be that prevalence of CTO differs between the countries due to variance in severity of coronary artery disease, treatment algorithms for acute coronary syndromes and organization of health care system [11].

Our study shows that CTO patients are a high-risk population with more traditional cardiovascular risk factors, multivessel disease, history of MI and PCI, which is in accordance with previous reports [1,6,9]. Furthermore, a substantial number (14%) of patients had multiple CTO's in separate vessels.

Majority of CTO patients had stable angina but approximately 40% had acute coronary syndrome at the time when CTO was diagnosed. Overall, 56% of the CTO patients were treated with medical treatment initially. The remaining patients were evenly distributed between percutaneous and surgical revascularization similar to the Canadian study [9]. The success rate for CTO procedures in all Swedish hospitals was 53% which is lower than 70% and 80% reported by others [2,6,12]. However, the success

Table 2. Baseline characteristics of patients from coronary segment subcohort with coronary artery disease, stratified for the presence of a CTO observed on angiography.

	CTO observed (n = 14,609)	Missing %	CTO not observed (n = 76,545)	Missing %	P-value
Male gender (%)	77.7	0	70.6	0.0	<0.01
Age (median, IQR)	68 (61–76)	0.2	68 (60–75)	0.2	<0.01
Diabetes (%)	24.0	1.0	18.6	0.8	<0.01
Hypertension (%)	62.0	2.4	52.5	2.0	<0.01
Hyperlipidemia (%)	61.9	2.8	44.4	2.5	<0.01
Smoking status (%)		5.8		5.5	<0.01
Current smoker	20.0		21.6		
Previous smoker	40.0		35.0		
Previous MI (%)	37.0	3.8	16.5	2.3	<0.01
Previous PCI (%)	17.5	0.1	10.7	0.05	<0.01
Cardiogenic shock(%)*	10.1	1.0	3.5	1.3	<0.01
Creatinine Clearance	80	28.2	81	34.2	<0.01
(ml/min)	(60–103)		(62–103)		
CCS class (%)**		6.9		5.5	0.19
I	9.3		9.6		
II	53.4		54.7		
III	36.0		34.5		
IV	1.3		1.2		
Indication (%)		0		0	<0.01
Stable CAD	44.5		17.1		
Unstable CAD/NSTEMI	26.3		49.6		
STEMI	15.1		26.0		
Other	14.0		7.3		
Extent of CAD (%)		1.5		1.2	<0.01
1 vessel	17.4		48.7		
2 vessel	35.1		25.9		
3 vessel	38.3		17.2		
Left main disease***	9.2		8.2		

CAD: coronary artery disease, CCS: Canadian cardiovascular society, CTO: chronic total occlusion, IQR: inter quartile range, MI: myocardial infarction, (N)STEMI: (non-)ST-elevation myocardial infarction, PCI: percutaneous coronary intervention.
* Cardiogenic shock only displayed for the indication STEMI.
**CCS class only displayed for the indication stable CAD.
*** Left main (LM) disease includes: LM+1 vessel, LM+2 vessel and LM+3 vessel.

rate in this study is based on all CTO procedures performed in our country rather than in a single hospital or smaller registries in other studies. The average success of 53% in SCAAR is unlikely to be representative for low- versus high-volume CTO centers [2,10]. Among the 30 hospitals reporting to SCAAR there are only a few high-volume centres with a dedicated CTO program and less than half of the CTO procedures in Sweden were performed at university hospitals. Some evidence suggest that procedural success is closely related to operator experience [13]. However, the recommendation that CTO procedures should be concentrated to dedicated high-volume hospitals needs stronger evidence.

Although CTO patients are common in clinical work, the evidence for the current guidelines and clinical practice is limited. The need for randomized clinical trials in this patient population is pressing; however, only a few such trials are initiated and on-going [12,14]. Until evidence from randomized trials becomes available we will need to identify and utilize the information available from

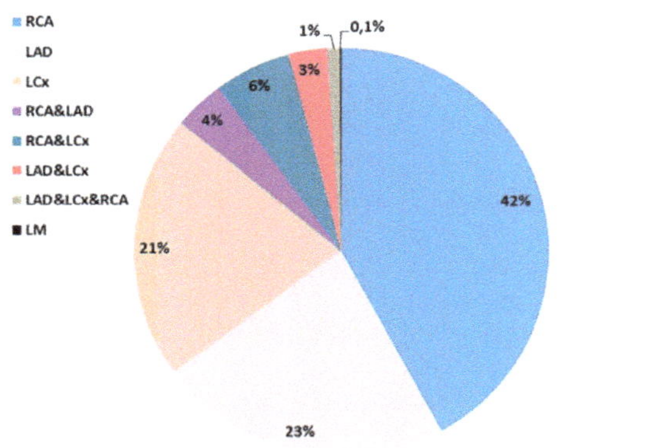

Figure 3. Coronary location of CTO observed at angiography. RCA = right coronary artery, LAD = left descending coronary artery, LCx = left circumflex coronary artery, LM = left main.

Table 3. Baseline characteristics of CTO patients from coronary segment subcohort according to the treatment strategy.

	No PCI of CTO (n = 8,182)		PCI of CTO (n = 3,251)		Referral for CABG (n = 3,172)		
	(%)	**Missing (%)**	**(%)**	**Missing (%)**	**(%)**	**Missing (%)**	**P-value**
Male gender	76.2	0	76.5	0	82.9	0	<0.01
Age (median, IQR)	69 (61–77)	0.2	66 (59–74)	0.2	68 (61–74)	0.2	<0.01
Diabetes	24.0	1.1	21.0	1.2	26.9	0.4	<0.01
Hypertension	61.6	3.0	59.8	2.3	65.2	1.5	<0.01
Hyperlipidemia	58.6	3.4	60.2	2.7	71.2	1.3	<0.01
Smoking status		7.0		5.0		3.6	<0.01
Current smoker	21.4		20.7		15.5		
Previous smoker	39.4		39.5		42.1		
Previous MI	41.3	4.1	33.4	3.5	29.4	3.2	<0.01
Previous PCI	19.9	0.1	20.3	0.2	8.3	0.03	<0.01
Cardiogenic Shock**	10.0	1.0	10.4	0.9	0	0	0.84
Creatinine Clearance (ml/min)	77 (57–101)	31.6	85 (65–109)	26.1	82 (64–102)	21.8	<0.01
CCS class*		7.1		4.6		7.8	<0.01
I	13.2		8.6		5.3		
II	55.2		56.3		49.8		
III	30.3		34.3		43.3		
IV	1.4		0.8		1.6		
Indication		0		0		0	<0.01
Stable CAD	33.1		41.3		77.4		
Unstable CAD/NSTEMI CAD/NSTEMI	31.1		39.8		0.4		
STEMI	21.7		13.5		0		
Other	14.2		5.5		22.2		
Extent of CAD (%)		1.2		1.3		1.3	<0.01
1 vessel	14.9		36.5		4.2		
2 vessel	40.9		39.6		15.8		
3 vessel	37.9		21.1		56.8		
Left main disease***	6.3		2.8		23.2		

CAD: coronary artery disease, CCS: Canadian cardiovascular society, CTO: chronic total occlusion, IQR: inter quartile range, MI: myocardial infarction, (N)STEMI: (non-)ST-elevation myocardial infarction, PCI: percutaneous coronary intervention.

* Cardiogenic shock only displayed for the indication STEMI.

**CCS class only displayed for the indication stable CAD.

*** Left main (LM) disease includes: LM+1 vessel, LM+2 vessel and LM+3 vessel.

Data about initial treatment strategy were missing in four CTO patients.

contemporary databases and quality registries. The SCAAR registry with its distinctive structure covering the whole Swedish nation provides unique possibility to study several important features of CTO's including epidemiology, patients characteristic as well as health outcomes. It contains information about both past and current treatment strategies of these complex patients not only from specialized centers, but also from all hospitals that preforms PCI. Given these circumstances, the SCAAR registry can be an important instrument to address many key questions in CTO.

The prevalence of CTO in Sweden decreased by one quarter during the study period. We hypothesize that this primarily reflects the increasing rate of timely revascularisation with PCI of patients with acute coronary syndrome – STEMI and non-STEMI. Because the prevalence decreased by 25% while the number of procedures remained unchanged, the proportion of CTO procedures increased by the same percentage. Besides the decreased prevalence, the relatively low annual rate of CTO procedures in Sweden may be related to improved treatment of symptoms, better quality of life, fear of complications, technical complexity, and low evidence-level.

There are some important limitations that need to be addressed. First, this is an observational study and as such it provides only associative evidence, not causative. Second, we cannot rule out the possibility of selection bias, as only hospitalized patients are included in the registry. Substantial proportion of missing data in the coronary segment subcohort may have resulted in biased estimate on CTO prevalence. Third, patients with missing data tend to have higher risk and their exclusion from the analysis might have produced biased results. Fourth, we cannot exclude the possibility that some occlusions had duration of less than three months, however the validation of CTO diagnosis and procedures in SCAAR have shown that only 3.8% were erroneously classified.

Conclusions

SCAAR is the largest database of CTO patients to date. CTO is a frequent finding in Swedish population and is diagnosed in every 10th patient undergoing coronary angiography. The prevalence of CTO has decreased by one quarter. Patients with a CTO represent a high risk subgroup of CAD patients. SCAAR may be a valuable source of data in the process of evidence-building in the CTO field.

Acknowledgments

We would like to acknowledge Rosie Perkins for excellent support and scientific editing.

Author Contributions

Conceived and designed the experiments: TR EO LH JPSH CD DI JO OA UJ MA RJ SJ BL GO JH PA GM. Analyzed the data: TR EO LH JPSH CD DI JO OA UJ MA RJ SJ BL GO JH PA GM. Wrote the paper: TR EO LH JPSH CD DI JO OA UJ MA RJ SJ BL GO JH PA GM.

References

1. Grantham JA, Marso SP, Spertus J, House J, Holmes DR Jr, et al. (2009) Chronic total occlusion angioplasty in the United States. JACC Cardiovascular Interventions 2: 479–486.
2. Galassi AR, Tomasello SD, Reifart N, Werner GS, Sianos G, et al. (2011) In-hospital outcomes of percutaneous coronary intervention in patients with chronic total occlusion: insights from the ERCTO (European Registry of Chronic Total Occlusion) registry. EuroIntervention 7: 472–479.
3. Task Force on Myocardial Revascularization of the European Society of C, the European Association for Cardio-Thoracic S, European Association for Percutaneous Cardiovascular I, Kolh P, Wijns W, et al. (2010) Guidelines on myocardial revascularization. Eur J Cardiothorac Surg 38 Suppl: S1–S52.
4. Members WC, Levine GN, Bates ER, Blankenship JC, Bailey SR, et al. (2011) 2011 ACCF/AHA/SCAI Guideline for Percutaneous Coronary Intervention: A Report of the American College of Cardiology Foundation/American Heart Association Task Force on Practice Guidelines and the Society for Cardiovascular Angiography and Interventions. Circulation 124: e574–e651.
5. Christofferson RD, Lehmann KG, Martin GV, Every N, Caldwell JH, et al. (2005) Effect of chronic total coronary occlusion on treatment strategy. AmJCardiol 95: 1088–1091.
6. Fefer P, Knudtson ML, Cheema AN, Galbraith PD, Osherov AB, et al. (2012) Current perspectives on coronary chronic total occlusions: the Canadian Multicenter Chronic Total Occlusions Registry. JAmCollCardiol 59: 991–997.
7. Kahn JK (1993) Angiographic suitability for catheter revascularization of total coronary occlusions in patients from a community hospital setting. AmHeart J 126: 561–564.
8. Angeras O, Albertsson P, Karason K, Ramunddal T, Matejka G, et al. (2013) Evidence for obesity paradox in patients with acute coronary syndromes: a report from the Swedish Coronary Angiography and Angioplasty Registry. Eur Heart J 34: 345–353.
9. Prasad A, Rihal CS, Lennon RJ, Wiste HJ, Singh M, et al. (2007) Trends in outcomes after percutaneous coronary intervention for chronic total occlusions: a 25-year experience from the Mayo Clinic. J Am Coll Cardiol 49: 1611–1618.
10. Mehran R, Claessen BE, Godino C, Dangas GD, Obunai K, et al. (2011) Long-term outcome of percutaneous coronary intervention for chronic total occlusions. JACC Cardiovasc Interv 4: 952–961.
11. Fox KA, Goodman SG, Klein W, Brieger D, Steg PG, et al. (2002) Management of acute coronary syndromes. Variations in practice and outcome; findings from the Global Registry of Acute Coronary Events (GRACE). Eur Heart J 23: 1177–1189.
12. Joyal D, Afilalo J, Rinfret S (2010) Effectiveness of recanalization of chronic total occlusions: a systematic review and meta-analysis. Am Heart J 160: 179–187.
13. Thompson CA, Jayne JE, Robb JF, Friedman BJ, Kaplan AV, et al. (2009) Retrograde techniques and the impact of operator volume on percutaneous intervention for coronary chronic total occlusions an early US experience. JACC Cardiovasc Interv 2: 834–842.
14. van der Schaaf RJ, Claessen BE, Hoebers LP, Verouden NJ, Koolen JJ, et al. (2010) Rationale and design of EXPLORE: a randomized, prospective, multicenter trial investigating the impact of recanalization of a chronic total occlusion on left ventricular function in patients after primary percutaneous coronary intervention for acute ST-elevation myocardial infarction. Trials 11: 89.

2

Epicardial Adipose Tissue Thickness Correlates with the Presence and Severity of Angiographic Coronary Artery Disease in Stable Patients with Chest Pain

Fabien A. Picard[1], Pascal Gueret[2], Jean-Pierre Laissy[3,4], Stéphane Champagne[2], Florence Leclercq[5], Didier Carrié[6], Jean-Michel Juliard[1], Patrick Henry[7], Ralph Niarra[8,9], Gilles Chatellier[8,9,10], Philippe Gabriel Steg[1,4,11]*

1 Cardiology Department, Assistance Publique-Hôpitaux de Paris, Hôpital Bichat, Université Paris-Diderot, Sorbonne-Paris Cité, Paris, France, **2** Cardiology Department, Assistance Publique-Hôpitaux de Paris, Hôpital Henri Mondor, Université Paris-Est-Créteil, Créteil, France, **3** Radiology Department, Assistance Publique-Hôpitaux de Paris, Hôpital Bichat, Université Paris-Diderot, Sorbonne-Paris Cité, Paris, France, **4** Département Hospitalo-Universitaire FIRE, INSERM U-1148, Assistance Publique-Hôpitaux de Paris, Hôpital Bichat, Université Paris-Diderot, Sorbonne-Paris Cité, Paris, France, **5** Cardiology Department, Centre Hospitalier Universitaire Arnaud de Villeneuve, Montpellier, France, **6** Cardiology Department, Centre Hospitalier Universitaire de Rangueil, Toulouse, France, **7** Cardiology Department, Assistance Publique-Hôpitaux de Paris, Hôpital Lariboisière, Université Paris-Diderot, Sorbonne-Paris Cité, Paris, France, **8** Epidemiology and Clinical Research Unit, Assistance Publique-Hôpitaux de Paris, Hôpital Européen Georges-Pompidou, Paris, France, **9** Unité INSERM Centre D'investigation Épidémiologique 4, Paris, France, **10** Université Paris Descartes, Sorbonne Paris Cité, Faculté de Médecine, Paris, France, **11** NHLI Imperial College, ICMS Royal Brompton Hospital, London, United Kingdom

Abstract

Objective: Epicardial adipose tissue (EAT) is suggested to correlate with metabolic risk factors and to promote plaque development in the coronary arteries. We sought to determine whether EAT thickness was associated or not with the presence and extent of angiographic coronary artery disease (CAD).

Methods: We measured epicardial fat thickness by computed tomography and assessed the presence and extent of CAD by coronary angiography in participants from the prospective EVASCAN study. The association of EAT thickness with cardiovascular risk factors, coronary artery calcification scoring and angiographic CAD was assessed using multivariate regression analysis.

Results: Of 970 patients (age 60.9 years, 71% male), 75% (n = 731) had CAD. Patients with angiographic CAD had thicker EAT on the left ventricle lateral wall when compared with patients without CAD (2.74 ± 2.4 mm vs. 2.08 ± 2.1 mm; $p = 0.0001$). The adjusted odds ratio (OR) for a patient with a LVLW EAT value ≥2.8 mm to have CAD was OR = 1.46 [1.03–2.08], $p = 0.0326$ after adjusting for risk factors. EAT also correlated with the number of diseased vessels ($p = 0.0001$ for trend). By receiver operating characteristic curve analysis, an EAT value ≥2.8 mm best predicted the presence of $>50\%$ diameter coronary artery stenosis, with a sensitivity and specificity of 46.1% and 66.5% respectively (AUC:0.58). Coronary artery calcium scoring had an AUC of 0.76.

Conclusion: Although left ventricle lateral wall EAT thickness correlated with the presence and extent of angiographic CAD, it has a low performance for the diagnosis of CAD.

Editor: Joseph Devaney, Children's National Medical Center, Washington, United States of America

Funding: The authors have no support or funding to report.

Competing Interests: The authors have declared that no competing interests exist.

* Email: gabriel.steg@bch.aphp.fr

Introduction

Epicardial adipose tissue (EAT) is a visceral adipose tissue surrounding the heart and the coronary arteries. Because of its endocrine and paracrine activity, secreting pro-inflammatory and anti-inflammatory cytokines and chemokines, it has been suggested to influence coronary atherosclerosis development [1–5]. The EVASCAN (EVAluation of CT SCANner) study [6] was recently performed to establish the diagnostic accuracy of computed tomography coronary angiography compared to conventional coronary angiography (CA) in a population of symptomatic patients with a clinical indication for anatomical coronary imaging.

Using EVASCAN data, which provided precise assessment of coronary artery disease by CA and the measure of EAT by cardiac computed tomography (CT) in a large cohort of patients, the current analysis was performed to clarify a possible link between EAT and CAD. Our hypothesis was that EAT, as measured by

CT scanner, was associated with the presence and extent of angiographic CAD.

Methods

Study population

We used EVASCAN data, which provided precise assessment of coronary artery disease by CA and the measure of EAT by cardiac CT to perform this study. Therefore, EVASCAN inclusion criteria were used. EVASCAN was a prospective study of correlation between CT angiography and conventional angiography in stable adults with chest pain referred for non-emergent invasive CA. Eligible patients were ≥18 years old with known or suspected CAD, able to undergo cardiac CT first, then CA within four days. The main exclusion criteria were: unstable clinical status, serum creatinine>150 μmol/L, atrial fibrillation, pregnancy and lactation. The protocol of this study complies with the Declaration of Helsinki, was approved by the institutional review board of Paris VI University and written informed consent was obtained from each patient. Classical CAD risk factors were recorded. The clinical characteristics of the patients are summarized in Table 1.

Cardiac CT and coronary angiography protocol

Patients underwent cardiac CT (684 (70.5%) patients had 64 row CT and 286 patients (29.5%) had 16 to 40 row CT) followed by conventional CA. Cardiac CT was performed using a standardized, optimized protocol for each system. All patients were in sinus rythm before cardiac CT. A beta-blocker was recommended if heart rate was>65 beats/minute.

Patients first underwent an unenhanced prospective ECG-gated acquisition for calcium scoring (Agatston score) and then a retrospective ECG-gated contrast-enhanced acquisition to explore the coronary tree and EAT. Scanning parameters varied according to the system used. Current intensity modulation was systematically applied to reduce radiation during systolic phases. The effective dose of the non-enhanced scan and the computed tomography coronary angiography was estimated from the product of the dose–length and a conversion coefficient ($k = 0.017 mSv/[mGy \times cm]$) for the chest as the investigated anatomic region [7].

A systematic reconstruction of the cardiac phases encompassing the RR interval (in 10% increments) was performed in all patients. Data were uploaded to dedicated workstations (Advantage Windows, GE; Brilliance, Philips; Leonardo, Siemens; Vitrea, Toshiba).

Conventional CA was performed using standard techniques via a femoral or radial approach [8]. All studies were performed using digital equipment. Multiple projections were obtained as deemed necessary by the angiographer.

Cardiac CT and CA interpretation

Cardiac CT and CA were analyzed visually in separate core laboratories in a blinded manner by experienced readers unaware of the patient's clinical information or the results of the other imaging technique.

For cardiac CT, EAT was defined as the adipose tissue between the surface of the heart and the visceral epicardium surrounding the 3 main coronary arteries. To determine EAT values, epicardial

Table 1. Population characteristics and comparison of the presence of significant angiographic coronary artery disease.

	All patients (n = 970)	Presence of significant coronary artery disease		
		No	Yes	
Characteristics		N = 239	N = 731	P
Men, n (%)	689 (71.03%)	122 (51.05%)	567 (77.56%)	**<0.0001**
Age (yrs), mean ± SD	60.85±11.36	57.19±12.29	62.05±10.77	**<0.0001**
BMI (kg/m2), mean ± SD	27.38±4.52	27.09±5.02	27.48±4.34	0.2614
Waist circumference (cm); mean ± SD	98.75±13.31	97.33±15.40	99.23±12.51	0.1601
Current smoker, n (%)	244 (25.15%)	59 (24.69%)	185 (25.31%)	0.8475
Diabetes, n (%)	244 (25.15%)	42 (17.57%)	181 (24.76%)	**0.0218**
Hypertension, n (%)	501 (51.65%)	95 (39.75%)	406 (55.54%)	**<0.0001**
Dyslipidemia, n (%)	427 (44.02%)	86 (35.98%)	341 (46.65%)	**0.0039**
Familial history of CAD; n (%)	660 (68.04%)	159 (66.53%)	501 (68.54%)	0.5631
Metabolic syndrome, n (%)	62 (6.39%)	11 (4.60%)	51 (6.98%)	0.1927
Total cholesterol (g/L), mean ± SD	2.09±1.04	2.09±0.92	2.09±1.07	0.9546
LDL cholesterol (g/L), mean ± SD	1.24±0.73	1.25±0.64	1.24±0.75	0.9163
HDL cholesterol (g/L), mean ± SD	0.54±0.29	0.59±0.32	0.53±0.28	**0.0255**
Calcium scoring, median [IQR]	15.50 [0.00; 331.00]	0.00 [0.00; 9.00]	82.00 [6.00; 626.00]	**<0.0001**
Calcium scoring; mean ± SD	379.72±840.59	72.43±275.58	539.28±980.08	**<0.0001**
LVLW EAT thickness (mm); mean ± SD	2.58±2.31	2.08±2.05	2.74±2.37	**0.0001**
RVLW EAT thickness (mm); mean ± SD	5.38±3.05	4.77±2.73	5.58±3.13	**0.0004**
LVLW EAT thickness ≥2.8 mm, n (%)	427 (44.02%)	83 (34.73%)	344 (47.06%)	**0.0009**
RVLW EAT thickness ≥5.3 mm, n (%)	405 (41.75%)	77 (32.22%)	328 (44.87%)	**0.0005**

BMI = body mass index; CAD = coronary artery disease; LDL = low-density lipoprotein; HDL = high-density lipoprotein; LVLW = left ventricle lateral wall; EAT = epicardial adipose tissue; RVLW = right ventricle lateral wall.

fat maximal thickness was measured at two different locations: on the left ventricle lateral free wall (LVLW) at the base of the ventricles in short-axis view and on the right ventricle lateral free wall (RVLW) at the base of the ventricles in short-axis view. Maximal thickness was measured from the visceral epicardium to the outside of the myocardium, and perpendicular to the surface of the heart. Maximal LVLW EAT thickness and maximal RVLW EAT thickness were used for analysis. EAT thickness was not measured at other sites (right atrioventricular groove, left atrioventricular groove, interventricular grooves...).

For CA, coronary arteries were scored using the American Heart Association coronary artery classification [9]. Each coronary segment was visually graded as: individually assessable or not; normal; non-significant stenosis (<50%); stenosis ≥50%; or total occlusion. In case of multiple lesions in a given segment or artery, the worst lesion was considered.

Baseline clinical and biological assessment

Baseline measurements were obtained for the following: total cholesterol, high-density lipoprotein cholesterol, low-density lipoprotein cholesterol, triglycerides; Body mass index (BMI) and waist circumference. Presence of high blood pressure, diabetes, coronary heredity and current or former smoker was recorded.

Biological samples were processed through local laboratories of each hospital.

Statistical analysis

Descriptive data are presented as frequencies and percentages. Continuous data are expressed as mean ± SD or median [IQR] according to the distribution of the parameter. Risk factors were compared between patients with and without CAD. Student's t test for independent groups was used to compare continuous variables, and chi-square test was used for categorical variables. The relation between cardiovascular risk factors and presence of CAD was assessed with univariate and multivariate logistic regression analysis. This relation was expressed by odds ratios (95% CIs). To determine the best cut-off of EAT thickness and calcium scoring, the Youden index (sensitivity + specificity −1) was calculated using the receiver operating characteristic (ROC) curve. The main aim of the Youden index is to find the best cut-off from the ROC curve, maximizing the difference between true positive rate (Sensitivity) and false positive rate (1-specificity). To determine the intra-observer variability of EAT measurements, one observer repeated the EAT data analysis for 25 randomly chosen CT-scanners on different days. Two observers measuring the already recorded image estimated inter-observer variability. The agreement for both intra- and inter-observer variability was evaluated by intra- and inter-class correlation coefficients (ICC). The ICC value is the ratio of the between-subject variance to the sum of the between-subject variance and the within-subject variance. The smaller the within-subject variance, the better the agreement and the higher the ICC. All statistical analyses were performed using SAS system version 9.2 (SAS Institute, Cary, NC, USA). A 2-tailed p-value <0.05 was considered statistically significant.

Results

Patients characteristics

Between June 2006 and June 2008, 40 centres prospectively enrolled 1254 patients; data from 970 were used in the present analysis. The patients excluded from the analysis had either incomplete, poor quality or missing Cardiac CT or CA, missing data for EAT thickness or withdrew consent. The baseline characteristics are shown in Table 1. The mean age was 61±11 years and 71% were male. The main cardiovascular risk factors were familial history of CAD in 68% of patients, treated hypertension in 52% of the patients, dyslipidaemia in 44% of the patients, current smoking in 25% of the patients and diabetes in 25% of the patients. Mean BMI was 27.4±4.5 kg/m2 and waist circumference was 99±13 cm.

EAT thickness measured by cardiac CT for the entire study sample was 2.58±2.31 mm for the LVLW and 5.38±3.05 mm for the RVLW.

The reproducibility of EAT measurements in our study was high both in terms of intra- and inter-observer variability (correlation coefficients: 0.89 and 0.74 respectively).

Epicardial fat thickness and presence of angiographic CAD

Seven hundred and thirty one patients (75%) were found to have significant CAD on coronary angiography. Their clinical and CT findings were compared to the remaining two hundred and thirty nine patients without significant CAD.

Baseline characteristics of the 2 groups (with or without CAD) are listed in Table 1.

Patients with angiographic evidence of CAD were more frequently males, older, with a higher prevalence of conventional risk factors (diabetes, hypertension, dyslipidaemia) although the prevalence of current smoking, the average BMI, waist circumference and metabolic syndrome were not different from patients without CAD. Total cholesterol and low-density lipoprotein cholesterol were similar among groups (probably because of a high prevalence of statin use). However, HDL levels were lower.

Patients with angiographic CAD had thicker EAT on both left and right ventricle lateral walls, when compared with patients without CAD (2.74±2.4 mm vs. 2.08±2.1 mm; p = 0.0001 for LVLW and 5.58±3.1 mm vs. 4.77±2.7 mm; p = 0.0004 for RVLW). Calcium scoring mean was also higher in patients with angiographic CAD (539.28±980.08 vs. 72.43±275.58; p< 0.0001). (Table 1).

The odds ratio (OR) for a patient with a LVLW EAT value ≥ 2.8 mm to have CAD was 1.67 (95%CI 1.23 to 2.26). This relation remained significant after adjusting for CAD risk factors (OR = 1.46 [1.03–2.08], p = 0.0326) (Table 2). Unlike LVLW EAT; the OR for a patient with a RVLW EAT value ≥5.3 mm to have CAD did not remain significant after adjusting for CAD risk factors (OR = 1.38 [0.97–1.98], p = 0.0757).

The probability of a stenosis on angiography increased with increasing LVLW EAT thickness. In the first tertile of EAT thickness, the prevalence of at least one significant coronary artery stenosis was 68.9% (n = 221). In the second and the third tertiles, the prevalence rose to 75.9% (n = 249) and 81.3% (n = 261), respectively (P for trend = 0.0002) (Table 3 and Figure 1).

Simple linear regression analysis demonstrated that epicardial fat thickness was correlated with degree of coronary stenosis OR = 1.67, p = 0.0009 but not with waist circumference: OR = 1.01, p = 0.16 and BMI: OR = 1.02, p = 0.26 in CAD subjects. The independent relation of epicardial fat thickness, waist circumference and BMI with coronary stenosis was then assessed by a multiple regression analysis in CAD subjects. Epicardial fat thickness was the most significant independent correlate of degree of coronary stenosis, dependent variable in CAD subjects. (Table 4).

Epicardial fat and extent of angiographic CAD

Increased LVLW EAT thickness correlated positively with the severity or extent of CAD (Figure 2): LVLW EAT thickness mean was 2.08±2.1 mm for the patients with no or minimal vessel

Table 2. Logistic regression analysis of the association between risk factors and presence of significant angiographic CAD.

	Univariate analysis			Multivariate analysis		
	OR	[95%CI]	P	OR	[95%CI]	P
Men	3.32	[2.44–4.51]	**<0.0001**	4.25	[2.98–6.05]	**<0.0001**
Age	1.04	[1.02–1.05]	**<0.0001**	1.04	[1.03–1.06]	**<0.0001**
BMI	1.02	[0.99–1.05]	0.2614	1.01	[0.98–1.05]	0.4632
Current smoker (yes vs. no)	1.03	[0.74–1.45]	0.8482	1.40	[0.92–2.14]	0.1139
Diabetes (yes vs. no)	1.54	[1.06–2.24]	**0.0226**	1.25	[0.79–1.98]	0.3469
Hypertension (yes vs. no)	1.90	[1.41–2.56]	**<0.0001**	1.89	[1.31–2.74]	**0.0007**
Dyslipidemia (yes vs. no)	1.56	[1.15–2.10]	**0.0041**	1.72	[1.22–2.42]	**0.0021**
Family history of CAD (yes vs. no)	1.10	[0.80–1.50]	0.5632	1.07	[0.75–1.53]	0.6985
Metabolic syndrome (yes vs. no)	1.55	[0.80–3.03]	0.1965	0.87	[0.39–1.92]	0.7241
LVLW EAT (≥2.8 vs. <2.8 mm)	1.67	[1.23–2.26]	**0.0009**	1.46	[1.03–2.08]	**0.0326**

OR = odds ratio; CI = confidence interval; other abbreviations as in Table 1.

disease, 2.43±2.4 mm for the patients with single vessel disease, 2.65±2.2 mm for patients with 2 vessel disease or left main disease and 2.95±2.5 mm for patients with 3 vessels disease or left main + right coronary artery disease (p for trend = 0.0001).

Moreover, patients with multivessel disease had more often a LV wall EAT thickness>2.8 mm. 83 (34.73%) patients with no or minimal vessel disease had LVLW EAT thickness>2.8 mm and 177 (51.45%) patients with three vessels disease had a LVLW EAT thickness>2.8 mm. This relation was better with calcium scoring (Figure 2).

Diagnostic performance of EAT and calcium scoring

On receiver operating characteristic (ROC) curve analysis, the best cut-off for LVLW EAT thickness to predict the presence of a significant coronary stenosis was 2.8 mm. LVLW EAT thickness ≥2.8 mm had a sensitivity of 46.1%, specificity of 66.5%, positive predictive value of 80%, and negative predictive value of 28.8%. The area under the curve was 0.58. The best cut-off for RVLW was 5.3 mm. RVLW EAT thickness ≥5.3 mm predicted the presence of significant coronary stenosis, with sensitivity of 45.1%, specificity of 67.9%, positive predictive value of 81.1%, and negative predictive value of 28.9%. The best cut-off for calcium scoring was 24 (Agatston score). Calcium scoring>24 predicted the presence of significant coronary stenosis, with sensitivity of 62.3%, specificity of 85.1%, positive predictive value of 89%, and negative predictive value of 54.2%. The area under the curve was 0.76 (Figure 3). Conventional cardiovascular risk factors ROC curve was determined and was added to LVLW EAT and calcium scoring measurement. Areas under the curve, sensibility, specificity, positive and negative predictive values are summarized in Table 5. LVLW EAT thickness and calcium scoring were statistically associated (p = 0.0125).

Discussion

The present study sought to determine the link between EAT and CAD using data from the EVASCAN study [6], a large multicenter prospective study originally performed to establish the diagnostic accuracy of CTCA compared to conventional coronary angiography in a population of symptomatic patients with a clinical indication for anatomical coronary imaging.

This study confirmed that EAT thickness of left ventricle wall was associated with CAD and an independent predictor of CAD. Interestingly, we found that, even though mean right ventricle wall EAT was thicker than left ventricle wall EAT, EAT of the left

Table 3. Association between angiographic coronary artery disease and left ventricle lateral wall EAT thickness tertiles.

	Tertile1	Tertile2	Tertile3	P
Men; n (%)	230 (71.65%)	223 (67.99%)	236 (73.52%)	0.2861
Age (yrs.); mean ± SD	57.34±11.77	61.36±10.92	63.91±10.38	**<0.0001**
BMI; mean ± SD	26.51±4.73	27.74±4.50	27.90±4.19	**0.0001**
Current smoker; n (%)	108 (33.64%)	67 (20.43%)	69 (21.50%)	**0.0001**
Diabetes; n (%)	66 (20.56%)	76 (23.17%)	81 (25.23%)	0.3700
Hypertension; n (%)	144 (44.86%)	179 (54.57%)	178 (55.45%)	**0.0170**
Dyslipidemia; n (%)	146 (45.48%)	149 (45.43%)	132 (41.12%)	0.4412
Metabolic syndrome; n (%)	14 (4.36%)	28 (8.54%)	20 (6.23%)	0.0931
Calcium scoring; median [IQR]	6.0 [0.0; 180.0]	24.0 [0.0; 422.0]	37.0 [0.0; 406.0]	**0.0024**
Presence of angiographic CAD; n (%)	221 (68.85%)	249 (75.91%)	261 (81.31%)	**0.0012**

Abbreviations as in Table 1 and 2.

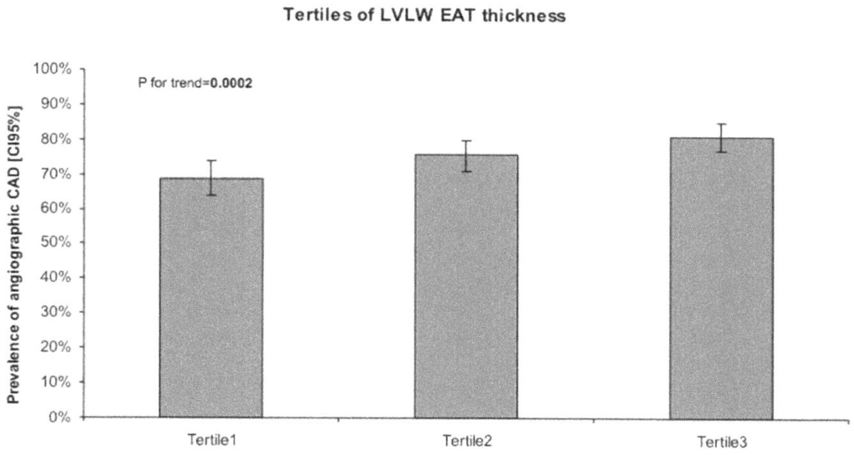

Figure 1. Association of angiographic coronary artery disease and left ventricle lateral wall (LVLW) epicardial adipose tissue (EAT) thickness tertile classification. CAD = coronary artery disease; LVLW = left ventricle lateral wall; EAT = epicardial adipose tissue. Prevalence of angiographic coronary artery disease and 95% confidence intervals [95% CIs] in LVLW EAT tertiles.

ventricle but not the right ventricle wall was associated to CAD. Whether this association is driven by a functional or mechanical cause is unclear and further physiopathological studies need to be done.

Second, EAT thickness was well correlated to the severity of angiographic CAD. The greater the LVLW EAT thickness, the greater the probability of multivessel disease. Thirdly, EAT thickness was not associated with BMI and waist circumference and was the best predictor of CAD. Finally, when studying EAT as a diagnostic screening tool, it had poor performance, lower than calcium scoring. Adding EAT measurement to calcium scoring did not improve significantly the ROC curve.

There are two main implications of the present results. First, from a pathophysiologic perspective, the association between EAT and angiographic CAD is consistent with the hypothesis that epicardial fat may play a role in the genesis of CAD. EAT is the visceral fat depot of the heart. It is a metabolically active organ with anatomical and functional contiguity to the myocardium as it is located along the coronary arteries on the surface of the ventricles and the apex of the heart [10]. Because of its close proximity, epicardial fat can locally affect the heart and coronary arteries through vasocrine or paracrine secretion of a number of bioactive molecules and pro-inflammatory cytokines [11–13]. In fact, excess accumulation of epicardial fat was reported to be a stronger coronary risk factor than the distribution of other body fat [14]. On the basis of these findings, several clinical studies have investigated EAT as a cause of CAD, finding that EAT thickness and volume strongly correlated with atherosclerosis and coronary artery calcium score, both of which are characteristic of plaques and CAD [1–5]. Echocardiographic studies have suggested that EAT was neither strongly associated with the incidence of major adverse cardiovascular events in patients with CAD, nor associated with coronary artery stenosis [15–17]. More recently, a meta-analysis by Xu et al. [18], of 15 case–control studies and one case sectional study (N = 2872 patients) found a positive association between EAT thickness and volume and the presence of CAD. Our study confirms this association.

In addition to being associated with the presence of CAD, EAT has also been associated with fatal and nonfatal coronary events in the general population, independently of conventional cardiovascular risk factors [19]. As such, the presence of EAT may complement information from cardiac computed tomography over and above the CAC scoring. These findings are consistent with the observation that EAT is strongly associated not only with the presence, but also with the severity of CAD. Whether this association is driven by functional or mechanical causes is still unclear and further physiopathological studies with molecular insights for this relation are needed. While additional information on the biological profile of our patients, including biomarkers of inflammation, would have been useful they were not available since our data were obtained in routine medical care. Nevertheless, recent studies have shown that increased EAT thickness was associated with low grade systemic *inflammation* [20] and that orosomucoid secretion by EAT could be a possible indicator of endothelial dysfunction in diabetes mellitus [21]. Moreover, Hirata et al. showed that inflammatory cell infiltration was

Table 4. Multivariable correlates of degree of coronary stenosis in CAD subjects.

	Univariate analysis			Multivariate analysis		
	OR	[95%CI]	P	OR	[95%CI]	P
BMI	1.02	[0.99–1.05]	0.2614	0.99	[0.92–1.06]	0.7239
Waist circumference	1.01	[0.99–1.03]	0.1604	1.01	[0.99–1.04]	0.3013
LVLW EAT (≥2.8 vs. 2.8 mm)	1.67	[1.23–2.26]	**0.0009**	1.67	[1.08–2.57]	**0.0197**

Abbreviations as in Table 1.

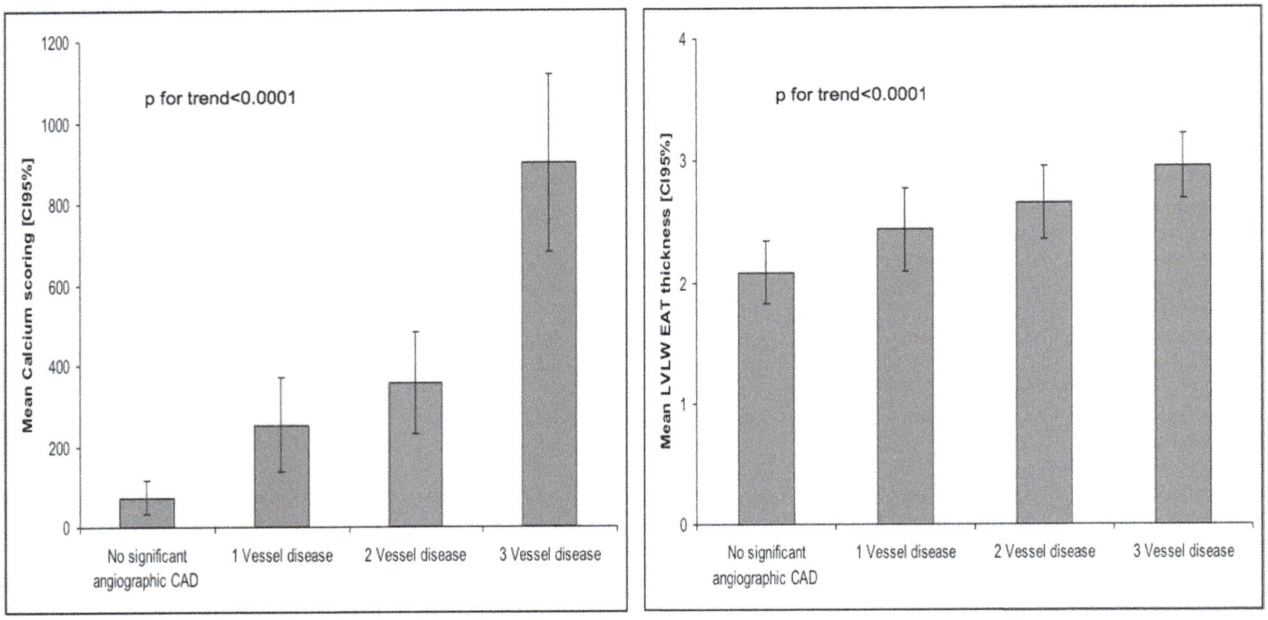

Figure 2. Association of left ventricle lateral wall (LVLW) epicardial adipose tissue (EAT) thickness and calcium scoring between patients with none or minimal coronary artery disease, 1, 2 or 3 vessel disease. Abbreviations as in Figure 1. Mean calcium scoring (Agatston score) and mean LVLW EAT thickness (mm) and 95% confidence intervals [95% CIs] in patients with no significant angiographic coronary artery disease, 1, 2 or 3 vessel disease.

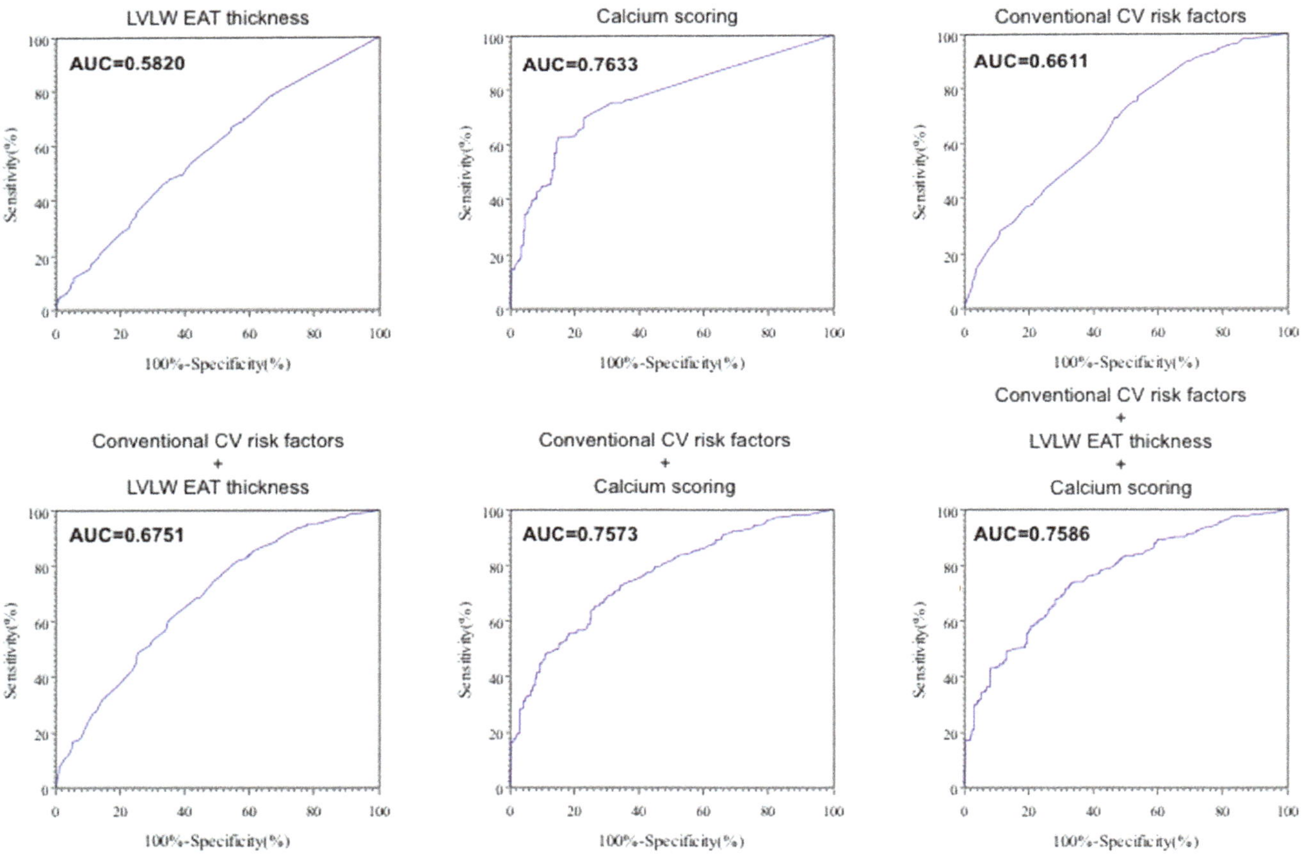

Figure 3. Receiver operating characteristic curves. Abbreviations as in Figure 1; CV = cardiovascular.

Table 5. Receiver operating characteristic curves: Areas under the curve, sensibility, specificity, positive and negative predictive values.

	AUC	Se	Sp	PPV	NPV
LVLW EAT thickness	0.5820	0.4610	0.6653	0.8081	0.2875
Calcium scoring	0.7633	0.6261	0.8514	0.8903	0.5418
Conventional CV risk factors	0.6611	0.7699	0.4635	0.8154	0.3956
Conventional CV risk factors + LVLW EAT thickness	0.6751	0.8061	0.4506	0.8187	0.4303
Conventional CV risk factors + calcium scoring	0.7573	0.6535	0.7352	0.8269	0.5230
Conventional CV risk factors + LVLW EAT thickness + calcium scoring	0.7586	0.7356	0.6706	0.8121	0.5672

AUC = area under the curve; Se = sensibility; Sp= specificity; PPV = positive predictive value; NPV = negative predictive value; CV = cardiovascular; other abbreviations as in Table 1.

enhanced in EAT, but not in subcutaneous fat, in patients with CAD [22]. Chronic inflammation in epicardial fat may participate in the pathogenesis of coronary atherosclerosis and therefore, it may be interesting to combine EAT abundance and biological markers to improve the identification of patient at risk of CAD events.

We reported an association between EAT and calcium scoring. Whether EAT could influence calcium scoring is unclear. Previous studies have shown that EAT correlates with the extent of CAC [23–25]. Alexopoulos et al. [3] found that larger EAT volumes were associated with the presence of plaques with a non-calcified component. However that study had a wide range of EAT volumes in patients with mixed plaques. Nevertheless, this observation suggests that the release of noxious agents from EAT may sustain an active atherosclerotic process as proven by the presence of non-calcified plaques. The presence of mere CAC, instead, could represent a more advanced and stable phase of the atherosclerotic process. In support of this hypothesis, Broedl et al. [26]. found that low levels of adiponectin, which is secreted locally by EAT, were associated with the presence of non-calcified or mixed coronary plaques, but not with the presence of calcified plaques. These concepts still remain speculative. It should also be noted that Greif et al. [27] found no relationship between EAT and any type of atherosclerotic plaque. However, these investigators did not adjust for differences in risk factor prevalence, likely confounding their ability to detect an effect of EAT volume.

The second important implication is that, although EAT is strongly correlated to the presence and extent of angiographic CAD, it is probably of little value as a diagnostic or screening tool since other methods such as calcium scoring or computed tomography coronary angiography have far superior sensibility and specificity. Moreover, adding EAT measurements to calcium scoring did not improve the diagnostic performance.

Limitations

The present study has some limitations. First, we measured EAT thickness rather than volume. However, even if multidetector CT measurements of volumetric EAT are considered more reproducible than multidetector CT measurements of EAT thickness [15,28], EAT thickness is easier to perform and less time-consuming compared to the labor-intensive work for measurements of volumetric EAT and therefore more suitable for research purposes. Consequently, we measured EAT thickness on the left and right ventricle free wall because of its accessibility and potential for use in clinical practice. We noted a strong positive association between EAT thickness and coronary atherosclerosis quantified by CA. Patients underwent mostly 64 row cardiac CT (684 (70.5%) patients) and the other 286 patients (29.5%) had 16 to 40 row CT. Nevertheless, even if 16 row cardiac CT are not used anymore (patients were included between June 2006 and June 2008), it does not affect EAT thickness measurement reliability. Second, this study was performed in symptomatic patients and not in an asymptomatic population undergoing screening, which could influence the results of EAT as a screening tool. However, this study was first performed on a pathophysiologic approach, not to prove the accuracy of EAT thickness measurement as a screening tool in an asymptomatic cohort. Thirdly, despite the independent association between epicardial thickness and CAD, our study did not provide direct molecular insights into this relation. Fourth, coronary angiography alone is not the most accurate method to estimate coronary stenosis degree and severity, especially in early lesions, due to outward remodeling of coronary vessels. However, coronary angiography represents the most widely used technique for assessing coronary anatomy. In the literature, significant stenosis is defined as>50% stenosis of the luminal diameter but this does not account for the presence of plaque instability, which may lead to acute coronary artery stenosis. Finally, we measured EAT in different parts of the heart, but the fact that it was not measured in right atrioventricular groove, left atrioventricular groove and interventricular groove could be a limitation.

Conclusions

From a pathophysiologic perspective, our study demonstrated a strong association between EAT and the presence and extent of angiographic CAD. It is consistent with the hypothesis that epicardial fat may play a role in the genesis of CAD, possibly due to paracrine or vasocrine mechanisms. Although EAT is correlated to CAD, it is probably of little value as a diagnostic or screening tool since other methods such as calcium scoring or computed tomography coronary angiography have far superior sensibility and specificity.

Author Contributions

Conceived and designed the experiments: FP PG PGS. Performed the experiments: JPL SC FL DC JMJ PH. Analyzed the data: RN GC. Contributed reagents/materials/analysis tools: FP PG PGS RN GC. Wrote the paper: FP PG PGS.

References

1. Wang TD, Lee WJ, Shih FY, Huang CH, Chen WJ, et al. (2010) Association of epicardial adipose tissue with coronary atherosclerosis is region-specific and independent of conventional risk factors and intra-abdominal adiposity. Atherosclerosis 213(1):279–87.
2. Bettencourt N, Toschke AM, Leite D, Rocha J, Carvalho M, et al. (2012) Epicardial adipose tissue is an independent predictor of coronary atherosclerotic burden. Int J Cardiol. 28;158(1):26–32.
3. Alexopoulos N, McLean DS, Janik M, Arepalli CD, Stillman AE, et al. (2010) Epicardial adipose tissue and coronary artery plaque characteristics. Atherosclerosis 210(1):150–4.
4. Oka T, Yamamoto H, Ohashi N, Kitagawa T, Kunita E, et al. (2012) Association between epicardial adipose tissue volume and characteristics of non-calcified plaques assessed by coronary computed tomographic angiography. Int J Cardiol. 161(1):45–9.
5. Eroglu S, Sade LE, Yildirir A, Bal U, Ozgul AS, et al. (2009) Epicardial adipose tissue thickness by echocardiography is a marker for the presence and severity of coronary artery disease. Nutr Metab Cardiovasc Dis. 19(3):211–7.
6. Gueret P, Deux JF, Bonello L, Sarran A, Tron C, et al. (2013) Diagnostic Performance of Computed Tomography Coronary Angiography (from the Prospective National Multicenter Multivendor EVASCAN Study). Am J Cardiol. 111(4):471–8.
7. Menzel HG, Shibilla H, Teunen D, editors (2000) European guidelines on quality criteria for computed tomography. Luxembourg: European Commission Publication. (No. EUR 16262 EN. 2000).
8. Smith SC, Feldman TE, Hirshfeld JW, Jacobs AK, Kern MJ, et al. (2006) ACC/AHA/SCAI 2005 guidelines update for percutaneous coronary intervention—summary article: a report of the American College of Cardiology/American Heart Association Task Force on Practice Guidelines (ACC/AHA/SCAI Writing Committee to Update the 2001 Guidelines for Percutaneous Coronary Intervention). J Am Coll Cardiol. 47(1):216–35.
9. Austen WG, Edwards JE, Frye RL, Gensini GG, Gott VL, et al. (1975) A reporting system on patients evaluated for coronary artery disease. Report of the Ad Hoc Committee for Grading of Coronary Artery Disease, Council on Cardiovascular Surgery, American Heart Association. Circulation 51(4 Suppl):5–40.
10. Sacks HS, Fain JN (2007) Human epicardial adipose tissue: A review. Am Heart J. 153(6):907–17.
11. Baker AR, Silva NF, Quinn DW, Harte AL, Pagano D, et al. (2006) Human epicardial adipose tissue expresses a pathogenic profile of adipocytokines in patients with cardiovascular disease. Cardiovasc Diabetol. 13;5: 1.
12. Rabkin SW (2007) Epicardial fat: properties, function and relationship to obesity. Obes Rev. 8(3):253–61.
13. Mazurek T, Zhang L, Zalewski A, Mannion JD, Diehl JT, et al. (2003) Human epicardial adipose tissue is a source of inflammatory mediators. Circulation 108(20):2460–6.
14. Taguchi R, Takasu J, Itani Y, Yamamoto R, Yokoyama K, et al. (2001) Pericardial fat accumulation in men as a risk factor for coronary artery disease. Atherosclerosis 157(1):203–9.
15. Chaowalit N, Somers VK, Pellikka PA, Rihal CS, Lopez-Jimenez F (2006) Subepicardial adipose tissue and the presence and severity of coronary artery disease. Atherosclerosis 186(2):354–9.
16. Albuquerque FN, Somers VK, Blume G, Miranda W, Korenfeld Y, et al. (2012) Usefulness of epicardial adipose tissue as a predictor of adverse cardiovascular events in patients with coronary artery disease. Am J Cardiol. 110(8):1100–5.
17. Parcon R, Kruk M, Kepka C, Pregowski J, Opolski MP, et al. (2011) Epicardial adipose tissue radiodensity is independently related to coronary atherosclerosis. A multidetector computed tomography study. Circ J. 75(2):391–7.
18. Xu Y, Cheng X, Hong K, Huang C, Wan L (2012) How to interpret epicardial adipose tissue as a cause of coronary artery disease: a meta-analysis. Coron Artery Dis. 23(4):227–33.
19. Mahabadi A, Berg M, Lehmann N, Kälsch H, Bauer M, et al. (2013) Association of Epicardial Fat With Cardiovascular Risk Factors and Incident Myocardial Infarction in the General Population: The Heinz Nixdorf Recall Study. J Am Coll Cardiol. 61(13):1388–95.
20. Tok D, Kadife I, Turak O, Ozcan F, Basar N, et al. (2012) Increased epicardial fat thickness is associated with low grade systemic inflammation in metabolic syndrome. Turk Kardiyol Dern Ars. 40(8):690–5.
21. Fandiño-Vaquero R, Fernández-Trasancos A, Alvarez E, Ahmad S, Batista-Oliveira AL, et al. (2014) Orosomucoid secretion levels by epicardial adipose tissue as possible indicator of endothelial dysfunction in diabetes mellitus or inflammation in coronary artery disease. Atherosclerosis 235(2):281–288.
22. Hirata Y, Kurobe H, Akaike M, Chikugo F, Hori T, et al. (2011) Enhanced inflammation in epicardial fat in patients with coronary artery disease. Int Heart J. 52(3):139–42.
23. Rosito GA, Massaro JM, Hoffmann U, Ruberg FL, Mahabadi AA, et al. (2008) Pericardial fat, visceral abdominal fat, cardiovascular disease risk factors, and vascular calcification in a community-based sample: the Framingham Heart Study. Circulation 117: 605–13.
24. de Vos AM, Prokop M, Roos CJ, Mejis MF, van der Schouw YT, et al. (2008) Peri-coronary epicardial adipose tissue is related to cardiovascular risk factors and coronary artery calcification in post-menopausal women. Eur Heart J. 29: 777–83.
25. Ding J, Kritchevsky SB, Harris TB, Burke GL, Detrano RC, et al. (2008) The association of pericardial fat with calcified coronary plaque. Obesity (Silver Spring) 16: 1914–9.
26. Broedl UC, Lebherz C, Lehrke M, Stark R, Greif M, et al. (2009) Low adiponectin levels are an independent predictor of mixed and non-calcified coronary atherosclerotic plaques. PLoS One 4:e4733.
27. Greif M, Becker A, von Ziegler F, Lebherz C, Lehrke M, et al. (2009) Pericardial adipose tissue determined by dual source CT is a risk factor for coronary atherosclerosis. Arterioscler Thromb Vasc Biol 29: 781–6.
28. Gorter PM, van Lindert AS, de Vos AM, Mejis MF, van der Graaf Y, et al. (2008) Quantification of epicardial and peri-coronary fat using cardiac computed tomography; reproducibility and relation with obesity and metabolic syndrome in patients suspected of coronary artery disease. Atherosclerosis 197(2):896–903.

Low-Density Lipoprotein Electronegativity Is a Novel Cardiometabolic Risk Factor

Jing-Fang Hsu[1], Tzu-Chieh Chou[2,3], Jonathan Lu[4], Shu-Hua Chen[4], Fang-Yu Chen[1], Ching-Chu Chen[5], Jeffrey L. Chen[6], MacArthur Elayda[7], Christie M. Ballantyne[8], Steven Shayani[9,10]*, Chu-Huang Chen[1,4,8,11]*

1 L5 Research Center, China Medical University Hospital, Taichung, Taiwan, **2** Department of Public Health, China Medical University, Taichung, Taiwan, **3** Department of Health Risk Management, China Medical University, Taichung, Taiwan, **4** Vascular and Medicinal Research, Texas Heart Institute, Houston, Texas, United States of America, **5** Department of Internal Medicine, China Medical University Hospital, Taichung, Taiwan, **6** Physical Medicine & Rehabilitation, Department of Orthopedic Surgery, University of California San Diego, San Diego, California, United States of America, **7** Biostatistics and Epidemiology, Texas Heart Institute, Houston, Texas, United States of America, **8** Department of Medicine, Baylor College of Medicine, Houston, Texas, United States of America, **9** Mount Sinai Medical Center, New York, New York, United States of America, **10** New York Heart Research Foundation, New York, New York, United States of America, **11** Department of Medicine, Kaohsiung Medical University, Kaohsiung, Taiwan

Abstract

Background: Low-density lipoprotein (LDL) plays a central role in cardiovascular disease (CVD) development. In LDL chromatographically resolved according to charge, the most electronegative subfraction–L5–is the only subfraction that induces atherogenic responses in cultured vascular cells. Furthermore, increasing evidence has shown that plasma L5 levels are elevated in individuals with high cardiovascular risk. We hypothesized that LDL electronegativity is a novel index for predicting CVD.

Methods: In 30 asymptomatic individuals with metabolic syndrome (MetS) and 27 healthy control subjects, we examined correlations between plasma L5 levels and the number of MetS criteria fulfilled, CVD risk factors, and CVD risk according to the Framingham risk score.

Results: L5 levels were significantly higher in MetS subjects than in control subjects (21.9±18.7 mg/dL vs. 11.2±10.7 mg/dL, *P*:0.01). The Jonckheere trend test revealed that the percent L5 of total LDL (L5%) and L5 concentration increased with the number of MetS criteria ($P<0.001$). L5% correlated with classic CVD risk factors, including waist circumference, body mass index, waist-to-height ratio, smoking status, blood pressure, and levels of fasting plasma glucose, triglyceride, and high-density lipoprotein. Stepwise regression analysis revealed that fasting plasma glucose level and body mass index contributed to 28% of L5% variance. The L5 concentration was associated with CVD risk and contributed to 11% of 30-year general CVD risk variance when controlling the variance of waist circumference.

Conclusion: Our findings show that LDL electronegativity was associated with multiple CVD risk factors and CVD risk, suggesting that the LDL electronegativity index may have the potential to be a novel index for predicting CVD. Large-scale clinical trials are warranted to test the reliability of this hypothesis and the clinical importance of the LDL electronegativity index.

Editor: Stefan Kiechl, Innsbruck Medical University, Austria

Funding: This work was supported by grants from the American Diabetes Association (1-04-RA-13), the National Institutes of Health (HL-63364), the National Science Council of Taiwan (NSC 100-2314-B-039-040-MY3), China Medical University and Hospital (CMU 100-TS-09), Taiwan Ministry of Health and Welfare Clinical Trial and Research Center of Excellence (DOH102-TD-B-111-004), and the Stroke Biosignature Project Grant of Academia Sinica, Taiwan (BM101100888, BM102021169, and BM103010096). The funders had no role in the study design, data collection and analysis, decision to publish, or preparation of the manuscript.

Competing Interests: The authors have declared that no competing interests exist.

* Email: steven.shayani@mountsinai.org (SS); cchen@texasheart.org (CHC)

These authors contributed equally to this work.

Introduction

Cardiovascular disease (CVD) is a significant public health problem and is a source of economic burden in the United States and globally [1,2]. The identification of major CVD risk factors is important for preventing, controlling, and treating this disease. Classic CVD risk factors include hypertension, dyslipidemia, diabetes mellitus, obesity, decreased physical exercise, and smoking [3–5]. Among these, the most evident causal disorder for CVD is dyslipidemia, or hypercholesterolemia [6,7].

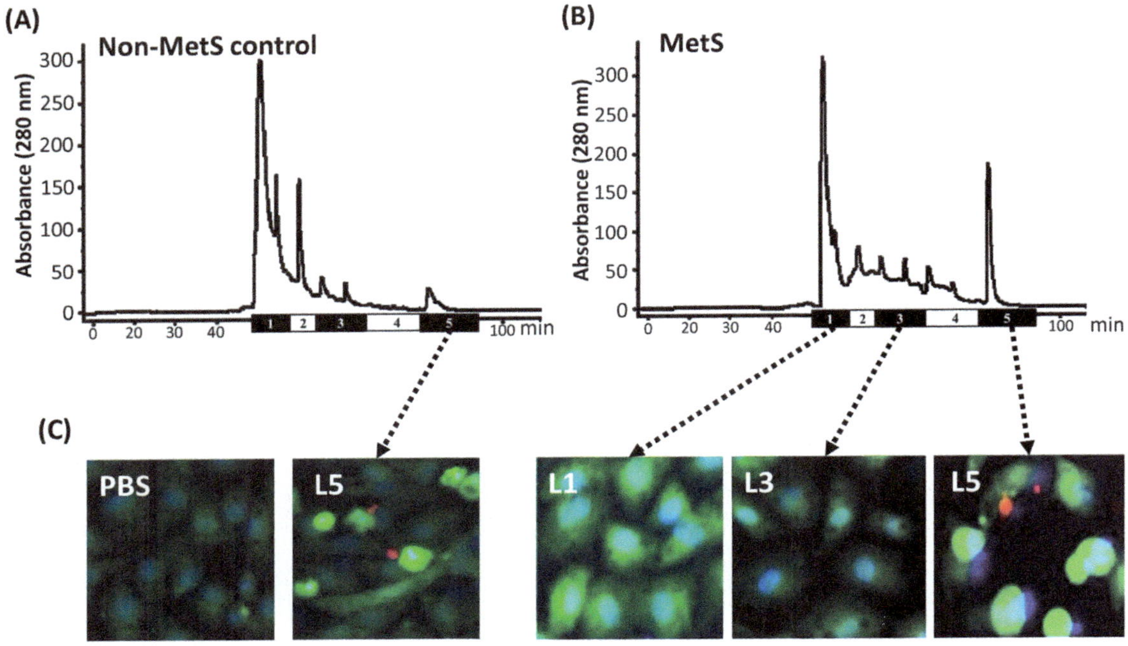

Figure 1. Distribution of LDL subfractions in metabolic syndrome (MetS) and healthy control subjects and the effects of LDL subfractions from MetS subjects on cell death. Representative chromatographs showing the distribution of LDL subfractions L1–L5 (labeled 1–5) in LDL from a (A) control subject and (B) MetS subject. (C) Effects of L1, L3, and L5 (50 µg/mL each) from MetS subjects and L5 (50 µg/mL) from non-MetS control subjects on bovine aortic endothelial cell (BAEC) death after 24 hours, as determined by staining with Hoechst 33342 (to assess nuclear morphology, blue) and calcein acetoxymethyl ester and propidium iodide (to assess membrane integrity, red). As a negative control, BAECs were incubated with phosphate-buffered saline (PBS) for 24 hours. BAECs that have condensed, fragmented nuclei were considered to be undergoing cell apoptosis.

Lipids, particularly low-density lipoprotein (LDL), are known to play a central role in CVD development. Avogaro and colleagues [8] were the first to report that LDL could be divided into electropositive [LDL (+)] and electronegative [LDL (–)] fractions by using ion-exchange chromatography. Since then, others have described the chemical and functional properties of these dichotomized LDL subfractions [9–12]. The proportion of plasma LDL(–) has been shown to be increased in patients with high cardiovascular risks [13] such as hyperlipidemia, diabetes, severe renal disease, and nonalcoholic steatohepatitis, as well as in patients with coronary syndromes when compared with healthy individuals. Thus, it has been suggested [13] that LDL(–) may be a useful biomarker for cardiovascular risks, but large-scale clinical trials are needed to test the reliability of this hypothesis. We have previously separated human plasma LDL according to charge into 5 subfractions (L1–L5) with increasing electronegativity by using anion-exchange chromatography [14]. Notably, plasma levels of the most electronegative LDL subfraction, L5, are moderately increased in patients with high cardiovascular risks such as hypercholesterolemia, type 2 diabetes mellitus, and smoking [14–16], as well as in patients with ST-segment elevation myocardial infarction, when compared with healthy individuals [17,18]. L5 has a chemical composition unique from that of other LDL subfractions, marked by decreased levels of apolipoprotein B and increased levels of other apolipoproteins [19]. In addition, L5 is not internalized by the normal LDL receptor but by the lectin-like oxidized LDL receptor- 1 (LOX-1), which in turn leads to endothelial cell apoptosis [20]. Circulating L5 has been shown to be pro-atherogenic [9] and is the only subfraction of human LDL that induces endothelial dysfunction and atherogenic responses in cultured vascular cells [14,15,21]. Although L5 has a role in promoting atherogenesis, it remains unknown whether L5 levels increase with the progression of CVD. Understanding the association between L5 and the progression of CVD may help clinicians counsel patients on lifestyle interventions while fueling research to identify preventions or interventions for CVD.

MetS is a clustering of metabolic abnormalities that are collectively associated with an increased risk of coronary heart disease, stroke, diabetes mellitus, CVD events, and cardiovascular mortality [22–25]. The combined presence of these abnormalities poses a greater risk than the presence of each component alone, which makes MetS useful for identifying high-risk individuals. Recently, we have shown that plasma L5 levels are elevated in individuals with MetS [26], suggesting that L5 levels may be associated with CVD progression and could be a novel CVD predictor. In this study, we examined plasma L5 levels in asymptomatic individuals with or without MetS and evaluated LDL electronegativity as an index for predicting CVD in these individuals by examining correlations between plasma L5 levels and the number of MetS criteria fulfilled, CVD risk factors, and CVD risk according to the Framingham risk score.

Methods

Study subjects

Between 2010 and 2012, we enrolled 57 asymptomatic individuals who had not received statin treatment or any other lipid-lowering therapy in the previous 3 months [27]. Patients who met the criteria for MetS, according to the 2009 Joint Interim Statement of the International Diabetes Federation Task Force on Epidemiology and Prevention (IDF), the National Heart, Lung, and Blood Institute (NHLBI), the American Heart Association

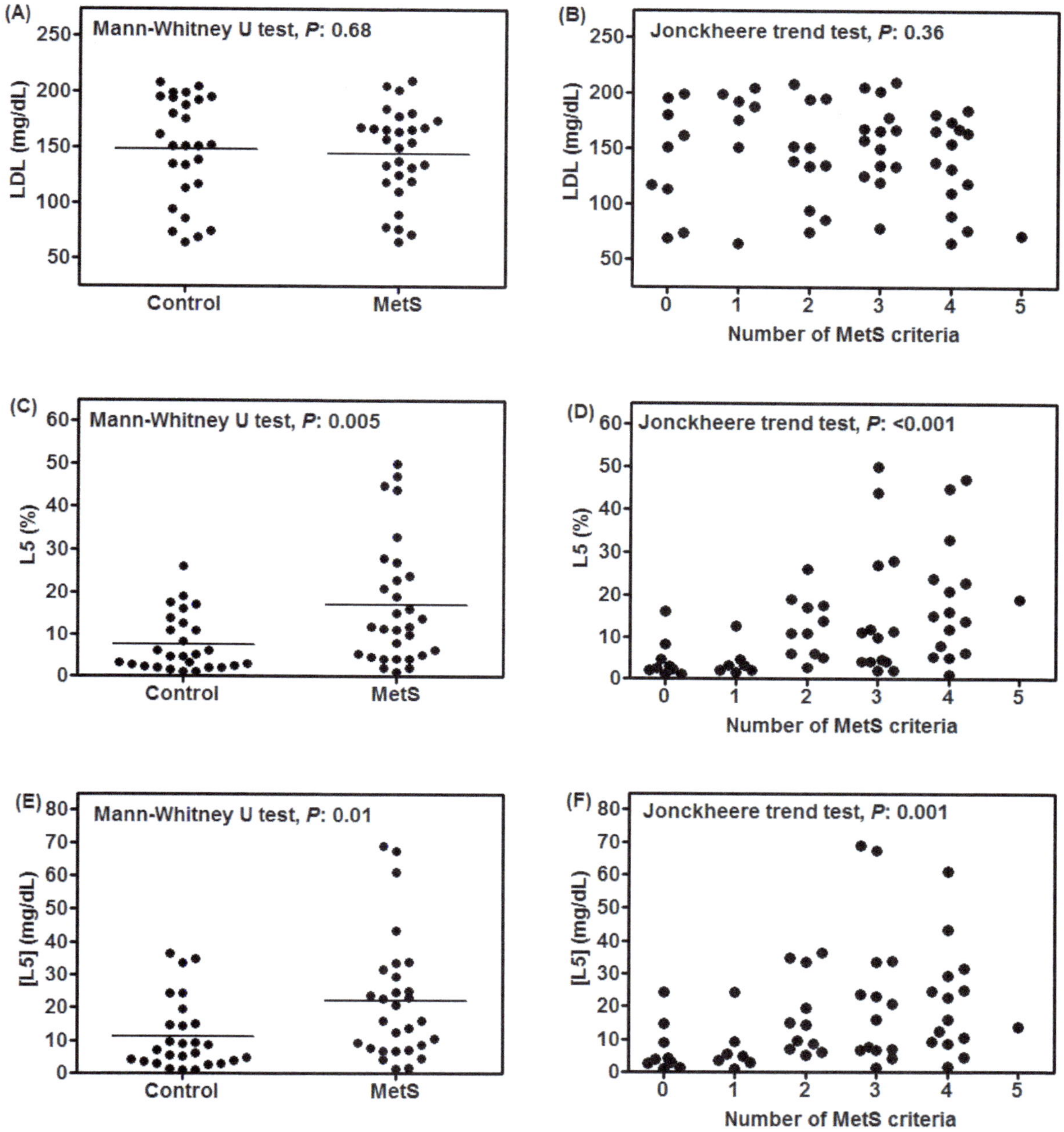

Figure 2. Correlation of low-density lipoprotein (LDL) concentration, L5 percentage (L5%), and L5 concentration ([L5]) with metabolic syndrome (MetS) and the number of MetS criteria. LDL concentration, L5%, and [L5] were plotted for MetS and control subjects and according to MetS criteria. Correlation of LDL concentration with (A) MetS and (B) the number of MetS criteria. Correlation of L5% with (C) MetS and (D) the number of MetS criteria. Correlation of [L5] with (E) MetS and (F) the number of MetS criteria.

(AHA), the World Heart Federation, the International Atherosclerosis Society, and the International Association for the Study of Obesity [28], composed the MetS group, and all other patients were healthy control subjects. All study subjects were seen by cardiologists at the Texas Heart Institute (Houston, Texas) or at the New York Heart Research Foundation (New York, New York). All participants provided written consent for the use of their plasma; the study protocol was approved by the medical ethics committee of Baylor College of Medicine (Houston, Texas) and the New York Heart Research Foundation. The study was conducted according to the principles in the Declaration of Helsinki.

Sample collection

All subjects were instructed to fast before blood sample collection so that lipid concentrations would represent stable lipid levels. Venous blood samples (30 mL) were drawn from each subject by using BD VACUETTE EDTA Blood Tubes (Becton, Dickinson and Company, UK) containing anti-coagulants. A questionnaire was administered to each subject that included a range of questions relating to personal characteristics (eg, age, sex)

Table 1. Characteristics of MetS and healthy control subjects[a].

	Control n = 27	MetS n = 30	P-value[c]
Gender (men:women)	8:19	11:19	0.57
Age (years)	48.8±10.9	55.4±8.7	**0.005**
DM drug treatment	0/27	5/30	**0.05**
Hypertension drug treatment	4/27	12/30	**0.04**
Smoker (no:yes)	13:14	9:21	0.16
Waist circumference (cm)	88.4±13.9	107.4±13.5	**<0.001**
Body mass index (kg/m^2)	27.0±5.9	33.7±6.2	**<0.001**
Waist-to-height (ratio)	0.56±0.08	0.65±0.08	**0.001**
Systolic blood pressure (mmHg)	119.2±20.8	133.8±14.8	**0.001**
Diastolic blood pressure (mmHg)	74.8±9.1	78.9±11.7	0.15
Pulse pressure (mmHg)[b]	44.4±17.3	54.9±14.7	**0.003**
Mean arterial pressure (mmHg)	89.6±11.6	97.2±10.8	**0.03**
Fasting plasma glucose (mg/dL)	90.8±17.2	117.8±45.5	**<0.001**
Total cholesterol (mg/dL)	227.7±60.5	224.4±46.2	0.61
Triglyceride (mg/dL)	118.0±73.9	178.8±108.0	**0.001**
HDL (mg/dL)	60.5±15.4	47.3±12.0	**<0.001**
LDL (mg/dL)	147.9±47.0	144.5±40.6	0.68
L5 (%)	7.6±6.2	17.0±14.5	**0.005**
[L5] (mg/dL)	11.2±10.7	21.9±18.7	**0.01**

[a]Data are expressed as the mean ± standard deviation or as a ratio.
[b]Pulse pressure is equal to systolic blood pressure minus diastolic blood pressure.
[c]The P-value was calculated by using the Mann-Whitney U test, excluding sex, hypertension drug treatment, and smoking status variables, which were subjected to the chi square test, and the DM drug treatment variable, which was subjected to the Fisher exact test.
DM, diabetes mellitus; HDL, high-density lipoprotein; LDL, low-density lipoprotein; L5%, percent L5 in total LDL; [L5], concentration of L5; MetS, metabolic syndrome.

and lifestyle (eg, tobacco usage, medical history). Information obtained from the questionnaire was used in the statistical analysis. For all study subjects, analysis of lipid levels and other biochemical parameters was performed in the Department of Laboratory Medicine at the Texas Heart Institute or at the New York Heart Research Foundation (accredited by the College of American Pathologists) according to standard operating procedures.

LDL isolation and separation of LDL subfractions

LDL (density = 1.063–1.019 g/cm^3) was isolated from whole blood samples (20 mL) by using sequential potassium bromide density centrifugation and was treated with 5 mmol/L EDTA and nitrogen to avoid ex vivo oxidation [29]. Isolated LDL was separated into 5 subfractions (L1, L2, L3, L4, and L5) with increasing negative charge on anion-exchange columns (Uno-Q12, BioRad, Hercules, CA) by using the ÄKTA fast protein liquid chromatography (FPLC) system (GE Healthcare Life Sciences, Pittsburgh, PA) as described previously [14,15]. The columns were equilibrated with buffer A (0.02 mol/L Tris–HCl, pH 8.0; 0.5 mmol/L EDTA). Subfractions were eluted with a multistep linear gradient of buffer B (1 mol/L NaCl in buffer A) at a flow rate of 2 mL/min and were monitored at 280 nm. LDL subfractions from subjects were individually concentrated by using Centriprep filters (YM-30; EMD Millipore Corp., Billerica, MA) and were sterilized by passage through 0.22-μm filters. Protein concentrations of LDL subfractions were measured by using the Lowry method [30].

Cell culture and cell apoptosis assays

Primary bovine aortic endothelial cells (BAECs; Cambrex, East Rutherford, NJ) were used after 3 or 4 passages and were maintained in Dulbecco's modified Eagle's medium (DMEM; Invitrogen, Carslbad, CA) containing 10% fetal bovine serum and antibiotics [14]. Subconfluent cultures washed and maintained in DMEM containing 5% serum were exposed for 24 hours to LDL subfractions (50 μg/mL each of L1, L3, or L5) from MetS or non-MetS control subjects. Generally, the percentage of L5 detected in LDL from healthy individuals is very low. Therefore, all of the LDL subfractions (L1, L3, or L5) were pooled from several MetS or non-MetS subjects to obtain the amount necessary for cell experiments. Treated cells were stained for 10 minutes with 1 mol/L Hoechst 33342 (Molecular Probes, Grand Island, NY) to assess nuclear morphology and with calcein acetoxymethyl ester and propidium iodide (Molecular Probes) to assess membrane integrity. Epifluorescence imaging (500 cells/well) was performed in triplicate by using a Zeiss inverted microscope (Axiovert; x400) with MetaView software (Universal Imaging Corp., Downington, PA).

CVD risk

Three CVD risks were calculated by using the Framingham risk score (developed by the large epidemiological Framingham Heart Study): the 10-year risk of "general" CVD [31], the 30-year risk of "general" CVD, and the 30-year risk of "hard" CVD [32]. The "general" CVD category included coronary death, myocardial infarction, coronary insufficiency, angina, ischemic stroke, hem-

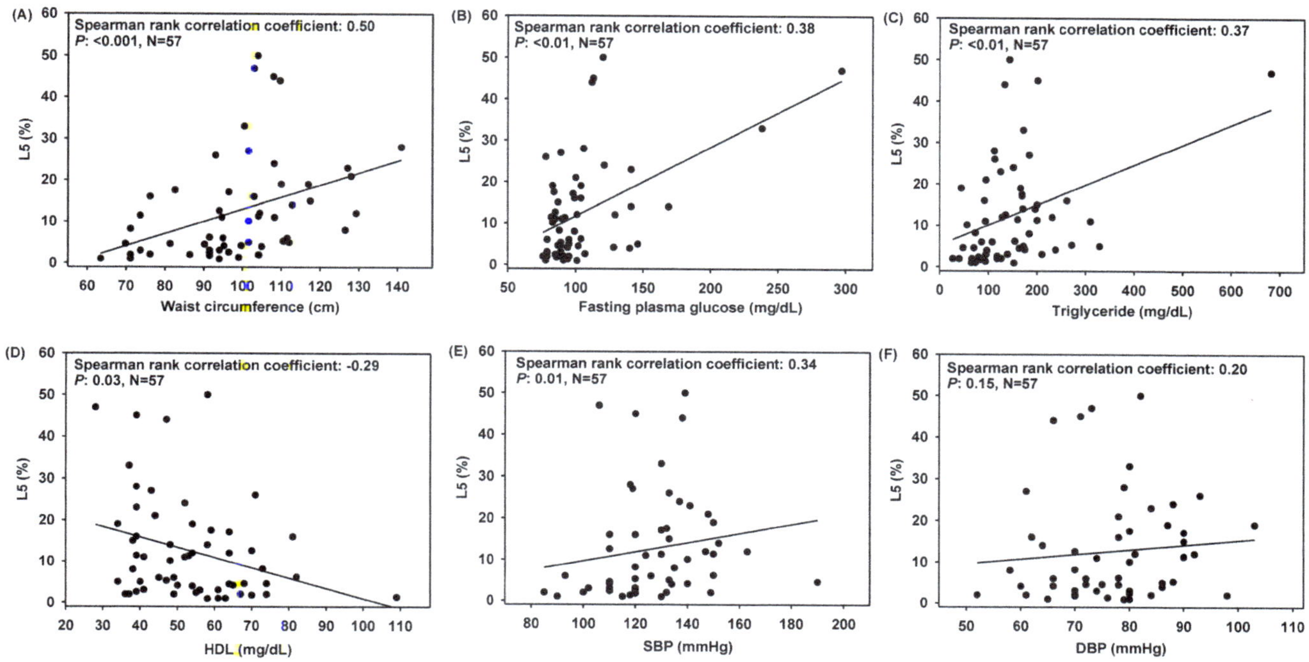

Figure 3. Correlation between L5 percentage (L5%) and various components of metabolic syndrome (MetS) criteria. L5% values were plotted against each component as indicated. Correlation between L5% and (A) waist circumference, (B) fasting plasma glucose, (C) triglyceride, (D) high-density lipoprotein (HDL), (E) systolic blood pressure (SBP), and (F) diastolic blood pressure (DBP).

orrhagic stroke, transient ischemic attack, peripheral artery disease, and heart failure. The "hard" CVD category included coronary death, myocardial infarction, and stroke. The predictors used to calculate the Framingham risk score included sex, age, blood pressure, information regarding the treatment of hypertension and diabetes mellitus, smoking status, body mass index (BMI), and levels of total cholesterol and high-density lipoprotein (HDL).

Statistical analysis

All data are presented as frequencies for discrete responses and as the mean ± standard deviation for continuous responses. For all parameters examined in this study, the Shapiro-Wilk normality test was used to determine whether a random sample of values followed a normal distribution. To compare differences between 2 groups, a nonparametric Mann-Whitney test was used for continuous data, and a chi square test or Fisher exact test was used for binary data. The Jonckheere trend test, a nonparametric test specifically designed to detect differences arising from ordered treatments [33], was used to compare the differences in the percent L5 of total LDL (L5%) and the L5 concentration ([L5]; L5% multiplied by LDL concentration) between 6 groups of subjects defined according to the number of MetS criteria met. More formally, the test considered the null hypothesis that, for 6 groups where $L5_i$ is an L5 level of the central tendency of the *i*th group, $L5_0 = L5_1 = L5_2 = L5_3 = L5_4 = L5_5$, against the alternative hypothesis that $L5_0 < L5_1 < L5_2 < L5_3 < L5_4 < L5_5$. If the results of the test were statistically significant (P: <0.05), the human plasma L5 level was believed to be associated with the progression of metabolic derangement in healthy individuals. The Jonckheere trend test was also used to compare the differences in the

Table 2. Correlation of L5% and various CVD risk factors.

	L5 (%)	
	Spearman Rank Correlation Coefficient (rho)	***P*-value**
Age (years)	0.08	0.57
Body mass index (kg/m²)	0.49	<0.001
Waist-to-height (ratio)	0.29	0.04
Pulse pressure (mmHg)[a]	0.31	0.02
Mean arterial pressure (mmHg)	0.29	0.03
Total cholesterol (mg/dL)	−0.08	0.58
LDL (mg/dL)	−0.08	0.54

[a]Pulse pressure is equal to systolic blood pressure minus diastolic blood pressure.
CVD, cardiovascular disease; LDL, low-density lipoprotein; L5%, percent of L5 in total LDL.

Table 3. Comparison of L5% in subjects grouped according to characteristics.

Characteristic	n	L5 (%)[a]	P-value[b]
Sex			0.37
Men	19	15.0±13.8	
Women	38	11.3±11.6	
DM drug treatment			0.26
No	52	11.7±11.5	
Yes	5	20.6±18.8	
Hypertension drug treatment			**0.006**
No	41	10.2±11.3	
Yes	16	18.4±13.4	
Smoker			**0.02**
No	22	6.9±5.2	
Yes	35	16.0±14.2	

[a]L5 (%) values are expressed as the mean ± standard deviation.
[b]The *P*-value was calculated by using the Mann-Whitney U test.
DM, diabetes mellitus.

concentration of LDL between 6 groups of subjects defined according to the number of MetS criteria met. The associations between L5% and other CVD risk factors, including waist circumference, systolic blood pressure (SBP), diastolic blood pressure (DBP), and levels of fasting plasma glucose, triglyceride, and HDL, were evaluated by using the Spearman rank correlation coefficient, a linear regression model, and a stepwise multiple regression model. Additionally, the association between L5% and CVD risk, as derived by the Framingham risk score [31,32], was evaluated by using the Spearman rank correlation coefficient and a stepwise multiple regression model. A *P*-value <0.05 was considered statistically significant. Statistical analysis was performed by using the Statistical Package for Social Science (version 19.0; SPSS Inc., Chicago, IL) software system.

Results

Clinical characteristics and biochemical parameters of study subjects

Of the 57 subjects enrolled in our study, 19 (33%) were men. The mean age of study subjects was 52.3±10.3 years (range, 32–86 years). Among the study subjects, 38/57 (66.7%) had a waist circumference above normal (≥88 cm for women and ≥102 cm for men), 26/57 (45.6%) had hypertriglyceridemia (triglyceride ≥ 150 mg/dL), 22/57 (38.6%) had low HDL levels (<50 mg/dL for women and <40 mg/dL for men), 28/57 (49.1%) had elevated SBP and/or DBP (SBP/DBP, ≥130/85 mmHg), and 22/57 (38.6%) had elevated fasting plasma glucose levels (≥100 mg/dL). Thirty study subjects (52.6%) were determined to have MetS; the remaining 27 subjects who did not meet the criteria for MetS were the healthy control subjects.

L5 levels in MetS and control subjects

In MetS subjects, the distribution of LDL subfractions L1–L5 was shifted more toward the most negatively charged subfractions (ie, L5) when compared with that of control subjects (Figure 1A and 1B). The percentage of L5 in MetS subjects was higher in men than in women (20.0±15.4% vs. 15.2±14.1%, respectively), but the difference was not statistically significant (*P*: 0.38, Mann-Whitney U test). For control subjects, the percentage of L5 was almost the same between men and women (8.0±7.4% vs. 7.4±6.8%, respectively). These findings indicate that among men and women with MetS, the effects of L5 may be more pronounced in men, which is consistent with the previously reported findings of Lee and colleagues [26]. To confirm the biologic effects of LDL subfractions, we examined cell apoptosis in BAECs treated with L1, L3, or L5 from MetS or non-MetS control subjects for 24 hours. L5 from MetS subjects and L5 from non-MetS control subjects each induced a marked increase in cell apoptosis, whereas L1 and L3 had negligible or mild effects,

Table 4. Multivariate analysis of L5% in terms of fasting plasma glucose level and body mass index (N = 57).

Independent Variable	Coefficients	P-value	Model R, P-value[a]
			0.53, <0.01
Constant	−20.03	<0.01	
Fasting glucose	0.14	0.02	
Body mass index	0.58	<0.01	

[a]Stepwise multiple regression analysis was used to select the independent variables in this model. The independent variables included age, sex, smoking status, body mass index, waist circumference, blood pressure, pulse pressure, mean arterial pressure, fasting plasma glucose level, total cholesterol level, triglyceride level, high-density lipoprotein level, and low-density lipoprotein level.

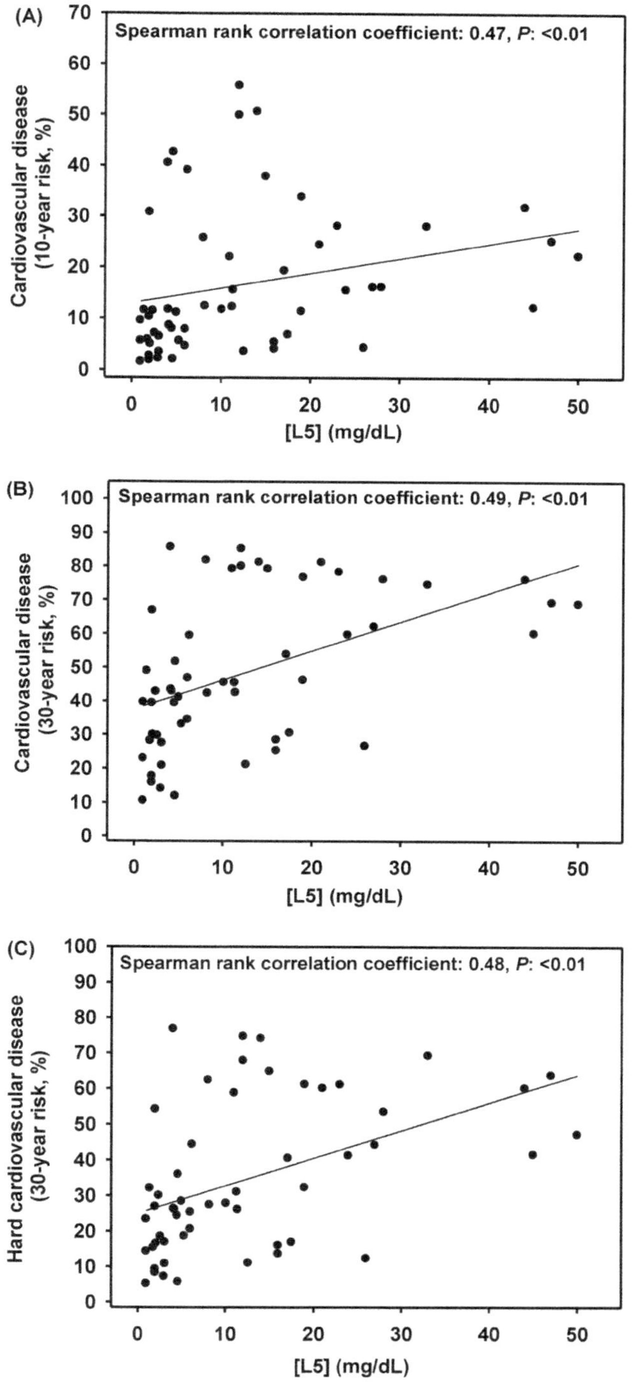

Figure 4. Correlation between L5 concentration ([L5]) and cardiovascular disease (CVD) risks. L5 concentration values are plotted against each risk as indicated. Correlation between [L5] and (A) 10-year general CVD risk, (B) 30-year general CVD risk, and (C) 30-year hard CVD risk.

respectively (Figure 1C). In addition, morphological changes were observed in BAECs treated with L5 and L3 but not in those treated with L1. When we compared the 5 interrelated risk factors for MetS (waist circumference, SBP, and levels of fasting plasma glucose, triglyceride, and HDL) between MetS and control subjects, we observed significant differences in all of these parameters (Table 1). Although total cholesterol and LDL levels were not significantly different between these groups (Table 1 and Figure 2A), the L5% and [L5] were significantly higher in MetS subjects than in control subjects (*P*: 0.005 for L5% and *P*: 0.01 for [L5], Figure 2C and 2E). Furthermore, the Jonckheere trend test revealed that L5% and [L5] increased with the number of MetS criteria (*P*: <0.001 for L5% and *P*: 0.001 for [L5], Figure 2D and 2F) but not with LDL level (*P*: 0.36, Figure 2B).

L5 levels and CVD risk factors

We evaluated the association between L5 and various CVD risk factors. For all study subjects, L5% increased with increasing waist circumference, SBP, and levels of fasting plasma glucose and triglyceride (Figure 3), as well as BMI, waist-to-height ratio, pulse pressure, and mean arterial pressure (Table 2, *P*: <0.05). HDL level was negatively associated with L5% (*P*: 0.03, Figure 3D). The subjects who were receiving drug treatment for hypertension or who were smokers had a significantly higher L5% than did those who were not receiving treatment or who were not smokers, respectively (Table 3, *P*: <0.05). No statistically significant association was observed between L5% and age, sex, DBP, total cholesterol, or LDL (*P*: >0.05, Tables 2 and 3 and Figure 3F). To evaluate the relationship between L5% and multiple CVD risk factors, we performed stepwise multiple regression analysis. As shown in Table 4, L5% was associated with fasting plasma glucose level and BMI (*P*: <0.05), and these 2 factors contributed to 28% of L5% variance (R^2:0.28, *P*: <0.01). The results of multiple regression analysis also revealed that L5% increased by 0.14% for every 1 mg/dL increase in fasting plasma glucose level and 0.58% for every 1 kg/m^2 increase in BMI (Table 4).

L5 levels and CVD risk

To further evaluate whether L5 levels have the potential to be a novel CVD predictor, we examined the relationship between [L5] and CVD risks, as calculated by using the Framingham risk score [31,32]. The 10- and 30-year risks of general CVD were highly correlated with [L5] (Spearman rank correlation coefficient: 0.47 and 0.49, respectively; *P*: <0.01, Figure 4). The 30-year risk of "hard" CVD was also highly correlated with [L5] (Spearman rank correlation coefficient: 0.42, *P*: <0.01). To extract the contribution of [L5] to CVD risk, we performed stepwise multiple regression analysis. As shown in Table 5, CVD risks were associated with [L5] and waist circumference. The [L5] and waist circumference contributed to a total of 23% (R^2:0.23, $P<0.01$), 59% (R^2:0.59, $P<0.01$), and 52% (R^2:0.52, $P<0.01$) of variance for 10-year general CVD risk, 30-year general CVD risk, and 30-year hard CVD risk, respectively. When we determined the contribution of [L5] to CVD risks when controlling the variance of waist circumference, we found that [L5] contributed to 11% of 30-year general CVD risk (partial r^2:0.11, *P*: 0.02) and 8% of 30-year hard CVD risk (partial r^2:0.08, *P*: 0.04) variances. No statistically significant association was observed between [L5] and 10-year general CVD risk (partial r^2:0.02, *P*: 0.28).

Discussion

Levels of total plasma triglycerides and cholesterol, as well as LDL and HDL, have traditionally been monitored as predictors of cardiovascular events [31,32]. In our study, we have investigated beyond total LDL levels and have examined whether plasma levels of electronegative L5 LDL may be a novel predictor of CVD. Similar to our previous findings, we showed that plasma L5 levels are increased in asymptomatic individuals with MetS [26].

Table 5. Multivariate analysis of CVD risks in terms of L5 concentration [L5] and waist circumference (N = 57).

	Coefficients	*P*-value	Partial correlation r	Model R, *P*-value[a]
Dependent variable: 10-year risk of cardiovascular disease				**0.48, <0.01**
Independent variable:				
Constant	−19.43	0.07		
[L5]	0.12	0.28	0.15	
Waist circumference	0.34	<0.01	0.40	
Dependent variable: 30-year risk of cardiovascular disease				**0.77, <0.01**
Independent variable:				
Constant	−44.04	<0.01		
[L5]	0.32	0.02	0.33	
Waist circumference	0.88	<0.01	0.70	
Dependent variable: 30-year risk of hard cardiovascular disease				**0.72, <0.01**
Independent variable:				
Constant	−45.91	<0.01		
[L5]	0.28	0.04	0.29	
Waist circumference	0.77	<0.01	0.65	

[a]Stepwise multiple regression analysis was used to select the independent variables used in this model. The independent variables included the plasma concentration of L5 ([L5]), waist circumference, diastolic blood pressure, total cholesterol level, triglyceride level, high-density lipoprotein level, and low-density lipoprotein level. CVD, cardiovascular disease.

Furthermore, we found that plasma L5 levels in asymptomatic MetS subjects were not only correlated with CVD risk factors and CVD risk but were also correlated with the number of MetS criteria fulfilled and, therefore, CVD progression. These strong correlations demonstrate that circulating L5 may have potential as a predictor of CVD progression and adverse cardiac events.

Several metabolic risk factors tend to cluster in middle-aged adults, including increased BMI and SBP, in addition to elevated levels of LDL, total cholesterol, triglycerides, and blood glucose. Each criterion of MetS is related to an increased risk of developing CVD, and some risk factors are related to a greater risk of coronary heart disease. In terms of attributable deaths, the leading CVD risk factor is elevated blood pressure (to which 13% of global deaths are attributed), followed by tobacco use (9%), elevated blood glucose (6%), physical inactivity (6%), and overweight/obesity (5%) [34]. Men with MetS have been shown to be 2.9 (95% confidence interval [CI], 1.2–7.2) to 4.2 (95% CI, 1.6–10.8) times more likely to die of coronary heart disease after adjusting for conventional cardiovascular risk factors [35]. Although the majority of CVD is caused by risk factors that can be controlled, treated, or modified [3–5], some major CVD risk factors may be unknown and thus cannot be controlled.

Both LDL (−) and L5 are naturally occurring forms of LDL [9,14]. LDL (−) can induce vascular endothelial cells and monocytes to release multiple cytokines, including interleukin-8, monocyte chemoattractant protein-1, tumor necrosis factor-α, and vascular cell adhesion molecule-1 [11,36–39]. Furthermore, L5 can induce endothelial cell apoptosis [14] and cardiomyocyte apoptosis indirectly through endothelial cell–released chemokines [38], which are both critical events in the development of atherothrombosis and CVD [40,41]. Thus, it has been suggested that elevated L5 levels may induce the development of atherothrombosis and CVD. In the current study, we showed that L5 but not L1 induced a marked increase in cell apoptosis and morphological changes in primary BAECs, which is consistent with previously reported findings [20]. L5 from non-MetS control subjects was as cytotoxic as L5 from MetS patients (both at a concentration of 50 μg/mL), indicating that increased concentrations of L5 in patients with MetS may contribute increased cytotoxicity in these individuals. The pathogenic role of L5 supports our present findings, indicating that L5 may be useful a predictor of CVD.

Modified LDL particles have been reported to play key roles in all stages of atherosclerosis. Oxidized LDL (oxLDL) and minimally modified LDL (mmLDL), a mildly oxidized LDL, are the most widely studied types of modified LDL [42]. Because LDL(−) and L5 are each pools of LDL particles modified by several mechanisms, oxLDL would account only for a variable small proportion of their composition [9,15]. The increased electronegativity and negative charge of these LDL particles are attributed to other non-oxidative causes [43]. In vitro and invivo studies have shown that oxLDL promotes endothelial cell toxicity and vasoconstriction [44], and oxLDL has been reported to be a predictor of secondary cardiovascular events. In a prospective study, baseline oxLDL levels were an independent predictor of cardiac death, nonfatal myocardial infarction, and unstable angina; patients in the highest quartile had a hazard ratio 3.15 times greater than did patients in the lowest quartile [45]. In addition, MetS subjects have higher levels of oxLDL than control subjects [46], although the number of MetS criteria was not shown to be associated with oxLDL levels [47]. Because the level of oxLDL circulating in the blood is very low, it is difficult to demonstrate its association with CVD risk factors; thus, the relationship between oxLDL and CVD risk factors has not been fully established [42]. Therefore, oxLDL may not be as useful as a biomarker in asymptomatic individuals with CVD.

Age is a CVD risk factor, as observed in previous studies [31,32]. In the present study, the mean age of MetS subjects was higher than that of control subjects (Table 1). However, the Spearman rank correlation coefficient revealed no association between age and L5% (Table 2). Thus, the L5 differential between the control and MetS groups can be attributed to the pathology of

CVD progression rather than the age difference between these groups, suggesting that L5 could potentially be considered a marker of CVD pathology.

The major limitation of this study was the cross-sectional study design, which was used because this was a discovery study. Although we are confident that our findings show an association between L5% and the progression of CVD, we cannot conclude from our data whether L5 plays a role in the causality of CVD. In addition, because we used questionnaires in our study, a Neyman bias may have affected our results. Although we believe our questionnaire was objectively and well written, the possibility remains that subject answers may have lacked accuracy, in turn minimizing or maximizing the effects of certain variables. Finally, because we did not obtain prospective follow-up data from these patients regarding CVD events, we estimated CVD risk according to the Framingham risk score.

In summary, we showed that L5% and [L5] was associated with the degree of MetS in asymptomatic individuals. Furthermore, L5% correlated strongly with various CVD risk factors, and fasting plasma glucose level and BMI explained 28% of the variation in L5%. Moreover, L5% was associated with CVD risk and contributed to 11% of the 30-year general CVD risk variance when controlling for waist circumference. Our findings indicate that LDL electronegativity was associated with multiple CVD risk factors and CVD risk, suggesting that the LDL electronegativity index may have the potential to be a novel index for predicting CVD. Future prospective studies will aim to identify a causal relationship between L5% and the progression of CVD and adverse cardiac events.

Acknowledgments

The authors thank Nicole Stancel, PhD, ELS, of the Texas Heart Institute in Houston, Texas, for editorial assistance in the preparation of this manuscript.

Author Contributions

Conceived and designed the experiments: JFH TCC SS CHC. Performed the experiments: JL SHC FYC. Analyzed the data: JFH TCC FYC MAE. Contributed reagents/materials/analysis tools: CCC SS CMB. Contributed to the writing of the manuscript: JFH TCC CHC. Manuscript revising and problem solving: CCC JLC JL MAE.

References

1. CDC (2011) Heart disease and stroke prevention, addressing the nation's leading killers. Chronic Disease Prevention and Health Promotion. United States.
2. Leal J, Luengo-Fernandez R, Gray A, Petersen S, Rayner M (2006) Economic burden of cardiovascular diseases in the enlarged European Union. Eur Heart J 27: 1610–1619.
3. Yeboah J, McClelland RL, Polonsky TS, Burke GL, Sibley CT, et al. (2012) Comparison of novel risk markers for improvement in cardiovascular risk assessment in intermediate-risk individuals. JAMA 308: 788–795.
4. Helfand M, Buckley DI, Freeman M, Fu R, Rogers K, et al. (2009) Emerging risk factors for coronary heart disease: a summary of systematic reviews conducted for the U.S. preventive services task force. Ann Intern Med 151: 496–507.
5. Gupta S, Gudapati R, Gaurav K, Bhise M (2013) Emerging risk factors for cardiovascular diseases: Indian context. Indian J Endocrinol Metab 17: 806–814.
6. Kashyap ML (1997) Cholesterol and atherosclerosis: a contemporary perspective. Ann Acad Med Singapore 26: 517–523.
7. Cziraky MJ, Watson KE, Talbert RL (2008) Targeting low HDL-cholesterol to decrease residual cardiovascular risk in the managed care setting. J Manag Care Pharm 14: S3–28; quiz S30–21.
8. Avogaro P, Bon GB, Cazzolato G (1988) Presence of a modified low density lipoprotein in humans. Arteriosclerosis 8: 79–87.
9. Sanchez-Quesada JL, Benitez S, Ordonez-Llanos J (2004) Electronegative low-density lipoprotein. Curr Opin Lipidol 15: 329–335.
10. Demuth K, Myara I, Chappey B, Vedie B, Pech-Amsellem MA, et al. (1996) A cytotoxic electronegative LDL subfraction is present in human plasma. Arterioscler Thromb Vasc Biol 16: 773–783.
11. Ziouzenkova O, Asatryan L, Sahady D, Orasanu G, Perrey S, et al. (2003) Dual roles for lipolysis and oxidation in peroxisome proliferation-activator receptor responses to electronegative low density lipoprotein. J Biol Chem 278: 39874–39881.
12. Benitez S, Sanchez-Quesada JL, Ribas V, Jorba O, Blanco-Vaca F, et al. (2003) Platelet-activating factor acetylhydrolase is mainly associated with electronegative low-density lipoprotein subfraction. Circulation 108: 92–96.
13. Sánchez-Quesada JL, Estruch M, Benítez S, Ordóñez-Llanos J (2012) Electronegative LDL: a useful biomarker of cardiovascular risk? Clinical Lipidology 7: 345–359.
14. Chen CH, Jiang T, Yang JH, Jiang W, Lu J, et al. (2003) Low-density lipoprotein in hypercholesterolemic human plasma induces vascular endothelial cell apoptosis by inhibiting fibroblast growth factor 2 transcription. Circulation 107: 2102–2108.
15. Yang CY, Raya JL, Chen HH, Chen CH, Abe Y, et al. (2003) Isolation, characterization, and functional assessment of oxidatively modified subfractions of circulating low-density lipoproteins. Arterioscler Thromb Vasc Biol 23: 1083–1090.
16. Tang D, Lu J, Walterscheid JP, Chen HH, Engler DA, et al. (2008) Electronegative LDL circulating in smokers impairs endothelial progenitor cell differentiation by inhibiting Akt phosphorylation via LOX-1. J Lipid Res 49: 33–47.
17. Chan HC, Ke LY, Chu CS, Lee AS, Shen MY, et al. (2013) Highly electronegative LDL from patients with ST-elevation myocardial infarction triggers platelet activation and aggregation. Blood 122: 3632–3641.
18. Chang PY, Chen YJ, Chang FH, Lu J, Huang WH, et al. (2013) Aspirin protects human coronary artery endothelial cells against atherogenic electronegative LDL via an epigenetic mechanism: a novel cytoprotective role of aspirin in acute myocardial infarction. Cardiovasc Res 99: 137–145.
19. Ke LY, Engler DA, Lu J, Matsunami RK, Chan HC, et al. (2011) Chemical composition-oriented receptor selectivity of L5, a naturally occurring atherogenic low-density lipoprotein. Pure Appl Chem 83: 1731–1740.
20. Lu J, Yang JH, Burns AR, Chen HH, Tang D, et al. (2009) Mediation of electronegative low-density lipoprotein signaling by LOX-1: a possible mechanism of endothelial apoptosis. Circ Res 104: 619–627.
21. Tang D, Lu J, Walterscheid JP, Chen H-H, Engler DA, et al. (2008) Electronegative LDL circulating in smokers impairs endothelial progenitor cell differentiation by inhibiting Akt phosphorylation via LOX-1. J Lipid Res 49: 33–47.
22. McNeill AM, Rosamond WD, Girman CJ, Golden SH, Schmidt MI, et al. (2005) The metabolic syndrome and 11-year risk of incident cardiovascular disease in the atherosclerosis risk in communities study. Diabetes Care 28: 385–390.
23. Mihic M, Modi P (2008) Metabolic syndrome–risk factors for atherosclerosis and diabetes. Curr Diabetes Rev 4: 122–128.
24. Gami AS, Witt BJ, Howard DE, Erwin PJ, Gami LA, et al. (2007) Metabolic syndrome and risk of incident cardiovascular events and death: a systematic review and meta-analysis of longitudinal studies. J Am Coll Cardiol 49: 403–414.
25. Mottillo S, Filion KB, Genest J, Joseph L, Pilote L, et al. (2010) The metabolic syndrome and cardiovascular risk a systematic review and meta-analysis. J Am Coll Cardiol 56: 1113–1132.
26. Lee AS, Chen WY, Chan HC, Hsu JF, Shen MY, et al. (2014) Gender disparity in LDL-induced cardiovascular damage and the protective role of estrogens against electronegative LDL. Cardiovasc Diabetol 13: 64–73.
27. Chu CS, Wang YC, Lu LS, Walton B, Yilmaz HR, et al. (2013) Electronegative low-density lipoprotein increases C-reactive protein expression in vascular endothelial cells through the LOX-1 receptor. PLoS One 8: e70533.
28. Alberti KG, Eckel RH, Grundy SM, Zimmet PZ, Cleeman JI, et al. (2009) Harmonizing the metabolic syndrome: a joint interim statement of the International Diabetes Federation Task Force on Epidemiology and Prevention; National Heart, Lung, and Blood Institute; American Heart Association; World Heart Federation; International Atherosclerosis Society; and International Association for the Study of Obesity. Circulation 120: 1640–1645.
29. Aviram M (1983) Plasma lipoprotein separation by discontinuous density gradient ultracentrifugation in hyperlipoproteinemic patients. Biochem Med 30: 111–118.
30. Chen CH, Cartwright J Jr, Li Z, Lou S, Nguyen HH, et al. (1997) Inhibitory effects of hypercholesterolemia and ox-LDL on angiogenesis-like endothelial growth in rabbit aortic explants. Essential role of basic fibroblast growth factor. Arterioscler Thromb Vasc Biol 17: 1303–1312.
31. D'Agostino RB Sr, Vasan RS, Pencina MJ, Wolf PA, Cobain M, et al. (2008) General cardiovascular risk profile for use in primary care: the Framingham Heart Study. Circulation 117: 743–753.
32. Pencina MJ, D'Agostino RB Sr, Larson MG, Massaro JM, Vasan RS (2009) Predicting the 30-year risk of cardiovascular disease: the framingham heart study. Circulation 119: 3078–3084.

33. Jonckheere AR (1954) A Distribution-Free k-Sample Test Against Ordered Alternatives. Biometrika 41: 133–145.
34. WHO (2009) Global health risks: mortality and burden of disease attributable to selected major risks. World Health Organization.
35. Lakka HM, Laaksonen DE, Lakka TA, Niskanen LK, Kumpusalo E, et al. (2002) The metabolic syndrome and total and cardiovascular disease mortality in middle-aged men. JAMA 288: 2709–2716.
36. De Castellarnau C, Sanchez-Quesada JL, Benitez S, Rosa R, Caveda L, et al. (2000) Electronegative LDL from normolipemic subjects induces IL-8 and monocyte chemotactic protein secretion by human endothelial cells. Arterioscler Thromb Vasc Biol 20: 2281–2287.
37. Abe Y, Fornage M, Yang CY, Bui-Thanh NA, Wise V, et al. (2007) L5, the most electronegative subfraction of plasma LDL, induces endothelial vascular cell adhesion molecule 1 and CXC chemokines, which mediate mononuclear leukocyte adhesion. Atherosclerosis 192: 56–66.
38. Lee AS, Wang GJ, Chan HC, Chen FY, Chang CM, et al. (2012) Electronegative low-density lipoprotein induces cardiomyocyte apoptosis indirectly through endothelial cell-released chemokines. Apoptosis 17: 1009–1018.
39. Benitez S, Bancells C, Ordonez-Llanos J, Sanchez-Quesada JL (2007) Pro-inflammatory action of LDL(-) on mononuclear cells is counteracted by increased IL10 production. Biochim Biophys Acta 1771: 613–622.
40. Guevara NV, Chen KH, Chan L (2001) Apoptosis in atherosclerosis: pathological and pharmacological implications. Pharmacol Res 44: 59–71.
41. Choy JC, Granville DJ, Hunt DW, McManus BM (2001) Endothelial cell apoptosis: biochemical characteristics and potential implications for atherosclerosis. J Mol Cell Cardiol 33: 1673–1690.
42. Fraley AE, Tsimikas S (2006) Clinical applications of circulating oxidized low-density lipoprotein biomarkers in cardiovascular disease. Current Opinion in Lipidology 17: 502–509.
43. Sanchez-Quesada JL, Camacho M, Anton R, Benitez S, Vila L, et al. (2003) Electronegative LDL of FH subjects: chemical characterization and induction of chemokine release from human endothelial cells. Atherosclerosis 166: 261–270.
44. Navab M, Ananthramaiah GM, Reddy ST, Van Lenten BJ, Ansell BJ, et al. (2004) The oxidation hypothesis of atherogenesis: the role of oxidized phospholipids and HDL. J Lipid Res 45: 993–1007.
45. Shimada K, Mokuno H, Matsunaga E, Miyazaki T, Sumiyoshi K, et al. (2004) Circulating oxidized low-density lipoprotein is an independent predictor for cardiac event in patients with coronary artery disease. Atherosclerosis 174: 343–347.
46. Pohjantahti-Maaroos H, Palomaki A, Kankkunen P, Laitinen R, Husgafvel S, et al. (2010) Circulating oxidized low-density lipoproteins and arterial elasticity: comparison between men with metabolic syndrome and physically active counterparts. Cardiovasc Diabetol 9: 41.
47. Pohjantahti-Maaroos H, Palomaki A, Kankkunen P, Husgafvel S, Knuth T, et al. (2012) Arterial elasticity and oxidized LDL among men with metabolic syndrome and different 10-year cardiovascular risk estimated by FINRISK and SCORE models. Ann Med 44: 503–512.

4

Using Multivariable Mendelian Randomization to Disentangle the Causal Effects of Lipid Fractions

Stephen Burgess*, Daniel F. Freitag, Hassan Khan, Donal N. Gorman, Simon G. Thompson

Cardiovascular Epidemiology Unit, Department of Public Health and Primary Care, University of Cambridge, Cambridge, Cambridgeshire, United Kingdom

Abstract

Background: Previous Mendelian randomization studies have suggested that, while low-density lipoprotein cholesterol (LDL-c) and triglycerides are causally implicated in coronary artery disease (CAD) risk, high-density lipoprotein cholesterol (HDL-c) may not be, with causal effect estimates compatible with the null.

Principal Findings: The causal effects of these three lipid fractions can be better identified using the extended methods of 'multivariable Mendelian randomization'. We employ this approach using published data on 185 lipid-related genetic variants and their associations with lipid fractions in 188,578 participants, and with CAD risk in 22,233 cases and 64,762 controls. Our results suggest that HDL-c may be causally protective of CAD risk, independently of the effects of LDL-c and triglycerides. Estimated causal odds ratios per standard deviation increase, based on 162 variants not having pleiotropic associations with either blood pressure or body mass index, are 1.57 (95% credible interval 1.45 to 1.70) for LDL-c, 0.91 (0.83 to 0.99, p-value =0.028) for HDL-c, and 1.29 (1.16 to 1.43) for triglycerides.

Significance: Some interventions on HDL-c concentrations may influence risk of CAD, but to a lesser extent than interventions on LDL-c. A causal interpretation of these estimates relies on the assumption that the genetic variants do not have pleiotropic associations with risk factors on other pathways to CAD. If they do, a weaker conclusion is that genetic predictors of LDL-c, HDL-c and triglycerides each have independent associations with CAD risk.

Editor: N. Charlotte Onland-Moret, University Medical Center Utrecht, The Netherlands

Funding: The authors received no specific funding for this work. Stephen Burgess is supported by a fellowship from the Wellcome Trust (100114). The funders had no role in study design, data collection and analysis, decision to publish, or preparation of the manuscript.

Competing Interests: The authors have declared that no competing interests exist.

* Email: sb452@medschl.cam.ac.uk

Introduction

Mendelian randomization employs genetic variants to estimate the causal effect of a risk factor on a disease. It is based on the principle that the distribution of a particular genetic variant in a population is analogous to the allocation of treatment in a randomized controlled trial [1]. For valid causal conclusions, each genetic variant used in a Mendelian randomization analysis must be only associated with the risk factor of interest, and be independent of all confounding variables. There must also be no causal pathway leading from the genetic variant to the disease, except for that through the risk factor of interest. These assumptions define an instrumental variable [2]. An association between such a genetic variant and the disease implies that the risk factor has a causal effect on the disease, analogous to inferring an intention-to-treat effect from an association between randomization and disease in a randomized controlled trial [3]. If the assumptions are violated, then a non-zero Mendelian randomization estimate still provides evidence that the risk factor and disease share common genetic predictors, but the estimated causal effect will be biased.

If there are several related risk factors, instrumental variable methods can be used to estimate the causal effects of each of the risk factors in a single analysis model [4]. Multiple genetic variants are required which are analogous to multiple treatment assignments in a factorial randomized trial, and have different magnitudes of association with each of the risk factors. Even if none of the variants show specific associations with any individual risk factor, causal assessments can be made by comparing the associations of the variants with each of the risk factors simultaneously. This approach has been referred to as 'multivariable Mendelian randomization' [5].

We consider 185 variants having known associations with at least one of low-density lipoprotein cholesterol (LDL-c), high-density lipoprotein cholesterol (HDL-c) and triglycerides in 188,578 participants reported by the Global Lipids Genetics Consortium [6]. We combine these with data on the associations of these variants with the risk of coronary artery disease (CAD) based on 22,233 cases and 64,762 controls taken from the CARDIoGRAM consortium [7]. The multivariable Mendelian randomization approach was taken as there are few genetic variants associated with one lipid fraction which are not also associated with a further lipid fraction, particularly for triglycerides. The data are displayed graphically in Figures 1–2.

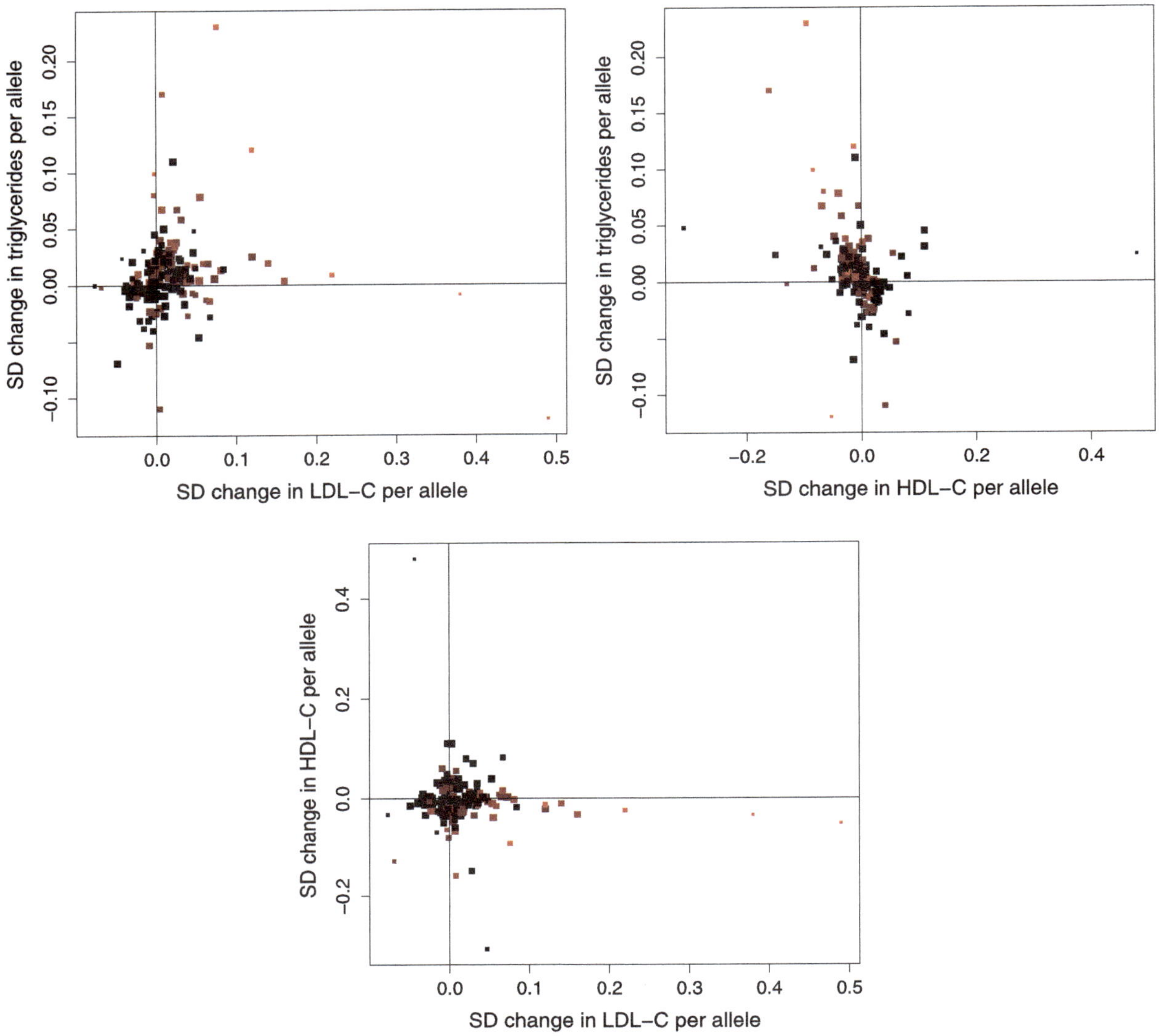

Figure 1. Associations of lipid-related genetic variants with lipid fractions. Association of coronary artery disease (CAD) risk-increasing alleles of 185 genetic variants with all pairs of low-density lipoprotein cholesterol (LDL-c), high-density lipoprotein cholesterol (HDL-c), and triglycerides (brightness and size of points: brighter points correspond to stronger associations with CAD risk, larger points correspond to more precise estimates). Note that some points are overlapping.

These data were previously investigated by Do et al., who performed a number of *ad hoc* analyses to try to disentangle the causal relationships of the lipid fractions [8]. These suggested that, while LDL-c and triglycerides are both causally related to CAD risk, HDL-c is not. However, their regression-based approaches do not account for statistical uncertainty in the reported genetic associations leading to potentially incorrect inference. They also allow information from each variant to receive an equal weight in the analysis, rather than the more common variants receiving a greater weight. This leads to potential bias and inefficiency in the causal estimates, as demonstrated in a simulation study [5]. Additionally, correlation between the genetic variants was not accounted for in the analysis. The conclusions of Do et al. are therefore in doubt.

A multivariable Mendelian randomization analysis requires that the genetic variants used are:

1) associated with the risk factors of interest (here LDL-c, HDL-c and triglycerides),
2) not associated with confounders of any of the associations of the risk factors of interest with the disease (here CAD),
3) not associated with the disease except via pathways through the risk factors of interest.

These assumptions (Figure 3), which are also implicit in the methods of Do et al., correspond with those of an instrumental variable in a conventional Mendelian randomization analysis. It is not necessary for each genetic variant to be associated with all of the risk factors of interest, but estimates of the causal effects of the risk factors will be imprecise unless there are a number of variants which have differing magnitudes of association with each of the risk factors.

We use a likelihood-based statistical method for analyzing summarized data on the genetic associations with the risk factors

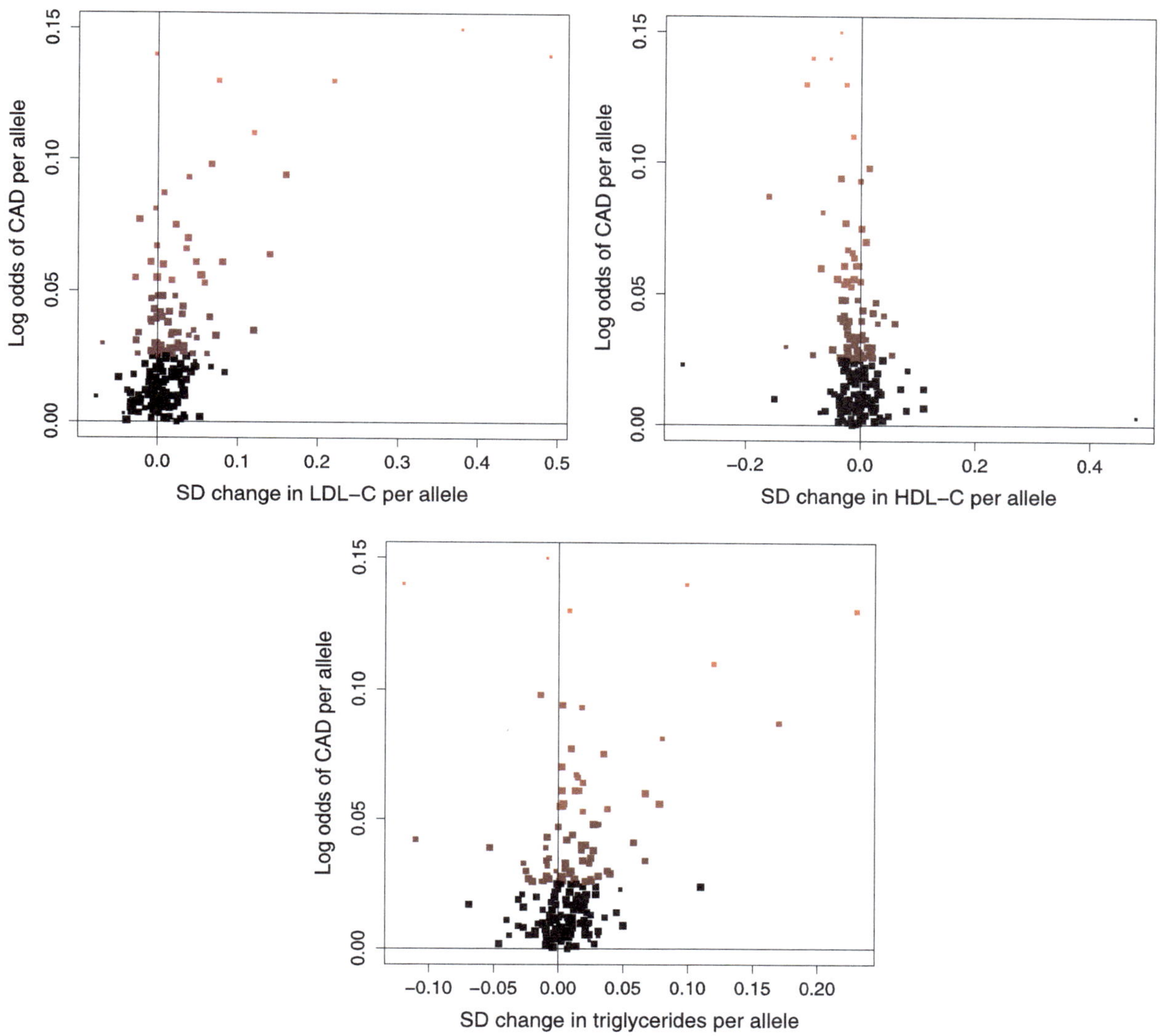

Figure 2. Associations of lipid-related genetic variants with lipid fraction and CAD risk. Association of coronary artery disease (CAD) risk-increasing alleles of 185 genetic variants with odds of CAD, and with each of low-density lipoprotein cholesterol (LDL-c), high-density lipoprotein cholesterol (HDL-c) and triglycerides in turn (brightness and size of points: brighter points correspond to stronger associations with CAD risk, larger points correspond to more precise estimates). Note that some points are overlapping.

and with disease [9] extended for application to multiple risk factors. The likelihood-based method was performed in a Bayesian analysis framework using WinBUGS v1.4.3 [10]. Further details of the analysis are provided in the Methods and Models section.

Results

The results of our likelihood-based method are contrasted with those from Do et al. in Table 1 (first two rows). Our results for LDL-c and triglycerides are qualitatively similar to those of Do et al., although the magnitude of the causal odds ratio for LDL-c is slightly greater and that for triglycerides slightly less. For HDL-c, however, we find a statistically significant inverse causal effect ($P = 0.008$) which Do et al. did not. Its magnitude is less than those for LDL-c and triglycerides, which may be why our more statistically rigorous analysis (which allows appropriate weighting of variants based on the precision of their associations with the risk factors and outcome) was able to identify it.

The crucial assumption necessary for a causal interpretation of our estimates is that the genetic variants used do not have pleiotropic effects with confounders on other pathways to CAD. It is never possible to fully investigate this assumption, but we have matched the 185 genetic variants used against the GWAS catalogue [11] and supplementary material provided by the Global Lipids Genetics Consortium [6] and identified 23 of them which have an association ($P<0.05$) with systolic or diastolic blood pressure, or with body mass index. Removing these 23 genetic variants, and repeating the multivariable Mendelian randomization analysis (Table 1, third row), gave similar estimates to our previous analysis, although the resulting p-value of 0.027 for HDL-c might not be regarded as definitively conclusive.

A heterogeneity test indicated that there was more variability in the genetic associations with the outcome than could be explained by chance alone (185 variants, $P = 2\times10^{-18}$, 162 variants $P = 1\times10^{-16}$). This test is analogous to an over-identification test

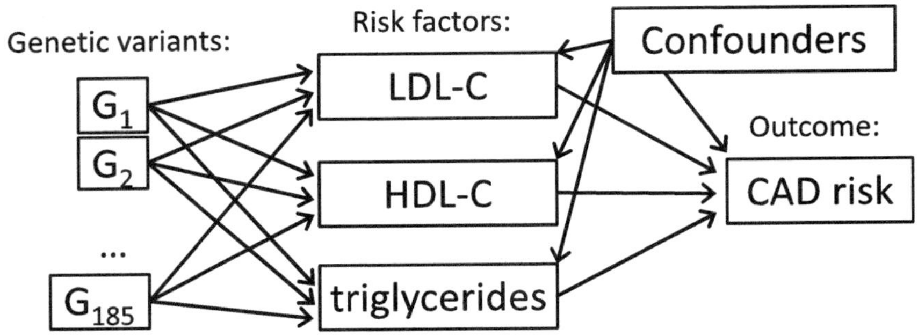

Figure 3. Causal assumptions as a directed acyclic graph. Diagram of causal relationships between genetic variants, risk factors (low-density lipoprotein cholesterol, LDL-c; high-density lipoprotein cholesterol, HDL-c; and triglycerides), confounders, and disease (coronary artery disease, CAD). Although confounders (common causes of a risk factor and the outcome) are represented as a single variable for simplicity, each risk factor may have a different set of confounders.

usually performed in a conventional instrumental variable analysis with individual-level data [12]. Such heterogeneity may partly be explained by misspecification of the model relating the risk factors and the outcome (for example, departure from linearity), but it is likely that there is residual pleiotropy in many of the genetic variants. Heterogeneity can also be assessed visually by plotting the observed and expected associations with CAD risk for each genetic variant using a lipid score based on the associations of the variant with the lipid fractions (Figure 4). The lipid score for a given variant is a linear function of the genetic associations with each of the lipid fractions multiplied by the relevant causal effect estimate. This reflects the expected association of each variant with CAD risk based on the causal effects of the lipid fractions. If the genetic variants are only associated with the outcome via the risk factors under analysis, this graph should (apart from random variation) be a straight-line through the origin; deviation from this is an indication of pleiotropy.

Post hoc analyses were also performed where genetic variants were removed from the analysis if their contribution to the heterogeneity test was greater than the 98th, 95th and 90th percentiles of the relevant chi-squared distribution. Pruning variants at the 98th percentile, 24 variants were excluded from the analysis; at the 95th percentile, 7 more variants were excluded; at the 90th percentile, 11 further variants were excluded. The heterogeneity test statistic was greatly reduced ($P = 0.16$, 0.62, 0.97 at 98th, 95th, 90th percentile). Similar results for the causal effect estimate of HDL-c were observed pruning at the 98th percentile (odds ratio 0.91, 95% credible interval 0.84 to 0.99, $P = 0.030$), although the estimate for HDL-c attenuated towards the null when pruning variants at the 95th (0.93, 0.85 to 1.01, $P = 0.086$) and 90th percentiles (0.94, 0.86 to 1.02, $P = 0.13$). The *post hoc* results show some robustness of the finding that HDL-c-associated variants predict CAD risk, although the strength of association reduces as more variants are excluded from the analysis.

Discussion

Mendelian randomization analyses that use a single genetic variant, for which the biological function is understood, are easily interpreted, as it is clear how the variant relates to the change in the risk factor. They are also valuable in that the function of the variant often provides a clue as to clinical or pharmaceutical interventions that may have a corresponding effect on the disease. When multiple variants for the same risk factor are used, each variant will have a specific functional pathway by which it is associated with the risk factor. The overall causal estimate reflects a weighted average change in the disease risk resulting from long-term interventions in the risk factor. However, it may be that not all ways of intervening on the risk factor result in the same magnitude of change in the disease. Therefore, it would be misleading to assume that all interventions on LDL-c, HDL-c and triglycerides would result in changes in the risk of CAD. As the functions of all the variants and the causal pathways between the risk factors (both measured and unmeasured) are unknown, we prefer to state that, for example, triglyceride-related pathways have a causal role in CAD risk, rather than necessarily triglycerides themselves.

If the extended instrumental variable assumptions necessary for multivariable Mendelian randomization are not satisfied for one or more of the variants, then the causal effect estimates may be biased. Systematic bias would not be expected if pleiotropic

Table 1. Causal odds ratios (95% confidence/credible intervals) of coronary artery disease per standard deviation increase in each lipid fraction (low-density lipoprotein cholesterol, LDL-c; high-density lipoprotein cholesterol, HDL-c; and triglycerides), with two-sided p-value for HDL-c.

Method	Number of variants	LDL-c	HDL-c	Triglycerides	p-value for HDL-c
Do et al. [a]	185	1.46 (1.37 to 1.57)	0.96 (0.89 to 1.03)	1.43 (1.28 to 1.61)	0.35
Multivariable MR	185	1.53 (1.42 to 1.66)	0.90 (0.82 to 0.97)	1.33 (1.20 to 1.47)	0.008
Multivariable MR	162 [b]	1.57 (1.45 to 1.70)	0.91 (0.83 to 0.99)	1.29 (1.16 to 1.43)	0.027

MR = Mendelian randomization.
[a]Derived from Table 3 of Do et al. [8]
[b]Removing 23 variants having known pleiotropic associations with blood pressure or body mass index.

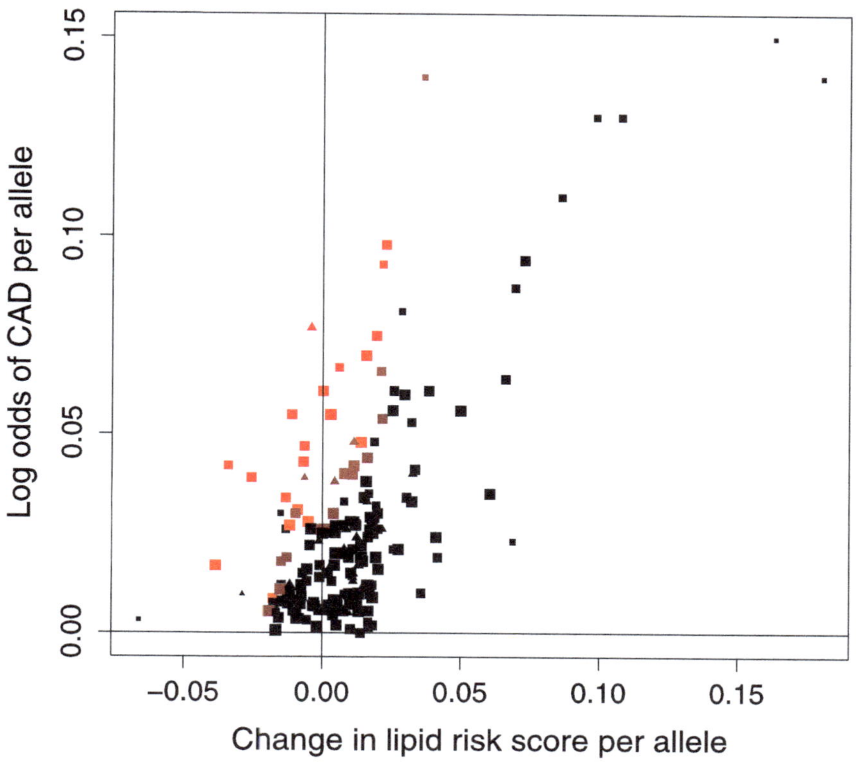

Figure 4. Association of lipid score for all lipid-related genetic variants with CAD risk. Association of coronary artery disease (CAD) risk-increasing alleles of 185 genetic variants with lipid risk score and odds of CAD (brightness corresponds to percentile of chi-squared distribution for heterogeneity test: 98th or higher [brightest red], 95th to 98th, 90th to 95th, below 90th [black]). Note that some points are overlapping. Variants associated with blood pressure or body mass index (P<0.05) are displayed as triangles.

associations of the variants (beyond those with LDL-c, HDL-c and triglycerides) are balanced between those which are beneficial and harmful for CAD risk [13]. However, even if the assumptions are violated and there is bias, this analysis still indicates a shared genetic architecture for CAD risk comprising independent components associated with each of LDL-c, HDL-c and triglycerides.

The interpretation of the causal estimates derived for each risk factor of interest on the disease also depends on whether or not the risk factors are themselves causally dependent. For example, if the effect of one risk factor on the disease is wholly or partially mediated by another risk factor, then they are causally dependent. In Figure 3, the lack of arrows between the risk factors indicates the assumption that these risk factors are causally independent. In fact, there is some biological and epidemiological evidence that the effect of triglycerides on CAD risk is mediated by HDL-c and LDL-c levels [14,15]. If there are causal effects between the risk factors, then estimates from a multivariable Mendelian randomization approach will represent the direct causal effects of each of the risk factors on the disease, not including indirect pathways via the other risk factors [5]. These will typically differ from the total effect of the risk factors. However, they still provide evidence on the causal involvement of the risk factors even if another part of the causal effect is mediated via another risk factor.

Additionally, the consideration of only three lipid categories is a simplification [16]. Some lipid fractions (for example, intermediate-density lipoprotein cholesterol) are omitted in the analysis, and the variability of particle size within the categories is ignored. If the associations with further lipid categories or a finer categorization of lipid fractions were measured, then these could be included in an analysis. However, the identification of the causal effects of precisely defined risk factors is only possible if the function of the genetic variants in the analysis is known. In this case, with multiple genetic variants having (in some cases) unknown functions, it is more appropriate to concentrate on whether the risk factor has a causal interpretation and the direction of the causal effect. For this reason, the division into a small number of clinically-relevant lipid categories is preferred.

Previous Mendelian randomization analyses for HDL-c have not reported statistically significant findings [17], although this may reflect a lack of statistical power due to the low proportion of variation in HDL-c explained by the limited number of genetic variants used. For example, the *LIPG* variant examined by Voight *et al.* was associated with a 0.29 standard deviation change in HDL-c and had a population frequency of 2.6%, so that the variant explained 0.2% of the variance of HDL-c ($R^2 = 0.002$). This translates to less than 10% power to detect an odds ratio of 0.90 per standard deviation increase in HDL-c even in the sample size of 20,913 cases and 95,407 controls considered by the authors [18]. Their analysis using 14 variants associated with HDL-c but not with LDL-c or triglycerides (P>0.05) gave an odds ratio estimate of 0.93 per standard deviation increase in HDL-c, although with a wide confidence interval (95% confidence interval 0.68, 1.26). Another recent study found that a genetic score for HDL-c calculated using all genetic variants associated with HDL-c at a GWAS level of significance was associated with CAD risk, while a similar score for HDL-c excluding those variants associated with LDL-c or triglycerides at a nominal level of significance (P>0.05) was not associated with CAD risk [19]. However, this restricted score explained only a small proportion of the variance in HDL-c (0.3%), and was also associated with LDL-c and triglycerides, limiting the utility of this analysis. Although the authors showed no association between the unrestricted genetic score for HDL-c and CAD risk on adjustment for LDL-c and triglycerides, these variables are on alternative causal pathways from the genetic variants to the outcome, meaning that such adjustment is inappropriate and may lead to bias [20].

Pharmaceutical agents which raise HDL-c levels have failed to show benefits for CAD and total mortality outcomes in clinical trials [21,22]. As our analysis uses many genetic variants with different functions, it is not specifically informative about the efficacy of an intervention for HDL-c on a particular causal pathway. Additionally, causal effect estimates from Mendelian randomization tend to overestimate the proportional effect of clinical interventions [23]. For example, statin therapy in the primary prevention of CAD over five years reduces LDL-c by around 30% and CAD risk by 27% (95% confidence interval 23, 30%) [24]. In contrast, genetic variants specifically associated with LDL-c predict a 67% (54, 76%) reduction in CAD risk for a 30% reduction in LDL-c [9]. Hence, even if HDL-c related pathways are causal for CAD, the expected magnitude of effect from clinical intervention may be much lower than the 9% decrease in CAD risk per 1 standard deviation predicted by the genetic analysis.

Multivariable Mendelian randomization is likely to be a promising design strategy for investigating the causal effects of closely-related risk factors with common genetic predictors. It enables a Mendelian randomization analysis of a risk factor even if there are no variants solely associated with it, such as triglycerides in this example. However, inference of a causal effect relies on the differential associations of multiple genetic variants with the disease, and so cannot be obtained from the distribution of a single genetic variant. Consequently, the intuitive appeal of using Mendelian randomization to infer a causal effect from a variant's sole associations with the risk factor and disease is somewhat reduced.

In conclusion, our analyses support the conclusions of Do et al. that LDL-c and triglycerides are independent risk factors for CAD, but additionally suggest that HDL-c-related pathways may also have a causal role in CAD.

Methods and Models

Estimates for the causal effects of LDL-c, HDL-c and triglycerides on the risk of CAD are obtained using data on the beta-coefficients and standard errors from the regression of the variables on each of the genetic variants in turn. These coefficients were taken from Do et al. [8], who reported the beta-coefficients from linear regression for the lipid fractions (scaled per 1 standard deviation increase in the lipid fraction) and from logistic regression for the disease outcome. Standard errors were obtained from the p-values cited in the paper; if the p-value was exactly 1 (which occurred 2 times out of 740 associations when the beta-coefficient was 0), the average of the standard errors for that variable across the other variants was taken. The standard errors were obtained using R [25], except when the p-value was lower than the smallest non-zero normalized floating-point number allowed in R (around 2×10^{-308}), in which case Wolfram Alpha was used (this occurred for 2 p-values) [26].

In the likelihood-based method, a multivariate normal distribution is assumed for the beta-coefficients representing the genetic associations with each of the risk factors and the disease. We assume that the estimate of association of genetic variant j, $j = 1, 2, \ldots, 185$ with LDL-c is X_{Lj} with standard error σ_{Lj}, and similarly with HDL-c (X_{Hj}, standard error σ_{Hj}), triglycerides (X_{Tj}, standard error σ_{Tj}) and with odds of CAD (Y_j, standard error σ_{Yj}):

$$(X_{Lj},\ X_{Hj},\ X_{Tj},\ Y_j)^T \sim \mathcal{N}_4\left((\xi_{Lj},\ \xi_{Hj},\ \xi_{Tj},\ \xi_{Yj})^T, \Sigma\right),$$

for $j = 1, \ldots, 185$

$$\text{where } \xi_{Yj} = \beta_L \xi_{Lj} + \beta_H \xi_{Hj} + \beta_T \xi_{Tj}$$

$$\text{and } \Sigma = \begin{pmatrix} \sigma_{Lj}^2 & \rho_{LH}\sigma_{Lj}\sigma_{Hj} & \rho_{LT}\sigma_{Lj}\sigma_{Tj} & \rho_{LY}\sigma_{Lj}\sigma_{Yj} \\ \rho_{LH}\sigma_{Lj}\sigma_{Hj} & \sigma_{Hj}^2 & \rho_{HT}\sigma_{Hj}\sigma_{Tj} & \rho_{HY}\sigma_{Hj}\sigma_{Yj} \\ \rho_{LT}\sigma_{Lj}\sigma_{Tj} & \rho_{HT}\sigma_{Hj}\sigma_{Tj} & \sigma_{Tj}^2 & \rho_{TY}\sigma_{Tj}\sigma_{Yj} \\ \rho_{LY}\sigma_{Lj}\sigma_{Yj} & \rho_{HY}\sigma_{Hj}\sigma_{Yj} & \rho_{TY}\sigma_{Tj}\sigma_{Yj} & \sigma_{Yj}^2 \end{pmatrix}$$

The parameters β_L, β_H, and β_T are the causal effects of LDL-c, HDL-c, and triglycerides on CAD risk. As the beta-coefficients for the disease (Y_j) are log odds ratios, the causal parameters represent log odds ratios for a unit increase (here, scaled to be a 1 standard deviation increase) in the risk factor. If the genetic variants were independent, then the overall likelihood would be the product of the above likelihood contributions for each genetic variant. As some of the genetic variants are correlated in their distributions (that is, in linkage disequilibrium), correlations are allowed in the likelihood contributions for these variants by assuming a multivariate normal distribution for all the coefficients of the correlated variants. The elements in the variance-covariance matrix are obtained using the correlations between genetic variants (as these correlations should be equal to the correlations between the beta-coefficients for the same variables). These correlations were taken from the 1000 Genomes Pilot 1 dataset and obtained from the SNP Annotation and Proxy Search (SNAP; http://www.broadinstitute.org/mpg/snap/ldsearchpw.php), and were all less than 0.25.

Causal estimates can be evaluated by numerical maximization of this likelihood function, or by Bayesian methods. Here, direct maximization of the likelihood is impractical, as there are 558 (= 185 × 3 + 3) parameters to optimize over. The analysis was therefore performed in a Bayesian framework using WinBUGS. Vague normal priors with mean zero and variance 10002 were used for each of the unknown parameters. Uniform priors for the β_L, β_H, and β_T parameters on [−3, +3] and on [−2, +2] were also considered; identical results were obtained. The use of vague priors corresponds to no external evidence being incorporated in the analysis, and means that the posterior distribution of the parameters approximates the frequentist likelihood function. The Bayesian method is undertaken purely for computational reasons, and does not correspond to a subjective Bayesian analysis.

Rather than maximizing the likelihood function, we take a sample from the posterior distribution using Monte Carlo Markov Chain (MCMC) sampling. We regard the mean and standard deviation of the posterior distribution as the 'estimate' and 'standard error (SE)'. Twice the tail probability from the posterior distribution for the parameter having the opposite sign to the point estimate is regarded as the two-sided 'p-value'. Further details of the method, including a simulation study, have been previously published [5].

Table 2. Sensitivity analysis for the correlation parameters ($\rho_{..}$) between beta-coefficients for genetic associations with LDL-c (ϑ_L), HDL-c (ϑ_H), triglycerides (ϑ_T) and CAD risk (ϑ_Y): estimates of causal log odds ratios ϑ_L, ϑ_H, and ϑ_T (with standard errors).

ρ_{LH}	ρ_{LT}	ρ_{LY}	ρ_{HT}	ρ_{HY}	ρ_{TY}	ϑ_L	ϑ_H	ϑ_T
−0.2	0.4	0.2	−0.2	−0.2	0.2	0.42 (0.04)	−0.10 (0.04)	0.28 (0.04)
−0.15	0.3	0.15	−0.15	−0.15	0.15	0.42 (0.04)	−0.11 (0.04)	0.28 (0.04)
−0.1	0.2	0.1	−0.1	−0.1	0.1	0.43 (0.04)	−0.11 (0.04)	0.28 (0.04)
−0.05	0.1	0.05	−0.05	−0.05	0.05	0.43 (0.04)	−0.11 (0.04)	0.28 (0.04)
0	0	0	0	0	0	0.43 (0.04)	−0.12 (0.04)	0.29 (0.04)
0.05	−0.1	−0.05	0.05	0.05	−0.05	0.43 (0.04)	−0.12 (0.04)	0.29 (0.04)
0.1	−0.2	−0.1	0.1	0.1	−0.1	0.44 (0.04)	−0.12 (0.04)	0.29 (0.04)

In the likelihood function, the correlation between the beta-coefficients for LDL-c and HDL-c (ρ_{LH}) was taken as −0.1, for LDL-c and triglycerides (ρ_{LT}) 0.2, for LDL-c and CAD risk (ρ_{LY}) 0.1, for HDL-c and triglycerides (ρ_{HT}) −0.1, for HDL-c and CAD risk (ρ_{HY}) −0.1, and for triglycerides and CAD risk (ρ_{TY}) 0.1. These values were taken as estimates of the correlations between the variables LDL-c, HDL-c, triglycerides, and the log odds of disease risk, which will be similar to the correlations between the beta-coefficients used in the likelihood-based analysis. A sensitivity analysis for the values of the correlation parameters ($\rho_{..}$) is given in Table 2. As well as the original parameter values (shown in italics), we take parameter values 2, 1.5, 0.5, 0, −0.5 and −1 times these values. We see that the causal estimates and standard errors are robust to different choices of these parameters.

To assess the homogeneity of the causal effects of the risk factors assessed using different genetic variants, we performed a likelihood-ratio test of the hypothesis that the causal effects of the risk factors were the same for each genetic variant (H_0: $\xi_{Yj} = \vartheta_L \xi_{Lj} + \vartheta_H \xi_{Hj} + \vartheta_T \xi_{Tj}$ for all j), versus the alternative hypothesis that the genetic associations with the outcome for each of the genetic variants were unrestricted (H_1: ξ_{Yj} unrestricted). The likelihood functions were calculated at the relevant point estimates (the mean of the posterior distribution); twice the difference in the log-likelihood function was then compared to a chi-squared distribution with the appropriate number of degrees of freedom. For the *post hoc* analysis, the likelihood contributions for each linkage disequilibrium-block of variants were considered separately and compared to the 98th, 95th, and 90th percentiles of the relevant chi-squared distribution. With 185 variants, the test statistic was 403.4 ($P = 8 \times 10^{-19}$ for a chi-squared distribution with 185−3 = 182 degrees of freedom); with 162 variants (excluding variants associated with blood pressure or body mass index), the test statistic was 352.2 ($P = 1 \times 10^{-16}$; 159 degrees of freedom).

In the *post hoc* analyses excluding variants having heterogeneous association with the outcome, the test statistics were 175.2 (P = 0.17; 158 degrees of freedom) pruning at the 98th percentile; 145.1 (P = 0.62; 151 degrees of freedom) pruning at the 95th percentile; and 111.1 (P = 0.97; 140 degrees of freedom) pruning at the 90th percentile.

The genetic variants omitted from the analysis due to possibly pleiotropic associations with either blood pressure or body mass index are: rs4660293, rs2710642, rs2290547, rs3822072, rs13107325, rs6450176, rs1800562, rs998584, rs702485, rs2293889, rs1883025, rs2068888, rs12801636, rs653178, rs4983559, rs2652834, rs3198697, rs2000999, rs2925979, rs731839, rs492602, rs181362, and rs5763662. These variants are displayed in Figure 4 as triangles.

The genetic variants omitted from the analysis on a *post hoc* basis due to heterogeneity are: rs10493326, rs4587594, rs2642438, rs903319, rs7422339, rs1250229, rs1515110, rs7640978, rs2240327, rs2602836, rs4976033, rs205262, rs12525163, rs17145738, rs799160, rs4921914, rs8176720, rs579459, rs653178, rs6489818, rs1186380, rs1169288, rs4465830, and rs3761445 in the analysis pruning at the 98th percentile; additionally rs17345563, rs998584, rs3996352, rs2412710, rs9930333, rs8077889, and rs4148005 in the analysis pruning at the 95th percentile; additionally rs2290547, rs9686661, rs4917014, rs2326077, rs4871137, rs7832643, rs1781930, rs10832962, rs12801636, rs8017377, and rs952044 in the analysis pruning at the 90th percentile. These variants are displayed in Figure 4 using different colours: the brightest points are those pruned at the 98th percentile.

Data visualization

To aid with visualizing the data, we provide several plots of the genetic associations with the lipid fractions and with CAD risk. Each of the genetic variants is orientated such that the "risk-increasing allele" (the allele associated with an increased risk of CAD) is displayed in each case. Figure 1 shows the per allele associations with each of the lipid fractions in pairs. Figure 2 shows the per allele associations with CAD risk and each of the lipid fractions. Figure 4 shows the association of a lipid score, calculated by multiplying the per allele associations with each of the lipid fractions by the causal effect estimate of the lipid fraction on CAD risk. The lipid score for variant j is therefore:

$$\text{Score}_j = \hat{\beta}_L X_{Lj} + \hat{\beta}_H X_{Hj} + \hat{\beta}_T X_{Tj}$$

If there is no pleiotropy and the causal effects corresponding to the different variants of each of the lipid fractions are homogeneous, then (apart from random variation) this graph should be a straight line through the origin.

Interactive versions of these graphs can be found and explored at http://www.phpc.cam.ac.uk/charttest3.html.

Acknowledgments

Stephen Burgess is funded by a fellowship from the Wellcome Trust (100114).

Author Contributions

Conceived and designed the experiments: SB SGT. Analyzed the data: SB. Wrote the paper: SB DFF HK DNG SGT.

References

1. Davey Smith G, Ebrahim S (2003) 'Mendelian randomization': can genetic epidemiology contribute to understanding environmental determinants of disease? International Journal of Epidemiology 32: 1–22.
2. Greenland S (2000) An introduction to instrumental variables for epidemiologists. International Journal of Epidemiology 29: 722–729.
3. Nitsch D, Molokhia M, Smeeth L, DeStavola B, Whittaker J, et al. (2006) Limits to causal inference based on Mendelian randomization: a comparison with randomized controlled trials. American Journal of Epidemiology 163: 397–403.
4. Angrist JD (2006) Instrumental variables methods in experimental criminological research: what, why and how. Journal of Experimental Criminology 2: 23–44.
5. Burgess S, Thompson SG (2014) Multivariable Mendelian randomization: the use of pleiotropic genetic variants to estimate causal effects. Submitted to American Journal of Epidemiology.
6. The Global Lipids Genetics Consortium (2013) Discovery and refinement of loci associated with lipid levels. Nature Genetics 45: 1274–1283.
7. Schunkert H, König IR, Kathiresan S, Reilly MP, Assimes TL, et al. (2011) Large-scale association analysis identifies 13 new susceptibility loci for coronary artery disease. Nature Genetics 43: 333–338.
8. Do R, Willer CJ, Schmidt EM, Sengupta S, Gao C, et al. (2013) Common variants associated with plasma triglycerides and risk for coronary artery disease. Nature Genetics 45: 1345–1352.
9. Burgess S, Butterworth A, Thompson S (2013) Mendelian randomization analysis with multiple genetic variants using summarized data. Genetic Epidemiology 37: 658–665.
10. Lunn D, Thomas A, Best N, Spiegelhalter D (2000) WinBUGS – A Bayesian modelling framework: Concepts, structure, and extensibility. Statistics and Computing 10: 325–337.
11. Hindorff L, MacArthur J, Morales J, Junkins H, Hall P, et al. (2013) A catalog of published genome-wide association studies. Technical report, European Bioinformatics Institute. Available: www.genome.gov/gwastudies. Accessed 14-March 2014.
12. Hansen L (1982) Large sample properties of generalized method of moments estimators. Econometrica: Journal of the Econometric Society 50: 1029–1054.
13. Davey Smith G (2011) Random allocation in observational data: how small but robust effects could facilitate hypothesis-free causal inference. Epidemiology 22: 460–463.
14. Sarwar N, Sattar N (2009) Triglycerides and coronary heart disease: have recent insights yielded conclusive answers? Current Opinion in Lipidology 20: 275–281.
15. Di Angelantonio E, Sarwar N, Perry P, Kaptoge S, Ray KK, et al. (2009) Major lipids, apolipoproteins, and risk of vascular disease. Journal of the American Medical Association 302: 1993–2000.
16. Würtz P, Kangas AJ, Soininen P, Lehtimäki T, Kähönen M, et al. (2013) Lipoprotein subclass profiling reveals pleiotropy in the genetic variants of lipid risk factors for coronary heart disease: a note on Mendelian randomization studies. Journal of the American College of Cardiology 62: 1906–1908.
17. Voight B, Peloso G, Orho-Melander M, Frikke-Schmidt R, Barbalic M, et al. (2012) Plasma HDL cholesterol and risk of myocardial infarction: a mendelian randomisation study. The Lancet 380: 572–580.
18. Burgess S (2014) Sample size and power calculations in Mendelian randomization with a single instrumental variable and a binary outcome. International Journal of Epidemiology 43: 922–929.
19. Holmes MV, Asselbergs FW, Palmer TM, Drenos F, Lanktree MB, et al. (2014) Mendelian randomization of blood lipids for coronary heart disease. European Heart Journal [epub ahead of print].
20. Christenfeld N, Sloan R, Carroll D, Greenland S (2004) Risk factors, confounding, and the illusion of statistical control. Psychosomatic Medicine 66: 868–875.
21. Barter PJ, Caulfield M, Eriksson M, Grundy SM, Kastelein JJ, et al. (2007) Effects of torcetrapib in patients at high risk for coronary events. New England Journal of Medicine 357: 2109–2122.
22. Schwartz GG, Olsson AG, Abt M, Ballantyne CM, Barter PJ, et al. (2012) Effects of dalcetrapib in patients with a recent acute coronary syndrome. New England Journal of Medicine 367: 2089–2099.
23. Burgess S, Butterworth A, Malarstig A, Thompson S (2012) Use of Mendelian randomisation to assess potential benefit of clinical intervention. British Medical Journal 345: e7325.
24. Taylor F, Ward K, Moore T, Burke M, Davey Smith G, et al. (2011) Statins for the primary prevention of cardiovascular disease. Cochrane Database of Systematic Reviews 1.
25. R Core Team (2014) R: A Language and Environment for Statistical Computing. R Foundation for Statistical Computing, Vienna, Austria. Available: http://www.R-project.org/.
26. Wolfram Alpha LLC Wolfram—Alpha. Available: http://www.wolframalpha.com. Accessed 28-June 2014.

5

Outcomes and Characteristics of Patients Undergoing Percutaneous Angioplasty Followed by Below-Knee or Above-Knee Amputation for Peripheral Artery Disease

Chun-Tai Mao[1,4], Ming-Lung Tsai[2,4], Chao-Yung Wang[2,4], Ming-Shien Wen[2,4], I-Chang Hsieh[2,4], Ming-Jui Hung[1,4], Chao-Hung Wang[1,4], Chun-Chi Chen[2,4], Tien-Hsing Chen[2,3,4]*

1 Heart Failure Center, Division of Cardiology, Department of Internal Medicine, Chang Gung Memorial Hospital, Keelung, Taiwan, **2** Division of Cardiology, Department of Internal Medicine, Chang Gung Memorial Hospital, Taipei, Taiwan, **3** Department of cardiology, Chang Gung Memorial Hospital, Xiamen, China, **4** College of Medicine, Chang Gung University, Taoyuan, Taiwan

Abstract

Objective: Little is known about long-term outcomes among patients who receive percutaneous angioplasty (PTA) for peripheral artery disease (PAD) then undergo below-knee or above-knee amputations. We sought to determine clinical outcomes associated with below-knee or above-knee amputation, along with possible explanatory factors and treatment strategies.

Methods: Using data from Taiwan's National Health Insurance Research Database from 1997 to 2010, 7,568 adult patients were divided into three groups: lower extremity preserved (LE), below-knee amputation (BK) and above-knee amputation (AK). We assessed outcomes including major adverse cardiovascular events (MACE) and associated risk factors.

Results: Overall MACE was significantly higher in the AK group compared to the LE and BK groups, over a mean follow-up of 2.45 years (hazard ratio [HR]: 1.81; 95% confidence interval [CI]: 1.50–2.18 for AK vs. LE; HR: 1.67; 95% CI: 1.36–2.06 for AK vs. BK). However MACE were similar for the BK and LE groups (HR: 1.08; 95% CI: 0.98–1.20). Overall mortality was highest in the AK group (HR: 1.65, 95% CI: 1.34–2.04 for AK vs. BK). As for patient characteristics, atrial fibrillation was more prevalent in the AK group than in the BK group (17% vs. 7%). Independent risk factors associated with death after above- or below-knee amputation included advanced age, heart failure, dialysis, male gender and high patient volume.

Conclusion: The MACE rate was highest in the AK group, whereas the LE and BK groups were similar in this regard. Furthermore, overall mortality increased with larger area of amputation.

Editor: Ryuichi Morishita, Osaka University Graduate School of Medicine, Japan

Funding: The authors have no support or funding to report.

Competing Interests: The authors have declared that no competing interests exist.

* Email: mr7599@outlook.com

These authors contributed equally to this work.

Introduction

As societies age, the incidence of peripheral artery disease (PAD) has been increasing, along with the increase in patients with risk factors for atherosclerosis, especially diabetes mellitus [1,2]. Patients with PAD have a high probability of suffering from critical limb ischemia (CLI) which may require major lower extremity amputation, including above-knee (AK) or below-knee (BK) amputations [2]. Prior studies have revealed that such patients face high morbidity and health costs [3–7]. Furthermore, major lower extremity amputations may contribute to high mortality [8–10]. Therefore revascularization, including bypass surgery and percutaneous angioplasty (PTA), should be considered before amputation, according to the American College of Cardiology/American Heart Association guideline recommendations [11]. In the real world, however, bypass surgery is rarely applied to patients with CLI, because such patients commonly have higher incidence of comorbidities and advanced age, making PTA the preferred treatment [2,12]. After PTA, patients may be able to keep their lower extremity, or they may receive BK or AK amputation. Little is known about long-term and short-term outcomes for these three groups of patients–those receiving only PTA, and those receiving PTA followed by BK, or receiving PTA followed by AK amputation. We evaluated the outcomes in terms of myocardial infarction (MI), stroke, and all causes of mortality. The clinical prognoses of these patients vary based on a number of factors, some of which are patient specific, but no comprehensive report thus far has evaluated the effect of such factors on cardiovascular outcomes.

To evaluate outcomes among PTA patients who kept their lower extremity or received AK or BK amputation, we analyzed data from Taiwan's National Healthcare Insurance (NHI) Program. Our specific aims were to (1) determine rates of death, MI, and stroke among patients who kept their leg or received AK or BK amputation following PTA; (2) determine factors associated with clinical outcomes in the three groups; and (3) determine the major causes of death.

Methods

1. Data source

We conducted a nationwide population-based cohort study using Taiwan's National Health Insurance Research Database (NHIRD), which consists of standard computerized claims documents submitted by medical institutions seeking reimbursement through the NHI Program. PTA is an option covered by the NHI, and patients with PAD who received PTA are recorded in the NHIRD.

The NHI program covers medical needs for 99.19% of the population in Taiwan, more than 25 million people. The accuracy and validation of NHIRD data is based on regular auditing of claims by the NHI Bureau [13–16]. False reimbursement claims result in substantial penalties. Minor infractions involve fines of 100 times the amount of the false claim, while serious infractions may result in revoking physicians' licenses or criminal charges.

This study was approved by the Ethics Institutional Review Board of Chang Gung Memorial Hospital. The information and records of patients were anonymized and de-identified prior to analysis.

2. Study Cohorts and Follow-up

We identified all patients in the NHIRD who received PTA between January 1, 1997 and December 31, 2010 and considered first time admission for PTA as the index hospitalization. The study excluded patients with arterio-venous shunt dysfunction in end stage renal disease who may have received PTA for this clinical event. After we selected this initial cohort of PAD patients receiving PTA, we divided them into three groups according to the results of their index hospitalization. The lower extremity preserved (LE) group consisted of patients whose lower extremity were preserved after PTA. The BK group included patients who received BK amputation following PTA. The AK group included patients receiving AK amputation after PTA (Fig. 1). Follow-up was from the date of index hospitalization to date of death or December 31th, 2010.

3. Outcomes and covariate measurements

Baseline comorbidities were identified by ICD-9-CM (International Classification of Diseases, 9th Revision, Clinical Modification) diagnosis codes and medication during index hospitalization. Primary outcomes were major adverse cardiovascular events (MACE) including death, MI and stroke.

4. Statistical methods

We used the chi-square test to examine the difference in proportions of categorical variables among the LE, AK and BK groups, and tested continuous variables by one-way ANOVA. Associations between the three groups and complications were identified by multivariate logistic regression analysis. We performed multivariate Cox regressions to reveal the association between the three groups and outcomes (prognoses). In a further subgroup analysis, we created a multivariate Cox model to identify the factors associated with overall mortality for patients receiving major amputations. The results are presented as adjusted odds ratios (OR) for logistic regression, or as adjusted hazard ratios (HR) for Cox regressions, with corresponding 95% confidence

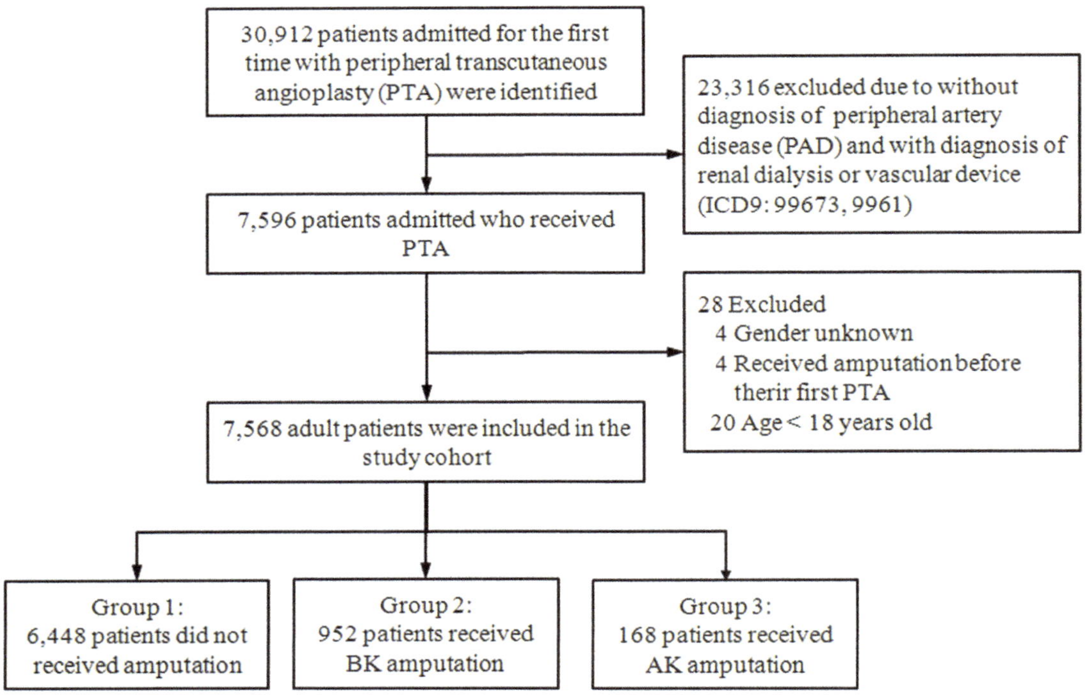

Figure 1. Enrollment flow chart.

Table 1. Clinical characteristics and comorbidities of the study patients.

Characteristics	All patients	Amputation at the admission LE group	BK group	AK group	*P*
Number of patients	7568	6448	952	168	–
Age, year	71.3±11.1	71.5±11.1	69.8±10.9	73.6±11.4	<0.001
Male sex	4694 (62)	4052 (63)	539 (57)	103 (61)	0.001
Indication					
Type2 DM foot	857 (11)	432 (7)	392 (41)	33 (20)	<0.001
Type1 DM foot	4 (0)	0 (0)	4 (0)	0 (0)	<0.001
Chronic ulceration	513 (7)	398 (6)	108 (11)	7 (4)	<0.001
Gangrene	1279 (17)	689 (11)	529 (56)	61 (36)	<0.001
Comorbidities					
Hypertension	6976 (92)	5927 (92)	884 (93)	165 (98)	0.008
Diabetes	5003 (66)	4040 (63)	845 (89)	118 (70)	<0.001
Dyslipidemia	2998 (40)	2655 (41)	304 (32)	39 (23)	<0.001
Gout	721 (10)	617 (10)	79 (8)	25 (15)	0.026
Stroke	2161 (29)	1830 (28)	277 (29)	54 (32)	0.524
Atrial fibrillation	855 (11)	756 (12)	71 (7)	28 (17)	<0.001
Malignancy	586 (8)	508 (8)	67 (7)	11 (7)	0.559
COPD	828 (11)	705 (11)	102 (11)	21 (13)	0.791
Uremia	1798 (24)	1440 (22)	314 (33)	44 (26)	<0.001
Congestive heart failure	1792 (24)	1501 (23)	242 (25)	49 (29)	0.083
Old myocardial infarction	1003 (13)	872 (14)	110 (12)	21 (13)	0.237
Coronary artery disease	3608 (48)	3194 (50)	349 (37)	65 (39)	<0.001
CABG	552 (7)	478 (7)	60 (6)	14 (8)	0.409
Carotid stenting	103 (1)	98 (2)	4 (0)	1 (1)	0.016
Dialysis	1348 (18)	1072 (17)	243 (26)	33 (20)	<0.001

Abbreviations: COPD = chronic obstructive pulmonary disease; CABG = coronary artery bypass graft; DM = diabetes; LE = Lower extremity preserved; BK = below knee; AK = above knee.

intervals (CI). All data analyses were conducted using SPSS software version 15 (SPSS Inc., Chicago, Illinois).

Results

1. Patient characteristics

For our study cohort, we identified a total of 7,588 patients diagnosed with PAD who underwent PTA. Twenty patients under age 18 when undergoing PTA were excluded, resulting in a total of 7,568 adult patients. In the whole cohort there were 4,694 (62%) male patients and 2,874 (38%) female ones. The mean age for the overall cohort was 71.3 years ($SD = 11.1$). The mean follow-up period was 2.45 years ($SD = 2.54$). At the index hospitalization where the patient received PTA, 6,448 patients who remained free of amputation were designated as the LE group, 952 patients who received BK amputation were designated as the BK group, and 168 patients who suffered AK amputation were designated as the AK group.

Table 1 shows the clinical characteristics and comorbidities of the patients. AK patients were older than patients in the two other groups. The prevalence of diabetes, dyslipidemia and end stage renal disease was substantially higher in the BK group compared to the AK group (89% *vs.* 70%; 32% *vs.* 23%; 26% *vs.* 20%, respectively). In contrast, the prevalence of atrial fibrillation was higher in the AK group when compared to the BK group (17% *vs.* 7%).

2. Events during index hospitalization

Table 2 shows the case number and proportion of various complications for the three groups. The risk of acute renal failure was higher in the AK group than the LE and BK groups (OR = 5.57, 3.90, $P<0.001$). Both the AK and BK groups had a higher risk of newly initiated dialysis compared to the LE group (OR = 1.79, $P = 0.003$, for BK; OR = 3.10, $P = 0.001$, for AK). A significantly higher risk of in-hospital mortality was observed for the AK group when compared to the LE and BK groups (OR = 4.18, 3.28, $P<0.001$). In contrast, these three groups did not differ in the risk of new occurrence of MI or stroke. Results for risk of MACE were similar to the pattern for in-hospital mortality.

3. Outcomes during Follow-up

Table 3 displays the numbers of cases and proportion of various prognoses one year after PTA and overall for the three groups. No risk of second amputation above the knee or newly initiated dialysis was found for the AK and BK groups. The BK group were at higher risk of suffering a second BK after PTA compared to the LE group (HR = 1.19, $P = 0.028$), whereas the AK group were less likely to suffer BK compared to the LE and BK groups (HR = 0.35, $P = 0.003$; HR = 0.30, $P = 0.001$). One year after

Table 2. The association of amputation status after PTA with complication at same admission.

	Number of event (%)			Adjusted odds ratio and 95% CI					
Variable	LE (*n*=6448)	BK (*n*=952)	AK (*n*=168)	BK *vs.* LE		AK *vs.* LE		AK *vs.* BK	
				OR (95% CI)	*P*	OR (95% CI)	*P*	OR (95% CI)	*P*
ARF	93 (1.4)	22 (2.3)	14 (8.3)	1.43 (0.88–2.32)	0.150	5.57 (3.04–10.20)	<0.001	3.90 (1.92–7.94)	<0.001
New onset of dialysis	113 (1.8)	38 (4.0)	10 (6.0)	1.79 (1.21–2.65)	0.003	3.10 (1.56–6.19)	0.001	1.73 (0.82–3.63)	0.147
MACE	498 (7.7)	69 (7.2)	25 (14.9)	1.00 (0.76–1.32)	0.991	2.11 (1.34–3.32)	0.001	2.11 (1.26–3.51)	0.004
In-hospital death	177 (2.7)	39 (4.1)	20 (11.9)	1.27 (0.88–1.84)	0.195	4.18 (2.52–6.94)	<0.001	3.28 (1.82–5.90)	<0.001
Myocardial infarction	124 (1.9)	17 (1.8)	4 (2.4)	1.08 (0.64–1.84)	0.767	1.33 (0.48–3.67)	0.584	1.23 (0.40–3.72)	0.718
Stroke	222 (3.4)	19 (2.0)	3 (1.8)	0.79 (0.47–1.32)	0.361	0.53 (0.16–1.77)	0.302	0.68 (0.19–2.44)	0.550

The odds ratio were adjusted for age, gender, diabetes, hypertension, dyslipidemia, previous cerebral vascular accident, heart failure, coronary artery disease, chronic kidney disease, gout, AF, malignancy, chronic obstructive pulmonary disease, center volume and level of hospital.

Abbreviations: ARF = acute renal failure; MACE = major adverse cardiac events; LE = Lower extremity preserved; BK = below knee; AK = above knee; OR = odds ratio; CI = confidence interval.

Table 3. The association of amputation status after PTA with prognoses.

Variable	Number of event (%)			Adjusted hazard ratio and 95% CI					
	LE (n=6448)	BK (n=952)	AK (n=168)	BK *vs.* LE		AK *vs.* LE		AK *vs.* BK	
				HR (95% CI)	P	HR (95% CI)	P	HR (95% CI)	P
Above knee amputation	236 (3.7)	48 (5.0)	9 (5.4)	1.23 (0.89–1.70)	0.206	1.83 (0.94–3.59)	0.077	1.49 (0.73–3.06)	0.276
Below knee amputation	945 (14.7)	216 (22.7)	8 (4.8)	1.19 (1.02–1.39)	0.028	0.35 (0.18–0.71)	0.003	0.30 (0.15–0.60)	0.001
New onset of dialysis	179 (2.8)	33 (3.5)	3 (1.8)	1.32 (0.89–1.94)	0.162	1.10 (0.35–3.48)	0.867	0.84 (0.26–2.75)	0.771
MACE (1 year)	1427 (22.1)	239 (25.1)	74 (44.0)	1.00 (0.87–1.15)	0.959	1.94 (1.53–2.45)	<0.001	1.93 (1.49–2.51)	<0.001
Death	1134 (17.6)	218 (22.9)	69 (41.1)	1.14 (0.98–1.32)	0.083	2.18 (1.70–2.78)	<0.001	1.91 (1.45–2.51)	<0.001
Myocardial infarction	122 (1.9)	12 (1.3)	3 (1.8)	0.70 (0.38–1.29)	0.253	1.15 (0.37–3.65)	0.807	1.64 (0.46–5.84)	0.444
Stroke	279 (4.3)	26 (2.7)	4 (2.4)	0.63 (0.42–0.95)	0.026	0.61 (0.23–1.63)	0.322	0.97 (0.34–2.78)	0.948
MACE (Overall)	2983 (46.3)	467 (49.1)	116 (69.0)	1.08 (0.98–1.20)	0.128	1.81 (1.50–2.18)	<0.001	1.67 (1.36–2.06)	<0.001
Death	2529 (39.2)	430 (45.2)	112 (66.7)	1.20 (1.08–1.33)	0.001	1.98 (1.63–2.40)	<0.001	1.65 (1.34–2.04)	<0.001
Myocardial infarction	310 (4.8)	38 (4.0)	8 (4.8)	1.00 (0.70–1.41)	0.985	1.49 (0.74–3.03)	0.265	1.50 (0.70–3.23)	0.301
Stroke	675 (10.5)	69 (7.2)	9 (5.4)	0.83 (0.64–1.07)	0.142	0.71 (0.37–1.37)	0.304	0.86 (0.43–1.72)	0.662

The hazard ratio were adjusted for age, gender, diabetes, hypertension, dyslipidemia, previous cerebral vascular accident, heart failure, coronary artery disease, chronic kidney disease, gout, AF, malignancy, chronic obstructive pulmonary disease, center volume and level of hospital.

Abbreviations: MACE = major adverse cardiac events; LE = Lower extremity preserved; BK = below knee; AK = above knee; HR = hazard ratio; CI = confidence interval.

Table 4. Cause of mortality ($n = 2531$).

	Overall	LE	BK	AK
Cause of mortality	*n* (%)	*n* (%)	*n* (%)	*n* (%)
Cannot be specified	258 (10.2)	216 (10.4)	36 (10.3)	6 (6.1)
DM and PAD related	435 (17.2)	331 (15.9)	74 (21.1)	30 (30.6)
Sepsis*	362 (14.3)	279 (13.4)	64 (18.3)	19 (19.4)
Pneumonia	290 (11.5)	240 (11.5)	39 (11.1)	11 (11.2)
COPD	20 (0.8)	18 (0.9)	2 (0.6)	0 (0.0)
Cardiovascular disease	395 (15.6)	340 (16.3)	41 (11.7)	14 (14.3)
Stroke	148 (5.8)	127 (6.1)	17 (4.9)	4 (4.1)
Respiratory failure	253 (10.0)	211 (10.1)	37 (10.6)	5 (5.1)
Renal failure	64 (2.5)	53 (2.5)	10 (2.9)	1 (1.0)
GI bleeding and GI system	75 (3.0)	60 (2.9)	11 (3.1)	4 (4.1)
Fall and related mortality	10 (0.4)	7 (0.3)	2 (0.6)	1 (1.0)
Malignancy	162 (6.4)	150 (7.2)	12 (3.4)	0 (0.0)
Others	59 (2.3)	51 (2.4)	5 (1.4)	3 (3.1)

*included UTI, septic septicemia, gangrene, decubitus ulcer.
Abbreviations: DM = diabetes; PAD = peripheral artery disease; COPD = chronic obstructive pulmonary disease; GI = Gastrointestinal; LE = Lower extremity preserved; BK = below knee; AK = above knee.

index hospitalization with PTA, the risk of death as well as MACE was significantly higher in the AK group than in the LE and BK groups. The BK group had a lower risk of stroke than the LE group (HR = 0.63, $P<0.05$), but there was no statistically significant difference in risk of MI among the three groups.

The AK group had higher risk of overall mortality and MACE than the other two groups. The rate of MACE was similar for the LE and BK groups, but the BK group had a higher risk of death than the LE group (HR = 1.20, $P<0.01$).

4. Death causes analysis

Table 4 tabulates the most common causes of death in PAD patients after PTA. For the whole cohort, the leading cause of death was diabetes mellitus (DM) and PAD-related complications (17.2%), followed by cardiovascular disease (15.6%), sepsis (14.3%), pneumonia (11.5%) and respiratory failure (10%), respectively. DM- and PAD-related death is defined as the death due to complications or sequelae induced or aggravated by DM and PAD, including gangrene-related sepsis and complications during PTA or amputation. Patients in the AK group were more

Table 5. Factors associated with death after major amputation of the lower extremity ($n = 1120$).

Variable	HR (95% CI)	*P*
Age (per 10 years)	1.38 (1.26–1.51)	<0.001
Male gender	1.19 (1.00–1.42)	0.049
Diabetes	1.13 (0.88–1.44)	0.342
Hypertension	1.10 (0.77–1.58)	0.606
Dyslipidemia	1.06 (0.86–1.29)	0.593
Previous stroke	1.08 (0.89–1.31)	0.428
Heart failure	1.62 (1.32–1.98)	<0.001
Coronary artery disease	0.98 (0.81–1.18)	0.837
Dialysis	1.98 (1.62–2.42)	<0.001
Gout	1.10 (0.82–1.46)	0.535
Atrial fibrillation	1.23 (0.92–1.64)	0.169
Malignancy	1.31 (0.98–1.77)	0.072
Chronic obstructive pulmonary disease	1.04 (0.79–1.37)	0.785
High center volume‡	1.23 (1.02–1.49)	0.029
Medical center	0.92 (0.77–1.11)	0.393

‡defined as greater than 27 procedures per year.
Abbreviations: HR = hazard ratio; CI = confidence interval.

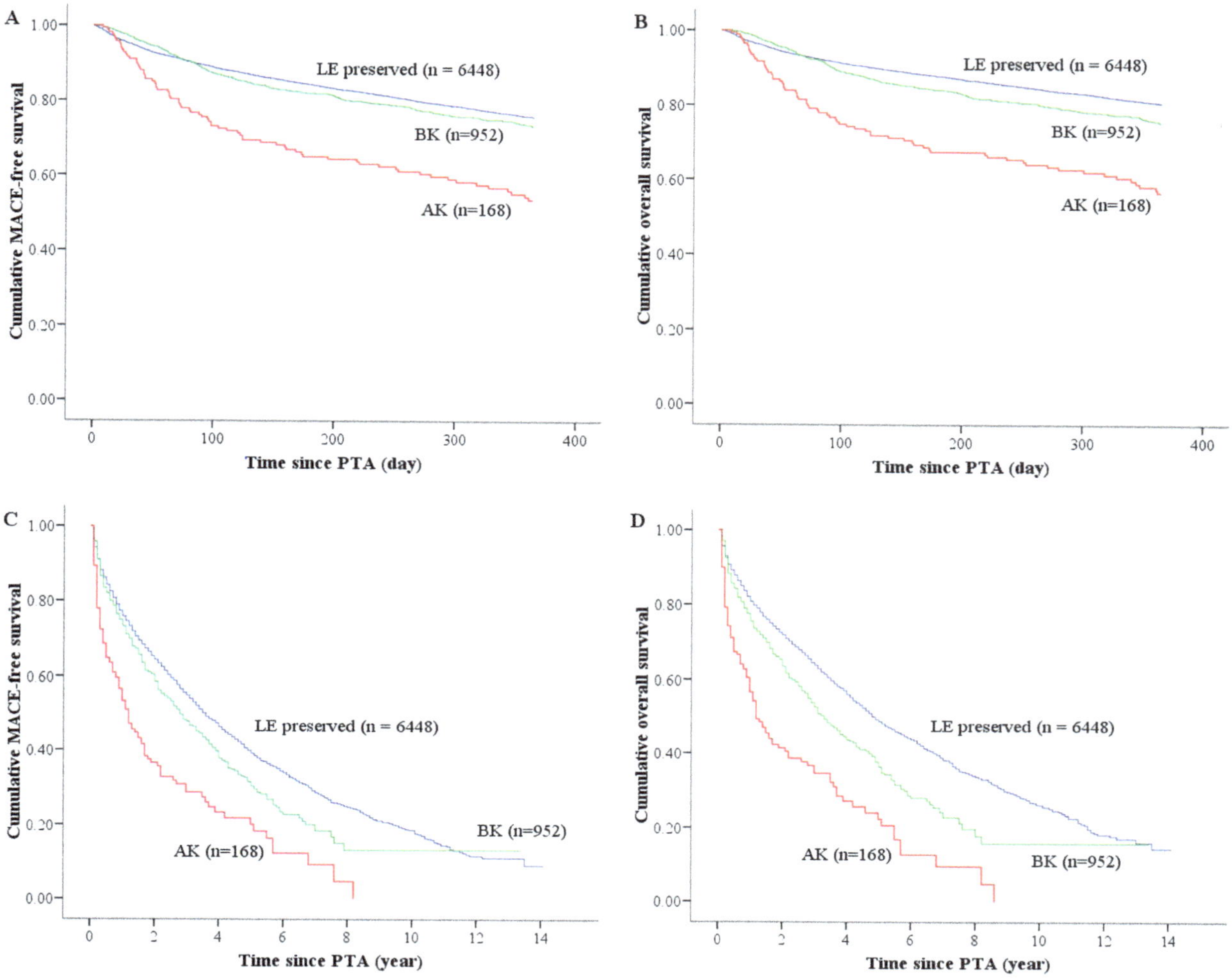

Figure 2. Comparison of prognostics among the study groups. (A) major adverse cardiac events in one year, (B) 1-year mortality, (C) overall major adverse cardiac events, and (D) overall mortality.

likely to expire due to DM and PAD-related complications (30.6%) and less likely to die of respiratory failure (5.1%) and malignancy (0%), when compared to the other groups. DM- and PAD-related complications and sepsis were substantially lower in the LE group (15.9%, 13.4%) compared to the AK and BK groups.

5. Clinical factors associated with death after major amputation of the lower extremity

Table 5 reveals the results of Cox models designed to identify the clinical predictors of overall mortality after BK or AK amputation. Older age (HR = 1.38, $P<0.001$), male gender (HR = 1.19, $P<0.05$), history of heart failure (HR = 1.62, $P<0.001$), history of dialysis (HR = 1.98, $P<0.001$) and receiving PTA in a hospital with high patient volume (HR = 1.23, $P<0.05$) were independently associated with higher risk of death after BK or AK amputation. In the subgroup analysis for patients receiving major amputation at large volume medical centers and low volume centers, the proportion of AK amputations at large volume centers is significantly higher than at low volume centers (19.7% vs. 11.3%, $p<0.001$). The baseline characteristics, including age and gender, were similar at large volume centers and low volume centers. The comorbidities, including hypertension, diabetes, stroke, malignancy, heart failure, coronary artery disease and myocardial infarction history, were not different between these two groups.

Discussion

The previous literature [10] demonstrated that the overall MACE rate was high in the AK and BK groups; however, in our study, the MACE rate was not significantly different for the LE and BK groups. Additionally, the incidence of atrial fibrillation (AF) was higher in the AK group than the two other groups, which may imply different disease mechanisms and treatment strategies for patients undergoing AK amputations.

1. Patient characteristics

In our cohort, patients with PAD undergoing PTA were predominantly male, consistent with findings from the previous study [17]. Because risk factors for PAD, such as smoking and hyperlipidemia, are more common among males, the incidence of PAD is higher for them. In addition, male gender was a predisposing factor for mortality in our cohort study. Meanwhile, comorbidities such as hypertension, stroke, coronary artery disease and myocardial infarction had the same prevalence across the three groups, which implied that atherosclerosis may be the common disease mechanism affecting those patients [8]. In coronary artery disease studies, many medications, including those for lipid profile modification [18], blood sugar control [19] or blood pressure control [20], have been used to promote atherosclerotic plaque regression. According to a previous study [21], regression of atherosclerotic coronary plaque volume may represent a surrogate for myocardial infarction and repeat revascularization. Medication that modifies lipid profiles, and those that act on blood sugar metabolism and blood pressure may also induce regression of atherosclerotic plaque in peripheral artery disease, consequently reducing the rate of re-stenosis in peripheral vessels and repeat revascularization.

2. Events during index hospitalization and outcomes after discharge

During the index hospitalization, the prevalence of acute renal failure was higher in the AK group than the BK and LE groups. Newly initiated dialysis occurred more frequently in the two amputation groups compared to the LE group (Table 2). However, after long-term follow up, the rate of new dialysis occurring was the same for the three groups (Table 3). So the transient renal function impairment showing in the AK group did not indicate increased risk of dialysis in the long term.

During following up, the frequency of a second amputation, BK, was much higher in the AK and BK groups than the LE group (Table 3). This result reveals that patients undergoing AK or BK amputation at index hospitalization are more likely to have the other leg amputated in the future. However MACE in the BK group was the same as in the LE group.

During one-year follow up, the incidence of stroke was a little lower in the BK group than the LE group, and a slightly higher mortality rate was noted in the BK group compared to the LE group, although the difference was not significant. Higher mortality rates may reduce the incidence of stroke due to the competitive outcome effect. The same scenario was also observed for the AK and LE groups, however the result was not statistically significant (HR: 0.61; 95% CI: 0.23–1.63) because of the relatively small sample size of the AK group.

Consistent with the previous literatures [9,10], despite undergoing PTA, high mortality among PAD patients was observed in our study, with or without major amputation. However it was surprising that all-cause mortality showed no statistically significant differences between the LE and BK groups at one-year follow up, but significantly higher mortality was observed in the AK group (Fig. 2B). In long-term follow up, mortality was higher in the BK group than the LE group, but it was highest in AK group (Fig. 2D). However there was no significant difference in MACE between the BK and LE groups in short-term (Fig. 2A) or long-term follow up (Fig. 2C). MACE was unequivocally highest in the AK group.

Although BK amputation, like AK amputation, has been defined as a major amputation [9,10,22], the outcomes were very different for those two groups. According to a previous study [23], survival among patients with BK amputations was not better than those with AK amputations, but our results show better outcomes for the BK amputation group and LE group than for the AK group. Our results are compatible with those from the latest study that has been done [10]. Our study shows that avoiding AK amputation should be a key treatment strategy for PAD patients who receive PTA.

3. Risk factors associated with outcomes and causes of death

Since avoiding AK amputation is the most important strategy following PTA, it is worth noting some different baseline characteristics of patients in the AK and BK groups. As mentioned previously, AF was more prevalent among the patients in the AK group compared to those in the BK group (17% vs. 7%, $p<0.001$), which could suggest that arterial embolisms induced by AF may be the cause of some severely ischemic legs needing AK amputation [8,17,24], On the other hand, the higher prevalence of DM and dyslipidemia among the patients in the BK group compared to the AK group (89% vs. 70%, $p<0.001$; 32% vs. 23%, $p<0.001$) may indicate that atherosclerosis may be a more important cause of PAD in the BK group than in the AK group. So anticoagulation and thrombolysis may be important treatment strategies for avoiding AK amputation in patients who have PAD and AF [22,25,26].

Consistent with findings from the existing literature [10,27], the factors associated with higher mortality included advanced age, heart failure, dialysis, and male gender, all of which could contribute to these extremely high short- and long-term event rates following AK or BK amputation. Unlike other study which revealed better outcomes at medical centers with higher patient volume [28], receiving PTA at high volume medical centers in Taiwan was associated with a higher risk of death after major amputation. According to subgroup analysis for large volume and low volume centers, the proportion of AK amputations in large volume centers is significantly greater than in low volume centers (19.7% vs. 11.3%, $p<0.001$). The baseline characteristics and comorbidities are similar for the two groups. This means that patients with more severe PAD are sent to large volume centers for peripheral angioplasty, so the proportion of AK amputations is higher in large volume centers, with the result that there seem to be more unfavorable outcomes in large volume centers.

Our study also reviewed the causes of mortality. DM or PAD was the most important cause of death in patients with PAD, even when they received aggressive treatment such as PTA. The risk of sepsis was higher in patients with PAD [29], and was an important cause of mortality. Consistent with previous literature [11,22], we found that cardiovascular disease is also a major cause of death in patients with PAD. Pneumonia also poses a threat to their lives. In order to reduce mortality among such patients, effective infection prevention and control are very important, in addition to treating the PAD itself. Some PAD patients may suffer walking impairment or even immobility due to lower limb dysfunction. As with stroke patients, immobility can predispose them to pneumonia [30]. Declining ability to walk is also known to affect mortality [31]. Rehabilitation to increase mobility may thus improve both daily activity levels and medical outcomes [32].

Study Limitations

Our study has a number of limitations. First, the NHI data do not include information about the severity of disease, such as the numbers of diseased vessels and TASC classifications, which may influence both the rate of AK or BK amputation and long-term outcomes following AK or BK amputation. Second, our study cannot distinguish whether new endovascular intervention devices such as stents or drug-eluting balloons, which may affect the prognosis of PAD, were used during PTA. Lastly, our study only suggests trends and possible treatment strategies for improving outcomes among patients with PAD. Randomized controlled trials should be designed to test these different treatment strategies.

Conclusion

Mortality rates among patients with PAD undergoing PTA remain high. MACE were much higher among patients receiving AK amputation than among those receiving BK amputation or those whose lower extremity were preserved, whether in both long-term or short-term follow up. Short-term and overall MACE were the same for the LE and BK groups. Furthermore, overall mortality increased with increasing area of amputation. Sepsis, cardiovascular disease and pneumonia are the major causes of mortality, in addition to DM and PAD-related complications.

Author Contributions

Conceived and designed the experiments: CTM MLT THC. Performed the experiments: CYW MSW. Analyzed the data: ICH MJH. Contributed reagents/materials/analysis tools: CHW CCC. Contributed to the writing of the manuscript: CTM MLT THC.

References

1. Tseng CH, Tai TY, Chen CJ, Lin BJ (1994) Ten-year clinical analysis of diabetic leg amputees. J Formos Med Assoc 93: 388–392.
2. Iida O, Nakamura M, Yamauchi Y, Kawasaki D, Yokoi Y, et al. (2013) Endovascular treatment for infrainguinal vessels in patients with critical limb ischemia: OLIVE registry, a prospective, multicenter study in Japan with 12-month follow-up. Circ Cardiovasc Interv 6: 68–76.
3. McDermott MM, Liu K, Greenland P, Guralnik JM, Criqui MH, et al. (2004) Functional decline in peripheral arterial disease: associations with the ankle brachial index and leg symptoms. JAMA 292: 453–461.
4. Margolis J, Barron JJ, Grochulski WD (2005) Health care resources and costs for treating peripheral artery disease in a managed care population: results from analysis of administrative claims data. J Manag Care Pharm 11: 727–734.
5. Hirsch AT, Criqui MH, Treat-Jacobson D, Regensteiner JG, Creager MA, et al. (2001) Peripheral arterial disease detection, awareness, and treatment in primary care. JAMA 286: 1317–1324.
6. Diehm C, Allenberg JR, Pittrow D, Mahn M, Tepohl G, et al. (2009) Mortality and vascular morbidity in older adults with asymptomatic versus symptomatic peripheral artery disease. Circulation 120: 2053–2061.
7. Peacock JM, Keo HH, Duval S, Baumgartner I, Oldenburg NC, et al. (2011) The incidence and health economic burden of ischemic amputation in Minnesota, 2005–2008. Prev Chronic Dis 8: A141.
8. Hirsch AT, Haskal ZJ, Hertzer NR, Bakal CW, Creager MA, et al. (2006) ACC/AHA 2005 guidelines for the management of patients with peripheral arterial disease (lower extremity, renal, mesenteric, and abdominal aortic): executive summary a collaborative report from the American Association for Vascular Surgery/Society for Vascular Surgery, Society for Cardiovascular Angiography and Interventions, Society for Vascular Medicine and Biology, Society of Interventional Radiology, and the ACC/AHA Task Force on Practice Guidelines (Writing Committee to Develop Guidelines for the Management of Patients With Peripheral Arterial Disease) endorsed by the American Association of Cardiovascular and Pulmonary Rehabilitation; National Heart, Lung, and Blood Institute; Society for Vascular Nursing; TransAtlantic Inter-Society Consensus; and Vascular Disease Foundation. J Am Coll Cardiol 47: 1239–1312.
9. Cruz CP, Eidt JF, Capps C, Kirtley L, Moursi MM (2003) Major lower extremity amputations at a Veterans Affairs hospital. Am J Surg 186: 449–454.
10. Jones WS, Patel MR, Dai D, Vemulapalli S, Subherwal S, et al. (2013) High mortality risks after major lower extremity amputation in Medicare patients with peripheral artery disease. Am Heart J 165: 809–815, 815 e801.
11. Rooke TW, Hirsch AT, Misra S, Sidawy AN, Beckman JA, et al. (2011) 2011 ACCF/AHA Focused Update of the Guideline for the Management of Patients With Peripheral Artery Disease (updating the 2005 guideline): a report of the American College of Cardiology Foundation/American Heart Association Task Force on Practice Guidelines. J Am Coll Cardiol 58: 2020–2045.
12. Goodney PP, Beck AW, Nagle J, Welch HG, Zwolak RM (2009) National trends in lower extremity bypass surgery, endovascular interventions, and major amputations. J Vasc Surg 50: 54–60.
13. Yang YW, Chen YH, Xirasagar S, Lin HC (2011) Increased risk of stroke in patients with bullous pemphigoid: a population-based follow-up study. Stroke 42: 319–323.
14. Wu CY, Wu MS, Kuo KN, Wang CB, Chen YJ, et al. (2010) Effective reduction of gastric cancer risk with regular use of nonsteroidal anti-inflammatory drugs in Helicobacter pylori-infected patients. J Clin Oncol 28: 2952–2957.
15. Wu CY, Chen YJ, Ho HJ, Hsu YC, Kuo KN, et al. (2012) Association between nucleoside analogues and risk of hepatitis B virus-related hepatocellular carcinoma recurrence following liver resection. JAMA 308: 1906–1914.
16. Cheng CL, Kao YH, Lin SJ, Lee CH, Lai ML (2011) Validation of the National Health Insurance Research Database with ischemic stroke cases in Taiwan. Pharmacoepidemiol Drug Saf 20: 236–242.
17. Chen JJ, Lin LY, Lee CH, Liau CS (2012) Age, male gender, and atrial fibrillation predict lower extremity amputation or revascularization in patients with peripheral artery diseases: a population-based investigation. Int J Angiol 21: 35–40.
18. Ballantyne CM, Raichlen JS, Nicholls SJ, Erbel R, Tardif JC, et al. (2008) Effect of rosuvastatin therapy on coronary artery stenoses assessed by quantitative coronary angiography: a study to evaluate the effect of rosuvastatin on intravascular ultrasound-derived coronary atheroma burden. Circulation 117: 2458–2466.
19. Nissen SE, Nicholls SJ, Wolski K, Nesto R, Kupfer S, et al. (2008) Comparison of pioglitazone vs glimepiride on progression of coronary atherosclerosis in patients with type 2 diabetes: the PERISCOPE randomized controlled trial. Jama 299: 1561–1573.
20. Hirohata A, Yamamoto K, Miyoshi T, Hatanaka K, Hirohata S, et al. (2010) Impact of olmesartan on progression of coronary atherosclerosis a serial volumetric intravascular ultrasound analysis from the OLIVUS (impact of OLmesarten on progression of coronary atherosclerosis: evaluation by intravascular ultrasound) trial. J Am Coll Cardiol 55: 976–982.
21. D'Ascenzo F, Agostoni P, Abbate A, Castagno D, Lipinski MJ, et al. (2013) Atherosclerotic coronary plaque regression and the risk of adverse cardiovascular events: a meta-regression of randomized clinical trials. Atherosclerosis 226: 178–185.
22. Kinlay S (2013) Outcomes for clinical studies assessing drug and revascularization therapies for claudication and critical limb ischemia in peripheral artery disease. Circulation 127: 1241–1250.
23. Harris JP, Page S, Englund R, May J (1988) Is the outlook for the vascular amputee improved by striving to preserve the knee? J Cardiovasc Surg (Torino) 29: 741–745.
24. Menke J, Luthje L, Kastrup A, Larsen J (2010) Thromboembolism in atrial fibrillation. Am J Cardiol 105: 502–510.
25. Ouriel K, Veith FJ, Sasahara AA (1998) A comparison of recombinant urokinase with vascular surgery as initial treatment for acute arterial occlusion of the legs. Thrombolysis or Peripheral Arterial Surgery (TOPAS) Investigators. N Engl J Med 338: 1105–1111.
26. Ouriel K, Veith FJ (1998) Acute lower limb ischemia: determinants of outcome. Surgery 124: 336–341; discussion 341–332.
27. Abou-Zamzam AM, Jr., Teruya TH, Killeen JD, Ballard JL (2003) Major lower extremity amputation in an academic vascular center. Ann Vasc Surg 17: 86–90.
28. Kontos MC, Wang Y, Chaudhry SI, Vetrovec GW, Curtis J, et al. (2013) Lower Hospital Volume Is Associated With Higher In-Hospital Mortality in Patients Undergoing Primary Percutaneous Coronary Intervention for ST-Segment-Elevation Myocardial Infarction: A Report From the NCDR. Circ Cardiovasc Qual Outcomes 6: 659–667.
29. Wang HE, Shapiro NI, Griffin R, Safford MM, Judd S, et al. (2012) Chronic medical conditions and risk of sepsis. PLoS One 7: e48307.
30. Westendorp WF, Nederkoorn PJ, Vermeij JD, Dijkgraaf MG, van de Beek D (2011) Post-stroke infection: a systematic review and meta-analysis. BMC Neurol 11: 110.
31. Jain A, Liu K, Ferrucci L, Criqui MH, Tian L, et al. (2013) Declining walking impairment questionnaire scores are associated with subsequent increased mortality in peripheral artery disease. J Am Coll Cardiol 61: 1820–1829.
32. Titsworth WL, Hester J, Correia T, Reed R, Guin P, et al. (2012) The effect of increased mobility on morbidity in the neurointensive care unit. J Neurosurg 116: 1379–1388.

6

Importance of Fatty Acid Compositions in Patients with Peripheral Arterial Disease

Milan Gautam[¶], **Atsushi Izawa***[¶], **Yuji Shiba, Hirohiko Motoki, Takahiro Takeuchi, Ayako Okada, Takeshi Tomita, Yusuke Miyashita, Jun Koyama, Uichi Ikeda**

Department of Cardiovascular Medicine, Shinshu University School of Medicine, Matsumoto, Nagano, Japan

Abstract

Objective: Importance of fatty acid components and imbalances has emerged in coronary heart disease. In this study, we analyzed fatty acids and ankle-brachial index (ABI) in a Japanese cohort.

Methods: Peripheral arterial disease (PAD) was diagnosed in 101 patients by ABI ≤0.90 and/or by angiography. Traditional cardiovascular risk factors and components of serum fatty acids were examined in all patients (mean age 73.2±0.9 years; 81 males), and compared with those in 373 age- and sex-matched control subjects with no evidence of PAD.

Results: The presence of PAD (mean ABI: 0.71±0.02) was independently associated with low levels of gamma-linolenic acid (GLA) (OR: 0.90; 95% CI: 0.85–0.96; $P = 0.002$), eicosapentaenoic acid:arachidonic acid (EPA:AA) ratio (OR: 0.38; 95% CI: 0.17–0.86; $P = 0.021$), and estimated glomerular filtration rate (OR: 0.97; 95% CI: 0.96–0.98; $P < 0.0001$), and with a high hemoglobin A1c level (OR: 1.34; 95% CI: 1.06–1.69; $P = 0.013$). Individuals with lower levels of GLA (≤7.95 μg/mL) and a lower EPA:AA ratio (≤0.55) had the lowest ABI (0.96±0.02, $N = 90$), while the highest ABI (1.12±0.01, $N = 78$) was observed in individuals with higher values of both GLA and EPA:AA ratio ($P < 0.0001$).

Conclusion: A low level of GLA and a low EPA:AA ratio are independently associated with the presence of PAD. Specific fatty acid abnormalities and imbalances could lead to new strategies for risk stratification and prevention in PAD patients.

Editor: Yan Gong, University of Florida, United States of America

Funding: The authors have no support or funding to report.

Competing Interests: The authors have declared that no competing interests exist.

* Email: izawa611@shinshu-u.ac.jp

¶ These authors contributed equally to this work.

Introduction

Peripheral arterial disease (PAD) is a manifestation of advanced systemic atherosclerosis, and is associated with high mortality and morbidity from cardiovascular disease (CVD) [1], [2]. The prevalence of PAD increases with age in both sexes, and affects 4.3% of individuals aged ≥40 years and 14.5% of those aged ≥70 years in the United States [3]. Although the prevalence of PAD in Japanese aged ≥40 years is lower, ranging from 1.5% to 2.7% [4], [5], [6], the number of Japanese PAD patients is anticipated to increase in the near future.

Traditional risk factors, such as diabetes mellitus (DM), hypertension, current smoking, and dyslipidemia, are strongly associated with the risk of PAD [3], [7]. In addition, other biomarkers, including homocysteine, C-reactive protein (CRP), lipoprotein(a), fibrinogen, and apolipoproteins (apo) A-I and B-100 have been examined for their association with PAD [7], [8], [9]. These biomarkers are not consistently and independently associated with the presence of PAD [8], [9], [10], [11]; therefore, it would be of great interest if new markers in addition to the traditional risk factors could contribute substantially to the diagnosis and the management of PAD.

A large scale cohort study spanning 30,829 person-years demonstrated that higher circulating components of omega-3 polyunsaturated fatty acid (PUFA) or the total omega-3 level were associated with lower total mortality, especially deaths from coronary heart disease in healthy older adults [12]. Likewise, low levels of omega-6 PUFAs (linoleic acid [13], [14] or dihomo-gamma-linolenic acid [15]) have been linked to the risk of coronary heart disease. Moreover, a reduced ratio of eicosapentaenoic acid (EPA), an omega-3 PUFA, to arachidonic acid (AA), an omega-6 PUFA (EPA:AA), has recently been highlighted as a risk predictor for secondary cardiovascular events [16], [17], [18], [19]. Importantly, these abnormalities and/or imbalances can be a therapeutic target to prevent future cardiovascular events; however, some controversy still exists regarding the efficacy of individual fatty acids in the prevention of adverse cardiovascular outcomes. Recently, one large-scale randomized clinical trial, as well as a systemic review and meta-analyses of randomized clinical trials, failed to show any efficacy of omega-3 PUFA supplementation in reducing cardiovascular mortality [20], [21]. Overall, the effects of omega-3 and omega-6 PUFAs in the PAD population have remained elusive.

Table 1. Baseline characteristics of the study population.

Patient's characteristics	PAD (N=101)	Controls (N=373)	P value*
Age (years)	73.2±0.9	72.4±0.4	0.243
Sex (male), N (%)	81 (80)	306 (82)	0.665
Body mass index (kg/m^2)	22.45±0.33	23.61±0.16	0.001
Triglycerides (mg/dL)	136.5±7.35	142.3±3.87	0.245
LDL-C (mg/dL)	95.67±3.26	98.76±1.57	0.245
HDL-C (mg/dL)	48.69±1.48	51.16±0.75	0.115
LDL:HDL ratio	2.14±0.10	2.03±0.04	0.702
ABI	0.71±0.02	1.12±0.005	<0.0001
CRP (mg/dL)	0.44±0.09	0.28±0.04	0.008
D-dimer (µg/mL)	2.16±0.33	1.80±0.19	<0.0001
HbA1c (%)	6.45±0.12	6.02±0.07	0.002
eGFR (mL/min/1.73 m^2)	49.96±2.37	64.57±0.95	<0.0001
Statin, N (%)	48 (48)	211 (57)	0.1153
Comorbidity, N (%)			
Coronary heart disease	61 (60)	245 (66)	0.349
Diabetes mellitus	46 (46)	123 (33)	0.025
CKD (eGFR <60 mL/min/1.73 m^2)	59 (58)	139 (37)	0.0002
Dyslipidemia	18 (18)	93 (25)	0.146

Abbreviations: PAD, peripheral artery disease; LDL-C, low-density lipoprotein cholesterol; HDL-C high-density lipoprotein cholesterol; ABI, ankle-brachial index; CRP, c-reactive protein; HbA1c, hemoglobin A1c; eGFR, estimated glomerular filtration rate; CKD, chronic kidney disease. Data are given as mean ± standard error of mean or n (%);

*The Mann–Whitney U test and Fisher's exact test were used to analyze differences in continuous and categorical variables, respectively.

The Framingham risk score [22] and the NIPPON DATA80 [23] chart in Japan have been used to assess the 10-year risk of cardiovascular mortality in the general population; however, factors associated with the presence of PAD have not been completely identified. In addition, current management is not sufficient to fully minimize future cardiovascular events in PAD patients. In this case-controlled study, we examined well-known cardiovascular risk factors and fatty acid composition in PAD patients, in an attempt to provide a new strategy for their risk management.

Methods

1. Study design

This case-control study enrolled adults aged 40 years and older with PAD. PAD was defined if a patient had a resting ankle-brachial index (ABI) ≤0.90 in at least one limb, and/or in claudicant patients who had one or more stenoses >75% in at least one leg artery on angiography. Patients receiving oral EPA supplements and patients with chronic kidney disease (CKD) undergoing hemodialysis were excluded from the study. Laboratory analyses and ABI levels of the cases were compared with those of age- and sex-matched control subjects who had ABI levels between 0.90 and 1.40 or no evidence of PAD. The presence of comorbid diseases was determined as follows: 1) coronary heart disease was diagnosed by coronary angiography, 2) diabetes mellitus by an elevation of fasting blood glucose level (≥126 mg/dL) or use of antidiabetic agents, 3) dyslipidemia by the criteria of the Japan Atherosclerosis Society [24] or use of lipid-lowering agents, and 4) CKD by estimated glomerular filtration rate (eGFR) <60 mL/min/1.73 m^2. Levels of eGFR were calculated using the Modified Diet in Renal Disease study equation, modified for Japanese patients with CKD: eGFR $= 194 \times$ Serum creatinine$^{-1.094} \times$Age$^{-0.287}$ (×0.739 if female) mL/min/1.73 m^2 [25].

The ethics committee of Shinshu University School of Medicine approved the protocol. The study was performed in accordance with the Declaration of Helsinki and with Good Clinical Practice. Patients were managed according to the recommended guidelines of the Japanese Circulation Society.

2. Laboratory analyses

Levels of low-density lipoprotein (LDL) cholesterol, high-density lipoprotein (HDL) cholesterol, triglycerides, hemoglobin A1c (HbA1c), CRP, and D-dimer were measured using routine laboratory tests in a hospital laboratory. Components of fatty acid levels were estimated from serum samples of fasting venous blood in all patients and control subjects using a gas chromatography technique, as described previously, at Special Reference Laboratories, Inc., Tokyo, Japan [16].

3. Measurements of ABI

Systolic blood pressures in upper extremities (brachial artery) and lower extremities (dorsalis pedis and posterior tibial artery) were measured using a FORM ABI/PWV device (Omron Colin Co., Tokyo, Japan), with the subjects resting in a supine position for at least 10 minutes. The ABI is the ratio of the systolic blood pressure in the leg to that in the arms. The ABI was calculated separately for each leg and the lower measurement was used in the analyses; an ABI ≤0.90 at rest represents clinically significant PAD.

4. Statistical analyses

Data were analyzed anonymously by using IBM SPSS Statistics version 18 (IBM Co.) and GraphPad Prism version 5.0f

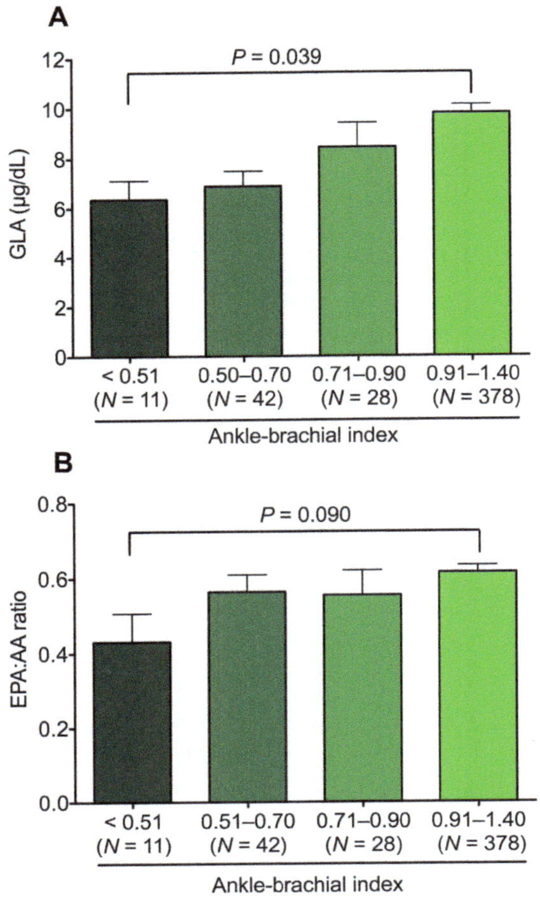

Figure 1. Distribution of levels of (A) gamma-linolenic acid (GLA) and (B) eicosapentaenoic acid:arachidonic acid (EPA:AA) ratio according to ankle-brachial index in 459 subjects.

(GraphPad Software, San Diego, California). Throughout the analysis, a two-tailed *P* value <0.05 was considered to be statistically significant. Differences in continuous variables were assessed by Mann–Whitney *U* tests, and Fisher's exact tests were used to examine differences in categorical variables between the cases and the controls. Univariable logistic regression analyses were performed on the significant variables in the non-parametric tests, and followed by multivariable-adjusted logistic regression analyses for significant variables in the univariable model. Odds ratios (OR) and their 95% confidence intervals (CI) were calculated, with adjustments for age, sex, body mass index, eGFR, HbA1c, gamma-linolenic acid (GLA), EPA:AA ratio, and docosahexaenoic:arachidonic acid (DHA:AA) ratio. Mann–Whitney *U* tests was used to calculate the distributions of GLA and EPA:AA ratio according to ABI levels. The areas under the receiver operating characteristic (ROC) curve were used to identify the sensitivity and specificity of cut-off points for the detection of PAD. We next calculated cut-off points at which the value of "sensitivity + specificity – 1" was maximum (Youden's Index). One way ANOVA with Tukey's multiple comparison test was used to compare ABI levels in individuals with lower or higher proportions of GLA and EPA:AA ratio using the cutoff values calculated from the ROC curve analyses.

Results

1. Characteristics of the study population

A total of 474 patients (101 cases with PAD and 373 controls without PAD) were enrolled. Among all subjects, mean age was 72.6±0.4 years, and 82% were male. The baseline characteristics are summarized in Table 1.

2. Conventional risk factors

There were no significant differences in the baseline serum levels of triglyceride, HDL cholesterol, LDL cholesterol, or LDL:HDL cholesterol ratio between the cases and the controls. No significant differences were observed between the cases and the controls in the numbers of patients with coronary heart disease and dyslipidemia. There was significantly higher morbidity from diabetes (46% versus 33%, *P* = 0.025) and CKD (58% versus 37%, *P* = 0.0002) in the PAD patients than in the controls. Levels of D-dimer and CRP were also significantly elevated in PAD patients compared to controls (*P*<0.05) (Table 1).

3. Fatty acid components

The PAD patients had significantly lower levels of docosapentaenoic acid (12%), docosahexaenoic acid (7%), GLA (27%), EPA:AA ratio (10%), and DHA:AA ratio (11%) than the controls. The lower levels of EPA:AA ratio and DHA:AA ratio were mainly due to lower EPA and DHA concentrations in PAD group. However, no significant differences were observed between the groups in saturated fatty acids, monosaturated fatty acids, alpha-linolenic acid, linoleic acid, dihomo-gamma-linolenic acid, AA, or eicosadienoic acid (Table 2). The distributions of GLA and EPA:AA ratio according to ABI levels were further examined (*N* = 459). The GLA level in patients with ABI<0.51 was 6.35±0.77, significantly lower than the 9.79±0.33 in patients with ABI>0.90 and ≤1.40 (*P* = 0.039; Fig. 1A). The EPA:AA ratio in patients with ABI<0.51 was 0.43±0.07, modestly lower than the 0.61±0.01 in patients with ABI>0.90 and ≤1.40 (*P* = 0.090; Fig. 1B).

4. Factors associated with the presence of PAD

Univariable logistic regression analyses showed that the presence of PAD was associated with low body mass index, reduced eGFR, elevated HbA1c and low levels of EPA, GLA, and EPA:AA ratio (*P*<0.05). In analyses using multivariable-adjusted logistic regression, the presence of PAD was independently associated with reduced eGFR, elevated HbA1c, and low GLA levels and EPA:AA ratio (*P*<0.05; Table 3). The areas under the ROC curve (95% CI) for eGFR, HbA1c, GLA, and EPA:AA ratio were 0.67 (0.60–0.73, *P*<0.0001), 0.59 (0.53–0.66, *P* = 0.002), 0.63 (0.57–0.69, *P*<0.0001), and 0.58 (0.51–0.64, *P* = 0.020), respectively. Based on the ROC curve analyses, the optimal cutoff values for eGFR, HbA1c, GLA, and EPA:AA ratio were 45.50 mL/min/1.73 m^2 (42.0% sensitivity, 86.92% specificity), 6.05% (60.0% sensitivity, 58.45% specificity), 7.95 μg/mL (67.33% sensitivity, 58.49% specificity), and 0.55 (66.34% sensitivity, 47.18% specificity), respectively. Using the optimal cutoff values for GLA and EPA:AA ratio, ABI levels were compared among the 4 subgroups (*N* = 90, GLA ≤7.95 μg/mL and EPA:AA ratio ≤0.55; *N* = 161, GLA >7.95 μg/mL and EPA:AA ratio ≤0.55; *N* = 123, GLA ≤7.95 μg/mL and EPA:AA ratio >0.55; *N* = 78, GLA >7.95 μg/mL and EPA:AA ratio > 0.55; Fig. 2). There was a significant difference in ABI levels among the 4 subgroups (*P*<0.0001). Furthermore, the mean level of ABI (0.96±0.02) was lowest in individuals with a lower GLA (≤ 7.95 μg/mL) and a lower EPA:AA ratio (≤0.55), as compared

Table 2. Serum fatty acid composition.

Fatty Acids (μg/mL)	PAD (*N*=101)	Controls (*N*=373)	*P* value*
Saturated			
Lauric acid (12:0)	5.1±1.45	4.45±0.40	0.644
Myristic acid (14:0)	31.59±2.49	33.23±1.10	0.090
Palmitic acid (16:0)	695.9±23.57	707.6±11.99	0.536
Stearic acid (18:0)	205.3±6.04	215.4±3.19	0.111
Behenic acid (22:0)	15.81±0.46	16.58±0.46	0.133
Lignoceric acid (24:0)	15.30±0.45	15.87±0.64	0.588
Monounsaturated			
Arachidic acid (20:0)	7.14±0.17	7.23±0.08	0.704
Palmitoleic acid (16:1)	70.60±4.12	69.65±1.97	0.833
Eicosenoic acid (20:1)	6.53±0.29	6.72±0.22	0.627
Olieic acid (18:1)	627.5±26.32	616.3±12.0	0.814
Erucic acid (22:1)	1.90±0.13	1.97±0.26	0.299
Polyunsaturated			
Omega-3			
Alpha-linolenic acid (18:3)	28.71±1.64	30.11±0.86	0.284
EPA (20:5)	76.71±4.32	89.81±2.44	0.008
DHA (22:6)	150.2±7.11	163.7±3.01	0.012
Docosapentaenoic acid (22:5)	21.60±0.98	23.77±0.51	0.024
Omega-6			
Linoleic acid (18:2)	772.8±25.55	775.2±11.13	0.490
GLA (18:3)	7.58±0.42	10.07±0.33	< 0.0001
Dihomo-gamma-linolenic acid (20:3)	31.66±1.23	33.57±0.65	0.128
AA (20:4)	155.6±5.04	157.1±2.55	0.652
Docosatetraenoic acid (22:4)	4.55±0.18	4.52±0.12	0.596
Eicosadienoic acid (20:2)	5.92±0.20	5.88±0.09	0.612
EPA:AA ratio	0.53±0.03	0.62±0.01	0.020
DHA:AA ratio	1.01±0.04	1.10±0.02	0.020

Abbreviations: PAD, peripheral artery disease; EPA, eicosapentaenoic acid; DHA, docosahexaenoic acid; GLA, gamma-linolenic acid; AA, arachidonic acid; EPA:AA, eicosapentaenoic acid to arachidonic acid ratio; DHA:AA, docosahexaenoic acid to arachidonic acid ratio. Numbers in parentheses show number of carbons and double bonds. Data are given as mean ± standard error of mean;
*Mann Whitney *U* test.

with the highest ABI levels (1.12±0.01) observed in individuals with higher values of both GLA and EPA:AA ratio ($P<0.001$).

Our results suggested that combined low GLA levels and low EPA:AA ratios were correlated with a potentially more advanced status of PAD. There were 90 enrolled patients with combined low GLA levels (≤7.95 μg/mL) and low EPA:AA ratios (≤0.55), and these patients had high morbidity of coronary heart disease (69%), chronic kidney disease (59%), diabetes mellitus (41%), and dyslipidemia (24%). Around 54% of these patients received statin treatment.

Discussion

This study showed that a low level of GLA and a low EPA:AA ratio were independently associated with the presence of PAD. Moreover, individuals with both a low GLA level and a low EPA:AA ratio had the lowest ABI levels, which suggest an advanced status of PAD. The areas under the ROC curves for CKD, DM, GLA, and EPA:AA ratio were comparable, suggesting that these values had equally important associations with the presence of PAD. In contrast, neither the other components of fatty acids nor the DHA:AA ratio had a significant association with PAD.

Background diseases in Japanese PAD patients have shown a high prevalence of DM (41.2%) [26] and CKD (60.7%) [27]. Similarly, high morbidities of DM and CKD were observed in PAD patients in this study. The average body mass index of our PAD patients was 5% lower than that of controls. This suggested the obesity paradox, which has been explained in part by malnutrition and/or systemic inflammation due to the severity of PAD and, more importantly, is associated with the high mortality of PAD patients [28], [29]. In fact, PAD patients in this study had significantly high CRP levels.

The following differences between EPA and AA have been demonstrated: EPA-derived eicosanoids decrease plasma triglyceride levels, improve endothelial function and arterial stiffness, inhibit platelet aggregation, attenuate inflammation, and stabilize atheromatous plaque [30], [31], [32], [33], [34], whereas AA derived eicosanoids are pro-inflammatory, pre-thrombotic, and vasoconstrictive [31], [32]. Importantly, the benefits of fish intake

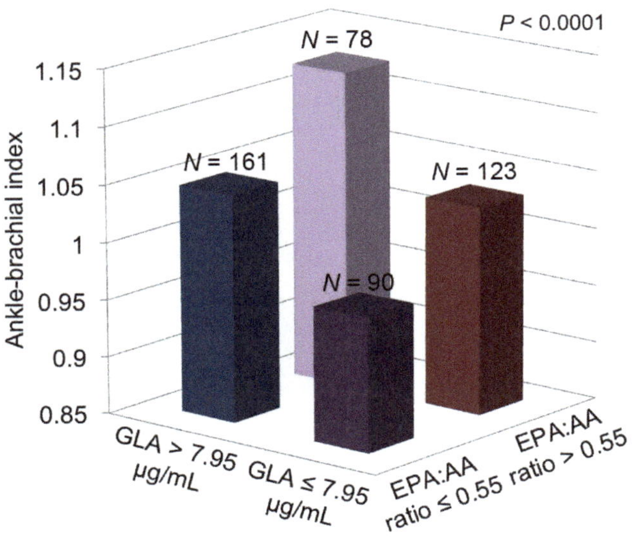

Figure 2. The association of serum levels of gamma-linolenic acid (GLA) and eicosapentaenoic acid:arachidonic acid (EPA:AA) ratio with ankle-brachial index levels. Study population was divided into 4 groups by using cut-off values at 7.95 μg/mL of GLA and at 0.55 of EPA:AA ratio. There was an association of low levels of GLA and low EPA:AA ratios with the presence of PAD.

or dietary supplements of omega-3 PUFAs [16], [35], [36], [37] have emerged in large-scale randomized clinical trials with EPA that reduced coronary events by 19% in Japanese hypercholesterolemic patients [37]. Additive administration of EPA to increase the EPA:AA ratio has reduced the incidence of secondary major adverse cardiovascular events in patients with either PAD [38] or established coronary artery disease [18].

Several findings that indicate favorable effects of GLA (omega-6 PUFA) on cardiovascular diseases have been reported. GLA supplementation was shown to have anti-inflammatory or immunomodulatory roles in patients with multiple sclerosis [39] or acne vulgaris [40], and also to promote vasodilation [41], reduce blood pressure [42], or to have an inhibitory effect on smooth muscle cell proliferation associated with the progression of atherosclerosis [43]. Combined treatment with GLA and EPA for 2 years in 120 patients with intermittent claudication showed a significant reduction in systolic blood pressure ($P \leq 0.05$), and modestly reduced non-fatal coronary events (10% vs. 15%, $P > 0.05$) [44]. These reports could support the results of this study, which suggest a potential role of GLA in inflammation mediating the development of peripheral atherosclerosis.

Current clinical guidelines recommend consumption of omega-3 PUFAs for secondary prevention [45], [46]. Japan has one of the highest mean dietary omega-3 PUFAs intake in the world [47]. More cardiovascular benefits of omega-3 PUFAs would be expected in countries with low omega-3 PUFAs consumption. In addition to the benefits of omega-3 PUFAs, an American Heart Association Science Advisory has recommended the consumption of omega-6 PUFAs of at least 5% to 10% of energy to reduce the risk of coronary artery disease [48]. In fact, a recent case control study demonstrated that patients with a recent myocardial infarction had lower total PUFA levels of both omega-3 and omega-6, as compared with those in control subjects [49]. In our study, however, only GLA levels, but no other PUFA components of omega-6 or the total level, were significantly associated with PAD. Further studies are required to clarify whether a lower GLA level has an exclusive role in the pathophysiology of PAD.

Lipid-lowering therapies with strong statins have been shown to modify the concentrations of omega-3 and omega-6 PUFAs [50], [51]; however, we observed no significant difference in the proportion of individuals receiving statin therapy or in lipid profiles between PAD patients and control subjects (Table 1). In

Table 3. Logistic regression analyses of 101 cases of PAD and 373 control subjects.

Variables	Univariable analysis		Multivariable analyses*	
	OR (95% CI)	P value	OR (95% CI)	P value
Age	1.01 (0.98–1.04)	0.386	0.99 (0.95–1.02)	0.532
Sex (male)	1.12 (0.64–1.96)	0.672	1.06 (0.56–1.99)	0.854
Body mass index	0.89 (0.83–0.96)	0.002	0.92 (0.85–1.002)	0.058
eGFR	0.96 (0.95–0.97)	<0.0001	0.97 (0.96–0.98)	<0.0001
HbA1c	1.28 (1.06–1.55)	0.009	1.34 (1.06–1.69)	0.013
CRP	1.19 (0.95–1.48)	0.199		
D-dimer	1.02 (0.96–1.08)	0.397		
EPA	0.99 (0.98–0.99)	0.013		
DHA	0.99 (0.99–1)	0.051		
Docosapentaenoic acid	0.97 (0.95–1)	0.054		
GLA	0.90 (0.85–0.95)	<0.0001	0.90 (0.85–0.96)	0.002
EPA:AA ratio	0.45 (0.22–0.91)	0.026	0.38 (0.17–0.86)	0.021
DHA:AA ratio	0.57 (0.33–1.005)	0.052	0.59 (0.31–1.11)	0.104

Abbreviations: PAD, peripheral artery disease; eGFR, estimated glomerular filtration rate; HbA1c, hemoglobin A1c; CRP, c-reactive protein; EPA, eicosapentaenoic acid; DHA, docosahexaenoic acid; GLA, gamma-linolenic acid; EPA:AA, eicosapentaenoic acid to arachidonic acid ratio; DHA:AA, docosahexaenoic acid to arachidonic acid ratio; OR, odds ratio; CI, confidence interval.

*Adjusted for age, sex, body mass index, eGFR, HbA1c, and GLA.

addition, neither GLA levels nor the EPA:AA ratio were significantly correlated with lipid profiles in our study.

There are some limitations to our study. First, the sample size was relatively small and the study was performed at a single facility using hospital controls to minimize confounding variables. Second, the attending physician based the diagnosis of PAD on the diagnostic criteria, while their clinical manifestations and disease severity were not reported. Third, this study was not designed to calculate the amount of fish consumption and/or omega-3 intake in the study population. Fourth, the mechanisms of action of fatty acid components in PAD and therapeutic strategies utilizing specific components were beyond the scope of our study. Further research is encouraged to establish risk management and treatment strategies for patients with PAD.

In conclusion, we found that low levels of GLA and a low EPA:AA ratio were significantly associated with the presence and advanced status of PAD in Japanese. These findings imply that, in addition to the well-known cardiovascular risk factors, abnormalities and imbalance of fatty acids play an important role in the pathophysiology of peripheral atherosclerosis, and may open new strategies for risk stratification and prevention for PAD patients.

Author Contributions

Conceived and designed the experiments: AI UI. Performed the experiments: MG AI YS HM TT AO TT YM JK. Analyzed the data: MG AI. Contributed reagents/materials/analysis tools: MG AI. Contributed to the writing of the manuscript: MG AI UI.

References

1. Criqui MH, Langer RD, Fronek A, Feigelson HS, Klauber MR, et al. (1992) Mortality over a period of 10 years in patients with peripheral arterial disease. N Engl J Med 326: 381–386.
2. Criqui MH, Ninomiya JK, Wingard DL, Ji M, Fronek A (2008) Progression of peripheral arterial disease predicts cardiovascular disease morbidity and mortality. J Am Coll Cardiol 52: 1736–1742.
3. Selvin E, Erlinger TP (2004) Prevalence of and risk factors for peripheral arterial disease in the United States: results from the National Health and Nutrition Examination Survey, 1999–2000. Circulation 110: 738–743.
4. Ohnishi H, Sawayama Y, Furusyo N, Maeda S, Tokunaga S, et al. (2010) Risk factors for and the prevalence of peripheral arterial disease and its relationship to carotid atherosclerosis: the Kyushu and Okinawa Population Study (KOPS). J Atheroscler Thromb 17: 751–758.
5. Fujiwara T, Saitoh S, Takagi S, Ohnishi H, Ohata J, et al. (2004) Prevalence of asymptomatic arteriosclerosis obliterans and its relationship with risk factors in inhabitants of rural communities in Japan: Tanno-Sobetsu study. Atherosclerosis 177: 83–88.
6. Usui T, Ninomiya T, Nagata M, Doi Y, Hata J, et al. (2011) Albuminuria as a risk factor for peripheral arterial disease in a general population: the Hisayama study. J Atheroscler Thromb 18: 705–712.
7. Fabsitz RR, Sidawy AN, Go O, Lee ET, Welty TK, et al. (1999) Prevalence of peripheral arterial disease and associated risk factors in American Indians: the Strong Heart Study. Am J Epidemiol 149: 330–338.
8. McDermott MM, Green D, Greenland P, Liu K, Criqui MH, et al. (2003) Relation of levels of hemostatic factors and inflammatory markers to the ankle brachial index. Am J Cardiol 92: 194–199.
9. Ridker PM, Stampfer MJ, Rifai N (2001) Novel risk factors for systemic atherosclerosis: a comparison of C-reactive protein, fibrinogen, homocysteine, lipoprotein(a), and standard cholesterol screening as predictors of peripheral arterial disease. JAMA 285: 2481–2485.
10. Folsom AR, Pankow JS, Tracy RP, Arnett DK, Peacock JM, et al. (2001) Association of C-reactive protein with markers of prevalent atherosclerotic disease. Am J Cardiol 88: 112–117.
11. Erren M, Reinecke H, Junker R, Fobker M, Schulte H, et al. (1999) Systemic inflammatory parameters in patients with atherosclerosis of the coronary and peripheral arteries. Arterioscler Thromb Vasc Biol 19: 2355–2363.
12. Mozaffarian D, Lemaitre RN, King IB, Song X, Huang H, et al. (2013) Plasma phospholipid long-chain ω-3 fatty acids and total and cause-specific mortality in older adults: a cohort study. Ann Intern Med 158: 515–525.
13. Harris WS, Poston WC, Haddock CK (2007) Tissue n-3 and n-6 fatty acids and risk for coronary heart disease events. Atherosclerosis 193: 1–10.
14. Laaksonen DE, Nyyssönen K, Niskanen L, Rissanen TH, Salonen JT (2005) Prediction of cardiovascular mortality in middle-aged men by dietary and serum linoleic and polyunsaturated fatty acids. Arch Intern Med 165: 193–199.
15. Wood DA, Butler S, Riemersma RA, Thomson M, Oliver MF, et al. (1984) Adipose tissue and platelet fatty acids and coronary heart disease in Scottish men. Lancet 2: 117–121.
16. Ninomiya T, Nagata M, Hata J, Hirakawa Y, Ozawa M, et al. (2013) Association between ratio of serum eicosapentaenoic acid to arachidonic acid and risk of cardiovascular disease: the Hisayama Study. Atherosclerosis 231: 261–267.
17. Fujihara M, Fukata M, Odashiro K, Maruyama T, Akashi K, et al. (2013) Reduced plasma eicosapentaenoic acid-arachidonic acid ratio in peripheral artery disease. Angiology 64: 112–118.
18. Matsuzaki M, Yokoyama M, Saito Y, Origasa H, Ishikawa Y, et al. (2009) Incremental effects of eicosapentaenoic acid on cardiovascular events in statin-treated patients with coronary artery disease. Circ J 73: 1283–1290.
19. Domei T, Yokoi H, Kuramitsu S, Soga Y, Arita T, et al. (2012) Ratio of serum n-3 to n-6 polyunsaturated fatty acids and the incidence of major adverse cardiac events in patients undergoing percutaneous coronary intervention. Circ J 76: 423–429.
20. Roncaglioni MC, Tombesi M, Avanzini F, Barlera S, Caimi V, et al. (2013) n-3 fatty acids in patients with multiple cardiovascular risk factors. N Engl J Med 368: 1800–1808.
21. Rizos EC, Ntzani EE, Bika E, Kostapanos MS, Elisaf MS (2012) Association between omega-3 fatty acid supplementation and risk of major cardiovascular disease events: a systematic review and meta-analysis. JAMA 308: 1024–1033.
22. Eichler K, Puhan MA, Steurer J, Bachmann LM (2007) Prediction of first coronary events with the Framingham score: a systematic review. Am Heart J 153: 722–31, 731.
23. NIPPON DATA80 Research Group (2006) Risk assessment chart for death from cardiovascular disease based on a 19-year follow-up study of a Japanese representative population. Circ J 70: 1249–1255.
24. Teramoto T, Sasaki J, Ishibashi S, Birou S, Daida H, et al. (2013) Executive summary of the Japan Atherosclerosis Society (JAS) guidelines for the diagnosis and prevention of atherosclerotic cardiovascular diseases in Japan -2012 version. J Atheroscler Thromb 20: 517–523.
25. Matsuo S, Imai E, Horio M, Yasuda Y, Tomita K, et al. (2009) Revised equations for estimated GFR from serum creatinine in Japan. Am J Kidney Dis 53: 982–992.
26. Yamazaki T, Goto S, Shigematsu H, Shimada K, Uchiyama S, et al. (2007) Prevalence, awareness and treatment of cardiovascular risk factors in patients at high risk of atherothrombosis in Japan. Circ J 71: 995–1003.
27. Endo M, Kumakura H, Kanai H, Araki Y, Kasama S, et al. (2010) Prevalence and risk factors for renal artery stenosis and chronic kidney disease in Japanese patients with peripheral arterial disease. Hypertens Res 33: 911–915.
28. Kumakura H, Kanai H, Aizaki M, Mitsui K, Araki Y, et al. (2010) The influence of the obesity paradox and chronic kidney disease on long-term survival in a Japanese cohort with peripheral arterial disease. J Vasc Surg 52: 110–117.
29. Golledge J, Cronin O, Iyer V, Bradshaw B, Moxon J V, et al. (2013) Body mass index is inversely associated with mortality in patients with peripheral vascular disease. Atherosclerosis 229: 549–555.
30. Thies F, Garry JMC, Yaqoob P, Rerkasem K, Williams J, et al. (2003) Association of n-3 polyunsaturated fatty acids with stability of atherosclerotic plaques: a randomised controlled trial. Lancet 361: 477–485.
31. Mozaffarian D, Wu JHY (2011) Omega-3 fatty acids and cardiovascular disease: effects on risk factors, molecular pathways, and clinical events. J Am Coll Cardiol 58: 2047–2067.
32. Schmitz G, Ecker J (2008) The opposing effects of n-3 and n-6 fatty acids. Prog Lipid Res 47: 147–155.
33. Harris WS, Miller M, Tighe AP, Davidson MH, Schaefer EJ (2008) Omega-3 fatty acids and coronary heart disease risk: clinical and mechanistic perspectives. Atherosclerosis 197: 12–24.
34. Tousoulis D, Plastiras A, Siasos G, Oikonomou E, Verveniotis A, et al. (2014) Omega-3 PUFAs improved endothelial function and arterial stiffness with a parallel antiinflammatory effect in adults with metabolic syndrome. Atherosclerosis 232: 10–16.
35. GISSI-Prevenzione Investigators (1999) Dietary supplementation with n-3 polyunsaturated fatty acids and vitamin E after myocardial infarction: results of the GISSI-Prevenzione trial. Gruppo Italiano per lo Studio della Sopravvivenza nell'Infarto miocardico. Lancet 354: 447–455.
36. Tavazzi L, Maggioni AP, Marchioli R, Barlera S, Franzosi MG, et al. (2008) Effect of n-3 polyunsaturated fatty acids in patients with chronic heart failure (the GISSI-HF trial): a randomised, double-blind, placebo-controlled trial. Lancet 372: 1223–1230.
37. Yokoyama M, Origasa H, Matsuzaki M, Matsuzawa Y, Saito Y, et al. (2007) Effects of eicosapentaenoic acid on major coronary events in hypercholesterolaemic patients (JELIS): a randomised open-label, blinded endpoint analysis. Lancet 369: 1090–1098.
38. Ishikawa Y, Yokoyama M, Saito Y, Matsuzaki M, Origasa H, et al. (2010) Preventive effects of eicosapentaenoic acid on coronary artery disease in patients with peripheral artery disease. Circ J 74: 1451–1457.

39. Rezapour-Firouzi S, Arefhosseini SR, Mehdi F, Mehrangiz E-M, Baradaran B, et al. (2013) Immunomodulatory and therapeutic effects of Hot-nature diet and co-supplemented hemp seed, evening primrose oils intervention in multiple sclerosis patients. Complement Ther Med 21: 473–480.
40. Jung JY, Kwon HH, Hong JS, Yoon JY, Park MS, et al. (2014) Effect of Dietary Supplementation with Omega-3 Fatty Acid and gamma-linolenic Acid on Acne Vulgaris: A Randomised, Double-blind, Controlled Trial. Acta Derm Venereol.
41. Takai S, Jin D, Kawashima H, Kimura M, Shiraishi-Tateishi A, et al. (2009) Anti-atherosclerotic effects of dihomo-gamma-linolenic acid in ApoE-deficient mice. J Atheroscler Thromb 16: 480–489.
42. Engler MM (1993) Comparative study of diets enriched with evening primrose, black currant, borage or fungal oils on blood pressure and pressor responses in spontaneously hypertensive rats. Prostaglandins Leukot Essent Fatty Acids 49: 809–814.
43. Fan YY, Ramos KS, Chapkin RS (1995) Dietary gamma-linolenic acid modulates macrophage-vascular smooth muscle cell interactions. Evidence for a macrophage-derived soluble factor that downregulates DNA synthesis in smooth muscle cells. Arterioscler Thromb Vasc Biol 15: 1397–1403.
44. Leng GC, Lee AJ, Fowkes FG, Jepson RG, Lowe GD, et al. (1998) Randomized controlled trial of gamma-linolenic acid and eicosapentaenoic acid in peripheral arterial disease. Clin Nutr 17: 265–271.
45. Smith SC, Benjamin EJ, Bonow RO, Braun LT, Creager MA, et al. (2011) AHA/ACCF Secondary Prevention and Risk Reduction Therapy for Patients with Coronary and other Atherosclerotic Vascular Disease: 2011 update: a guideline from the American Heart Association and American College of Cardiology Foundation. Circulation 124: 2458–2473.
46. Perk J, De Backer G, Gohlke H, Graham I, Reiner Z, et al. (2012) European Guidelines on cardiovascular disease prevention in clinical practice (version 2012). The Fifth Joint Task Force of the European Society of Cardiology and Other Societies on Cardiovascular Disease Prevention in Clinical Practice (constituted by representatives of nine societies and by invited experts). Eur Heart J 33: 1635–1701.
47. Micha R, Khatibzadeh S, Shi P, Fahimi S, Lim S, et al. (2014) Global, regional, and national consumption levels of dietary fats and oils in 1990 and 2010: a systematic analysis including 266 country-specific nutrition surveys. BMJ 348: g2272.
48. Harris WS, Mozaffarian D, Rimm E, Kris-Etherton P, Rudel LL, et al. (2009) Omega-6 fatty acids and risk for cardiovascular disease: a science advisory from the American Heart Association Nutrition Subcommittee of the Council on Nutrition, Physical Activity, and Metabolism; Council on Cardiovascular Nursing; and Council on Epidemiology and Prevention. Circulation 119: 902–907.
49. Marangoni F, Novo G, Perna G, Perrone Filardi P, Pirelli S, et al. (2014) Omega-6 and omega-3 polyunsaturated fatty acid levels are reduced in whole blood of Italian patients with a recent myocardial infarction: the AGE-IM study. Atherosclerosis 232: 334–338.
50. Harris JI, Hibbeln JR, Mackey RH, Muldoon MF (2004) Statin treatment alters serum n-3 and n-6 fatty acids in hypercholesterolemic patients. Prostaglandins Leukot Essent Fatty Acids 71: 263–269.
51. Nozue T, Yamamoto S, Tohyama S, Fukui K, Umezawa S, et al. (2013) Effects of statins on serum n-3 to n-6 polyunsaturated fatty acid ratios in patients with coronary artery disease. J Cardiovasc Pharmacol Ther 18: 320–326.

7

The Plasma B-Type Natriuretic Peptide Levels Are Low in Males with Stable Ischemic Heart Disease (IHD) Compared to Those Observed in Patients with Non-IHD

Kosuke Minai*, Takayuki Ogawa, Makoto Kawai, Kimiaki Komukai, Toshikazu Tanaka, Kazuo Ogawa, Tomohisa Nagoshi, Satoshi Arase, Satoshi Morimoto, Yasunori Inoue, Hiroshi Sekiyama, Akihiro Urabe, Seiichiro Matsuo, Kenichi Hongo, Michihiro Yoshimura

Division of Cardiology, Department of Internal Medicine, The Jikei University School of Medicine, Tokyo, Japan

Abstract

Objective: Although the plasma B-type natriuretic peptide (BNP) level is a marker of heart failure, it is unclear whether BNP *per se* plays a pivotal role for pathogenic mechanisms underlying the development of ischemic heart disease (IHD). In this study, we retrospectively examined the plasma BNP levels in stable patients with IHD and compared to stable patients with cardiovascular diseases other than IHD.

Methods: The study population was 2088 patients (1698 males and 390 females) who were admitted to our hospital due to IHD (n = 1,661) and non-IHD (n = 427) and underwent cardiac catheterization. Measurements of the hemodynamic parameters and blood sampling were performed.

Results: The plasma BNP levels were significantly lower in the IHD group than in the non-IHD group ($p<0.001$). The multiple regression analysis examining the logBNP values showed that age, a male gender, low left ventricular ejection fraction, low body mass index, serum creatinine, atrial fibrillation and IHD *per se* were significant explanatory variables. When the total study population was divided according to gender, the plasma BNP levels were found to be significantly lower in the IHD group than in the non-IHD group among males ($p<0.001$), but not females (p = NS). Furthermore, a multiple logistic regression analysis of IHD showed the logBNP value to be a significant explanatory variable in males (regression coefficient: −0.669, $p<0.001$), but not females (p = NS).

Conclusions: The plasma BNP levels were relatively low in stable patients with IHD compared with those observed in stable patients with non-IHD; this tendency was evident in males. Perhaps, the low reactivity of BNP is causally associated with IHD in males. We hope that this study will serve as a test of future prospective studies.

Editor: Yasuhiro Ikeda, Mayo Clinic, United States of America

Funding: The authors received no specific funding for this work.

Competing Interests: The authors have declared that no competing interests exist.

* Email: heart@jikei.ac.jp

Introduction

A-type natriuretic peptide and B-type natriuretic peptide (BNP), also known as atrial and brain natriuretic peptides, respectively, are cardiac hormones with a wide range of potent biological effects, including vasodilation, natriuresis and inhibition of the renin-angiotensin-aldosterone and sympathetic nervous systems [1–8]. BNP is selectively secreted from the ventricles, and the magnitude of secretion also varies as a function of the severity of heart failure. The BNP value is thus used as a biochemical marker of heart failure.

In addition, we previously reported that, in patients with acute myocardial infarction (AMI), the time course of the changes in the plasma BNP levels just after the onset of AMI exhibited a biphasic pattern, with the first peak occurring approximately 24 hours after the onset and the second peak 3–5 days after the onset. The second peak of plasma BNP was more marked in severe cases of AMI with heart failure [9].

The plasma immunoreactive BNP level is a sensitive biochemical marker of heart failure; although the precise molecular forms of BNP and its precursors have been discussed from different angles [10,11]. BNP increases the cyclic guanosine monophosphate (cGMP) levels [1]. cGMP activated by BNP is protective against cellular injury as it increase particulate guanylate cyclases [12]. BNP may also be beneficial for suppressing the progression of heart failure and atherosclerosis [13,14]. If the plasma BNP level is insufficiently increased for any reason, heart failure and atherosclerosis are likely

Table 1. Baseline characteristics and the past medical history and medication regimen of the study subjects.

	Total			Female			Male		
	Non-IHD (n = 427)	IHD (n = 1,661)	P Value	Non-IHD (n = 144)	IHD (n = 246)	P-Value	Non-IHD (n = 283)	IHD (n = 1,415)	P-Value
Age (yrs ± SD)	63.1±13.1	65.2±10.5	P<0.01	67.5±13.5	70.4±10.2	P<0.05	60.9±12.3	64.4±10.3	P<0.001
Male (%)	66.3	85.1	P<0.001						
Body mass index (kg/m2 ± SD)	23.2±3.6	24.3±3.4	P<0.001	21.9±3.2	23.0±3.5	P<0.01	23.7±3.6	24.5±3.4	P<0.001
Current smoker (%)	21.8	23.2	NS	8.3	12.6	NS	28.6	25.1	NS
Current+past smoker (%)	53.4	69.8	P<0.001	19.4	28.5	P<0.05	70.7	77.0	P<0.05
Hypertension (%)	64.6	76.5	P<0.001	66.0	77.6	P<0.05	64.0	76.3	P<0.001
Diabetes Mellitus (%)	28.8	45.1	P<0.001	27.1	42.7	P<0.01	29.7	45.5	P<0.001
Dyslipidemia (%)	45.7	75.9	P<0.001	43.1	74.0	P<0.001	47.0	76.3	P<0.001
s-Cr (mg/dl ± SD)	1.6±2.4	1.6±2.3	P = 0.001	1.6±2.5	1.5±2.3	NS	1.6±2.3	1.6±2.3	NS
HbA1c (% ± SD)	5.8±1.1	6.0±1.1	P<0.001	5.7±1.1	5.9±0.8	NS	5.8±1.1	6.1±1.1	P<0.001
BNP (pg/ml ± SD)	310.2±650.0	157.6±401.1	P<0.001	319.5±650.4	303.2±668.2	NS	305.5±650.9	132.3±327.4	P<0.001
HD & CAPD (%)	10.8	9.3	NS	13.2	13.0	NS	9.5	8.7	NS
LVEF (% ± SD)	56.0±14.4	57.7±10.8	P<0.05	59.3±12.3	59.5±11.6	NS	54.4±15.1	57.4±10.7	P = 0.001
Heart rate (beat/min ± SD) (At LVG)	74.0±16.4	70.6±13.5	P<0.001	73.3±14.0	72.5±14.3	NS	74.4±17.6	70.3±13.4	P<0.001
LVEDP (mmHg ± SD) (At PreLVG)	16.5±7.2	15.5±6.3	P<0.05	16.4±7.0	16.1±6.9	NS	16.6±7.3	15.5±6.1	P<0.05
LVESVI (ml/m^2 ± SD)	36.5±25.1	28.9±16.3	P<0.001	31.7±19.8	27.3±17.0	P<0.05	39.0±27.2	29.1±16.2	P<0.001
Prior MI (%)	0	38.5	P<0.001	0	35.8	P<0.001	0	38.9	P<0.001
Prior PCI (%)	0	44.6	P<0.001	0	35.8	P<0.001	0	46.1	P<0.001
Prior CABG (%)	0	12.5	P<0.001	0	15.9	P<0.001	0	12.0	P<0.001
Coronary spastic angina	0	8.5	P<0.001	0	12.6	P<0.001	0	7.8	P<0.001
Prior valve repair (%)	4.9	0.7	P<0.001	7.6	1.6	P<0.01	3.5	0.5	P<0.001
Valvular heart disease (%)	30.2	3.4	P<0.001	38.2	6.9	P<0.001	26.1	2.8	P<0.001
Congenital heart disease (%)	5.2	0.36	P<0.001	8.3	0.4	P<0.001	3.5	0.4	P<0.001
Cardiomyopathy (%)	22.7	2.0	P<0.001	20.8	3.3	P<0.001	23.7	1.8	P<0.001
AF (%)	20.6	5.5	P<0.001	19.4	4.9	P<0.001	21.2	5.7	P<0.001
Calcium-channel blockers (%)	39.1	60.6	P<0.001	43.1	59.8	P = 0.001	37.1	60.8	P<0.001
ACE-inhibitors (%)	15.0	21.3	P<0.01	14.6	18.3	NS	15.2	21.8	P<0.05
Angiotensin Receptor Blockers (%)	37.9	41.0	NS	44.4	42.7	NS	34.6	40.7	NS (P = 0.056)
Nitrates (%)	9.1	26.6	P<0.001	8.3	28.5	P<0.001	9.5	26.2	P<0.001
Nicorandil (%)	4.2	20.4	P<0.001	4.2	23.2	P<0.001	4.2	19.9	P<0.001

Table 1. Cont.

	Total			Female			Male		
	Non-IHD (n = 427)	IHD (n = 1,661)	P Value	Non-IHD (n = 144)	IHD (n = 246)	P-Value	Non-IHD (n = 283)	IHD (n = 1,415)	P-Value
Beta-blockers (%)	18.7	34.4	P<0.001	20.8	28.9	NS (P = 0.081)	17.7	35.3	P<0.001
Statins (%)	23.0	59.3	P<0.001	29.9	57.7	P<0.001	19.4	59.6	P<0.001
Fibrates (%)	3.3	3.4	NS	1.4	1.2	NS	4.2	3.8	NS
Diuretics (%)	32.1	19.1	P<0.001	38.2	28.5	P<0.05	29.0	17.5	P<0.001
Oral Hypoglycemic Agents (%)	11.5	23.5	P<0.001	9.7	18.3	P<0.05	12.4	24.5	P<0.001
insulin (%)	5.2	9.9	P<0.01	6.9	10.6	NS	4.2	9.8	P<0.01
Number of vessels disease (0–3)	0	0.95±0.97		0	0.96±0.96		0	0.95±0.97	

s-Cr, Serum creatinine; BNP, B-type natriuretic peptide; HD & CAPD, Hemodialysis & continuous ambulatory peritoneal dialysis; LVEF, Left ventricular ejection fraction; LVEDP, Left ventricular end-diastolic pressure; LVESVI, Left ventricular end-systolic volume Index; MI, Myocardial Infarction; PCI, Percutaneous coronary intervention; CABG, Coronary artery bypass graft; AF, Atrial Fibrillation.

to advance; therefore, low plasma BNP level, even in patients with high risk factors, may play a causative role in the pathogenetic mechanisms underlying the development of IHD and heart failure. However, the discussion regarding this issue has been insufficient to date, although genetic variations of BNP and related molecules have previously been reported [15–21]. It is also unclear whether the plasma BNP level actually varies according to the individual and whether individual changes in this parameter are associated with disease. Nevertheless, there were a few early reports showing dysregulation of ANP and BNP in patients prone to developing hypertension and other cardiovascular disease [22–24].

Here, we hypothesized that BNP contributes to a pathogenetic mechanism of IHD, and retrospectively examined a possible contribution by comparing the BNP levels between stable patients with IHD and stable patients with cardiovascular diseases other than IHD.

Methods

Study design

The study population was 2088 consecutive patients admitted to the Jikei University Hospital from January 2008 through January 2012 in whom cardiac catheterization, including left ventriculography, and blood sampling for the plasma BNP levels were performed and reviewed. The baseline patient characteristics, including the clinical parameters and the biochemical data, were collected retrospectively from the medical records. The study protocol was approved by the ethics committee of the Jikei University School of Medicine (24–355; 7121).

Recruitment of stable IHD patients and non-IHD patients in this study

The stable IHD patients consisted of 1,661 patients who had coronary stenosis newly diagnosed by angiography, or who had a medical history of coronary artery disease, such as previous myocardial infarction, post-percutaneous coronary intervention and coronary artery bypass graft. A total of 762 patients underwent only one cardiac catheterization, while 359 patients underwent catheterization twice, 50 patients three times, five patients four times, one patient five times and one patient underwent catheterization six times. In order to avoid a selection bias by choosing among the plural data in one patient, we used all consecutive data in this analysis (n = 1661). Patients with coronary spastic angina were included in the stable IHD group if the disease activity of coronary spasm was not clinically high. Coronary spasm was diagnosed by the acetylcholine provocation test. Patients with previously diagnosed coronary spastic angina were also included in the stable IHD group. In contrast, patients requiring urgent catheter intervention for AMI were excluded from this study because the plasma BNP levels are rapidly and extensively changes during the acute phase of AMI [9]. Similarly, patients with acute coronary syndrome were excluded from the stable IHD group in this study. In addition, Also, patients with chest pain syndrome of unknown origin and those with suspected microvascular angina were excluded from the stable IHD group because we were unable to appropriately define cardiac ischemia in such patients. Detailed information of the patients in the stable IHD group were summarized in Table 1.

The non-IHD group consisted of 427 patients; all of those had organic heart diseases such as valvular heart diseases, cardiomyopaty, congenital heart disease and others. All non-IHD patients were clinically stable and admitted to the hospital for evaluation of their underlying cardiac disease. A total of 406 patients underwent cardiac catheterization one time, while nine patients were

Table 2. Comparisons between female and male with and without IHD.

	Non-IHD			IHD		
	Female (n = 144)	**Male (n = 283)**	**P-Value**	**Female (n = 246)**	**Male (n = 1,415)**	**P-Value**
Age (yrs ± SD)	67.5±13.5	60.9±12.3	P<0.001	70.4±10.2	64.4±10.3	P<0.001
Body mass index (kg/m2 ± SD)	21.9±3.2	23.7±3.6	P<0.001	23.0±3.5	24.5±3.4	P<0.001
Current smoker (%)	8.3	28.6	P<0.001	12.6	25.1	P<0.001
Current+past smoker (%)	19.4	70.7	P<0.001	28.5	77.0	P<0.001
Hypertension (%)	66.0	64.0	NS	77.6	76.3	NS
Diabetes Mellitus (%)	27.1	29.7	NS	42.7	45.5	NS
Dyslipidemia (%)	43.1	47.0	NS	74.0	76.3	NS
s-Cr (mg/dl ± SD)	1.6±2.5	1.6±2.3	P<0.001	1.5±2.3	1.6±2.3	P<0.001
HbA1c (% ± SD)	5.7±1.1	5.8±1.1	NS	5.9±0.8	6.1±1.1	P<0.05
BNP (pg/ml ± SD)	319.5±650.4	305.5±650.9	P<0.05	303.2±668.2	132.3±327.4	P<0.001
HD & CAPD (%)	13.2	9.5	NS	13.0	8.7	P<0.05
LVEF (% ± SD)	59.3±12.3	54.4±15.1	P<0.001	59.5±11.6	57.4±10.7	P<0.01
Heart rate (beat/min ± SD) (At LVG)	73.3±14.0	74.4±17.6	NS	72.5±14.3	70.3±13.4	P<0.05
LVEDP (mmHg ± SD) (At Pre LVG)	16.4±7.0	16.6±7.3	NS	16.1±6.9	15.5±6.1	NS
LVESVI (ml/m² ± SD)	31.7±19.8	39.0±27.2	P<0.01	27.3±17.0	29.1±16.2	NS
Prior myocardial infarction (%)	0	0		35.8	38.9	NS
Prior PCI (%)	0	0		35.8	46.1	P<0.01
Prior CABG	0	0		15.9	12.0	NS
Coronary spastic angina	0	0		12.6	7.8	P<0.05
Prior valve repair (%)	7.6	3.5	NS	1.6	0.5	P<0.05
Valvular heart disease (%)	38.2	26.1	P = 0.01	6.9	2.8	P = 0.001
Congenital heart disease (%)	8.3	3.5	P<0.05	0.4	0.4	NS
Cardiomyopathy (%)	20.8	23.7	NS	3.3	1.8	NS
AF (%)	19.4	21.2	NS	4.9	5.7	NS
Calcium-channel blockers (%)	43.1	37.1	NS	59.8	60.8	NS
ACE-inhibitors (%)	14.6	15.2	NS	18.3	21.8	NS
Angiotensin Receptor Blockers (%)	44.4	34.6	P<0.05	42.7	40.7	NS
Nitrates (%)	8.3	9.5	NS	28.5	26.2	NS
Nicorandil (%)	4.2	4.2	NS	23.2	19.9	NS
Beta-blockers (%)	20.8	17.7	NS	28.9	35.3	P<0.05
Statins (%)	29.9	19.4	P<0.05	57.7	59.6	NS
Fibrates (%)	1.4	4.2	NS	1.2	3.8	P<0.05
Diuretics (%)	38.2	29.0	NS	28.5	17.5	P<0.001
Oral Hypoglycemic Agents (%)	9.7	12.4	NS	18.3	24.5	P<0.05
insulin (%)	6.9	4.2	NS	10.6	9.8	NS
Number of vessels disease (0–3)	0	0		0.96±0.96	0.95±097	NS

s-Cr, Serum creatinine; BNP, B-type natriuretic peptide; HD & CAPD, Hemodialysis & continuous ambulatory peritoneal dialysis; LVEF, Left ventricular ejection fraction; LVEDP, Left ventricular end-diastolic pressure; LVESVI, Left ventricular end-systolic volume Index; PCI, Percutaneous coronary intervention; CABG, Coronary artery bypass graft;AF, Atrial Fibrillation.

catheterized twice and one patient was catheterized three times. We used all consecutive data in this analysis just as we did in the IHD group (n = 427). We excluded patients suffering from acute heart failure at the time of cardiac cathetherization and blood sampling. Precise information including underlying cardiac disorders was also summarized in Table 1.

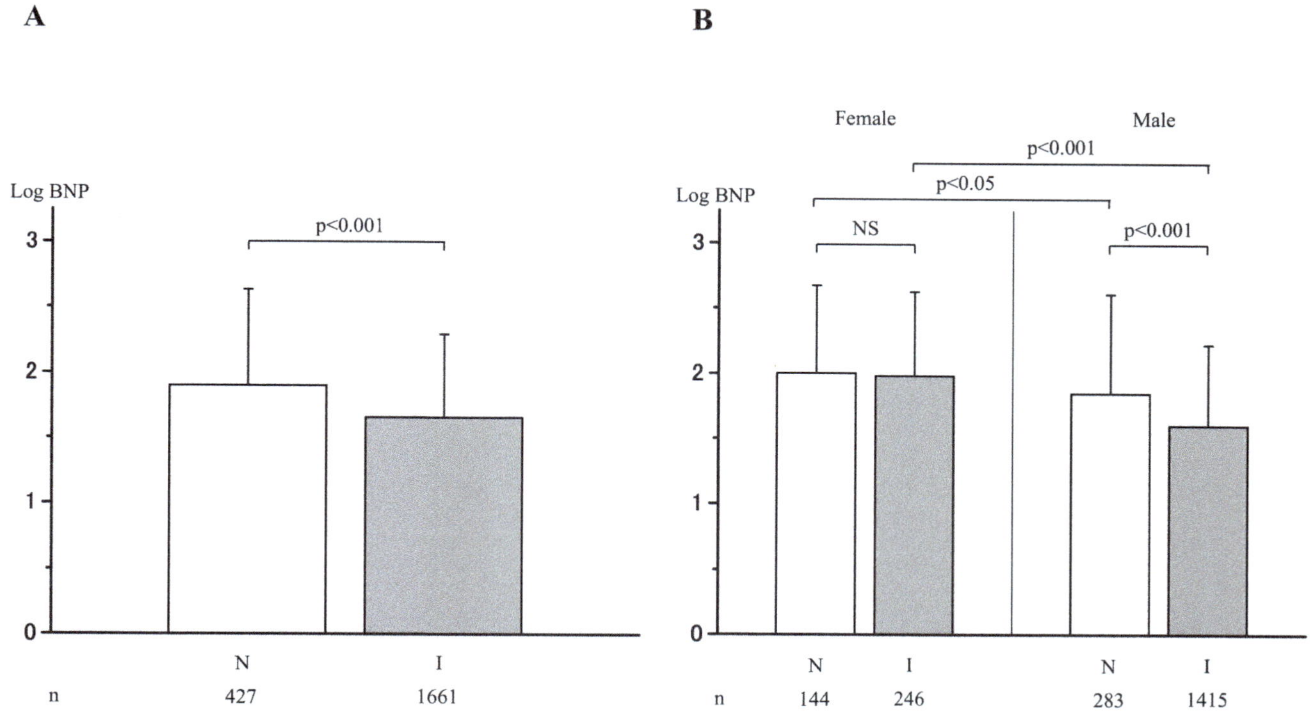

Figure 1. Comparison of the logBNP levels between the non-IHD and IHD groups. A: In the overall population. B: In males and females. N: non-ischemic heart disease group (non-IHD); I: ischemic heart disease group (IHD). BNP: B-type natriuretic peptide.

Measurement of the plasma BNP levels and other parameters

Whole blood (5 ml) was collected in tubes containing potassium EDTA (1 mg/ml blood). The plasma BNP level was determined by an enzyme-linked immunosorbent assay (non-extracted) using an antibody against human BNP (Shionogi Co. Ltd., Tokyo, Japan). Blood sampling was performed immediately before and after the cardiac catheterization whenever possible. The average interval between catheterization and blood sampling was 5.21±8.94 days; 1384 (66.3%) of patients had blood collected for BNP within 72 hours post catheterization. Of these patients, 830 underwent blood collection at the time of the procedure (during, immediately before or just after cardiac catheterization), 1185 underwent blood collection within 24 hours, and 1342 underwent blood collection within 48 hours.

The BMI was calculated as the body weight (kg) divided by the square of the height (m). Hypertension, diabetes mellitus and dyslipidemia were defined as described previously [25].

Statistical analysis

Continuous variables were expressed as the means ± SD. Categorical variables were expressed as percentages. Comparisons between groups were performed using Pearson's chi-square test for categorical variables and the Mann-Whitney U test or Student's t-test for continuous variables, where appropriate. To achieve a normal distribution, the BNP value was log-transformed before the analysis. To assess the dependent determinants of the log BNP, a multiple regression analysis was performed after the simple regression analysis. Age, gender (0 for females and 1 for males), IHD (0 for non-IHD and 1 for IHD), atrial fibrillation (0 for non-AF and 1 for AF), the LVEF, age, BMI, and s-Cr were included as

Table 3. The results of the simple regression analyses for the log BNP in all patients (n = 2088).

Explanatory variable	Regression coefficient	Standard regression coefficient	P	95%CI
Age	0.016	0.270	<0.001	0.014~0.019
Gender	−0.348	−0.203	<0.001	−0.420~−0.276
BMI	−0.047	−0.247	<0.001	−0.055~−0.039
s-Cr	0.119	0.415	<0.001	0.108~0.130
LVEF	−0.027	−0.478	<0.001	−0.030~−0.025
AF	0.597	0.251	<0.001	0.499~0.696
IHD	−0.243	−0.147	<0.001	−0.314~−0.173

BMI, Body mass index; s-Cr, Serum creatinine; LVEF, Left ventricular ejection fraction; AF, Atrial fibrillation; IHD, Ischemic heart disease.

Table 4. The results of the multiple regression analyses for the log BNP in all patients (n = 2088).

Explanatory variable	Regression coefficient	Standard regression coefficient	P	95%CI	VIF
Age	0.015	0.249	<0.001	0.013~0.017	1.125
Gender	−0.272	−0.159	<0.001	−0.327~−0.217	1.120
BMI	−0.015	−0.081	<0.001	−0.022~−0.009	1.128
s-Cr	0.095	0.333	<0.001	0.086~0.104	1.061
LVEF	−0.024	−0.414	<0.001	−0.026~−0.022	1.097
AF	0.325	0.137	<0.001	0.249~0.401	1.107
IHD	−0.115	−0.069	<0.001	−0.168~−0.061	1.131

BMI, Body mass index; s-Cr, Serum creatinine; LVEF, Left ventricular ejection fraction; AF, Atrial fibrillation; IHD, Ischemic heart disease.

variables in the multiple regression analysis. In addition, a gender-segregated multiple logistic regression analysis was performed to determine predictive factors for IHD using age, LVEF, BMI, s-Cr, atrial fibrillation (0 for non-AF and 1 for AF), and logBNP. A value of $p<0.05$ was considered to be statistically significant for all data that were statistically analyzed using the SPSS software package, version 21.0 (SPSS Inc., Chicago, IL).

Results

Clinical characteristics of the study subjects

Table 1 shows the clinical characteristic and the past medical history and medication regimen of the total 2088 patients.

High age, male gender, high BMI, smoking, hypertension, diabetes mellitus and dyslipidemia were more frequently seen in the IHD group than in the non-IHD group. The s-Cr was significantly higher in the non-IHD group than in the IHD group. The heart rate, LVESVI and LVEDP were lower in the IHD group than in the non-IHD group. The LVEF was slightly higher in the IHD group than in the non-IHD group. In this study, AF was more frequently detected in the non-IHD group than in the IHD group, which was due to the higher prevalence of valvular heart disease and cardiomyopathy in the non-IHD groups (precise data not shown in the Results).

The clinical characteristics are shown by gender in Table 2. It is important to compare the clinical characteristics between the females and males in the IHD group. For example, the LVEF was lower and the s-Cr was higher in males, whereas the age was lower and BMI values were higher in this group. With regard to the medical treatments, diuretics were used more frequently in females, and beta-blockers were used more frequently in males, while angiotensin-converting enzyme inhibitors/angiotensin II receptor blockers (ARBs) were used equally in females and males. Every patient had been prescribed the classes and doses of drugs based on his or her individual condition; therefore, it is difficult to compare the drugs more precisely. Nevertheless, the frequency in use and the amount used of major drugs such as enalapril, cavedilol or spironolactones was equivalent between females and males with or without IHD, while only the frequency of use and amount used of furosemide was significantly higher in males than in females (precise data not shown).

Comparison of the plasma BNP levels between the non-IHD and IHD groups and statistical analysis of the logBNP values in the total study population

The plasma BNP levels were significantly lower in the IHD group than in the non-IHD group as shown in Figure 1-A. In order to identify factors contributing to the difference in the plasma BNP levels between the IHD and non-IHD groups among the total study population, statistical analyses was performed, as shown in Table 3 and Table 4. Table 3 is the results of the simple regression analysis of the logBNP values using clinical factors as explanatory variables. Table 4 shows the results of the subsequent multiple regression analysis. Consequently, age, gender, BMI, s-Cr, LVEF, AF, and IHD were found to be significant determinants of the logBNP value. Among these factors, it is noteworthy that IHD *per se* was significantly and inversely correlated with the logBNP value.

Comparison of the plasma BNP levels between the non-IHD and IHD groups based on gender

Figure 1B shows that females with and without IHD had higher levels of plasma BNP compared to males with and without IHD.

Table 5. The results of the logistic regression analysis for IHD in females.

Explanatory variable	Regression coefficient	P	Odds ratio	Odds 95% CI
Log BNP	−0.085	NS (p = 0.719)	0.919	0.579~1.457
LVEF	−0.014	NS (p = 0.232)	0.986	0.963~1.009
Age	0.027	<0.01	1.028	1.007~1.048
BMI	0.101	<0.01	1.106	1.034~1.183
AF	−1.703	<0.001	0.182	0.086~0.388
s-Cr	−0.002	NS (p = 0.965)	0.998	0.901~1.105

BNP, B-type natriuretic peptide; LVEF, Left ventricular ejection fraction; BMI, Body mass index; AF, Atrial fibrillation; IHD, Ischemic heart disease; s-Cr, Serum creatinine.

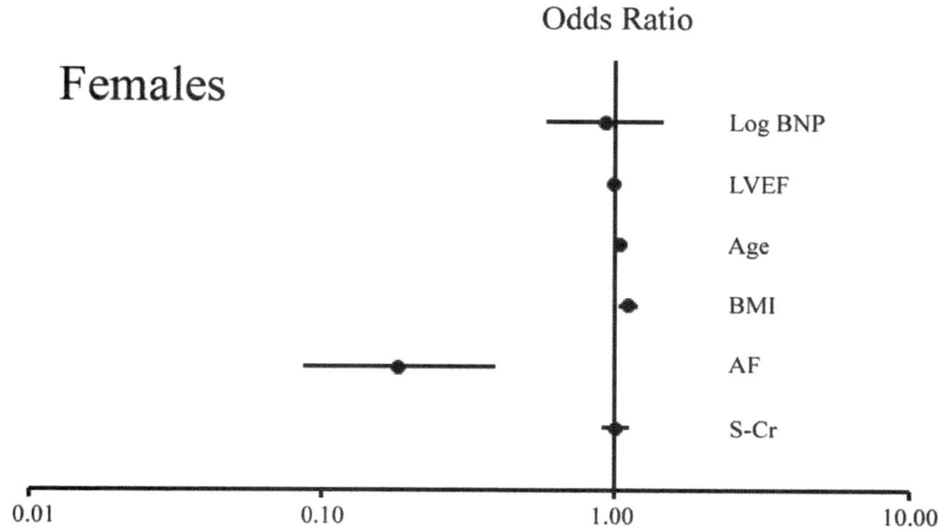

Figure 2. The Forest Plot displaying the odds ratio about risk of IHD in a females. BNP, B-type natriuretic peptide; LVEF, Left ventricular ejection fraction; BMI, Body mass index; AF, Atrial fibrillation; IHD, Ischemic heart disease; s-Cr, Serum creatinine.

The plasma BNP levels were similar in females with and without IHD ($p = NS$, actually $p = 0.725$). In contrast, the plasma BNP level was lower in males with IHD compared to males without IHD ($p<0.001$).

The results of the multiple logistic regression analysis for the determination of IHD

We finally examined the factors determining the presence of IHD; a multiple logistic regression analysis was performed for the determination of IHD by using the logBNP, LVEF, age, BMI, AF and s-Cr as explanatory variables in females and males. As shown in Tables 5 and Figure 2 (Females), and Table 6, and Figure 3 (Males), the trend between females and males was similar for age (significant in each gender), BMI (significant in each gender), AF (significant in each gender) and LVEF (not significant in each gender); however, the s-Cr was not significant in females ($p = NS$) but was significant in males ($p<0.05$). This result may suggest that chronic kidney disease is a more important risk factor for IHD in males than in females. It is noteworthy that the logBNP was not significantly associated with IHD in females ($p = NS$, actually $p = 0.719$), but was significantly and inversely associated with IHD in males (Regression coefficient: −0.669, $p < 0.001$). Thus, the logBNP may only correlate with IHD in males, and may have a possible causative role, although it is difficult to distinguish between cause and effect based on the present analysis.

Sub-analysis based on the presence or absence of AF

AF was found to be significantly associated with non-IHD in both females and males, as shown in Table 5 and Figure 2 (Females) and Table 6 and Figure 3 (Males). Therefore, an additional analysis would be necessary, and the study population was subsequently divided based on the presence or absence of AF: the AF (+) group and the AF (−) group. There were no significant differences in the plasma BNP levels between the non-IHD and IHD groups among the AF (+) or AF (−) females; however, the plasma BNP levels were significantly lower in the IHD group than in the non-IHD group among AF(+) or AF(−) males. The subgroup analysis of AF therefore suggested that the tendency toward a low plasma BNP level in IHD males was not affected by AF.

Discussion

In the beginning of the study, we found the plasma BNP levels to be specifically lower in the stable patients with IHD than in the stable patients with non-IHD among the total study population. In addition, the multiple regression analysis clearly showed for the

Table 6. The results of the logistic regression analysis for IHD in males.

Explanatory variable	Regression coefficient	P	Odds ratio	Odds 95% CI
Log BNP	−0.669	<0.001	0.512	0.388~0.677
LVEF	−0.007	NS (p = 0.318)	0.993	0.981~1.006
Age	0.049	<0.001	1.050	1.037~1.064
BMI	0.080	<0.001	1.083	1.039~1.128
AF	−1.351	<0.001	0.259	0.172~0.389
s-Cr	0.087	0.01	1.091	1.021~1.167

BNP, B-type natriuretic peptide; LVEF, Left ventricular ejection fraction; BMI, Body mass index; AF, Atrial fibrillation; IHD, Ischemic heart disease; s-Cr, Serum creatinine.

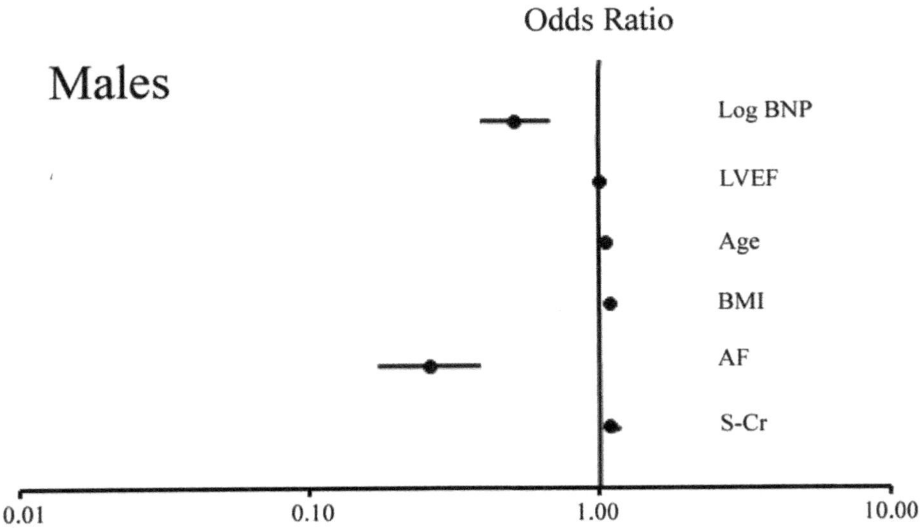

Figure 3. The Forest Plot displaying the odds ratio about risk of IHD in a males. BNP, B-type natriuretic peptide; LVEF, Left ventricular ejection fraction; BMI, Body mass index; AF, Atrial fibrillation; IHD, Ischemic heart disease; s-Cr, Serum creatinine.

first time that IHD *per se* is an independent determinant of the plasma BNP level, in addition to other known factors, such as age, male gender, low BMI, s-Cr, low LVEF and AF [26–31]. Furthermore, when the total study population was divided by gender, significant differences were identified between females and males. For example, it is noteworthy that the plasma BNP levels were significantly lower in the IHD group than in the non-IHD group among males only. In this analysis, the gender-difference observed in the plasma BNP levels in the IHD group was prominent even in consideration of the diverse clinical backgrounds. Therefore, unknown factors likely contributed to the observed gender difference. Next, by a multiple logistic regression analysis conversely performed using IHD as an objective variable and the logBNP as one of the explanatory variables, IHD was inversely determined by the logBNP only in males, but not in females. Hence the statistical analysis clarified that there is a substantial association between IHD *per se* and low plasma BNP level in males only. It is difficult to distinguish between cause and effect based on the present analyses; however, low plasma levels of BNP may be causally associated with IHD in males. In other words, the factor 'low reactivity of the plasma BNP level' may be a new risk factor for IHD in males. This way of thinking is supported by the previous reports showing that a deficiency of ANP and BNP was causatively associated with hypertension and other cardiovascular diseases [22–24].

BNP is biologically active and increases the cGMP levels. BNP is thus beneficial for suppressing the progression of heart failure, and probably atherosclerosis [13,14]. If the BNP level is insufficiently increased, low plasma BNP levels may have a causative role in IHD and heart failure. The reasons for the comparatively low plasma BNP levels or deteriorated response of BNP in IHD are unknown at present. Various factors such as neurohormones or genetic factors associated with gender differences may be linked to the current results. In addition, it is unknown whether a reduction of the synthesis or an augmented clearance of BNP affected the current results. As a next step, we need to examine the precise mechanisms responsible for the low plasma BNP levels seen only in male patients with IHD. The findings of the present and future studies may be able to provide a new strategy to prevent IHD and heart failure by increasing the endogenous natriuretic peptides using agents such as neutral endopeptidase inhibitors.

It is interesting to note a gender difference in the contribution of the plasma BNP level to the pathogenesis of IHD, as a gender difference have generally been reported to be negligible in patients with heart failure to date [27]. The results of this study may therefore help to answer the remaining questions regarding the impact of gender differences in the setting of IHD [32–37]. At present, it remains unknown whether IHD is the only or one of several cardiovascular diseases associated with the gender difference in the plasma BNP levels.

In general, the measurement of the plasma BNP levels is useful for early monitoring of asymptomatic ventricular dysfunction in patients with high risk factors. A value <18.4 pg/ml is considered to be ideal, and less than 40 pg/ml is considered to be within the normal range for patients without cardiac organic disorders visiting the hospital [27]. However, in this study, a considerable number of patients with a low EF (<55%) and low plasma BNP levels (<40 pg/ml) was seen in the IHD group compared with the non-IHD group among males; 153 patients (10.81%) vs. 16 patients (5.65%), $p<0.01$. On the other hand, there were few female patients with the same conditions; only two patients (0.81%) in the IHD group and nine patients (6.25%) in the non-IHD group, $p<0.01$ (precise data not shown in the Results). This indicates that clinicians should take care not to underestimate the degree of heart failure even if the plasma BNP levels are relatively low (less than 40 pg/ml) in male patients with IHD.

It is known that the BNP level increases with inflammation [38]. In this study, we examined the serum C-reactive protein (CRP) levels between 396 patients with IHD and 136 patients with non-IHD via blood samples obtained on the day of the catheterization. The average CRP level was 0.670±1.653 (95%CI: 0.390–0.950) in the non-IHD group and 0.521±1.109 (95%CI: 0.412–0.631) in the IHD group, which was not significantly different ($p=0.239$) (precise data not shown in the Results). Therefore, we thought that the inflammation status would not have influenced the present results.

To avoid a selection bias, the study population was consecutively and non-selectively recruited; therefore, all plural data from one patient were used in this analysis. We essentially performed the analysis by using 1,661 IHD patients and 427 non-IHD patients. However, by way of caution, we performed a similar statistical analysis by using only one dataset from each patient (1178 IHD patients and 416 non-IHD patients) who underwent cardiac catheterization for the first time during this protocol. As a result, the plasma BNP levels were found to be significantly lower in the IHD group than in the non-IHD group ($p<0.001$), the same as in the full dataset. In addition, when the total study population was divided by gender, the plasma BNP levels were significantly lower in the IHD group than in the non-IHD group only in males ($p<0.001$), but not in females ($p = NS$). Thus, the findings of the full dataset and the data from just individual cases were the same.

Finally, this is only a pilot retrospective study of the possible contribution of a low plasma BNP level to the pathogenesis of IHD. Therefore, a prospective study is needed to examine whether male patients with very low levels of plasma BNP, even under conditions of high risk factors, are more likely to develop IHD, for example, by comparing the rates of acute ischemic attack, the progression of IHD and the severity of stenosis in IHD patients grouped by the plasma BNP level.

Study Limitation

First, the number of females was small compared with that of males (1698 males and 390 females); thus, it is difficult to draw any definitive conclusions regarding the gender difference in the contribution of the plasma BNP level to IHD. A larger study including more females is required to arrive at an absolute conclusion. Second, while the plasma BNP level was the primary outcome measurement of the study, the samples were collected on a wide range intervals, and up to 33.7% of the subjects underwent blood collection more than 72 hours after cardiac catheterization. It is ideal to perform simultaneous sampling with hemodynamic measurements during cardiac catheterization; however, this was a retrospective study, and blood sampling for the purpose of measuring the plasma BNP levels was performed in the clinical setting based on the discretion of the attending physician. For this reason, there was a time delay in blood sampling in some patients. However, no statistical differences were noted in the timing of sampling between females and males; the patients who underwent blood sampling after more than 72 hours included 125 females (32.1% of the total 390 females) and 579 males (34.1% of the total 1,698 males) ($P = NS$). Therefore, we do not believe that the time lag in sampling in some cases largely affected the present findings.

Conclusions

The plasma BNP levels were relatively low in stable patients with IHD compared with that observed in the stable patients with non-IHD; this tendency was more evident in males. Perhaps, the low reactivity of BNP is causally associated with IHD in males. We hope this study serves as a test of a prospective study in the future.

Acknowledgments

We thank Mr. Brian Quinn (Japan Medical Communication) for his kind advice regarding the use of the English language.

Author Contributions

Conceived and designed the experiments: KM MY. Performed the experiments: KM TO TT KO TN SA S. Morimoto YI HS AU. Analyzed the data: KM TO MK KK TT S. Matsuo KH MY. Contributed reagents/materials/analysis tools: KM MK MY. Wrote the paper: KM TO KK TT MY.

References

1. Sudoh T, Kangawa K, Minamino N, Matsuo H (1988) A new natriuretic peptide in porcine brain. Nature 332: 78–81.
2. Mukoyama M, Nakao K, Hosoda K, Suga S, Saito Y, et al. (1991) Brain natriuretic peptide as a novel cardiac hormone in humans. Evidence for an exquisite dual natriuretic peptide system, atrial natriuretic peptide and brain natriuretic peptide. J Clin Invest 87: 1402–1412.
3. Yasue H, Yoshimura M, Sumida H, Kikuta K, Kugiyama K, et al. (1994) Localization and mechanism of secretion of B-type natriuretic peptide in comparison with those of A-type natriuretic peptide in normal subjects and patients with heart failure. Circulation 90: 195–203.
4. Omland T, Aakvaag A, Bonarjee VV, Caidahl K, Lie RT, et al. (1996) Plasma brain natriuretic peptide as an indicator of left ventricular systolic function and long-term survival after acute myocardial infarction. Comparison with plasma atrial natriuretic peptide and N-terminal proatrial natriuretic peptide. Circulation 93: 1963–1969.
5. Tsutamoto T, Wada A, Maeda K, Hisanaga T, Maeda Y, et al. (1997) Attenuation of compensation of endogenous cardiac natriuretic peptide system in chronic heart failure: prognostic role of plasma brain natriuretic peptide concentration in patients with chronic symptomatic left ventricular dysfunction. Circulation 96: 509–516.
6. Richards AM, Nicholls MG, Espiner EA, Lainchbury JG, Troughton RW, et al. (2003) B-type natriuretic peptides and ejection fraction for prognosis after myocardial infarction. Circulation 107: 2786–2792.
7. Suzuki S, Yoshimura M, Nakayama M, Mizuno Y, Harada E, et al. (2004) Plasma level of B-type natriuretic peptide as a prognostic marker after acute myocardial infarction: a long-term follow-up analysis. Circulation 110: 1387–1391.
8. Wang TJ, Larson MG, Levy D, Benjamin EJ, Leip EP, et al. (2004) Plasma natriuretic peptide levels and the risk of cardiovascular events and death. N Engl J Med 350: 655–663.
9. Morita E, Yasue H, Yoshimura M, Ogawa H, Jougasaki M, et al. (1993) Increased plasma levels of brain natriuretic peptide in patients with acute myocardial infarction. Circulation 88: 82–91.
10. Hawkridge AM, Heublein DM, Bergen HR III, Cataliotti A, Burnett JC Jr, et al. (2005) Quantitative mass spectral evidence for the absence of circulating brain natriuretic peptide (BNP-32) in severe human heart failure. Proc Natl Acad Sci U S A 102: 17442–17447.
11. Nishikimi T, Okamoto H, Nakamura M, Ogawa N, Horii K, et al. (2013) Direct immunochemiluminescent assay for proBNP and total BNP in human plasma proBNP and total BNP levels in normal and heart failure. PLoS One 8: e53233.
12. Gorbe A, Giricz Z, Szunyog A, Csont T, Burley DS, et al. (2010) Role of cGMP-PKG signaling in the protection of neonatal rat cardiac myocytes subjected to simulated ischemia/reoxygenation. Basic Res Cardiol 105: 643–650.
13. Ogawa Y, Itoh H, Tamura N, Suga S, Yoshimasa T, et al. (1994) Molecular cloning of the complementary DNA and gene that encode mouse brain natriuretic peptide and generation of transgenic mice that overexpress the brain natriuretic peptide gene. J Clin Invest 93: 1911–1921.
14. Nishikimi T, Maeda N, Matsuoka H (2006) The role of natriuretic peptides in cardioprotection. Cardiovasc Res 69: 318–328.
15. Costello-Boerrigter LC, Boerrigter G, Ameenuddin S, Mahoney DW, Slusser JP, et al. (2011) The effect of the brain-type natriuretic peptide single-nucleotide polymorphism rs198389 on test characteristics of common assays. Mayo Clin Proc 86: 210–218.
16. Szabo G, Molvarec A, Stenczer B, Rigo J Jr, Nagy B (2011) Natriuretic peptide precursor B gene (TTTC)(n) microsatellite polymorphism in pre-eclampsia. Clin Chim Acta 412: 1371–1375.
17. Ellis KL, Newton-Cheh C, Wang TJ, Frampton CM, Doughty RN, et al. (2011) Association of genetic variation in the natriuretic peptide system with cardiovascular outcomes. J Mol Cell Cardiol 50: 695–701.
18. Choquet H, Cavalcanti-Proenca C, Lecoeur C, Dina C, Cauchi S, et al. (2009) The T-381C SNP in BNP gene may be modestly associated with type 2 diabetes: an updated meta-analysis in 49 279 subjects. Hum Mol Genet 18: 2495–2501.
19. Poreba R, Poczatek K, Gac P, Poreba M, Gonerska M, et al. (2009) SNP rs198389 (T-381 C) polymorphism in the B-type natriuretic peptide gene promoter in patients with atherosclerotic renovascular hypertension. Pol Arch Med Wewn 119: 219–224.
20. Weber M, Burian M, Dragutinovic I, Moellmann H, Nef H, et al. (2008) Genetic polymorphism of the type A human natriuretic peptide receptor (NPR-A) gene contributes to the interindividual variability in the BNP system. Eur J Heart Fail 10: 482–489.

21. Vassalle C, Andreassi MG, Prontera C, Fontana M, Zyw L, et al. (2007) Influence of ScaI and natriuretic peptide (NP) clearance receptor polymorphisms of the NP System on NP concentration in chronic heart failure. Clin Chem 53: 1886–1890.
22. Ferrari P, Weidmann P, Ferrier C, Dietler R, Hollmann R, et al. (1990) Dysregulation of atrial natriuretic factor in hypertension-prone man. J Clin Endocrinol Metab 71: 944–951.
23. Belluardo P, Cataliotti A, Bonaiuto L, Giuffre E, Maugeri E, et al. (2006) Lack of activation of molecular forms of the BNP system in human grade 1 hypertension and relationship to cardiac hypertrophy. Am J Physiol Heart Circ Physiol 291: H1529–1535.
24. Macheret F, Boerrigter G, McKie P, Costello-Boerrigter L, Lahr B, et al. (2011) Pro-B-type natriuretic peptide(1-108) circulates in the general community: plasma determinants and detection of left ventricular dysfunction. J Am Coll Cardiol 57: 1386–1395.
25. Komukai K, Ogawa T, Yagi H, Date T, Sakamoto H, et al. (2008) Decreased renal function as an independent predictor of re-hospitalization for congestive heart failure. Circ J 72: 1152–1157.
26. Nakane T, Kawai M, Komukai K, Kayama Y, Matsuo S, et al. (2012) Contribution of extracardiac factors to the inconsistency between plasma B-type natriuretic peptide levels and the severity of pulmonary congestion on chest X-rays in the diagnosis of heart failure. Intern Med 51: 239–248.
27. Kawai M, Yoshimura M, Harada M, Mizuno Y, Hiramitsu S, et al. (2013) Determination of the B-type natriuretic peptide level as a criterion for abnormalities in japanese individuals in routine clinical practice: the J-ABS Multi-Center Study (Japan Abnormal BNP Standard). Intern Med 52: 171–177.
28. Cataliotti A, Malatino LS, Jougasaki M, Zoccali C, Castellino P, et al. (2001) Circulating natriuretic peptide concentrations in patients with end-stage renal disease: role of brain natriuretic peptide as a biomarker for ventricular remodeling. Mayo Clin Proc 76: 1111–1119.
29. Redfield MM, Rodeheffer RJ, Jacobsen SJ, Mahoney DW, Bailey KR, et al. (2002) Plasma brain natriuretic peptide concentration: impact of age and gender. J Am Coll Cardiol 40: 976–982.
30. Wang TJ, Larson MG, Levy D, Leip EP, Benjamin EJ, et al. (2002) Impact of age and sex on plasma natriuretic peptide levels in healthy adults. Am J Cardiol 90: 254–258.
31. Knudsen CW, Riis JS, Finsen AV, Eikvar L, Muller C, et al. (2004) Diagnostic value of a rapid test for B-type natriuretic peptide in patients presenting with acute dyspnoe: effect of age and gender. Eur J Heart Fail 6: 55–62.
32. Njolstad I, Arnesen E, Lund-Larsen PG (1996) Smoking, serum lipids, blood pressure, and sex differences in myocardial infarction. A 12-year follow-up of the Finnmark Study. Circulation 93: 450–456.
33. Jousilahti P, Vartiainen E, Tuomilehto J, Puska P (1999) Sex, age, cardiovascular risk factors, and coronary heart disease: a prospective follow-up study of 14 786 middle-aged men and women in Finland. Circulation 99: 1165–1172.
34. Yarnell JW, Beswick AD, Sweetnam PM, Riad-Fahmy D (1993) Endogenous sex hormones and ischemic heart disease in men. The Caerphilly prospective study. Arterioscler Thromb 13: 517–520.
35. Malkin CJ, Pugh PJ, Jones TH, Channer KS (2003) Testosterone for secondary prevention in men with ischaemic heart disease? Qjm 96: 521–529.
36. Schuit SC, Oei HH, Witteman JC, Geurts van Kessel CH, van Meurs JB, et al. (2004) Estrogen receptor alpha gene polymorphisms and risk of myocardial infarction. Jama 291: 2969–2977.
37. Rod NH, Kristensen TS, Diderichsen F, Prescott E, Jensen GB, et al. (2010) Cortisol, estrogens and risk of ischaemic heart disease, cancer and all-cause mortality in postmenopausal women: a prospective cohort study. Int J Epidemiol 39: 530–538.
38. Inoue T, Kawai M, Nakane T, Nojiri A, Minai K, et al. (2010) Influence of low-grade inflammation on plasma B-type natriuretic peptide levels. Intern Med 49: 2659–2668.

8

NSFC Health Research Funding and Burden of Disease in China

Gelin Xu, Zhizhong Zhang, Qiushi Lv, Yun Li, Ruidong Ye, Yunyun Xiong, Yongjun Jiang, Xinfeng Liu*

Department of Neurology, Jinling Hospital, Nanjing University School of Medicine, Nanjing, Jiangsu Province, China

Abstract

Background: Allocation of health research funds among diseases has never been evaluated in China. This study aimed to examine the relationship between disease-specific funding levels of National Nature Science Foundation of China (NSFC), the main governmental resource for health research in China, and burden of disease.

Methods: Funding magnitudes for 53 diseases or conditions were obtained from the website of NSFC. Measures of disease burden, mortality, years of life lost (YLLs) and disability-adjusted life years (DALYs), were derived from the Global Burden of Disease Study 2010. The relationship between NSFC funding and disease burden was analyzed with univariate linear regression. For each measure associated with funding, regression-derived estimates were used to calculate the expected funds for each disease. The actual and expected funds were then compared. We also evaluated the impacts of changes of disease burden metrics since 1990, and differences from the world averages on NSFC funding.

Results: NSFC health research funding was associated with disease burden measured in mortality ($R = 0.33$, $P = 0.02$), YLLs ($R = 0.39$, $P = 0.004$), and DALYs ($R = 0.40$, $P = 0.003$). But none of the changes of mortality ($R = 0.22$, $P = 0.12$), YLLs ($R = -0.04$, $P = 0.79$) and DALYs ($R = -0.003$, $P = 0.98$) since 1990 was associated with the funding magnitudes. None of the differences of mortality ($R = -0.11$, $P = 0.45$), YLLs ($R = -0.11$, $P = 0.43$) and DALYs ($R = -0.12$, $P = 0.38$) from that of the concurrent world averages were associated with the funding magnitudes. Measured by DALY, stroke and COPD received the least funding compared to expected; while leukemia and diabetes received the most funding compared to expected.

Conclusion: Although NSFC funding were roughly associated with disease burden as measured in mortality, YLLs and DALYs. Some major diseases such as stroke were underfunded; while others such as leukaemia were overfunded. Change of disease burden during the last 20 years and country-specialized disease burden were not reflected in current allocation of NSFC funds.

Editor: Guangyuan He, Huazhong University of Science and Technology, China

Funding: This study was sponsored by Nature Science Foundation of Jiangsu (BE2013713) to GX. The funders had no role in study design, data collection and analysis, decision to publish, or preparation of the manuscript.

Competing Interests: The authors have declared that no competing interests exist.

* Email: xfliu2@vip.163.com

Introduction

In recent years, China is pouring cash into science and technology faster than its economy has expanded [1]. The total research and development (R&D) expenditure in China has increased by 23% annually on average over the past decade [2]. The central government's budget on science and technology reached 267.4 billion yuan renminbi (RMB), or US $43.6 billion, in 2014 [2]. Consistent with this trend, the governmental funding for health research is also increasing. Although still dwarfed by that of US (US $ 3.1 billion for National Natural Science Foundation of China (NSFC) against US $ 30 billion for US National Institute of Health (NIH) in 2014), China's governmental funds, principally NSFC, are becoming an important supporter for health research in the world [3].

However, the allocation of research funds among diseases, and its rationality has never been evaluated in China. The disbursement of grant money has been criticized for lack of transparency, and funding tends to go to eminent scientists and safe projects [4,5]. There are short-term (annual) and long-term (5 years) national priorities for health researches, but they are merely results of government decisions based on politic will, public opinions, extemporaneous expert comments and immediate experience from western countries, rather than on systematic analysis of China's own disease burden. Considering the limited resources, it is important for China to optimize the process for health fund allocation with disease burden as a reference, as did in USA and other countries [6–8].

NSFC is a centre goverment agency specialized in administrating basic research funds, and it is the main source for the health research funds. Utilizing the design and methods in previous studies for evaluating association of NIH funding level and disease burden in USA [6,7], this study evaluated the relationship between NSFC funding levels and measures of disease burden. We also

Table 1. Funding levels of NSFC and disease burden in China.

Condition or disease	NSFC research fund	Measure of disease burden in 2010					
		thousands (rank)					
	thousands in RMB (% of total)	Mortality	Mortality change since 1990	YLLs	YLLs change since 1990	DALYs	DALYs change since 1990
Leukaemia	327854 (12.8)	58 (17)	5 (25)	2390 (15)	−366 (40)	2418 (19)	−354 (42)
Diabetes	176635 (6.9)	160 (11)	90 (5)	3173 (13)	1251 (5)	7835 (9)	2989 (4)
Ischemic heart disease	169185 (6.6)	949 (2)	499 (1)	16084 (3)	7093 (1)	17886 (3)	7759 (1)
Dementia	115785 (4.5)	50 (20)	24 (11)	616 (30)	159 (17)	1593 (23)	636 (13)
Liver cancer	114225 (4.5)	370 (6)	131 (4)	10014 (6)	2684 (4)	10089 (7)	2718 (5)
Injury	103560 (4.0)	796 (4)	−56 (47)	31759 (1)	−12827 (51)	40804 (1)	−10386 (51)
Breast cancer	95360 (3.7)	53 (19)	23 (12)	1563 (17)	645 (8)	1671 (22)	716 (10)
Asthma	80060 (3.1)	20 (32)	−32 (45)	358 (37)	−173 (38)	1095 (30)	−143 (39)
Colorectal cancer	75990 (3.0)	150 (12)	57 (6)	3305 (11)	901 (7)	3423 (15)	975 (8)
Chronic kidney diseases	75389 (2.9)	82 (15)	28 (9)	2054 (16)	413 (11)	2782 (17)	696 (11)
Cirrhosis	68085 (2.7)	114 (13)	−61 (48)	3180 (12)	−2095 (47)	3316 (16)	−2088 (47)
Neonatal disorders	63730 (2.5)	83 (14)	−260 (52)	7173 (7)	−22334 (53)	8679 (8)	−22534 (53)
Lung cancer	63580 (2.5)	513 (5)	253 (3)	11197 (5)	4943 (2)	11318 (6)	5013 (3)
Hypertensive heart disease	61463 (2.4)	173 (10)	39 (7)	2734 (14)	458 (10)	2767 (18)	460 (15)
Stroke	55330 (2.2)	1727 (1)	387 (2)	29173 (2)	4829 (3)	30139 (2)	5262 (2)
Stomach cancer	53610 (2.1)	297 (7)	0 (38)	6523 (8)	−849 (43)	6616 (10)	−825 (43)
Hepatitis	53245 (2.1)	44 (23)	11 (16)	1319 (19)	−48 (34)	1443 (28)	−38 (37)
Brain cancers	52610 (2.1)	49 (21)	13 (14)	1473 (18)	232 (14)	1497 (26)	240 (19)
Depression	51335 (2.0)	0 (53)	0 (36)	0 (53)	0 (30)	11767 (5)	2297 (6)
Pneumonia	46600 (1.8)	195 (8)	−197 (51)	4771 (9)	−20173 (52)	5135 (11)	−20166 (52)
Schizophrenia	43260 (1.7)	9 (42)	−4 (40)	279 (39)	−171 (37)	3472 (14)	918 (9)
HIV-AIDS	40075 (1.6)	36 (24)	36 (8)	1111 (23)	1100 (6)	1752 (20)	1739 (7)
Peptic ulcer	39870 (1.6)	19 (33)	−36 (46)	382 (35)	−942 (45)	453 (41)	−958 (45)
Atrial fibrillation and flutter	39150 (1.5)	13 (37)	8 (18)	154 (47)	91 (22)	596 (39)	259 (18)
Prostate cancer	34530 (1.3)	11 (39)	7 (19)	165 (45)	97 (21)	178 (50)	109 (25)
Nasopharynx cancer	31250 (1.2)	34 (26)	12 (15)	1046 (24)	314 (13)	1060 (31)	320 (17)
Epilepsy	31240 (1.2)	12 (38)	−7 (42)	559 (32)	−424 (41)	1507 (25)	−216 (40)
Maternal disorders	30260 (1.2)	5 (49)	−16 (43)	272 (40)	−911 (44)	546 (40)	−855 (44)
COPD	29450 (1.2)	934 (3)	−493 (53)	12995 (4)	−10808 (50)	16724 (4)	−9746 (50)
Parkinson disease	29160 (1.1)	7 (47)	3 (30)	121 (49)	25 (28)	265 (44)	91 (28)
Tuberculosis	26710 (1.0)	45 (22)	−124 (50)	1172 (22)	−4059 (49)	1733 (21)	−4418 (49)
Cervical cancer	26245 (1.0)	25 (29)	5 (26)	727 (28)	180 (16)	742 (35)	185 (21)

Table 1. Cont.

Condition or disease		NSFC research fund	Measure of disease burden in 2010					
			thousands (rank)					
		thousands in RMB (% of total)	Mortality	Mortality change since 1990	YLLs	YLLs change since 1990	DALYs	DALYs change since 1990
Pancreatic cancer		24051 (0.9)	58 (16)	26 (10)	1315 (20)	551 (9)	1322 (29)	555 (14)
Ovarian cancer		22270 (0.9)	21 (31)	6 (23)	594 (31)	141 (19)	603 (38)	145 (23)
Mouth cancer		19970 (0.8)	14 (36)	7 (21)	351 (38)	150 (18)	361 (43)	156 (22)
Oesophageal cancer		19480 (0.8)	176 (9)	7 (20)	3824 (10)	−15 (32)	3858 (12)	−10 (34)
Multiple sclerosis		18085 (0.7)	2 (51)	−2 (39)	50 (51)	−60 (35)	149 (52)	−26 (36)
Lymphoma		16400 (0.6)	29 (28)	6 (22)	835 (26)	40 (26)	854 (33)	50 (31)
Malaria		15050 (0.6)	0 (52)	0 (37)	2 (52)	−6 (31)	12 (53)	−4 (33)
Schistosomiasis		14650 (0.6)	9 (43)	0 (35)	222 (42)	−34 (33)	251 (45)	−23 (35)
Bladder cancer		13280 (0.5)	23 (30)	8 (17)	399 (34)	106 (20)	411 (42)	115 (24)
Pancreatitis		13110 (0.5)	8 (44)	2 (32)	188 (44)	25 (29)	205 (48)	27 (32)
Anaemias		12860 (0.5)	15 (35	−5 (41)	420 (33)	−494 (42)	1513 (24)	−346 (41)
Cardiomyopathy and myocarditis		12710 (0.5)	35 (25)	3 (31)	985 (25)	−125 (36)	1013 (32)	−127 (38)
Alcohole Chinae disorders		10720 (0.4)	5 (50)	1 (33)	163 (46)	32 (27)	3489 (13)	688 (12)
Kidney cancer		10020 (0.4)	32 (27)	18 (13)	823 (27)	400 (12)	837 (34)	384 (16)
Melanoma		8330 (0.3)	7 (48)	4 (28)	153 (48)	75 (24)	156 (51)	77 (29)
Gallbladder cancer		7560 (0.3)	18 (34)	0 (34)	637 (29)	225 (15)	644 (37)	229 (20)
Peripheral vascular disease		6990 (0.3)	9 (41)	6 (24)	119 (50)	−346 (39)	182 (49)	100 (26)
Thyroid cancer		6660 (0.3)	8 (45)	3 (29)	201 (43)	67 (25)	213 (47)	76 (30)
Meningitis		5350 (0.2)	8 (46)	−23 (44)	358 (36)	−1488 (46)	675 (36)	−1555 (46)
Rheumatic heart disease		4470 (0.2)	57 (18)	−74 (49)	1270 (21)	−2581 (48)	1487 (27)	−2654 (48)
Multiple myeloma		1710 (0.1)	9 (40)	4 (27)	246 (41)	90 (23)	250 (46)	93 (27)
Association with NSFC research fund	R		0.33	0.22	0.39	−0.04	0.40	−0.003
	P		0.02	0.12	0.004	0.79	0.003	0.98

discussed the differences of health research system in China and USA and the possible factors influencing the health fund allocation among diseases.

Methods

The budgets for NSFC are determined at least one year before each fiscal year, and some major research plans are made even five years ago. To reflect this time lag, data of 2010 disease burden and 2012 NSFC funding were chose to evaluate the relationship between disease burden and magnitude of research funding. Diseases were included in this study if 1) they were defined in *International Classification of Diseases, 9th revision, Clinical Modification (ICD-9-CM);* 2) their funding levels of NSFC were available; and 3) their measures of the burden of disease were available in Global Burden of Disease (GBD) Study 2010 [9].

Data Sources

NSFC has eight departments responsible for funding researches in different scientific subjects: mathematics, chemistry, life science, geoscience, engineering and material science, information science, management science and health. Before 2010, health research was included in the life science department, which also involved specialties of biology, botany, ecology, zoology, forestry, microbiology, immunology, psychology, agronomy and veterinary medicine. In 2010, health research was separated from life science department as a separate department.

The health department of NSFC has a similar framework to NIH, but with fewer "institutes" (currently eight compared with 27 institutes and centers in NIH), and endued with less functions. Applicants submit their protocols to different institutes according to target disease. For example, No.1 institute is responsible for diseases in circulatory, respiratory, blood and digestive systems. No.2 institute is responsible for disease in urinary, genital and endocrine systems, and diseases of ophthalmology, otolaryngology and dentistry. No. 3 institute is responsible for diseases of neurology and psychology. No.4 institute is responsible for diseases of skin, locomotor system and injury. No. 5 institute is responsible for cancer. No. 6 institute is responsible for communicable diseases and occupational diseases. No. 7 institute is responsible for pharmacology and pharmaceutics. No. 8 institute is responsible for Traditional Chinese Medicine.

Data concerning the funding levels for specific diseases or conditions in 2012 fiscal year were obtained from the NSFC website (http://isisn.nsfc.gov.cn/egrantweb/). The funding data were updated annually by NSFC. Data concerning disease burden were derived from GBD Study 2010 [9].

Three measures were chose to reflect disease burden from the GBD Study 2010: mortality, years of life lost (YLLs), and disability-adjusted life years (DALYs). In GBD Study, YLLs are calculated by multiplying the number of deaths in each age group by a reference life expectancy at that age. YLDs are calculated from the prevalence of a sequela multiplied by the disability weight for that sequela. Disability weights are based on surveys of general population. DALYs are the sum of YLLs and YLDs [10].

Due to the rapid population ageing and widespread westernized lifestyle changing, there is a remarkable change of disease

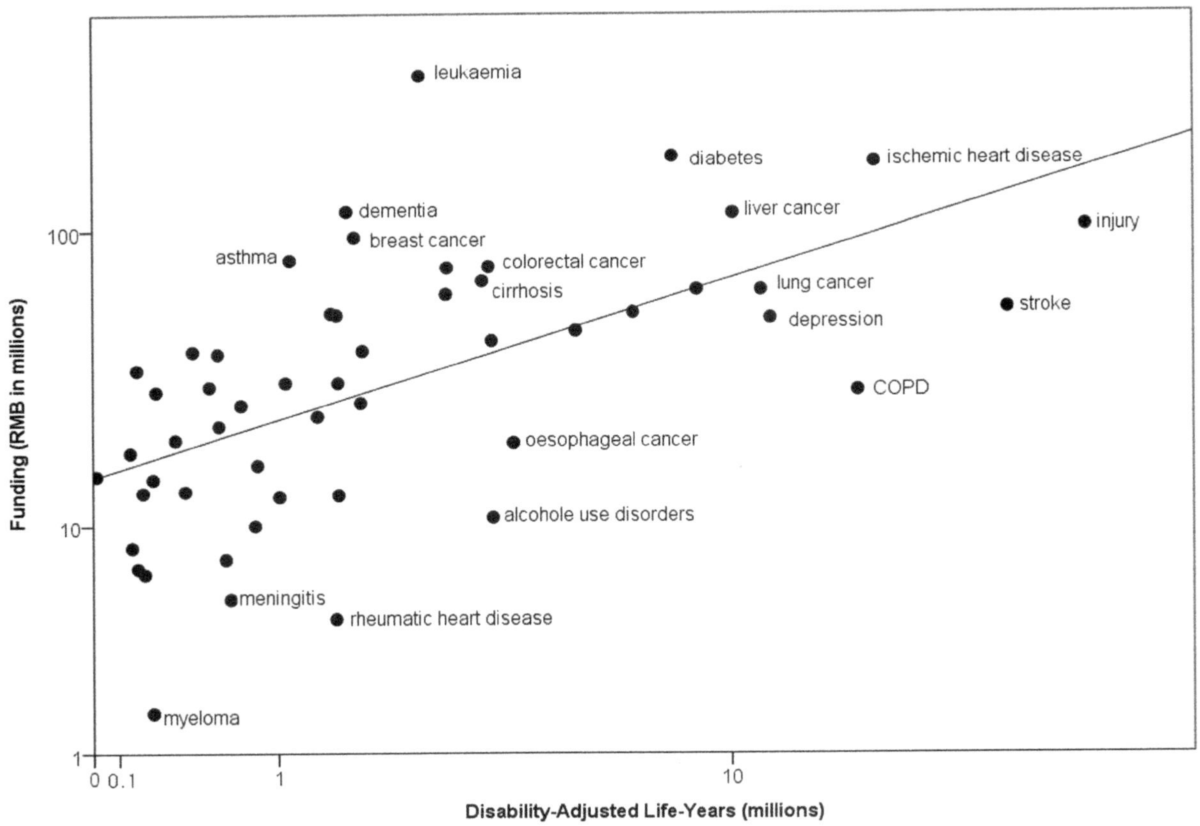

Figure 1. Relationship between NSFC disease-specific funding in 2012 and disability-adjusted life-years (DALYs) in 2012. Both X and Y axes are submitted to logarithmic scale. The line represents funding predicted on the basis of a linear regression with DALYs.

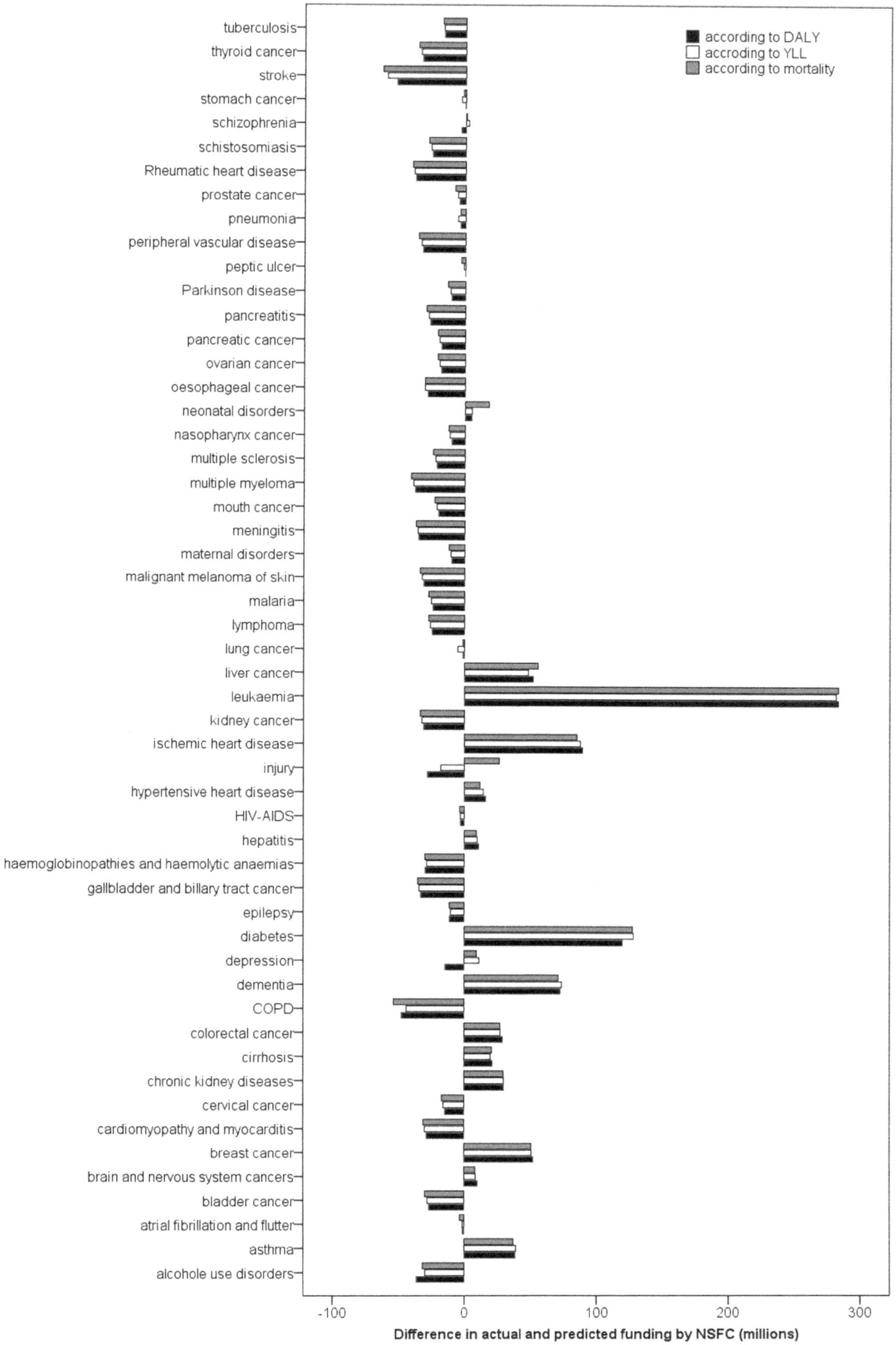
according to DALY
accroding to YLL
according to mortality
tuberculosis
thyroid cancer
stroke
stomach cancer
schizophrenia
schistosomiasis
Rheumatic heart disease
prostate cancer
pneumonia
peripheral vascular disease
peptic ulcer
Parkinson disease
pancreatitis
pancreatic cancer
ovarian cancer
oesophageal cancer
neonatal disorders
nasopharynx cancer
multiple sclerosis
multiple myeloma
mouth cancer
meningitis
maternal disorders
malignant melanoma of skin
malaria
lymphoma
lung cancer
liver cancer
leukaemia
kidney cancer
ischemic heart disease
injury
hypertensive heart disease
HIV-AIDS
hepatitis
haemoglobinopathies and haemolytic anaemias
gallbladder and billary tract cancer
epilepsy
diabetes
depression
dementia
COPD
colorectal cancer
cirrhosis
chronic kidney diseases
cervical cancer
cardiomyopathy and myocarditis
breast cancer
brain and nervous system cancers
bladder cancer
atrial fibrillation and flutter
asthma
alcohole use disorders
-100
0
100
200
300
Difference in actual and predicted funding by NSFC (millions)

Figure 2. Differences between actual and expected disease-specific NSFC funding as predicted by mortality, YLLs and DALYs. Negative values indicates underfunded, and positive values indicates overfunded.

spectrum in China in recent 20 years. These trends may have influenced the allocation of research resources, because some disease may become more, while others less prevalent. We, therefore, evaluated the impacts of changes of mortality, YLLs, DALYs between 1990 and 2010 on disease funding. Data of disease burden, mortality, YLLs and DALYs for China in 1990, were also retrieved from GBD Study [9].

Some diseases are more prevalent, and pose an extra burden in China compared to the world average level. These diseases deserve extra research resource to accelerate improvements in prevention and management. Therefore, we evaluated the differences of mortality, YLLs and DALYs of each disease between China and the world average level. Data of mortality, YLLs and DALYs for the world average level in 2010 were retrieved from GBD Study [11–13].

Statistic Analysis

Univariate linear regression was performed to assess the relationship between funding levels and disease burden metrics. For each measure that had a significant association with funding, regression-derived estimates were used to calculate the expected NSFC funding for each disease. The expected and the actual funding magnitudes were then compared. In univaritate regression analyses, we also evaluated the association of funding levels with changes of disease burden during 1990 and 2010, and with differences of disease burden between China and the worldwide average. The SPSS statistical package (Version 16, Chicago, Ill) was used for all statistic analyses.

Results

The total NSFC budget of 2012 fiscal year was 16.93 billion RMB (US $2.69 billion), with 4.12 billion RMB allocated to health research (disease targeted), of which 2.57 billion RMB (62.4%) was devoted to the 53 diseases included in this study. Disease funding ranged from about 2 million RMB for multiple myeloma, to 328 million for leukemia, with a median of 31 million RMB (4.8±5.5 million RMB, **Table 1**).

In the univariate regression analysis, NSFC health funding was associated with burden of disease measured in mortality ($R = 0.33$, $P = 0.02$), YLLs ($R = 0.39$, $P = 0.004$), and DALYs ($R = 0.40$, $P = 0.003$, **Table 1**).

Since 1990, the burdens decreased in some diseases, while increased in others in large extents (**Table 1**). The mortality of chronic obstructive pulmonary disorder (COPD) decreased from 1427 thousand in 1990 to 934 thousand in 2010, with a decrement of 493 thousand which ranked top among diseases. The mortality of neonatal disorders decreased from 343 thousand to 83 thousand, with a decrement of 260 thousand which ranked second among diseases. Progress in neonatal disorders contributed the largest reduction of DALYs (a decrement of 22534), followed by pneumonia (a decrement of 20166). On the other hand, ischemic heart disease induced the largest increment of mortality (499 thousand) during 1990 to 2010, followed by stroke (387 thousand). Ischemic heart disease also induced the largest increment of DALYs (7759 thousand), followed by stroke (5262 thousand). Because these transitional trends of disease burden may be a reflection of past research strength, and could have been used as indicators for allocating research resources, we analyzed the changes of disease burdens during 1990 to 2010. But none of the changes of mortality ($R = 0.22$, $P = 0.12$), YLLs ($R = -0.04$, $P = 0.79$) and DALYs ($R = -0.003$, $P = 0.98$) was associated with NSFC funding magnitudes (**Table 1**).

Some diseases pose extra burden in China compare to the world averages, while others pose less burden. Of note, stroke demonstrated the largest extra mortality (126.1/100000 higher), YLLs (614/100000 higher) and DALYs (618/100000 higher) than the world averages. Ischemic heart disease induced the least extra mortality than the world average (35.6/100000 lower), and neonatal disorders induced the least extra YLLs (1985/100000 lower) and DALYs (2004/100000 lower) than the world averages. We analyzed differences of disease burden metrics in 2010 between China and world averages. But none of the differences of mortality ($R = -0.11$, $P = 0.45$), YLLs ($R = -0.11$, $P = 0.43$) and DALYs ($R = -0.12$, $P = 0.38$) to the world averages were associated with NFSC funding magnitudes (**Table 2**).

In standard multivariable analysis, DALYs became the only significant predictor for NSFC funding. The amount of predicted and actual NSFC funding as a function of DALYs is shown in **Figure 1**. The line represents the predicted funding levels if DALYs were the sole criterion for funding.

The difference between actual and predicted funding for each disease, with mortality, YLLs and DALYs as explanatory variables, is shown in **Figure 2**. Stroke, and COPD received the least funding compared to expected, while the leukemia and diabetes received the most funding compared to expected.

Discussion

In this study we analyzed the relationship between NSFC funding and burden of disease measured in mortality, YLLs and DALYs. Although the NSFC health funding was associated with disease burden, measured in mortality ($R = 0.33$, $P = 0.02$), YLLs ($R = 0.39$, $P = 0.004$), and DALYs ($R = 0.40$, $P = 0.003$), there exist significant differences between the actual and expected funding in some diseases according to these measures.

The relationship between disease research funding and burden of disease has been investigated in US National Institute of Health (NIH) system in several studies [6,7,14]. Disease incidence and prevalence were unrelated to funding, while mortality and YLLs weakly correlated with funding. DALYs were more strongly predictive [6,7]. In this study, mortality also weakly correlated with funding. Both YLLs and DALYs correlated significantly with NSFC funding. Although NSFC has a smaller total funding budget for health research, and is more inclusive and involves several subjects other than health, its organization is roughly similar to those of NIH. So it is not surprise that the overall profiles of NSFC funding distribution among diseases are similar to that of NIH.

The funding programs in NSFC can be classified as three types: free-applying, predetermined and investigator-targeted programs, which accounts for about 93%, 5% and 2% of the total budget respectively. For free-applying programs, there is no preset research scope, so applicants can choose any health research topics. For predetermined programs, every year one or two research topics were preset in each institute according to expertise and scientific needs. For the investigator-targeted programs, prominent investigators younger than 45 years were selected base on their previous academic achievements, and 1.5–3.0 million RMB was arranged to each awarder. With the money, they can choose any health research topics in five years. These arrange-

Table 2. Funding levels of NSFC and disease burden of world.

Condition or disease	NSFC research fund	Measure of disease burden in 2010					
		Age-standardized rate per 100000 (rank)					
	thousands in RMB (% of total)	Mortality,	Mortality,	YLLs,	YLLs,	DALYs,	DALYs,
		World	China-World	World	China-World	World	China-World
Leukaemia	327854 (12.8)	4.2(27)	0.0 (12)	137(23)	45 (7)	139(31)	46 (7)
Diabetes	176635 (6.9)	19.5(9)	−8.0 (46)	378(13)	−160 (43)	680(11)	−148 (41)
Ischemic heart disease	169185 (6.6)	105.7(1)	−35.6 (53)	1757(3)	−636 (48)	1884(3)	−642 (48)
Dementia	115785 (4.5)	7.1(18)	−3.2 (39)	66(34)	−20 (27)	165(28)	−46 (33)
Liver cancer	114225 (4.5)	11.5(14)	13.5 (4)	275(14)	379 (2)	277(17)	382 (2)
Injury	103560 (4.0)	74.3(3)	−17.6 (49)	3347(1)	−1024 (50)	4058(1)	−1118 (50)
Breast cancer	95360 (3.7)	6.6(19)	−3.1 (38)	161(21)	−62 (36)	174(27)	−67 (35)
Asthma	80060 (3.1)	5.2(23)	−3.7 (42)	125(27)	−100 (41)	326(15)	−242 (44)
Colorectal cancer	75990 (3.0)	10.8(17)	−0.2 (18)	201(19)	22 (9)	209(25)	21 (9)
Chronic kidney diseases	75389 (2.9)	11.1(16)	−5.3 (43)	249(15)	−108 (42)	307(16)	−116 (39)
Cirrhosis	68085 (2.7)	15.6(12)	−7.9 (45)	441(11)	−233 (45)	450(13)	−233 (43)
Neonatal disorders	63730 (2.5)	31.0(6)	−21.6 (51)	2794(2)	−1985 (53)	2931(2)	−2004 (53)
Lung cancer	63580 (2.5)	23.4(7)	12.4 (5)	465(10)	287 (3)	470(12)	290 (3)
Hypertensive heart disease	61463 (2.4)	13.1(13)	−0.3 (19)	216(17)	−23 (29)	222(23)	−28 (27)
Stroke	55330 (2.2)	88.4(2)	38.5 (1)	1421(5)	614 (1)	1484(5)	618 (1)
Stomach cancer	53610 (2.1)	11.5(15)	17.3 (3)	235(16)	204 (5)	238(20)	207 (4)
Hepatitis	53245 (2.1)	4.6(26)	−1.6 (33)	185(20)	−97 (40)	192(26)	−95 (37)
Brain cancers	52610 (2.1)	3(33)	0.3 (9)	87(32)	14 (10)	88(37)	14 (10)
Depression	51335 (2.0)	0(53)	0.0 (14)	0(53)	0 (16)	1078(9)	−260 (45)
Pneumonia	46600 (1.8)	41(5)	−25.1 (52)	1639(4)	−1204 (52)	1672(4)	−1208 (52)
Schizophrenia	43260 (1.7)	0.3(50)	0.3 (10)	9(49)	10 (12)	218(24)	8 (11)
HIV-AIDS	40075 (1.6)	21.4(8)	−19.0 (50)	1121(7)	−1010 (49)	1184(7)	−1065 (49)
Peptic ulcer	39870 (1.6)	3.7(29)	−2.3 (36)	93(28)	−67 (37)	98(33)	−67 (34)
Atrial fibrillation and flutter	39150 (1.5)	1.7(40)	−0.7 (25)	17(46)	−6 (21)	52(41)	−10 (21)
Prostate cancer	34530 (1.3)	3.8(28)	−2.9 (37)	48(38)	−36 (31)	55(39)	−42 (30)
Nasopharynx cancer	31250 (1.2)	1(46)	1.3 (7)	29(43)	39 (8)	29(47)	40 (8)
Epilepsy	31240 (1.2)	2.6(34)	−1.7 (35)	126(26)	−84 (39)	253(19)	−141 (40)
Maternal disorders	30260 (1.2)	3.7(30)	−3.4 (40)	208(18)	−189 (44)	234(21)	−196 (42)
COPD	29450 (1.2)	43.8(4)	26.8 (2)	687(8)	250 (4)	1114(8)	77 (6)
Parkinson disease	29160 (1.1)	1.7(41)	−1.2 (30)	19(45)	−11 (23)	28(48)	−9 (20)
Tuberculosis	26710 (1.0)	18(10)	−14.9 (47)	619(9)	−538 (47)	717(10)	−599 (47)

Table 2. Cont.

Condition or disease		NSFC research fund	Measure of disease burden in 2010					
			Age-standardized rate per 100000 (rank)					
		thousands in RMB (% of total)	Mortality,	Mortality,	YLLs,	YLLs,	DALYs,	DALYs,
			World	China-World	World	China-World	World	China-World
Cervical cancer		26245 (1.0)	3.4(32)	−1.7 (34)	92(30)	−45 (34)	94(35)	−46 (31)
Pancreatic cancer		24051 (0.9)	4.7(25)	−0.7 (24)	89(31)	−1 (18)	89(36)	−1 (15)
Ovarian cancer		22270 (0.9)	2.4(37)	−1.0 (28)	59(35)	−20 (26)	60(38)	−21 (25)
Mouth cancer		19970 (0.8)	1.9(39)	−0.9 (27)	45(39)	−22 (28)	47(43)	−23 (26)
Oesophageal cancer		19480 (0.8)	6.1(20)	6.2 (6)	129(24)	128 (6)	130(32)	129 (5)
Multiple sclerosis		18085 (0.7)	0.3(51)	−0.2 (17)	8(50)	−5 (20)	16(51)	−6 (18)
Lymphoma		16400 (0.6)	3.5(31)	−1.4 (31)	93(29)	−33 (30)	94(34)	−34 (29)
Malaria		15050 (0.6)	16.7(11)	−16.7 (48)	1141(6)	−1141 (51)	1200(6)	−1199 (51)
Schistosomiasis		14650 (0.6)	0.2(52)	0.4 (8)	5(52)	10 (11)	48(42)	−31 (28)
Bladder cancer		13280 (0.5)	2.6(35)	−0.9 (26)	42(41)	−14 (24)	44(45)	−15 (22)
Pancreatitis		13110 (0.5)	1.2(44)	−0.6 (23)	31(42)	−19 (25)	34(46)	−20 (24)
Anaemias		12860 (0.5)	1.7(42)	−0.5 (22)	79(33)	−46 (35)	227(22)	−105 (38)
Cardiomyopathy/myocarditis		12710 (0.5)	6.1(21)	−3.6 (41)	156(22)	−84 (38)	162(29)	−87 (36)
Alcohole Chinae disorders		10720 (0.4)	1.7(43)	−1.4 (32)	55(36)	−45 (33)	256(18)	−20 (23)
Kidney cancer		10020 (0.4)	2.5(36)	−0.3 (20)	52(37)	5 (13)	53(40)	4 (12)
Melanoma		8330 (0.3)	0.7(47)	−0.2 (16)	16(47)	−6 (22)	17(50)	−6 (19)
Gallbladder cancer		7560 (0.3)	2.3(38)	−0.2 (15)	44(40)	0 (17)	44(44)	0 (14)
Peripheral vascular disease		6990 (0.3)	0.7(48)	0.0 (13)	8(51)	0 (15)	14(52)	−1 (16)
Thyroid cancer		6660 (0.3)	0.5(49)	0.1 (11)	11(48)	2 (14)	12(53)	2 (13)
Meningitis		5350 (0.2)	6.1(22)	−5.5 (44)	389(12)	−357 (46)	426(14)	−372 (46)
Rheumatic heart disease		4470 (0.2)	5.2(24)	−1.2 (29)	127(25)	−41 (32)	147(30)	−46 (32)
Multiple myeloma		1710 (0.1)	1.1(45)	−0.4 (21)	21(44)	−4 (19)	21(49)	−4 (17)
Association with NSFC research fund	R		0.33	−0.11	0.24	−0.11	0.25	−0.12
	P		0.02	0.45	0.09	0.43	0.07	0.38

ments made the distribution of NSFC health research fund among diseases largely determined by numbers of applications and applicants' interests in individual disease, which may be further influenced by international research trends, governmental policies and public opinions.

Based on the limited data of the present study, it is unlikely to determine why some diseases were underfunded, while others overfunded relative to disease burden. The over-funding of leukemia in China may be explained by the governmental reinforce of children health after the implementation of One-Child Policy in 1978. Successes in treating some types of leukemia in resent years, arsenic trioxide for acute promyelocytic leukemia as an example, which was originally discovered by Chinese researchers and they also contributed remarkably in the subsequent studies [15,16], may have further incited the enthusiasm for leukemia research in China. On the other hand, stroke and COPD remained as the most underfunded diseases. The limited data suggested that incidence, prevalence of stroke, COPD and several other chronic diseases are increasing rapidly in China in recent year due to population ageing, lifestyle transition and environment pollution [17,18]. These rapid changes in disease burdens have not reflected in the current NSFC funding assignment, possibly due to the unawareness of impact of these changes to public health or delayed responses to these changes. Furthermore, lack of major progress in managing stroke and COPD in recent years probably have depressed the interests for studying these chronic diseases.

Given the limited resource for health research, developing countries like China should allocate more research fund to their country-specific diseases–those with extra burden than other countries [19]. But in analyzing NCSF allocation, we failed to find this association. Measured by mortality, YLLs or DALYs, stroke poses the heaviest disease burden in China. The mortality, YLLs and DALYs of stroke in China is 38.5/100000, 614/100000 and 618/100000 higher than the world average level respectively, and all of these differences rank first among diseases. On the other hand, mortality, YLLs and DALYs of ischemic heart disease is 35.6/100000, 636/100000 and 642/100000 lower than the world average level respectively, which make it one of the least country-specific diseases in China. Although DALYs caused by stroke in 2010 (30139 thousand) is about two times of DALYs caused by ischemic heart disease (17886 thousand), the NSFC fund allocated for stroke is only one third of that for ischemic heart disease (55 vs 169 million RMB). This phenomenon of disproportionally underfunding of stroke and overfunding of ischemic heart disease in reference to disease burden was not observed in the recent NIH fund allocation [7].

The disease spectrum in China has changed significant in recent 20 years. Measured by DALYs, the disease burden of neonatal disorders and pneumonia decreased with the largest extent (22534/100000 and 20166/100000) during 1990 to 2010; while DALYs due to ischemic heart disease and stroke increased with the largest extent (7759/100000 and 5262/100000) [9]. Theoretically, those with disease burden increased rapidly deserve more research resources to find approach for counteracting the trends. But we failed to find this association in NCSF allocation.

There are several limitations in this study which should be addressed when interpreting the results. First, we did not evaluate other sources, such as health research funds from government agencies other than NSFC. Other national funds, such as 863 projects, 973 projects, and National Supporting Programs administrated by Ministry of Science and Technology (MOST), account for about 10% of all governmental funds dedicated to health research in 2012 [20]. Funds from provincial government account for about 20% of all governmental funds dedicated to health research. Thus, contribution of resources other than NSFC for health research is unremarkable. Second, we did not include prevalence and incidence as measures for disease burden due to lack of recent data. In the previous studies, prevalence and incidence were not associated with NIH funding levels. We presume this is also the case in NSFC funding. Third, there may be fluctuation of funding magnitudes for a given diseases over years. The annual fluctuation of funding may be more predominant in less common diseases, for which the number of applicants is relatively small.

In conclusion, although the funding levels of NSFC were roughly associated with diseases burden as measured with mortality, YLLs and DALYs, some major diseases such as stroke were underfunded; with others such as leukemia were overfunded. Changes of disease burden during the past 20 years, and differences of disease burden from the world average have not been considered in allocating the current NSFC health funds.

Acknowledgments

This study was sponsored by Nature Science Foundation of Jiangsu (BE2013713) to GX. Authors thank Dr. Heqin Cao from NSFC for providing the annual funding data of NSFC, and for his suggestions in the study design and manuscript revision.

Author Contributions

Conceived and designed the experiments: GX ZZ QL YL RY YX YJ XL. Performed the experiments: GX ZZ QL YL. Analyzed the data: GX ZZ. Contributed reagents/materials/analysis tools: GX ZZ QL YJ XL. Wrote the paper: GX ZZ XL.

References

1. Van Noorden R (2014) China tops Europe in R&D intensity. Nature 505:144–145.
2. Qiu J (2014) China goes back to basics on research funding. Nature 507:148–149.
3. Morello L, Morrison J, Reardon S, Tollefson J, Witze A (2014) Obama's budget request falls flat. Nature 507:147–148.
4. Shi Y, Rao Y (2010) China's research culture. Science 329:1128.
5. Cao C, Li N, Li X, Liu L (2013) Science and Government. Reforming China's S&T system. Science 341:460–462.
6. Gross CP, Anderson GF, Powe NR (1999) The relation between funding by the National Institutes of Health and the burden of disease. N Engl J Med 340:1881–1887.
7. Gillum LA, Gouveia C, Dorsey ER, Pletcher M, Mathers CD, et al. (2011) NIH disease funding levels and burden of disease. PLoS One 6:e16837.
8. McCarthy M, Harvey G, Conceição C, la Torre G, Gulis G (2009) Comparing public-health research priorities in Europe. Health Res Policy Syst 7:17.
9. Yang G, Wang Y, Zeng Y, Gao GF, Liang X, et al. (2013) Rapid health transition in China, 1990–2010: findings from the Global Burden of Disease Study 2010. Lancet 381:1987–2015.
10. Murray CJ, Ezzati M, Flaxman AD, Lim S, Lozano R, et al. (2012) GBD 2010: design, definitions, and metrics. Lancet 380:2063–2066.
11. Lozano R, Naghavi M, Foreman K, Lim S, Shibuya K, et al. (2012) Global and regional mortality from 235 causes of death for 20 age groups in 1990 and 2010: a systematic analysis for the Global Burden of Disease Study 2010. Lancet 380:2095–2128.
12. Murray CJ, Vos T, Lozano R, Naghavi M, Flaxman AD, et al. (2012) Disability-adjusted life years (DALYs) for 291 diseases and injuries in 21 regions, 1990–2010: a systematic analysis for the Global Burden of Disease Study 2010. Lancet 380:2197–2223.
13. Vos T, Flaxman AD, Naghavi M, Lozano R, Michaud C, et al. (2012) Years lived with disability (YLDs) for 1160 sequelae of 289 diseases and injuries 1990–2010: a systematic analysis for the Global Burden of Disease Study 2010. Lancet 380:2163–2196.

14. Sampat BN, Buterbaugh K, Perl M (2013) New evidence on the allocation of NIH funds across diseases. Milbank Q 91:163–185.
15. Rao Y, Li R, Zhang D (2013) A drug from poison: how the therapeutic effect of arsenic trioxide on acute promyelocytic leukemia was discovered. Sci China Life Sci 56:495–502.
16. Wang ZY, Chen Z (2008) Acute promyelocytic leukemia: from highly fatal to highly curable. Blood 111:2505–2515.
17. Liu M, Wu B, Wang WZ, Lee LM, Zhang SH, et al. (2007) Stroke in China: epidemiology, prevention, and management strategies. Lancet Neurol 6:456–464.
18. Fang X, Wang X, Bai C (2011) COPD in China: the burden and importance of proper management. Chest 139:920–929.
19. Viergever RF, Olifson S, Ghaffar A, Terry RF (2010) A checklist for health research priority setting: nine common themes of good practice. Health Res Policy Syst 8:36.
20. National Bureau of Statistics Ministry of Science and Technology (2013) China Statistical Yearbook on Science and Technology. China Statistics Press. Beijing.

Dietary Protein Intake and Coronary Heart Disease in a Large Community Based Cohort: Results from the Atherosclerosis Risk in Communities (ARIC) Study

Bernhard Haring[1]*, Noelle Gronroos[2], Jennifer A. Nettleton[3], Moritz C. Wyler von Ballmoos[4], Elizabeth Selvin[5], Alvaro Alonso[2]

1 Department of Internal Medicine I, Comprehensive Heart Failure Center, University of Würzburg, Würzburg, Bavaria, Germany, 2 Division of Epidemiology and Community Health, University of Minnesota, Minneapolis, Minnesota, United States of America, 3 Division of Epidemiology, Human Genetics and Environmental Sciences, School of Public Health, University of Texas Health Science Center at Houston, Houston, Texas, United States of America, 4 Department of Surgery & Division of Cardiothoracic Surgery, Froedtert Memorial Hospital & Medical College of Wisconsin, Milwaukee, Wisconsin, United States of America, 5 Department of Epidemiology and the Welch Center for Prevention, Epidemiology and Clinical Research, Johns Hopkins Bloomberg School of Public Health, Baltimore, Maryland, United States of America

Abstract

Background: Prospective data examining the relationship between dietary protein intake and incident coronary heart disease (CHD) are inconclusive. Most evidence is derived from homogenous populations such as health professionals. Large community-based analyses in more diverse samples are lacking.

Methods: We studied the association of protein type and major dietary protein sources and risk for incident CHD in 12,066 middle-aged adults (aged 45–64 at baseline, 1987–1989) from four U.S. communities enrolled in the Atherosclerosis Risk in Communities (ARIC) Study who were free of diabetes mellitus and cardiovascular disease at baseline. Dietary protein intake was assessed at baseline and after 6 years of follow-up by food frequency questionnaire. Our primary outcome was adjudicated coronary heart disease events or deaths with following up through December 31, 2010. Cox proportional hazard models with multivariable adjustment were used for statistical analyses.

Results: During a median follow-up of 22 years, there were 1,147 CHD events. In multivariable analyses total, animal and vegetable protein were not associated with an increased risk for CHD before or after adjustment. In food group analyses of major dietary protein sources, protein intake from red and processed meat, dairy products, fish, nuts, eggs, and legumes were not significantly associated with CHD risk. The hazard ratios [with 95% confidence intervals] for risk of CHD across quintiles of protein from poultry were 1.00 [ref], 0.83 [0.70–0.99], 0.93 [0.75–1.15], 0.88 [0.73–1.06], 0.79 [0.64–0.98], P for trend =0.16). Replacement analyses evaluating the association of substituting one source of dietary protein for another or of decreasing protein intake at the expense of carbohydrates or total fats did not show any statistically significant association with CHD risk.

Conclusion: Based on a large community cohort we found no overall relationship between protein type and major dietary protein sources and risk for CHD.

Editor: Antony Bayer, Cardiff University, United Kingdom

Funding: The Atherosclerosis Risk in Communities Study is carried out as a collaborative study supported by National Heart, Lung, and Blood Institute contracts (HHSN268201100005C, HHSN268201100006C, HHSN268201100007C, HHSN268201100008C, HHSN268201100009C, HHSN268201100010C, HHSN268201100011C, and HHSN268201100012C). There are no relationships with industry to declare. Open Access publication was funded by the German Research Foundation (DFG) and the University of Würzburg in the funding program Open Access Publishing. The funders had no role in study design, data collection and analysis, decision to publish, or preparation of the manuscript.

Competing Interests: The authors have declared that no competing interests exist.

* Email: Haring_B@ukw.de

Introduction

The relationship of dietary protein distinguished by animal versus vegetable origin with risk of coronary heart disease (CHD) has shown conflicting results [1,2,3,4,5,6]. This is surprising since the type of protein has been shown to influence cardiovascular risk factors such as hypertension [7,8,9,10,11,12]. Various observational studies [7,8,10,13] and feeding trials [9,11,12] have associated dietary protein of vegetable type inversely with blood pressure. To elucidate this apparent paradox, Bernstein et al. have focused on the effect of various food groups as major sources of dietary protein rather than on protein type in the Nurses' Health Study [2]. Greater consumption of red meat or processed meat products was associated with a higher risk of CHD, while higher intakes of poultry, fish and nuts were associated with lower risk [2]. These findings are again in contrast with other results that showed no association of red meat with CHD [14] or that showed beneficial effects of animal protein on vascular health [15,16]. The discordance in findings may be explained by several factors including research design and study populations. Large randomized controlled feeding trials on this topic are sparse and current evidence is mostly derived from observational studies which used nurses or health professionals as study populations [1,2,4,5]. Community based analyses are mostly missing [6,17]. Thus, conclusions regarding the relation of various sources of protein intake with cardiovascular health are difficult to draw. Analyses conducted in large general communities are warranted as these may provide greater exposure variability with more generalizable results.

In this study, we aimed to investigate the associations between total, animal, and plant-based dietary protein, as well as individual protein-rich food groups, and the risk for CHD in a large, community-based cohort of middle-aged adults. We hypothesized that intake of animal protein and proteins from processed meats would be associated with a higher risk of CHD and vegetable proteins and corresponding food groups with a lower CHD risk.

Methods

Study Population

The Atherosclerosis Risk in Communities Study (ARIC) is a community-based prospective cohort study of 15,792 middle-aged adults (aged 45–64 years at baseline) from four U.S. communities (Washington County, Md; Forsyth County, NC; Jackson, Miss; and suburbs of Minneapolis, Minn.) [18]. The first examination (visit 1) of participants occurred during 1987–1989, with three follow-up visits taking place each approximately every 3 years; response rates were 93%, 86%, and 81% at visits 2 (1990 to 1992), 3 (1993 to 1995), and 4 (1996 to 1998), respectively. A fifth exam (visit 5) took place in 2011–2013 among surviving participants. At all visits, participants received an extensive examination, including collection of medical, social, and demographic data [18]. For this analysis, only white and black adults were included; blacks from the Minneapolis and Washington County field centers were excluded due to small numbers. Individuals with self-reported diabetes, fasting blood glucose ≥126 mg/dL, non-fasting blood glucose ≥200 mg/dL or use of diabetes medication, a history of myocardial infarction, stroke, heart failure, coronary bypass surgery, angioplasty or with missing data on covariates of interest were excluded. Our final sample size included 12,066 persons.

The ARIC study was approved by the Institutional Review Boards (IRB) of all participating institutions, including the IRBs of the University of Minnesota, Johns Hopkins University, University of North Carolina, University of Mississippi Medical Center, and Wake Forest University. Written informed consent at each clinical site was obtained from all participants.

Assessment of protein intake

Protein intake was assessed using an interviewer-administered, 66-item food frequency questionnaire (FFQ) adapted from the 61-item FFQ developed by Willett et al. [19]. The FFQ was administered to all subjects at visit 1 at baseline (1987–1989) and at visit 3 (1993–1995). The usual frequency of food consumption was reported in 9 categories, from never or less than once a month to>6 times per day. The major contributors to protein intake included: unprocessed red meat, processed red meat, poultry, high-fat dairy, low-fat dairy, fish & seafood, eggs, nuts, and legumes. Average daily intake of nutrients was calculated by multiplying the frequency of consumption of each food item by its nutrient content and adding up the nutrient intake for all of the items. Vegetable protein intake was defined as the difference of total and animal protein intake. The residual method was used to adjust for total energy intake [20]. For assessing dietary behaviour, participants were divided into quintiles of cumulative average intake of various protein sources. Cumulative updating of the FFQ (i.e. visit 1 FFQ for follow-up between visit 1 and visit 3 and the average of visits 1 and 3 FFQ afterwards for those who attended both examinations, or visit 1 FFQ for those who did not attend visit 3) was used to reduce within-person variation and best represent long-term dietary behavior [2]. Participants with incomplete dietary information or with extreme calorie intake (<600 kcal or>4200 kcal per day for men, <500 kcal or> 3600 kcal per day for women) were excluded from further analysis. We stopped updating a participant's cumulative average intake when the participant of our study was diagnosed with an intermediate variable on the causal pathway between diet and CHD such as hypercholesterolemia, hypertension, stroke and diabetes. This was done to avoid exposure misclassification due to short-term changes in dietary patterns.

Assessment of coronary heart disease

The primary end point for this study was CHD occurring after the completion of the first FFQ (between 1987 and 1989). CHD was defined as a definite or probable myocardial infarction or a death from coronary heart disease. CHD events were identified and adjudicated using information from study visits, yearly telephone follow-up calls, review of hospital discharge lists and medical charts, death certificates, next-of-kin interviews, and physician-completed questionnaires [18,21]. Follow-up for CHD was available until December 31, 2010.

Covariates

Height, weight, and waist circumference were measured following a standardized protocol [18,21]. ARIC participants underwent fasting venipuncture at each examination [18]. Diabetes was defined as current use of glucose-lowering medications, fasting blood glucose ≥126 mg/dL, non-fasting blood glucose ≥200 mg/dL or self-reported history of diabetes. Hypertension was defined as the average of the last two of three blood-pressure readings at the first visit (using 140 mmHg or higher for systolic and 90 mmHg or higher for diastolic as cut-off points). Current smoking, ethanol intake, education, intake of antihypertensive or lipid lowering medication were derived from standardized questionnaires [18]. Sports-related physical activity and leisure related physical activity were assessed with the use of Baecke's questionnaire and scoring systems [22].

Statistical Analysis

To assess the association of CHD and average cumulative intake of protein by quintiles, we calculated incidence rates (IR) of CHD events per 1000 person-years as the number of diagnosed cases of CHD occurring during the entire follow-up period divided by person-years of follow-up. Person-years of follow up were defined as time from the baseline examination to the date of the first coronary event, death, lost to follow-up, or December 31, 2010, whichever occurred earlier. Thereafter, corresponding rate ratios were calculated by dividing the rate among participants in each specific intake quintile by the rate among participants in the lowest quintile of intake (reference). Cox proportional hazards regression models were used to account for potential confounding. An initial model adjusted for age, race, sex, ARIC study center,

Table 1. Unadjusted baseline characteristics according to quintiles of total protein intake, ARIC 1987–1989.

	Q 1 (low)	Q 2	Q 3	Q 4	Q5 (high)	p-trend[a]
N	2412	2414	2413	2414	2413	
Protein intake, g/day (SD)	49.3 (10.2)	62.9 (3.9)	70.2(3.9)	77.8 (4.0)	93.5 (12.6)	<0.0001
Protein intake, % of total energy	12.4 (1.7)	15.7 (1.0)	17.8 (1.5)	19.8 (2.0)	22.8 (3.4)	<0.0001
Age, years (SD)	53.4 (5.7)	54.0 (5.7)	54.0 (5.8)	53.8 (5.7)	53.8 (5.7)	0.11
Women, %	55.9	55.8	55.8	55.8	55.8	0.99
Black, %	24.8	24.5	21.9	21.6	22.4	0.005
High school graduate, %	72.1	77.7	80.7	82.6	84.0	<0.0001
Current smoker, %	32.3	28.8	24.7	22.5	21.6	<0.0001
Hypertension, %	29.9	27.5	29.1	28.0	28.8	0.57
Body Mass Index, kg/m^2 (SD)	26.6 (5.1)	26.8 (4.9)	27.0 (5.0)	27.4 (5.0)	27.7 (5.1)	<0.0001
Waist-to-hip ratio (SD)	0.9 (0.1)	0.9 (0.1)	0.9 (0.1)	0.9 (0.1)	0.9 (0.1)	0.19
Baecke Sport Activity Score (SD)	2.4 (0.8)	2.4 (0.8)	2.5 (0.8)	2.5 (0.8)	2.6 (0.8)	<0.0001
Baecke Leisure Index (SD)	2.3 (0.6)	2.3 (0.6)	2.4 (0.6)	2.4 (0.6)	2.5 (0.6)	<0.0001
Systolic blood pressure, mmHg (SD)	120.7 (18.7)	119.9 (17.5)	119.9 (17.6)	119.2 (17.6)	119.4 (18.2)	0.004
Serum HDL, mmol/L (SD)	1.4 (0.4)	1.4 (0.4)	1.4 (0.4)	1.4 (0.5)	1.4 (0.4)	0.27
Serum cholesterol, mmol/L (SD)	5.5 (1.0)	5.5 (1.1)	5.6 (1.1)	5.5 (1.1)	5.5 (1.1)	0.23
Use of antihypertensive medication, %	19.4	18.3	20.4	18.4	19.6	0.89
Use of lipid lowering medication, %	1.3	1.7	2.2	3.2	2.7	<0.0001
Carbohydrate intake, g/day (SD)	231.2 (57.6)	208.0 (31.4)	197.8 (31.3)	188.5 (32.3)	172.4 (38.4)	<0.0001
Carbohydrate intake, % of total energy (SD)	56.2 (9.5)	51.3 (7.9)	48.3 (7.7)	45.8 (7.5)	42.8 (7.8)	<0.0001
Fiber intake, g/day (SD)	15.5 (7.4)	16.7 (5.6)	17.3 (5.6)	17.6 (5.9)	18.3 (7.0)	<0.0001
Magnesium intake, g/day (SD)	217.0 (66.1)	240.7 (52.5)	253.5 (53.9)	267.0 (57.9)	288.4 (65.6)	<0.0001
Alcohol intake, g/week (SD)	68.7 (148.7)	43.9 (89.0)	40.7 (78.9)	36.9 (70.4)	32.7 (65.4)	<0.0001
Total energy intake, kcal/day (SD)	1818.1 (693.9)	1488.7 (555.6)	1489.7 (538.1)	1565.9 (537.1)	1802.8 (606.7)	0.23
Total fat Intake (g/d) (Median ±SD)	53.9 (16.0)	59.9 (11.7)	61.4 (12.0)	62.6 (12.8)	63.4 (15.4)	<0.0001
Total fat intake, % of total energy (SD)	30.0 (7.2)	32.5 (6.2)	33.4 (6.3)	34.2 (6.2)	34.5 (6.5)	<0.0001

Values are % for categorical variables and mean (SD) for continuous variables.
[a]p-values from general linear models for continuous variables and Mantel-Haenszel 1-degree of freedom chi-square statistic.

and total energy intake (minimally adjusted model). A second model additionally adjusted for smoking (current, former, never), pack years of smoking, education (less than high school, high school, more than high school), systolic blood pressure (mmHg), use of antihypertensive medication, HDLc (mmol/l), total cholesterol (mmol/l), use of lipid lowering medication, body mass index (kg/m^2), waist-to-hip ratio, alcohol intake (g/week), Baecke's physical activity score, leisure-related physical activity, carbohydrate intake (quintiles), fiber intake (quintiles), and magnesium intake (quintiles) (fully adjusted model). Median protein intake of each quintile (g/d) modeled as a continuous variable was used to test for linear trend.

We further conducted food substitution analyses based on the fully adjusted model. Hazard ratios of CHD associated with increasing 1 serving/day in the consumption of protein sources at the expense of decreasing 1 serving/day in a different protein source were calculated. Similarly, we conducted nutrient substitution analyses by examining the risk for CHD when increasing 10% energy from carbohydrates or fat while decreasing 10% of energy from protein. Tests of the proportional hazards assumption were evaluated. All p-values were 2-tailed. Data were analyzed with SAS 9.3 (SAS Corp, Cary, NC).

Results

Baseline characteristics of the study participants according to quintiles of total protein intake at baseline are shown in Table 1. Compared with participants with low protein consumption, individuals with high protein consumption were less likely to be current smoker, to drink less alcohol per week, and more likely to conduct physical activity and to have graduated from high school. Furthermore, participants with high protein intake had higher BMI levels, higher intakes of fiber, magnesium and fat whereas decreased intake of carbohydrates.

During a median follow-up of 22 years, there were 1,147 CAD events among the 12,066 participants at baseline. In age, sex, race, study center and total energy adjusted analyses (minimally adjusted model) animal protein intake was not associated with an increased risk for CHD (Table 2). These results did not change significantly after full adjustment. In the minimally adjusted model, total and vegetable protein were associated with a significantly lower risk of CHD (Table 2, Model 1). This relationship was considerably attenuated and became non-significant after full adjustment (Table 2, Model 2).

In food-group analyses of major dietary protein sources using our minimally adjusted model, higher intake of red or processed meat was significantly associated with increased risk for CHD,

Table 2. Association of total, animal and vegetal protein intake with coronary heart disease incidence, ARIC 1987–2010.

	Q 1	Q 2	Q 3	Q 4	Q 5	p-trend
Total Protein Intake						
Events, n	241	230	231	230	215	
Person-time	46149	46720	46725	46991	47102	
Incidence, per 1000 py	5.2	4.9	4.9	4.9	4.6	
HR (95%CI)*	1 (ref)	0.84 (0.70, 1.01)	0.86 (0.72, 1.03)	0.89 (0.74, 1.06)	0.79 (0.66, 0.95)	0.04
HR (95%CI)**	1 (ref)	0.91 (0.75, 1.11)	0.93 (0.76, 1.14)	1.00 (0.80, 1.24)	0.84 (0.66, 1.07)	0.34
Animal Protein Intake						
Events, n	236	240	212	238	221	
Person-time	46175	46781	46915	47067	46750	
Incidence, per 1000 py	5.1	5.1	4.5	5.1	4.7	
HR (95%CI)*	1 (ref)	1.05 (0.88, 1.26)	0.97 (0.80, 1.17)	1.01 (0.84, 1.21)	0.95 (0.79, 1.15)	0.56
HR (95%CI)**	1 (ref)	1.16 (0.96, 1.40)	1.01 (0.82, 1.24)	1.11 (0.90, 1.37)	1.00 (0.79, 1.26)	0.94
Vegetable Protein Intake						
Events, n	247	228	253	215	204	
Person-time	45991	46902	46518	47070	47207	
Incidence, per 1000 py	5.4	4.9	5.4	4.6	4.3	
HR (95%CI)*	1 (ref)	0.92 (0.77, 1.10)	0.91 (0.76, 1.09)	0.82 (0.68, 0.98)	0.71 (0.59, 0.85)	0.0001
HR (95%CI)**	1 (ref)	1.08 (0.89, 1.31)	1.15 (0.94, 1.40)	1.04 (0.84, 1.29)	0.87 (0.68, 1.10)	0.17

*adjusted for age, sex, race, study, center, and total energy intake.
** adjusted for age, sex, race, study center, total energy intake, smoking, education, systolic blood pressure, use of antihypertensive medication, HDLc, total cholesterol, use of lipid lowering medication, body mass index, waist-to-hip ratio, alcohol intake, sports-related physical activity, leisure-related physical activity, carbohydrate intake, fiber intake, and magnesium intake.

whereas low-fat dairy, poultry and nuts consumption were significantly associated with decreased risk for CHD (Table 3, Model 1). After adjustment for potential confounders, only higher poultry intake remained associated with a lower risk of CHD (Table 3, Model 2).

Last, we conducted replacement analysis evaluating the association of substituting one source of dietary protein for another and of decreasing protein intake at the expense of carbohydrates or total fats (Table 4). Overall, these results did not show any statistically significant association with CHD risk, although they suggested that decreasing red meat and increasing intake of any other protein source was associated with non-significant lower risk of CHD (10–20% reduction per 1 serving/day change).

Discussion

In this prospective community based study with 22 years of follow-up, neither total, animal or vegetable protein intake was associated with risk of CHD. In food group analyses of major dietary protein sources, we found no significant trend between various sizes of intake of meat products, poultry, dairy, eggs, nuts, fish, or legumes and risk for CHD. Our results are contrary to our initial hypothesis as we expected food groups based on animal protein such as red or processed meat products to be significantly associated with an increased risk for CHD.

Thus far, the largest cohort analyses to examine an association between protein intake and coronary heart disease were undertaken using data from the Nurses' Health Study with 14, 16 and 26 years of follow up [2,5,23]. Interestingly, similar to our results it was found that after 14 to 16 years of follow-up, neither animal protein nor vegetable protein were associated with CHD [5,24]. Results from the Health Professional Follow-up Study also indicate no association between dietary protein and risk of coronary heart disease after 18 years of follow-up [4]. In a later analysis of the Nurses' Health Study spanning 26 years of follow-up higher intakes of red meat, red meat excluding processed meat, and high-fat dairy were indeed found to be significantly associated with an elevated risk of CHD while higher intakes of poultry, fish, and nuts were significantly associated with lower risk [2]. Other prospective studies using California Seventh Day Adventists or the NIH-AARP Diet and Health cohort as study base also report a positive association between (red) meat consumption and CHD risk [6,25]. Nonetheless, generalizability of the existing data is limited as the respective cohorts are characterized by well-educated, ethnically homogenous study populations. A recent meta-analysis summarizing 9 studies on red and processed meat consumption and risk for CHD found processed meats (RR 1.42, 95%CI 1.07, 1.89), but not red meats (RR 1.00, 95% CI 0.81,1.23) to increase incident coronary events [14]. The effects of other dietary protein sources or type of protein were not addressed in this analysis. Moreover all included studies were observational and among included studies only one was based in a general community setting in the UK [17]. Interventional studies such as the Bold Study suggest that dietary protein, also of animal origin, can exert positive effects on biomarkers of CHD [15,16]. Lean beef in an optimal lean diet has been shown to exhibit beneficial effects on systolic blood pressure and vascular elasticity [15,16].

In spite of the lack of strong epidemiologic evidence for an association between animal derived protein sources (in particular meat products) and risk for CHD, several arguments mainly based on contents of sodium and saturated fat have been previously made to potentially explain a harmful effect of animal derived protein products on the risk of CHD. Processed meats are known

Table 3. Association of major dietary protein sources with coronary heart disease, ARIC 1987–2010.

	Q 1	Q 2	Q 3	Q 4	Q 5	p-trend
Processed Meat						
Median svg/day	0	0.1	0.4	0.5	1.1	
HR (95%CI)*	1 (ref)	1.04 (0.86, 1.25)	1.22 (1.01, 1.49)	1.28 (1.06, 1.553)	1.40 (1.15, 1.71)	0.003
HR (95%CI)**	1 (ref)	0.95 (0.78. 1.15)	1.02 (0.84, 1.24)	1.04 (0.85, 1.265)	1.04 (0.85, 1.29)	0.49
Red Meat						
Median svg/day	0.1	0.3	0.5	0.6	1.1	
HR (95%CI)*	1 (ref)	1.00 (0.83, 1.21)	1.11 (0.93, 1.33)	1.18 (0.98, 1.43)	1.30 (1.06, 1.59)	0.004
HR (95%CI)**	1 (ref)	0.92 (0.76, 1.12)	1.02 (0.85, 1.24)	1.10 (0.90, 1.35)	1.13 (0.89, 1.44)	0.13
Red Meat & Processed Meat						
Median svg/day	0.2	0.5	0.8	1.2	1.9	
HR (95%CI)*	1 (ref)	1.15 (0.95, 1.40)	1.32 (1.09, 1.60)	1.51 (1.24, 1.84)	1.53 (1.23, 1.90)	<0.0001
HR (95%CI)**	1 (ref)	1.00 (0.82, 1.23)	1.084 (0.88, 1.33)	1.18 (0.95, 1.46)	1.15 (0.89, 1.48)	0.21
Poultry						
Median svg/day	0.1	0.1	0.3	0.4	0.8	
HR (95%CI)*	1 (ref)	0.80 (0.67, 0.95)	0.83 (0.67, 1.03)	0.75(0.63, 0.90)	0.67 (0.55, 0.82)	0.0007
HR (95%CI)**	1 (ref)	0.83 (0.70, 0.99)	0.93 (0.75, 1.15)	0.88 (0.73, 1.06)	0.79 (0.64, 0.98)	0.16
Dairy						
Median svg/day	0.1	0.6	1.1	1.5	2.9	
HR (95%CI)*	1 (ref)	0.88 (0.73, 1.05)	0.99 (0.83, 1.18)	0.72 (0.59, 0.87)	0.88 (0.72, 1.08)	0.24
HR (95%CI)**	1 (ref)	0.96 (0.80, 1.16)	1.14 (0.95, 1.37)	0.85 (0.69, 1.04)	1.04 (0.84, 1.29)	0.77
High-Fat Dairy						
Median svg/day	0.1	0.1	0.4	0.8	1.2	
HR (95%CI)*	1 (ref)	1.09 (0.91, 1.31)	0.96 (0.80, 1.16)	1.04 (0.86, 1.27)	1.1 (0.90, 1.34)	0.56
HR (95%CI)**	1 (ref)	1.16 (0.96, 1.39)	1.03 (0.86, 1.25)	1.13 (0.93, 1.38)	1.14 (0.93, 1.39)	0.47
Low-Fat Dairy						
Median svg/day	0	0.1	0.4	1	2.5	
HR (95%CI)*	1 (ref)	0.93 (0.77, 1.12)	0.73 (0.61, 0.87)	0.73 (0.61, 0.87)	0.75 (0.62, 0.90)	0.007
HR (95%CI)**	1 (ref)	1.04 (0.86, 1.25)	0.86 (0.72, 1.03)	0.90 (0.75, 1.08)	0.91 (0.74, 1.12)	0.39
Fish & seafood						
Median svg/day	0	0.1	0.2	0.3	0.6	
HR (95%CI)*	1 (ref)	0.98 (0.81, 1.17)	1.05 (0.85, 1.29)	0.95 (0.77, 1.16)	0.90 (0.74, 1.10)	0.20
HR (95%CI)**	1 (ref)	1.04 (0.87, 1.25)	1.17 (0.95, 1.44)	1.07 (0.87, 1.32)	1.06 (0.86, 1.31)	0.81
Eggs						
Median svg/day	0	0.1	0.1	0.4	1.0	
HR (95%CI)*	1 (ref)	0.90 (0.74, 1.09)	0.86 (0.72, 1.03)	0.84 (0.70, 1.01)	1.09 (0.88, 1.34)	0.20
HR (95%CI)**	1 (ref)	0.92 (0.76, 1.12)	0.88 (0.73, 1.06)	0.83 (0.69, 0.99)	0.96 (0.77, 1.19)	0.89
Nuts						
Median svg/day	0	0.1	0.2	0.4	1.0	
HR (95%CI)*	1 (ref)	0.83 (0.70, 0.99)	0.74 (0.60, 0.90)	0.71 (0.59, 0.87)	0.73 (0.60, 0.89)	0.02
HR (95%CI)**	1 (ref)	0.89 (0.75, 1.06)	0.86 (0.71, 1.05)	0.83 (0.68, 1.01)	0.91 (0.74, 1.12)	0.67
Legumes						
Median svg/day	0.1	0.1	0.2	0.3	0.6	
HR (95%CI)*	1 (ref)	1.01 (0.84, 1.20)	1.04 (0.83, 1.32)	0.98 (0.82, 1.17)	1.04 (0.85, 1.26)	0.64
HR (95%CI)**	1 (ref)	1.07 (0.89, 1.27)	1.16 (0.92, 1.46)	1.05 (0.87, 1.27)	1.159 (0.93, 1.44)	0.18

*adjusted for age, sex, race, study, center, and total energy intake.
** adjusted for age, sex, race, study center, total energy intake, smoking, education, systolic blood pressure, use of antihypertensive medication, HDLc, total cholesterol, use of lipid lowering medication, body mass index, waist-to-hip ratio, alcohol intake, sports-related physical activity, leisure-related physical activity, carbohydrate intake, fiber intake, and magnesium intake.

to have high sodium contents. High sodium intake is strongly correlated with the development of hypertension and CHD

Table 4. Food substitution analysis.

Increase 1 svg/d → Decrease 1 svg/d ↓	Red meat	Poultry	High-fat dairy	Low-fat dairy	Fish/seafood	Eggs	Nuts	Legumes
Processed meat	1.14 (0.90–1.44)	0.93 (0.73–1.18)	1.04 (0.90–1.20)	0.96 (0.84–1.11)	0.98 (0.74–1.15)	0.92 (0.74–1.15)	0.94 (0.79–1.10)	0.97 (0.74–1.27)
Red meat	-	0.81 (0.62–1.07)	0.91 (0.74–1.12)	0.84 (0.68–1.05)	0.86 (0.65–1.13)	0.81 (0.63–1.05)	0.81 (0.65–1.02)	0.85 (0.61–1.18)
Poultry	-	-	1.12 (0.90–1.40)	1.04 (0.83–1.30)	1.05 (0.76–1.45)	0.99 (0.77–1.29)	1.00 (0.79–1.27)	1.04 (0.76–1.44)
High-fat dairy	-	-	-	0.93 (0.84–1.02)	0.94 (0.75–1.19)	0.89 (0.75–1.06)	0.90 (0.78–1.03)	0.93 (0.73–1.19)
Low-fat dairy	-	-	-	-	1.02 (0.80–1.28)	0.96 (0.81–1.14)	0.97 (0.84–1.11)	1.01 (0.79–1.28)
Fish/seafood	-	-	-	-	-	0.94 (0.72–1.24)	0.95 (0.74–1.22)	0.99 (0.72–1.38)
Eggs	-	-	-	-	-	-	1.01 (0.83–1.22)	1.05 (0.79–1.39)
Nuts	-	-	-	-	-	-	-	1.04 (0.81–1.34)

Nutrient substitution analysis:
- Increasing 10% energy from carbohydrates, decreasing 10% from protein: HR 0.96 (95% CI 0.82–1.14).
- Increasing 10% energy from fats, decreasing 10% from protein: HR 0.99 (95% CI 0.80–1.24).

*adjusted for age, sex, race, study center, total energy intake, smoking, education, systolic blood pressure, use of antihypertensive medication, HDLc, total cholesterol, use of lipid lowering medication, body mass index, waist-to-hip ratio, alcohol intake, sports-related physical activity, leisure-related physical activity, carbohydrate intake, fiber intake, magnesium intake, and all the food items in the table (continuous variables, in servings/day).
Hazard ratios (95% confidence intervals) of CHD associated with increasing 1 serving/day in the consumption of protein sources (rows) at the expense of decreasing 1 serving/day in a different protein source (columns).* For example, the orange shaded cell can be interpreted as the HR (95% CI) of CHD increasing poultry consumption 1 serving/day and reducing red meat by the same amount, keeping all other sources of dietary protein constant.

[26,27]. On the other hand, high animal protein as provided by dark meat intake often accompanies large intakes of saturated fat intake which has been linked to increased cardiovascular risk [23,28,29]. In contrast to animal protein diets consisting of vegetable protein have been associated with cardiovascular and overall health benefits because of their high content of mono- and polyunsaturated fats, fiber, vitamins and minerals and low content of sodium [30]. These lines of argumentation are supported by current dietary recommendations [31], however, the role of saturated fat on the risk of CHD has been subject to controversial debates most recently [32,33]. Further research is warranted to elucidate the mechanisms of action of protein on the risk of CHD.

The absence of an association between major dietary protein sources and risk for CHD in our population may be explained in part by limited variation in consumptions of these food groups. Our study participants reported low meat intake whereas consumption of eggs, nuts, fish and dairy consumption were similar to other study populations [2]. Therefore, our observation suggesting a protective association of high poultry intake with lower CHD risk has to be interpreted with caution as this singular result may be spurious.

Other reasons that explain inconsistent findings and reports between dietary protein sources, food groups and CHD can be found in differences in study design, follow-up and assessment of outcomes and covariates. Similar to previous reports of the Nurses' Health Study and the Health Professional Study a follow-up period of 22 years may not have been long enough to detect significant differences between various dietary intake levels and risk for CHD events [2,4,5]. Second, our dietary data assessment was imperfect and incomplete. Although repeated dietary data measurements may take changing dietary patterns into account and thus serve to reduce intra-individual error, exposure variability of our study population was limited as protein intake was only assessed at two time-points. Changing dietary habits may not have been covered adequately by our FFQs with time-points only 6 years apart. On the other hand, it is well known that behavioral dietary changes are very challenging to accomplish and to maintain on the individual level and thus great changes in the overall population are unlikely to occur [34,35]. Last, dietary substitution effects as well as different characteristics of particular food group (e.g fat content, micronutrient content) may limit our analyses. Strengths of our study include the sample size, a large community based cohort with two different races in the setting of the general US population and a prospective design with long follow-up. CHD and several confounding factors were assessed using standardized protocols whereas other studies were based on self-report data [2,5].

In conclusion, using a large community based cohort study we found neither total nor animal or vegetable protein to be associated with CHD. In detailed food group analyses of major protein sources, no statistically significant trends between animal or vegetable-based food groups and risk for CHD were observed. Individuals should continue to make appropriate dietary modifications following current guidelines and recommendations for cardiovascular disease risk reduction [16,36].

Acknowledgments

The authors thank the staff and participants of the ARIC study for their important contributions. AA, BH and NG had full access to all of the data in the study and take responsibility for the integrity of the data and the accuracy of the data analysis.

Author Contributions

Conceived and designed the experiments: BH NG JN MWvB ES AA. Performed the experiments: ES JN BH AA. Analyzed the data: AA NG BH. Contributed reagents/materials/analysis tools: JN NG ES BH MWvB AA. Wrote the paper: BH NG JN MWvB ES AA.

References

1. Halton TL, Willett WC, Liu S, Manson JE, Albert CM, et al. (2006) Low-carbohydrate-diet score and the risk of coronary heart disease in women. N Engl J Med 355: 1991–2002.
2. Bernstein AM, Sun Q, Hu FB, Stampfer MJ, Manson JE, et al. (2010) Major dietary protein sources and risk of coronary heart disease in women. Circulation 122: 876–883.
3. Kelemen LE, Kushi LH, Jacobs DR Jr, Cerhan JR (2005) Associations of dietary protein with disease and mortality in a prospective study of postmenopausal women. Am J Epidemiol 161: 239–249.
4. Preis SR, Stampfer MJ, Spiegelman D, Willett WC, Rimm EB (2010) Dietary protein and risk of ischemic heart disease in middle-aged men. Am J Clin Nutr 92: 1265–1272.
5. Hu FB, Stampfer MJ, Manson JE, Rimm E, Colditz GA, et al. (1999) Dietary protein and risk of ischemic heart disease in women. Am J Clin Nutr 70: 221–227.
6. Sinha R, Cross AJ, Graubard BI, Leitzmann MF, Schatzkin A (2009) Meat intake and mortality: a prospective study of over half a million people. Arch Intern Med 169: 562–571.
7. Stamler J, Elliott P, Kesteloot H, Nichols R, Claeys G, et al. (1996) Inverse relation of dietary protein markers with blood pressure. Findings for 10,020 men and women in the INTERSALT Study. INTERSALT Cooperative Research Group. INTERnational study of SALT and blood pressure. Circulation 94: 1629–1634.
8. Iseki K, Iseki C, Itoh K, Sanefuji M, Uezono K, et al. (2003) Estimated protein intake and blood pressure in a screened cohort in Okinawa, Japan. Hypertens Res 26: 289–294.
9. Stamler J, Caggiula A, Grandits GA, Kjelsberg M, Cutler JA (1996) Relationship to blood pressure of combinations of dietary macronutrients. Findings of the Multiple Risk Factor Intervention Trial (MRFIT). Circulation 94: 2417–2423.
10. Stamler J, Liu K, Ruth KJ, Pryer J, Greenland P (2002) Eight-year blood pressure change in middle-aged men: relationship to multiple nutrients. Hypertension 39: 1000–1006.
11. Wang YF, Yancy WS Jr, Yu D, Champagne C, Appel LJ, et al. (2008) The relationship between dietary protein intake and blood pressure: results from the PREMIER study. J Hum Hypertens 22: 745–754.
12. Appel LJ, Sacks FM, Carey VJ, Obarzanek E, Swain JF, et al. (2005) Effects of protein, monounsaturated fat, and carbohydrate intake on blood pressure and serum lipids: results of the OmniHeart randomized trial. JAMA 294: 2455–2464.
13. Elliott P, Stamler J, Dyer AR, Appel L, Dennis B, et al. (2006) Association between protein intake and blood pressure: the INTERMAP Study. Arch Intern Med 166: 79–87.
14. Micha R, Wallace SK, Mozaffarian D (2010) Red and processed meat consumption and risk of incident coronary heart disease, stroke, and diabetes mellitus: a systematic review and meta-analysis. Circulation 121: 2271–2283.
15. Roussell MA, Hill AM, Gaugler TL, West SG, Heuvel JP, et al. (2012) Beef in an Optimal Lean Diet study: effects on lipids, lipoproteins, and apolipoproteins. Am J Clin Nutr 95: 9–16.
16. Roussell MA, Hill AM, Gaugler TL, West SG, Ulbrecht JS, et al. (2014) Effects of a DASH-like diet containing lean beef on vascular health. J Hum Hypertens.
17. Whiteman D, Muir J, Jones L, Murphy M, Key T (1999) Dietary questions as determinants of mortality: the OXCHECK experience. Public Health Nutr 2: 477–487.
18. (1989) The Atherosclerosis Risk in Communities (ARIC) Study: design and objectives. The ARIC investigators. Am J Epidemiol 129: 687–702.
19. Willett WC, Sampson L, Stampfer MJ, Rosner B, Bain C, et al. (1985) Reproducibility and validity of a semiquantitative food frequency questionnaire. Am J Epidemiol 122: 51–65.
20. Willett W, Stampfer MJ (1986) Total energy intake: implications for epidemiologic analyses. Am J Epidemiol 124: 17–27.
21. White AD, Folsom AR, Chambless LE, Sharret AR, Yang K, et al. (1996) Community surveillance of coronary heart disease in the Atherosclerosis Risk in Communities (ARIC) Study: methods and initial two years' experience. J Clin Epidemiol 49: 223–233.
22. Richardson MT, Ainsworth BE, Wu HC, Jacobs DR Jr, Leon AS (1995) Ability of the Atherosclerosis Risk in Communities (ARIC)/Baecke Questionnaire to assess leisure-time physical activity. Int J Epidemiol 24: 685–693.
23. Hu FB, Stampfer MJ, Manson JE, Ascherio A, Colditz GA, et al. (1999) Dietary saturated fats and their food sources in relation to the risk of coronary heart disease in women. Am J Clin Nutr 70: 1001–1008.
24. Hu FB, Bronner L, Willett WC, Stampfer MJ, Rexrode KM, et al. (2002) Fish and omega-3 fatty acid intake and risk of coronary heart disease in women. JAMA 287: 1815–1821.
25. Snowdon DA, Phillips RL, Fraser GE (1984) Meat consumption and fatal ischemic heart disease. Prev Med 13: 490–500.
26. Appel LJ, Moore TJ, Obarzanek E, Vollmer WM, Svetkey LP, et al. (1997) A clinical trial of the effects of dietary patterns on blood pressure. DASH Collaborative Research Group. N Engl J Med 336: 1117–1124.
27. Sacks FM, Campos H (2010) Dietary therapy in hypertension. N Engl J Med 362: 2102–2112.
28. Hu FB, Stampfer MJ, Manson JE, Rimm E, Colditz GA, et al. (1997) Dietary fat intake and the risk of coronary heart disease in women. N Engl J Med 337: 1491–1499.
29. Oh K, Hu FB, Manson JE, Stampfer MJ, Willett WC (2005) Dietary fat intake and risk of coronary heart disease in women: 20 years of follow-up of the nurses' health study. Am J Epidemiol 161: 672–679.
30. Vega-Lopez S, Lichtenstein AH (2005) Dietary protein type and cardiovascular disease risk factors. Prev Cardiol 8: 31–40.
31. Lichtenstein AH, Appel LJ, Brands M, Carnethon M, Daniels S, et al. (2006) Diet and lifestyle recommendations revision 2006: a scientific statement from the American Heart Association Nutrition Committee. Circulation 114: 82–96.
32. Chowdhury R, Warnakula S, Kunutsor S, Crowe F, Ward HA, et al. (2014) Association of dietary, circulating, and supplement fatty acids with coronary risk: a systematic review and meta-analysis. Ann Intern Med 160: 398–406.
33. Ramsden CE, Zamora D, Leelarthaepin B, Majchrzak-Hong SF, Faurot KR, et al. (2013) Use of dietary linoleic acid for secondary prevention of coronary heart disease and death: evaluation of recovered data from the Sydney Diet Heart Study and updated meta-analysis. BMJ 346: e8707.
34. Kumanyika SK, Van Horn L, Bowen D, Perri MG, Rolls BJ, et al. (2000) Maintenance of dietary behavior change. Health Psychol 19: 42–56.
35. Luepker RV, Murray DM, Jacobs DR, Jr., Mittelmark MB, Bracht N, et al. (1994) Community education for cardiovascular disease prevention: risk factor changes in the Minnesota Heart Health Program. Am J Public Health 84: 1383–1393.
36. Perk J, De Backer G, Gohlke H, Graham I, Reiner Z, et al. (2012) European Guidelines on cardiovascular disease prevention in clinical practice (version 2012). The Fifth Joint Task Force of the European Society of Cardiology and Other Societies on Cardiovascular Disease Prevention in Clinical Practice (constituted by representatives of nine societies and by invited experts). Eur Heart J 33: 1635–1701.

10

Replication of the 4p16 Susceptibility Locus in Congenital Heart Disease in Han Chinese Populations

Bijun Zhao[1,☯], Yuan Lin[2,3,☯], Jing Xu[4], Bixian Ni[3], Min Da[5], Chenyue Ding[6], Yuanli Hu[5], Kai Zhang[2,3], Shiwei Yang[7], Xiaowei Wang[4], Shiqiang Yu[1], Yijiang Chen[4], Xuming Mo[5], Jiayin Liu[2,6], Hongbing Shen[2,3], Jiahao Sha[2,8], Hongxia Ma[3]*

1 Department of Cardiovascular Surgery, Xijing Hospital, The Fourth Military Medical University, Xi'an, China, **2** State Key Laboratory of Reproductive Medicine, Nanjing Medical University, Nanjing, China, **3** Department of Epidemiology and Biostatistics and Key Laboratory of Modern Toxicology of Ministry of Education, School of Public Health, Nanjing Medical University, Nanjing, China, **4** Department of Thoracic and Cardiovascular Surgery, The First Affiliated Hospital of Nanjing Medical University, Nanjing, China, **5** Department of Cardiothoracic Surgery, Nanjing Children's Hospital, Nanjing Medical University, Nanjing, China, **6** Center of Clinical Reproductive Medicine, First Affiliated Hospital, Nanjing Medical University, Nanjing, China, **7** Department of Cardiology, Nanjing Children's Hospital, Nanjing Medical University, Nanjing, China, **8** Department of Histology and Embryology, Nanjing Medical University, Nanjing, China

Abstract

Congenital heart disease (CHD) is the most common form of congenital human birth anomalies and a leading cause of perinatal and infant mortality. Some studies including our published genome-wide association study (GWAS) of CHD have indicated that genetic variants may contribute to the risk of CHD. Recently, Cordell *et al.* published a GWAS of multiple CHD phenotypes in European Caucasians and identified 3 susceptibility loci (rs870142, rs16835979 and rs6824295) for ostium secundum atrial septal defect (ASD) at chromosome 4p16. However, whether these loci at 4p16 confer the predisposition to CHD in Chinese population is unclear. In the current study, we first analyzed the associations between these 3 single nucleotide polymorphisms (SNPs) at 4p16 and CHD risk by using our existing genome-wide scan data and found all of the 3 SNPs showed significant associations with ASD in the same direction as that observed in Cordell's study, but not with other subtypes- ventricular septal defect (VSD) and ASD combined VSD. As these 3 SNPs were in high linkage disequilibrium (LD) in Chinese population, we selected one SNP with the lowest *P* value in our GWAS scan (rs16835979) to perform a replication study with additional 1,709 CHD cases with multiple phenotypes and 1,962 controls. The significant association was also observed only within the ASD subgroup, which was heterogeneous from other disease groups. In combined GWAS and replication samples, the minor allele of rs16835979 remained significant association with the risk of ASD ($OR = 1.22$, 95% $CI = 1.08–1.38$, $P = 0.001$). Our findings suggest that susceptibility loci of ASD identified from Cordell's European GWAS are generalizable to Chinese population, and such investigation may provide new insights into the roles of genetic variants in the etiology of different CHD phenotypes.

Editor: Kelvin Yuen Kwong Chan, Hospital Authority, China

Funding: This work was supported by the following sources: National Key Basic Research Program Grant (2011CB944300, 2013CB911400 and 2012CB944902), the National Science Foundation for Distinguished Young Scholars of China (81225020), the New Century Excellent Talents in University (NCET-10-0178), the Organization Department of the CPC Central Committee, the Jiangsu Outstanding Youth Science Foundation (BK2012042), Jiangsu Province Clinical Science and Technology Projects (BL2012008), the Priority Academic Program for the Development of Jiangsu Higher Education Institutions (Public Health and Preventive Medicine) and Collaborative Innovation Center For Cancer Personalized Medicine in Jiangsu Province. The funders had no role in study design, data collection and analysis, decision to publish, or preparation of the manuscript.

Competing Interests: The authors have declared that no competing interests exist.

* Email: hongxiama@njmu.edu.cn

☯ These authors contributed equally to this work.

Introduction

Congenital heart disease (CHD) usually refers to abnormalities in the heart's structure or function that arise before birth [1]. As the most frequent birth defect, CHD affects about 0.8% of live births [2,3], and it is also a leading cause of perinatal and infant mortality, causing more than 220,000 deaths globally every year [4]. In China, epidemiological studies suggest an obvious increasing trend of CHD mortality with the overall mortality rate increasing from 141 in 2003 to 229 in 2010 per 10,000,000 person-years [5]. CHD can be classified into three broad categories: cyanotic heart disease, left-sided obstruction defects and septation defects [1]. Among them, septation defects are most common and can affect septation of the atria (atrial septal defect, ASD), septation of the ventricle (ventricular septal defect, VSD) or formation of structures in the central part of the heart (atrioventricular septal defect, AVSD) [1]. CHD may occur as part of recognized chromosomal and Mendelian syndromes [6,7]; however, it manifests as a non-syndromic, non-Mendelian condition in 80% of cases and may result from a multifactorial inheritance model that involves environmental factors and genetic predisposition [8]. In the past years, several genes linked to CHD have been identified, including T-box transcription factors (*TBX1*, *TBX5* and *TBX20*), homobox transcription factors (*NKX2.5* and *NKX2.6*), basic helix-loop-helix transcription factors (*HAND1* and *HAND2*), and GATA binding protein 4 (*GATA4*) [9].

More recently, genome-wide association studies (GWAS) have emerged as a powerful tool to identify novel susceptibility loci or genes of disease [10]. In May 2013, our research group conducted a GWA scan with 945 patients of ASD, VSD and ASD combined VSD cases and 1,246 non-CHD controls, followed by a two-stage validation with 2,160 ASD, VSD and ASD combined VSD cases and 3,866 controls [11]. We identified 2 loci at 1p12 (rs2474937 near *TBX15* gene, odds ratio (OR) = 1.40, $P = 8.44 \times 10^{-10}$) and 4q31.1 (rs1531070 in *MAML3* gene, OR = 1.40, $P = 4.99 \times 10^{-12}$) associated with CHD significantly ($P < 5.0 \times 10^{-8}$). However, these variants may represent only a very small proportion of SNPs contributing to CHD risk because of the strict criteria of the GWAS significance level ($P = 10^{-7}$ or $P = 10^{-8}$). Simultaneously, a GWAS of multiple CHD phenotypes in European Caucasians was conducted by Cordell *et al.* In that GWAS, when all CHD phenotypes were considered together, no region achieved genome-wide significant association. However, 3 SNPs were identified to be associated with ASD risk significantly after the stratification analysis was performed in different diagnostic groups (rs870142, $P_{combined} = 2.61 \times 10^{-10}$, odds ratio (OR) = 1.456; rs16835979, $P_{combined} = 2.94 \times 10^{-10}$, OR = 1.452 and rs6824295, $P_{combined} = 9.73 \times 10^{-10}$, OR = 1.437) [12]. However, it is uncertain whether these associations could be applicable to diverse populations. Therefore, we first investigated the association between the 3 SNPs (rs870142, rs16835979 and rs6824295) and CHD risk by using our existing genome-wide scan data and then performed a replication study with additional 1,709 CHD cases with multiple phenotypes and 1,962 controls.

Materials and Methods

Ethics Statement

This study was approved by the institutional review board of Nanjing Medical University. The design and performance of current study involving human subjects were clearly described in a research protocol. All participants over the age of 18 would complete the informed consent in writing before taking part in this research. For the participants under the age of 18, parental written consent was obtained.

Study populations

Study population of GWAS scan has been described previously [11]. For the replication stage, 1,709 CHD cases and 1,962 controls were recruited from the First Affiliated Hospital of Nanjing Medical University and the Affiliated Nanjing Children's Hospital of Nanjing Medical University, Nanjing, China, between March 2009 and May 2013. CHD were diagnosed based on echocardiography, some of which were further confirmed by cardiac catheterization and/or surgery. Cases that had clinical features of developmental syndromes, multiple major developmental anomalies or known chromosomal abnormalities were excluded. Exclusion criteria also included a positive family history of CHD in a first-degree relative (parents, siblings and children), maternal diabetes mellitus, phenylketonuria, maternal teratogen exposures (e.g., pesticides and organic solvents), and maternal therapeutic drugs exposures during the intrauterine period. Controls were non-CHD outpatients from the same geographic areas. They were recruited from the hospitals listed above during the same time period. Controls with congenital anomalies or cardiac disease were excluded. For each participant, approximately 2-ml whole blood was obtained to extract genomic DNA for genotyping analysis.

Quality control for GWAS scan and genotyping of replication study

The GWA scan was conducted using Illumina Omni zhonghua chips followed by a systematic quality control before association analysis [11]. In brief, we removed samples with low call rates, ambiguous gender, familial relationships, and extreme heterozygosity rate. We also detected population outliers and stratification using a PCA-based method. Our PCA analysis showed that the cases and controls were genetically matched, and the genomic control inflation factor (λ) was 1.065 [11]. SNPs were excluded if they are not mapped on autosomal chromosomes, or have a call rate <95%, minor allele frequency (MAF)<0.05 or $P < 1.00 \times 10^{-5}$ for Hardy-Weinberg equilibrium. After quality control procedures, a total of 708,275 SNPs in 945 CHD cases and 1,246 controls were included in the final GWA analysis [11]. The genotyping analyses in the replication study were performed by using the TaqMan allelic discrimination Assay (Applied Biosystems, Inc, USA). The information of the primers and probes were provided in **Table 1**. A series of methods were used to control the quality of genotyping: (i) case and control samples were mixed on each plate; (ii) genotyping was performed without knowing the case or control status; (iii) two water controls were used in each plate as blank control; (iv) five percent of the samples were randomly selected for repeat genotyping. The accurate concordance rate of genotyping for the SNP rs16835979 was 100.00% in the replication stage.

Statistical analysis

Population structure was evaluated by PCA as implemented in the software package EIGENSTRAT 3.1. The significant ($P < 0.05$) top eigenvector was included in the logistic regression model as a covariate for genetic association analysis [11]. Hardy-Weinberg equilibrium was evaluated using the $\chi 2$ test in all of the controls. The genome-wide association analysis was performed using an additive model in a logistic regression analysis in PLINK 1.07 (http://pngu.mgh.harvard.edu/~purcell/plink/). The statistical significance was declared at $\alpha = 0.05$. *P* values were two-sided, and ORs were estimated with an additive model by logistic regression analyses. The linkage disequilibrium (LD) analysis of the 3 SNPs (rs870142, rs16835979 and rs6824295) was performed in the controls of GWAS by using PLINK 1.07. Other analyses were performed using Stata version 9.2 (StataCorp LP, TX). The Chi-squared based Cochran's Q statistic was calculated to test for heterogeneity between groups in stratified analysis. We used inverse-variance-weighted model for meta-analysis when performing combined analysis. Random-effects model was used when heterogeneity between studies exists, that is, *P* value for heterogeneity test was less than 0.05; otherwise, fixed-effect model was used.

Results

The characteristics of the 945 CHD cases and the 1,246 non-CHD controls in GWA scan have been described previously [11]. Moreover, selected characteristics of the 1,709 cases and 1,962 non-CHD controls in the replication study were shown in **Table 2** and there were similar distributions of age and sex between cases and controls ($P = 0.221$ and 0.870, respectively).

The genotype distributions of these 3 SNPs in cases and controls of GWA scan were shown in **Table 3**. The observed genotype frequencies were all in Hardy-Weinberg equilibrium in controls ($P = 0.337$ for rs870142, $P = 0.370$ for rs16835979 and $P = 0.385$ for rs6824295). Logistic regression analyses showed that no obvious associations were found between the 3 SNPs and overall

Table 1. Primers and probes of rs16835979.

rs16835979	
F-primer	TGTGGACTCTAGAATGGACTTCCA
R-primer	TGTCAGATTAGGACCATCTCCATCT
FAM-probe	FAM-AGTGACTTTACTGTCCTC-MGB
HEX-probe	HEX-AAGTGACTTTAATGTCC-MGB

risk of CHD in an additive model (**Table 3**). Then, we performed stratification analysis by different diagnostic groups (ASD, VSD and ASD combined VSD) and found that all 3 SNPs showed significant associations with ASD risk (N = 334 cases) in the same direction as that observed in Cordell's study (rs870142: OR = 1.24, 95% CI = 1.04–1.49, $P = 0.016$; rs16835979: OR = 1.25, 95% CI = 1.05–1.50, $P = 0.014$; rs6824295: OR = 1.24, 95% CI = 1.04–1.48, $P = 0.019$). However, no significant association was observed in the other two disease groups (**Table 3**).

As these 3 SNPs were in high LD ($r^2 = 0.86$–0.99) in Chinese population, we selected one SNP with the lowest P value in our GWAS scan (rs16835979) to perform a replication study with additional 1,709 CHD cases of multiple phenotypes (ASD: N = 367; VSD: N = 432, Tetralogy of Fallot (TOF): N = 211, other CHDs: N = 699) and 1,962 controls. Similarly, no significant association was observed when all phenotypes were combined together. In the stratification analysis by disease groups, rs16835979 only showed significant association with the risk of ASD (OR = 1.20, 95% CI = 1.02–1.42, $P = 0.030$), which was heterogeneous from the other subgroups significantly (P for heterogeneity = 0.046) (**Table 4**). In combined GWAS and replication samples, the minor allele of rs16835979 remained significantly associated with ASD risk (OR = 1.22, 95%CI = 1.08–1.38, $P = 0.001$) (**Table 5**).

Discussion

In this study, we attempted to replicate the 4p16 ASD susceptibility loci in Han Chinese population and found that our results were consistent with the results presented by Cordell *et al* to a certain extent. These findings suggest that the susceptibility loci of diseases may have some similarities among different races and ethnicities.

In Cordell's study, 3 SNPs (rs870142, rs16835979 and rs6824295) were identified to be significantly associated with ASD risk [12]. We performed a LD analysis among the 3 SNPs by the online software of SNAP (http://www.broadinstitute.org/mpg/snap/ldsearchpw.php) and found strong LD between them ($r^2 = 0.89$ to 0.96) in CEU (CEPH- Utah residents with European ancestry). After evaluating the LD between the 3 SNPs in the controls of our GWAS samples, we found that they were also in high LD in Chinese populations ($r^2 = 0.86$–0.99). There were 28 other SNPs in the LD plot of the region containing the 3 mentioned SNPs (chr4:4665181-4698948) and we found that most SNPs were in high LD with the 3 SNPs in European population, while only about half of them were in high LD with the 3 SNPs in Chinese population. Although we included 701 ASD cases and 3,208 controls in this study (334 cases and 1,246 controls in our GWA scan and 367 ASD cases and 1,962 controls in the replication study), the sample size, especially the case sample size was relatively smaller compared to the original Cordell's GWAS. After performing multiple testing corrections with the Bonferroni single-step method (corrected α: $0.05/3 = 0.017$), we found the SNPs rs870142 and rs16835979 remained association with ASD risk; however, the SNP rs6824295 lost its association with ASD. Given the high LD of the 3 SNPs, Bonferroni correction might be too strict. Additionally, owing to the genetic heterogeneity, the allele frequency of the SNP rs16835979 in both populations was different (Chinese population: MAF = 0.380 in cases, MAF = 0.334 in controls; European population: MAF = 0.314 in cases, MAF = 0.235 in controls) and the effect size in the current study was weaker than that in European population (OR = 1.22 in

Table 2. Characteristics of CHD cases in validation stage.

Variables	Case (N = 1,709)	Control (N = 1,962)	*P*
Age (mean±SD)	3.21±8.70	3.45±7.93	0.221
Sex			
Male	738 (43.2%)	842 (42.9%)	0.870
Female	971 (56.8%)	1,120 (57.1%)	
Phenotype			
ASD	367		
VSD	432		
TOF	211		
Other CHDs	699		

ASD: ostium secundum atrial septal defect; VSD: ventricular septal defect; TOF: tetralogy of fallot; Other CHDs included patent ductus arteriosus, ebstein anomaly, double-chambered right ventricle, bicuspid aortic valve, aortic insufficiency, aortic stenosis, mitral insufficiency, rupture of valsalva sinus aneurysm, etc.
P-values were derived from the $\chi 2$ test for the categorical variable (sex) and t-test for the continuous variable (age).

Table 3. Associations of the 3 SNPs with CHD in our GWA scan.

Chr. (cytoband)	Position (bp)	SNP	Study	Cases[b]	Controls[b]	MAF[c] (Cases)	MAF[c] (Controls)	OR (95% CI)[d]	P^d
4p16.2	4698948	rs870142	Combined All (945 cases, 1,246 controls)	116/428/399	145/534/558	0.35	0.33	1.08 (0.95–1.22)	0.259
		G/A[a]	ASD (334 cases, 1,246 controls)	45/164/123	145/534/558	0.38	0.33	**1.24 (1.04–1.49)**	**0.016**
			VSD (534 cases, 1,246 controls)	63/230/241	145/534/558	0.33	0.33	1.00 (0.86–1.17)	0.969
			ASD/VSD (77 cases, 1,246 controls)	8/34/35	145/534/558	0.32	0.33	0.97 (0.69–1.38)	0.876
4p16.2	4686177	rs16835979	Combined All (945 cases, 1,246 controls)	116/426/396	144/536/560	0.35	0.33	1.08 (0.95–1.23)	0.212
		C/A[a]	ASD (334 cases, 1,246 controls)	44/164/121	144/536/560	0.38	0.33	**1.25 (1.05–1.50)**	**0.014**
			VSD (534 cases, 1,246 controls)	64/228/241	144/536/560	0.33	0.33	1.01 (0.87–1.18)	0.896
			ASD/VSD (77 cases, 1,246 controls)	8/34/34	144/536/560	0.33	0.33	1.00 0.70–1.41)	0.986
4p16.2	4665181	rs6824295	Combined All (945 cases, 1,246 controls)	127/445/372	163/554/525	0.37	0.35	1.07 (0.94–1.21)	0.298
		G/A[a]	ASD (334 cases, 1,246 controls)	46/177/111	163/554/525	0.40	0.35	**1.24 (1.04–1.48)**	**0.019**
			VSD (534 cases, 1,246 controls)	71/232/230	163/554/525	0.35	0.35	0.99 (0.85–1.15)	0.878
			ASD/VSD (77 cases, 1,246 controls)	10/36/31	163/554/525	0.36	0.35	1.05 (0.75–1.48)	0.765

[a]major/minor alleles.
[b]variant homozygote/heterozygote/wild type homozygote.
[c]minor allele frequency (MAF).
[d]OR and *P* were derived from logistic regression analysis in additive model adjusting for the first principal component in GWAS.

Table 4. Associations of rs16835979 with CHD in replication study.

Chr. (cytoband)	Position (bp)	SNP	Study	Cases[b]	Controls[b]	MAF[c] (Cases)	MAF[c] (Controls)	OR (95% CI)[d]	P^d	P^f
4p16.2	4686177	rs16835979	ASD (367 cases, 1,962 controls)	52/165/139	215/888/859	0.38	0.34	**1.20 (1.02–1.42)**	**0.030**	0.046
		C/A[a]	VSD (432 cases, 1,962 controls)	56/178/187	215/888/859	0.34	0.34	1.04 (0.89–1.22)	0.635	
			TOF (211 cases, 1,962 controls)	23/76/110	215/888/859	0.29	0.34	0.81 (0.65–1.02)	0.070	
			Other CHDs (699 cases, 1,962 controls)	91/312/287	215/888/859	0.36	0.34	1.10 (0.97–1.26)	0.136	
			Combined subjects[e] (1,709 cases, 1,962 controls)	222/731/723	215/888/859	0.35	0.34	1.05 (0.91–1.20)	0.521	

[a]major/minor alleles.
[b]variant homozygote/Heterozygote/Wild type homozygote.
[c]minor allele frequency (MAF).
[d]estimated in additive model.
[e]combined via random-effects meta-analysis.
[f]*P* values for heterogeneity test between groups.

Table 5. Associations of rs16835979 with ASD.

Chr. (cytoband)	Position (bp)	SNP	Study	Cases[b]	Controls[b]	MAF[c] (Cases)	MAF[c] (Controls)	OR (95% CI)[d]	P^d	P^e
4p16.2	4686177	rs16835979	**GWAS** (334 ASD cases, 1,246 controls)	44/164/121	144/536/560	0.38	0.33	**1.25 (1.05–1.50)**	**0.014**	0.742
		C/A[a]	**Replication** (367 ASD cases, 1,962 controls)	52/165/139	215/888/859	0.38	0.34	**1.20 (1.02–1.42)**	**0.030**	
			Combined analysis (combined via fixed-effects meta-analysis)	96/329/260	359/1424/1419	0.38	0.33	**1.22 (1.08–1.38)**	**0.001**	

[a]major/minor alleles.
[b]variant homozygote/heterozygote/wild type homozygote.
[c]minor allele frequency (MAF).
[d]estimated in additive model.
[e]*P* values for heterogeneity test between group.

Chinese population vs. OR = 1.46 in European population). Using Levin's formula [13], we also found that the population-attributable risk of ASD for the SNP rs16835979 was relatively lower in Chinese (7%) than that in Caucasian (9%).

All 3 SNPs locate within an intron of the noncoding RNA gene *LOC100507266* with unknown function. Meanwhile, they also lie in the 320-kb interval between *STX18* (syntaxin 18) and *MSX1* (msh homeobox 1) and locate upstream of both genes. The long non-coding RNA gene *LOC100507266* is known as *STX18* antisense RNA 1 (STX18-AS1). *STX18* is principally located in the endoplasmic reticulum, and it plays roles in transport between the endoplasmic reticulum and Golgi [14]; however, no data are available for its function in heart development. *MSX1* has been showed to be expressed in mesenchymal structures, including the limb buds, pharyngeal arches, neural crest, and endocardial cushions of the heart [15,16]. In Cordell's study, *MSX1* was showed to be expressed in the atrial septum during development, both in mouse and chick [12]. *MSX1* and *MSX2*, which belong to the highly conserved *Nk* family of homeobox genes, display overlapping expression patterns and redundant functions in multiple tissues and organs during vertebrate development [15,16]. The functions of *Msx1* and *Msx2* in endocardial activation prior to EMT via upregulation of *NFATc1* expression have been documented [15]. In addition, *Msx1* has a well-documented role as both a downstream effector and an upstream regulator of Bmp signaling. It has been implicated in regulating epithelial-mesenchymal transition (EMT) during cardiac valve and septa formation [15,17]. *Hand1* and *Hand2* are also candidate target genes regulated by *Msx1* and *Msx2* [18]. Since myocardium-specific *Hand1* deficiency leads to thickened atrioventricula (AV) valves, which is associated with impaired valve remodeling [19–21], decreasing *Hand1* expression in the *Msx1/2* double mutant AV myocardium may be associated with defects in remodeling of the AV cushions into mature valve leaflets [15]. In the mouse, loss both of Msx1 and Msx2 leads to a severe endocardial cushion and conotruncal defects [15,18]. In humans, mutations in *MSX1* cause orofacial clefting and tooth agenesis [22,23]. It is speculated that these 3 SNPs may affect the regulation of above genes and thus have associations with the development of ASD; however, the specific mechanisms of the 3 SNPs affecting the risk of ASD still need to be further investigated.

Like Cordell's study, we did not observe genome-wide significant associations of 4p16 loci with overall CHD risk in our GWAS as well as replication study. The findings suggested that genetic etiology of CHD could have a considerable degree of phenotypic specificity, which was also identified by some recent studies [24,25]. For the various phenotypes of CHD originated from different part of heart, we believe different genetic factors are involved in their pathogenic process.

Interestingly, our previous GWAS has identified 2 susceptibility loci (rs2474937 at 1p12 and rs1531070 at 4q31.1) for CHD in Han Chinese. However, these variants may contribute to the risk of CHD through different pathways. As described previously, the SNP rs2474937 may affect the expression of *TBX15*, a member of T-box transcription factors that have key roles in the development of the embryonic mesoderm, including of the heart and skeleton. Another SNP rs1531070 is in a LD region overlapping the *MAML3* (mastermind-like 3) gene and mastermind (Mam) is one of the essential components of Notch signaling pathway. In the current study, we confirmed the ASD-specific association of SNP rs16835979 in Chinese. This SNP may influence *MSX1* (msh homeobox 1), which belongs to the highly conserved *Nk* family of homeobox genes. *MSX1* has functions in endocardial activation prior to epithelial-mesenchymal transition (EMT) as well as Bmp signaling. Thus, the findings in the current study supplemented the existing results of our GWAS.

In conclusion, we present evidence for association between the common SNP rs16835979 at 4p16 and the ASD-specific risk in Han Chinese, which extends Cordell's results in different populations and suggests that the susceptibility loci of disease indeed have some similarities among different races and ethnicities.

Author Contributions

Conceived and designed the experiments: HM JS HS JL. Performed the experiments: YL BN MD CD YH KZ. Analyzed the data: BZ YL. Contributed reagents/materials/analysis tools: JX YC XM S. Yang XW. Wrote the paper: BZ YL. Oversaw the study design: S. Yu JS HS JL. Contributed to interpretation of results: S. Yu JS HS JL.

References

1. Bruneau BG (2008) The developmental genetics of congenital heart disease. Nature 451: 943–948.
2. van der Linde D, Konings EE, Slager MA, Witsenburg M, Helbing WA, et al. (2011) Birth prevalence of congenital heart disease worldwide: a systematic review and meta-analysis. J Am Coll Cardiol 58: 2241–2247.
3. Reller MD, Strickland MJ, Riehle-Colarusso T, Mahle WT, Correa A (2008) Prevalence of congenital heart defects in metropolitan Atlanta, 1998–2005. J Pediatr 153: 807–813.
4. Lozano R, Naghavi M, Foreman K, Lim S, Shibuya K, et al. (2013) Global and regional mortality from 235 causes of death for 20 age groups in 1990 and 2010: a systematic analysis for the Global Burden of Disease Study 2010. Lancet 380: 2095–2128.
5. Hu Z, Yuan X, Rao K, Zheng Z, Hu S (2014) National trend in congenital heart disease mortality in China during 2003 to 2010: A population-based study. J Thorac Cardiovasc Surg 148: 596–602 e591.
6. Pierpont ME, Basson CT, Benson DW Jr, Gelb BD, Giglia TM, et al. (2007) Genetic basis for congenital heart defects: current knowledge: a scientific statement from the American Heart Association Congenital Cardiac Defects Committee, Council on Cardiovascular Disease in the Young: endorsed by the American Academy of Pediatrics. Circulation 115: 3015–3038.
7. Weismann CG, Gelb BD (2007) The genetics of congenital heart disease: a review of recent developments. Curr Opin Cardiol 22: 200–206.
8. Ware SM, Jefferies JL (2012) New Genetic Insights into Congenital Heart Disease. J Clin Exp Cardiolog S8.
9. Wessels MW, Willems PJ (2010) Genetic factors in non-syndromic congenital heart malformations. Clin Genet 78: 103–123.
10. Shen H, Jin G (2013) Human genome epidemiology, progress and future. J Biomed Res 27: 167–169.
11. Hu Z, Shi Y, Mo X, Xu J, Zhao B, et al. (2013) A genome-wide association study identifies two risk loci for congenital heart malformations in Han Chinese populations. Nat Genet 45: 818–821.
12. Cordell HJ, Bentham J, Topf A, Zelenika D, Heath S, et al. (2013) Genome-wide association study of multiple congenital heart disease phenotypes identifies a susceptibility locus for atrial septal defect at chromosome 4p16. Nat Genet 45: 822–824.
13. Rückinger S, von Kries R, Toschke AM (2009) An illustration of and programs estimating attributable fractions in large scale surveys considering multiple risk factors. BMC Med Res Methodol 9: 7.
14. Hatsuzawa K, Hirose H, Tani K, Yamamoto A, Scheller RH, et al. (2000) Syntaxin 18, a SNAP receptor that functions in the endoplasmic reticulum, intermediate compartment, and cis-Golgi vesicle trafficking. J Biol Chem 275: 13713–13720.
15. Chen YH, Ishii M, Sucov HM, Maxson RE Jr (2008) Msx1 and Msx2 are required for endothelial-mesenchymal transformation of the atrioventricular cushions and patterning of the atrioventricular myocardium. BMC Dev Biol 8: 75.
16. Davidson D (1995) The function and evolution of Msx genes: pointers and paradoxes. Trends Genet 11: 405–411.
17. Bei M, Maas R (1998) FGFs and BMP4 induce both Msx1-independent and Msx1-dependent signaling pathways in early tooth development. Development 125: 4325–4333.
18. Chen YH, Ishii M, Sun J, Sucov HM, Maxson RE Jr (2007) Msx1 and Msx2 regulate survival of secondary heart field precursors and post-migratory proliferation of cardiac neural crest in the outflow tract. Dev Biol 308: 421–437.
19. Iwamoto R, Mekada E (2006) ErbB and HB-EGF signaling in heart development and function. Cell Struct Funct 31: 1–14.

20. Jackson LF, Qiu TH, Sunnarborg SW, Chang A, Zhang C, et al. (2003) Defective valvulogenesis in HB-EGF and TACE-null mice is associated with aberrant BMP signaling. EMBO J 22: 2704–2716.
21. Schroeder JA, Jackson LF, Lee DC, Camenisch TD (2003) Form and function of developing heart valves: coordination by extracellular matrix and growth factor signaling. J Mol Med (Berl) 81: 392–403.
22. Blanco R, Chakraborty R, Barton SA, Carreno H, Paredes M, et al. (2001) Evidence of a sex-dependent association between the MSX1 locus and nonsyndromic cleft lip with or without cleft palate in the Chilean population. Hum Biol 73: 81–89.
23. Vastardis H, Karimbux N, Guthua SW, Seidman JG, Seidman CE (1996) A human MSX1 homeodomain missense mutation causes selective tooth agenesis. Nat Genet 13: 417–421.
24. Soemedi R, Topf A, Wilson IJ, Darlay R, Rahman T, et al. (2012) Phenotype-specific effect of chromosome 1q21.1 rearrangements and GJA5 duplications in 2436 congenital heart disease patients and 6760 controls. Hum Mol Genet 21: 1513–1520.
25. Ching YH, Ghosh TK, Cross SJ, Packham EA, Honeyman L, et al. (2005) Mutation in myosin heavy chain 6 causes atrial septal defect. Nat Genet 37: 423–428.

11

Plasma PCSK9 Levels Are Elevated with Acute Myocardial Infarction in Two Independent Retrospective Angiographic Studies

Naif A. M. Almontashiri[1,2,3], Ragnar O. Vilmundarson[1,2], Nima Ghasemzadeh[4], Sonny Dandona[5], Robert Roberts[1,6], Arshed A. Quyyumi[5], Hsiao-Huei Chen[6,7]*, Alexandre F. R. Stewart[1,2,6]*

1 Ruddy Canadian Cardiovascular Genetics Centre, University of Ottawa Heart Institute, Ottawa, Ontario, Canada, **2** Department of Biochemistry, Microbiology and Immunology, University of Ottawa, Ottawa, Ontario, Canada, **3** Center for Genetics and Inherited Diseases, Taibah University, Almadina, Saudi Arabia, **4** Department of Medicine, Emory University, Atlanta, Georgia, United States of America, **5** Department of Medicine, McGill University, Montreal, Canada, **6** Department of Medicine, University of Ottawa, Ottawa, Ontario, Canada, **7** Ottawa Hospital Research Institute, Ottawa, Ontario, Canada

Abstract

Objective: Proprotein convertase subtilisin/kexin type 9 (PCSK9) is a circulating protein that promotes degradation of the low density lipoprotein (LDL) receptor. Mutations that block PCSK9 secretion reduce LDL-cholesterol and the incidence of myocardial infarction (MI). However, it remains unclear whether elevated plasma PCSK9 associates with coronary atherosclerosis (CAD) or more directly with rupture of the plaque causing MI.

Methods and Results: Plasma PCSK9 was measured by ELISA in 645 angiographically defined controls (<30% coronary stenosis) and 3,273 cases of CAD (>50% stenosis in a major coronary artery) from the Ottawa Heart Genomics Study. Because lipid lowering medications elevated plasma PCSK9, confounding association with disease, only individuals not taking a lipid lowering medication were considered (279 controls and 492 with CAD). Replication was sought in 357 controls and 465 with CAD from the Emory Cardiology Biobank study. PCSK9 levels were not associated with CAD in Ottawa, but were elevated with CAD in Emory. Plasma PCSK9 levels were elevated in 45 cases with acute MI (363.5 ± 140.0 ng/ml) compared to 398 CAD cases without MI (302.0 ± 91.3 ng/ml, $p=0.004$) in Ottawa. This finding was replicated in the Emory study in 74 cases of acute MI (445.0 ± 171.7 ng/ml) compared to 273 CAD cases without MI (369.9 ± 139.1 ng/ml, $p=3.7\times10^{-4}$). Since PCSK9 levels were similar in CAD patients with or without a prior (non-acute) MI, our finding suggests that plasma PCSK9 is elevated either immediately prior to or at the time of MI.

Conclusion: Plasma PCSK9 levels are increased with acute MI.

Editor: Michael Lipinski, Washington Hospital Center, United States of America

Funding: This work was supported by grants from the Canadian Institutes of Health Research, CIHR #MOP82810 (RR), CIHR #MOP77682 (AFRS), CIHR #MOP179197 (HHC), the Canada Foundation for Innovation, CFI #11966 (RR), a student scholarship from Taibah University, Saudi Arabia, and a University of Ottawa Endowed Graduate Award at the Heart Institute (NAMA). The Emory Cardiovascular Biobank was supported by National Institutes of Health (NIH) Grant R01 HL89650-01, Robert W. Woodruff Health Sciences Center Fund, Emory Heart and Vascular Center Funds, and supported in part by NIH Grant UL1 RR025008 from the Clinical and Translational Science Award Program. These funding agencies played no part in the study's design, conduct, and reporting.

Competing Interests: The authors have declared that no competing interests exist.

* Email: hchen@uottawa.ca (HHC); astewart@ottawaheart.ca (AFRS)

Introduction

By promoting the degradation of low density lipoprotein (LDL) receptors (LDL-R) in the liver, proprotein convertase subtilisin/kexin type 9 (PCSK9) elevates plasma levels of LDL-cholesterol (LDL–C) [1]. In African Americans, loss-of-function mutations in PCSK9 that prevent its secretion are associated with a 30%–40% reduction in plasma levels of LDL-C, but surprisingly reduce events associated with coronary atherosclerosis (CAD, coronary artery disease) by 88% over a 15 year period [2]. A similar level of reduced LDL-C attained by statins would be associated with only a 25% reduction in the risk of coronary events. This observation has also been confirmed in individuals of European ancestry for the R46L PCSK9 variant. The MIGen consortium found markedly reduced risk of MI associated with this allele [3]. In another independent study, a large meta-analysis of several Danish cohorts found that carriers of the 46L allele had a 12% reduction in LDL-C that predicted a 5% reduction, but that was in fact associated with a 28% reduction, in ischemic heart disease [4]. These similar findings have been hypothesized to result from a lifetime reduction in LDL-C, reducing the burden of atherosclerosis, but could also be explained if PCSK9 does more than control LDL-R levels. Overall, plasma PCSK9 accounts for less than 8% of the variance of plasma LDL-C [5].

Statins, while lowering LDL-C, markedly elevate plasma PCSK9, most likely due to increased expression of the PCSK9 activating transcription factors SREBP2 and HNF1α [6]. It would appear that the LDL-C lowering effect of statins outweighs the risk associated with elevated PCSK9, because statins dose-dependently lower LDL-C in both men and women [7] and reduce cardiovascular events in women just as well as in men [8]. _ENREF_13_ENREF_14_ENREF_15Recent clinical trials using antibodies against PCSK9 that block PCSK9 interaction with the LDL-R were successful at lowering LDL-C below the levels obtained with statins over several weeks [9,10] As a proof of concept, this approach has generated considerable excitement [11]. It remains to be seen whether therapies that lower plasma PCSK9 will lower the incidence of MI. Since MI occurs on a substrate of coronary atherosclerosis, whether elevated plasma PCSK9 increases MI risk through increased coronary atherosclerosis or by additional mechanisms remains unclear. Genetic studies have shown that variants contributing to the risk of coronary atherosclerosis can be distinguished from variants contributing to the risk of MI [12,13]. If elevated plasma PCSK9 contributes to the risk of thrombosis and MI, rather than or in addition to the risk of atherosclerosis, then this could also account for the disproportionate reduction in MI risk associated with genetic variants that lower plasma PCSK9 levels. Importantly, if elevated plasma PCSK9 carries risk beyond its effect on LDL-C, there may be an additional benefit to lowering plasma PCSK9 in individuals treated with statins. Here, we asked whether elevated plasma PCSK9 is associated with MI or angiographically-defined CAD in two independent retrospective angiographic studies, the Ottawa Heart Genomics Study (OHGS) [14] and the Emory Cardiology Biobank (EmCB) study [15].

Materials and Methods

Study design

Plasma PCSK9 levels were measured by ELISA and tested for association with angiographic CAD and MI in two independent angiographic cross-sectional studies, the OHGS [14] with replication in a subset of the EmCB study [15].

Study participants

For the OHGS, the Research Ethics Board of the University of Ottawa Heart Institute approved this study and written informed consent was obtained from all study participants. The OHGS excluded individuals with diabetes mellitus to ensure that the genetic risk primarily associated with coronary artery disease would not be confounded by the risk associated with diabetes, as described previously [16]. In addition, diabetes is known to elevate plasma PCSK9 levels [5], and a priori exclusion of diabetics in the OHGS study design removes this confounding variable.

CAD cases were identified by angiography as having a stenosis of greater than 50% in a major coronary artery, whereas angiographic controls had less than 30% stenosis. Severity of CAD was ranked according to the number of coronary arteries with stenosis, as described previously [16]. Patients were further stratified as having had an acute MI, according to elevated troponin and/or ST-elevation, if it was documented at the time of catheterization. Acute MI samples were obtained within 24–48 hours of the onset of symptoms, prior to the initiation of statin therapy. Otherwise, CAD cases were classified as having prior (or historical) MI or as having no MI from chart review. Controls were individuals who underwent coronary angiography prior to heart valve surgery or symptomatic individuals but with minimal (<30%) stenosis. Individuals with intermediate stenoses between 30% and 50% were excluded. Information regarding statin use, medication to treat hypertension, and recent (at the time of recruitment or within 12 months prior to recruitment) plasma LDL-C, HDL-C, and triglycerides was measured by colorimetric assays on a Roche Modular Analytics P Module clinical chemistry analyzer (Roche Diagnostics Inc., Laval, Quebec, Canada). Plasma samples were obtained at the time of cardiac catheterization from fasting individuals, stored at −80°C and thawed once for assessment of plasma PCSK9 levels. Of note, plasma samples were drawn at various times randomly distributed throughout the day.

The EmCB study was approved by the Institutional Review Board at Emory University, Atlanta, GA, USA. All subjects provided written informed consent at the time of enrollment. For the present study, 822 plasma samples were selected from 2,357 individuals of the EmCB study who underwent elective or emergent cardiac catheterization and who were not taking a statin or fibrate nor were diabetic at the time of recruitment. CAD cases were defined as having greater than 50% stenosis whereas controls had less than 20% stenosis, as described previously [15]. Similar criteria as in the OHGS were used to define CAD cases with acute, prior or no MI in the EmCB study.

PCSK9 ELISA

Plasma levels of PCSK9 were measured by ELISA using a commercial assay (Quantikine ELISA, R&D Systems, Minneapolis, MN) that has been previously validated [17,18]. Plasma samples were diluted 1:20 in dilution buffer. The minimal detectable dose of PCSK9 was 0.1 ng/ml, with a typical range of 39 to 1,400 ng/ml in human plasma. We were concerned that plasma LDL-C might affect the measurement of plasma PCSK9 using the PCSK9 ELISA assay, since PCSK9 interacts with LDL-C [19]. The PCSK9 protein standard was diluted and incubated at 37°C for 30 minutes without or with the addition of LDL-C to a concentration of 2.6 mmol/L and no difference in PCSK9 levels was detected (data not shown). Thus, LDL-C does not interfere with the ELISA. PCSK9 levels in 12 individuals were tested in 6 replicates in one assay and again in a separate assay. Several different lots of the assay were used to measure PCSK9 in the OHGS samples, whereas a single lot was used for the EmCB study. The intra-assay coefficient of variance was 8.9% and between assays was 12%.

Statistical analysis

Continuous variables are presented as mean ± standard deviation (SD) and categorical variables are presented as N (%). To determine whether differences between CAD cases and controls were significant for continuous and categorical variables the Student's t-test and χ^2 test were used, respectively. To determine whether mean plasma PCSK9 levels differed between 0, 1, 2 or 3 vessel disease a one-way analysis of variance (ANOVA) was used. Multiple logistic regression analysis was used to examine whether PCSK9 was associated with CAD or acute MI when correcting for known risk factors (age, male sex, BMI, smoking, antihypertensive medication use, LDL-C, HDL-C, and TG). The acute MI variable compared CAD cases with no MI to those with acute MI, excluding CAD cases with prior MI except when an individual who had suffered a prior MI had also suffered an acute MI, in which case they were labeled as having an acute MI. Spearman's rank correlation was used to determine whether plasma PCSK9 and LDL-C levels are correlated. All statistical analyses were two-sided and performed with SPSS (version 19.0, SPSS Inc., Chicago IL, USA), SAS Enterprise Guide (v. 4.3, SAS Institute Inc., Cary NC, USA) and R (v. 3.0.2, The R Foundation for Statistical Computing, Vienna, Austria). One-way ANCOVA was used to determine whether PCSK9 levels differed between controls, CAD cases with no MI, CAD cases with acute MI and CAD cases with prior MI and post-hoc tests were adjusted for multiple comparisons by Sidak correction. The threshold for significance was set at $p<0.05$ for all analyses performed.

Results

Statins elevate plasma PCSK9

The clinical characteristics of the OHGS [14] samples are presented in Table 1, stratified by statin use because of the marked effect of statins to elevate plasma PCSK9 levels [6]. Plasma PCSK9 levels were not different between cases or controls in either those taking or not taking a statin. Linear regression analysis confirmed that plasma PCSK9 is elevated by statin use as well as by young age and female sex (Table 2). Smoking, antihypertensive medication and CAD were also independent predictors of PCSK9.

Plasma PCSK9 levels are not associated with coronary atherosclerosis in the OHGS for individuals not taking a statin

To determine whether PCSK9 levels are associated with CAD, we performed a logistic regression analysis correcting for known CAD risk factors (Table 3). However, given the known marked effect of statins [6,20] and fibrates [21,22] to elevate PCSK9 levels, also seen in our study (Table 2), we stratified the analysis by statin use. PCSK9 levels were only associated with CAD in individuals taking a statin (Table 3, $p=0.0003$), suggesting that the observed effect of CAD on PCSK9 levels (Table 2) is driven by higher statin use among CAD cases. Similarly, no association between PCSK9 levels and severity of CAD, assessed by the number of diseased vessels, was observed in the OHGS by ANOVA in individuals not taking a statin (Figure 1). Given that plasma PCSK9 levels did not associate with CAD in individuals not taking a statin, we asked whether plasma PCSK9 levels might instead be associated with acute or prior MI.

Plasma PCSK9 levels are elevated with acute MI, but not with prior MI, in the OHGS

Out of the 3,273 CAD patients in the OHGS, 1,371 had an MI (799 with prior history of MI and 572 with acute MI), and of those with an MI, 94 were not taking a statin (6.8%); 45 had acute MI and 49 had prior MI. Plasma PCSK9 levels were markedly elevated in 45 individuals with acute MI (363.5±140.0 ng/ml) compared to 398 CAD cases without MI (302.0±91.3 ng/ml, $p=0.004$), adjusted for age at consent, male sex, BMI, smoking, and antihypertensive meds (Figure 2). In contrast, no difference in PCSK9 levels was seen between 49 individuals with a prior MI (315.9±107.5 ng/ml) and 398 CAD cases without an MI ($p=0.977$). A mean of 11.4 ± 8.1 years separated the occurrence of MI from the time of recruitment in this group. Elevated PCSK9 levels seen with acute MI were not accompanied by elevated LDL-C levels (3.051±0.090 mmol/L for acute MI, 3.322±0.914 mmol/L for CAD no MI, $p=0.12$). Logistic regression analysis confirmed that PCSK9 levels are an independent predictor of acute MI in CAD cases not taking a statin in the OHGS (Table 4).

PCSK9 levels are associated with coronary atherosclerosis in the EmCB study

We next sought "a priori" confirmation of our findings in an independent cohort. The Emory Cardiology Biobank (EmCB)

Table 1. Clinical characteristics of OHGS CAD cases and controls.

	Total			On Statin			Not taking statin		
Variable	Cases (N = 3273)	Controls (N = 645)	p	Cases (N = 2781)	Controls (N = 366)	p	Cases (N = 492)	Controls (N = 279)	p
Age, (years)	64±11	63±11	0.367	63±11	64± 11	0.665	65±11	63±12	0.003
Male sex, N (%)	2503 (76.5)	302 (46.8)	<0.001	2169 (78.0)	170 (46.4)	<0.001	334 (67.9)	132 (47.3)	<0.001
BMI, kg/m²	28.0±4.9	28.7±5.8	0.003	28.1±4.9	28.9±5.8	0.007	27.4±5.0	28.4±5.7	0.014
Smoking, N (%)	2354 (71.9)	374 (58.0)	<0.001	2009 (72.2)	233 (63.7)	<0.001	345 (70.1)	141 (50.5)	<0.001
HTN, N (%)	2029 (62.0)	514 (79.9)	<0.001	1784 (64.1)	307 (83.9)	<0.001	245 (49.8)	207 (74.2)	<0.001
Total-C, mmol/L	4.53±1.24	4.83±1.04	<0.001	4.43±1.22	4.64±1.03	0.002	5.26±1.08	5.15±0.98	0.246
LDL-C, mmol/L	2.61±1.05	2.79±0.87	<0.001	2.51±1.02	2.62±0.87	0.057	3.29±0.95	3.05±0.80	0.004
HDL-C, mmol/L	1.16±0.41	1.37±0.47	<0.001	1.15±0.41	1.32±0.44	<0.001	1.25±0.43	1.47±0.51	<0.001
TG, mmol/L	1.69±1.09	1.52±0.88	0.001	1.70±1.10	1.58±0.95	0.135	1.62±1.00	1.41±0.74	0.015
PCSK9, ng/mL	375.5±131.2	349.7±143.2	<0.001	387.3±132.6	374.6±146.5	0.117	309.0±99.7	317.1±131.9	0.376

Continuous variables presented as mean ± SD and categorical variables as N (%). Abbreviations: BMI, body mass index; HTN, anithypertensive medication, Total-C, total-cholesterol; LDL-C, Low density lipoprotein-cholesterol, HDL-C, high density lipoprotein-cholesterol, TG, triglycerides.

Table 2. Linear regression analysis of the relationships between explanatory variables and the level of PCSK9 in the OHGS.

Variable	β	p
Age, (years)	−0.086	<0.001
Male sex	−0.151	<0.001
BMI, kg/m^2	0.024	0.127
Smoking	0.033	0.033
HTN	−0.050	0.002
Statin (including fibrates)	0.225	<0.001
CAD	0.041	0.013

Abbreviations: BMI, body mass index; HTN, anithypertensive medication. N = 3,918.

study is another large angiographic cohort consisting of more than 2,400 individuals [15]. To avoid the confounding effect of statins and to replicate the selection criteria of the OHGS cohort (non-diabetic), we measured plasma PCSK9 levels in 465 CAD cases and 357 controls without diabetes mellitus and not taking a statin or fibrate at the time of recruitment (see Table 5). Linear regression analysis also showed that CAD was significantly associated with elevated plasma PCSK9 (Table 6). In contrast to the subset of individuals not taking a statin or fibrate in the OHGS, plasma PCSK9 levels were elevated in angiographic CAD cases (385.0±146.9 ng/ml) compared to controls (340.4±125.2 ng/ml, p<0.001) in the EmCB sample. Logistic regression confirmed that plasma PCSK9 levels are an independent predictor of CAD in the EmCB sub-study (Table 7). The overall higher PCSK9 values in the EmCB study likely reflect a lot-specific variation in the PCSK9 ELISA.

Plasma PCSK9 levels are also elevated with acute MI, but not with prior MI, in the EmCB study

Similar to the OHGS sample, plasma PCSK9 levels were elevated in the 74 individuals with acute MI (445.0±171.7 ng/mL) compared to the 273 individuals with CAD but no MI (369.9±139.1 ng/mL, $p = 3.7\times10^{-4}$, after adjusting for variables, Figure 2). Here too, elevated plasma PCSK9 levels with acute MI were not associated with LDL-C levels (2.94±1.28 mmol/L for acute MI and 2.75±1.00 mmol/L for CAD no MI, p = 0.423). Also similar to the OHGS, no difference was seen between the 118 individuals with prior MI (382.3±139.1 ng/mL) and 273 CAD cases without MI (369.9±139.13 ng/mL, p = 0.0.954). An average of 10.1 ± 9.3 years elapsed between the MI and the time of recruitment for CAD cases of prior MI in the EmCB study. Logistic regression analysis confirmed that PCSK9 levels are an independent predictor of acute MI in CAD cases in the EmCB sub-study (Table 8).

In individuals taking statins, there was no correlation between PCSK9 levels and plasma LDL-C ($r_s = -0.0288$, p = 0.158, N = 2,410) in the OHGS. In individuals not taking statins, there was also no correlation between PCSK9 levels and LDL cholesterol ($r_s = 0.0813$, p = 0.0754, N = 479). When the analysis is stratified by CAD, a weak positive correlation between the levels of PCSK9 and LDL cholesterol ($r_s = 0.176$, p = 0.0257, N = 160) was observed in controls not taking statins. No correlation was seen in CAD cases not taking statins, nor in CAD cases ($r_s = -0.0268$, p = 0.214, N = 2155) or controls ($r_s = -0.0114$, p = 0.856, N = 225) taking statins. Similarly, in the EmCB sub-study of individuals not taking statins, there was no correlation between PCSK9 levels and LDL cholesterol in either those with CAD ($r_s = -0.00840$, p = 0.862, N = 429) or controls ($r_s = -0.00742$, p = 0.895, N = 322).

Table 3. Logistic regression analysis of the association of PCSK9 with CAD in the OHGS cohort, stratified by statin use.

	On statin		Not taking statin	
Variable	β or OR (95% CI)	p	β or OR (95% CI)	p
Age, (years)	0.004 (−0.009, 0.018)	0.530	0.013 (−0.007, 0.034)	0.210
Male sex	2.776 (2.075, 3.714)	6.10E-12	1.382 (0.875, 2.184)	0.166
BMI, kg/m^2	−0.033 (−0.059, −0.006)	0.015	−0.035 (−0.076, 0.006)	0.091
Smoking	1.261 (0.946, 1.68)	0.113	3.343 (2.156, 5.184)	7.00E-08
HTN	0.379 (0.267, 0.538)	5.92E-08	0.442 (0.282, 0.694)	3.88E-04
LDL, mmol/L	−0.125 (−0.259, 0.009)	0.068	0.251 (−0.004, 0.506)	0.053
HDL, mmol/L	−0.612 (−0.916, −0.308)	7.86E-05	−0.887 (−1.396, −0.378)	0.001
TG, mmol/L	0.366 (−0.319, 1.050)	0.295	0.733 (−0.331, 1.797)	0.177
PCSK9, ng/mL	0.002 (0.001, 0.003)	0.0004	−0.001 (−0.002, 0.001)	0.505

Results given as beta for continuous variables and odds ratio (OR) for categorical variables. Abbreviations: BMI, body mass index; HTN, anithypertensive medication; Total-C, total-cholesterol; LDL-C, Low density lipoprotein-cholesterol; HDL-C, high density lipoprotein-cholesterol; TG, triglycerides. On statin, N = 2,396; Not taking statin, N = 478. Samples with missing values for variables were excluded.

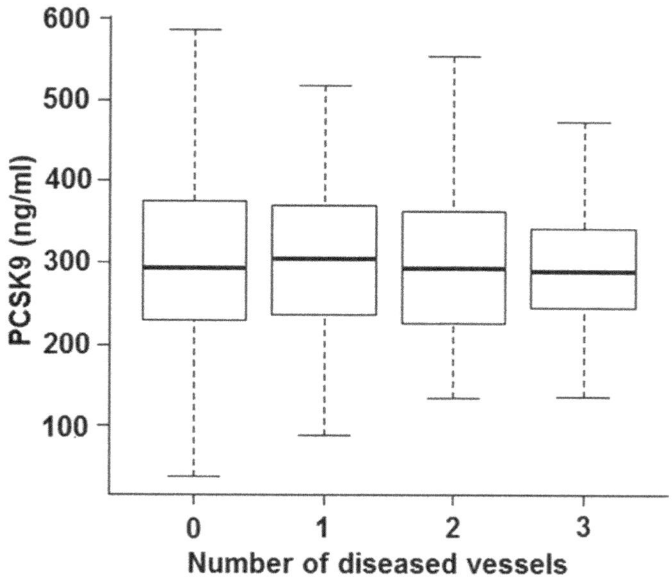

Figure 1. Mean PCSK9 levels do not differ with atherosclerosis burden. A Tukey's boxplot displaying PCSK9 levels in OHGS CAD controls (0 diseased vessels) and cases (1, 2 or 3 diseased vessels) in individuals not taking statins. The median is the line in the box, the 1st and 3rd quartiles are the upper and lower edges of the boxes and 1.5 interquartile range (IQR) is displayed as whiskers. Outliers have been removed. (0 vessel disease, N = 280; 1-vessel disease, N = 126; 2-vessel disease, N = 102; 3-vessel disease, N = 104).

Discussion

Here, for the first time to our knowledge, we found that plasma PCSK9 is elevated with acute MI in non-diabetic individuals who are not taking a statin and have angiographically proven CAD. A strength of our study is that this finding was replicated in a second independent cohort, an EmCB sub-study. Furthermore, our observation that plasma PCSK9 levels are not elevated in individuals with prior MI compared to those with angiographic CAD that did not have an MI argues that PCSK9 levels are transiently elevated with acute MI.

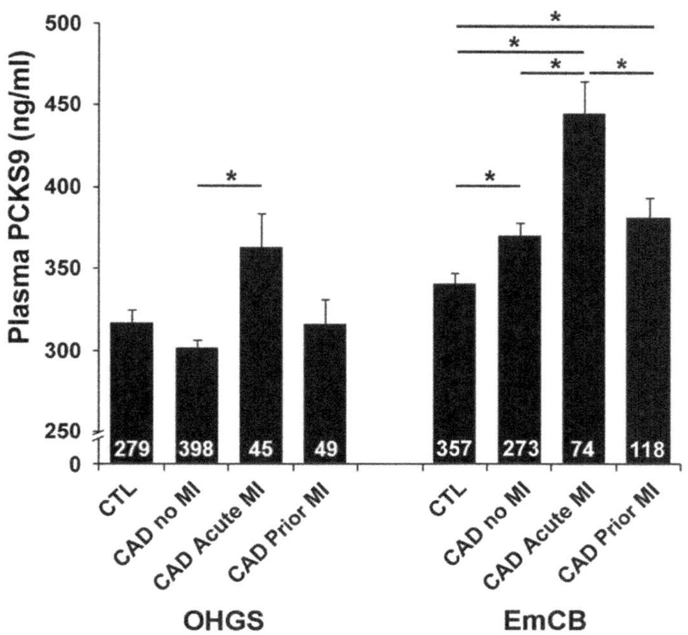

Figure 2. Plasma PCSK9 levels are increased with acute MI. Numbers in columns reflect sample size per group for individuals not taking a lipid-lowering medication (statin or fibrate) at the time of recruitment. Values are mean±SEM. Asterisks indicate significantly elevated PCSK9 by ANCOVA, $p < 0.05$ after adjusting for variables (age, male sex, BMI, antihypertensive medication use, and smoking) and correcting for multiple comparisons.

Table 4. Logistic regression analysis of the association of PCSK9 with acute MI in the OHGS cohort, stratified by statin use.

	On statin		Not taking statin	
Variable	**β or OR (95% CI)**	**p**	**β or OR (95% CI)**	**p**
Age, (years)	−0.024 (−0.036, −0.012)	4.79E-05	−0.013 (−0.052, 0.027)	0.523
Male sex	0.876 (0.655, 1.172)	0.374	0.692 (0.268, 1.786)	0.447
BMI, kg/m^2	−0.039 (−0.065, −0.013)	0.003	0.015 (−0.063, 0.093)	0.705
Smoking	1.287 (0.9997, 1.658)	0.050	0.94 (0.369, 2.391)	0.896
HTN	0.752 (0.594, 0.953)	0.019	0.643 (0.277, 1.49)	0.303
LDL, mmol/L	−0.049 (−0.163, 0.065)	0.403	−0.346 (−0.836, 0.143)	0.166
HDL, mmol/L	−1.068 (−1.470, −0.665)	1.97E-07	−2.038 (−3.455, −0.622)	0.005
TG, mmol/L	−0.139 (−0.751, 0.472)	0.655	−1.093 (−3.143, 0.956)	0.296
PCSK9, ng/ml	0.0004 (−0.0004, 0.001)	0.307	0.005 (0.002, 0.009)	0.002

Results given as beta for continuous variables and odds ratio (OR) for categorical variables. Abbreviations: BMI, body mass index; HTN, anithypertensive medication; Total-C, total-cholesterol; LDL-C, Low density lipoprotein-cholesterol; HDL-C, high density lipoprotein-cholesterol; TG, triglycerides. On statin, N = 1,568; Not taking statin, N = 287.

Since lipid lowering medications elevate plasma PCSK9 [6,20,22]_ENREF_20, it is necessary to exclude individuals on lipid lowering medications to avoid possible spurious associations due to medication. However, given the high prevalence of cholesterol-lowering prescriptions in older Americans [23], as high as 44.9% in persons over age 60, it is a challenge to obtain a large sample size. Nevertheless, we were able to identify 45 individuals in the OHGS and 74 in the EmCB study with acute MI that were not taking a lipid-lowering medication at the time of recruitment. It is likely that individuals with CAD and prior MI not taking a statin may have been intolerant to statins, since statin-induced myopathy is estimated to affect 10–15% of statin users [24].

Our findings are consistent with genetic studies that have demonstrated a causal link between lower plasma PCSK9 levels and reduced risk of MI [2–4,25]. The mechanism whereby PCSK9 contributes to the risk of MI has been attributed largely to its effect on degrading the LDL-R, thereby elevating LDL-C and promoting atherosclerosis. Indeed, MI occurs on a foundation of coronary atherosclerosis, and most genetic factors that contribute to the elevation of coronary atherosclerosis risk were discovered through their association with the increased risk of MI [26]. However, our finding that elevated plasma PCSK9 is associated with acute MI, rather than prior MI or with coronary atherosclerosis cautions that the relationship of PCSK9 to MI risk may be more complex than previously thought.

It is well recognized that elevated LDL-C is one of the most significant risk factors of atherosclerosis. Intriguingly, among the top 10 genetic variants associated with elevated LDL-C, a PCSK9 variant had the weakest association with elevated LDL-C but had the third strongest effect on the risk of MI [27]. In other words, the effect of PCSK9 on MI risk far exceeds its effect on plasma LDL-C levels and on coronary atherosclerosis risk. It is noteworthy that in the present study, in individuals not taking a statin, only a weak (OHGS) or no correlation was seen between plasma PCSK9 levels and LDL-C.

PCSK9 might increase the risk of MI by a mechanism distinct from its well-known effect on LDL–C. We observed a weak correlation between plasma PCSK9 levels and LDL-C only in controls not taking a lipid lowering medication in the OHGS but

Table 5. Clinical characteristics of CAD cases and controls from the EmCB sub-study.

Variable	Cases (N = 465)	Controls (N = 357)	p
Age, (years)	65±12	56±12	<0.001
Male sex, N (%)	352(75.7)	193 (54.1)	<0.001
BMI, kg/m^2	28.3±5.5	29.8±6.8	<0.001
Smoking, N (%)	92 (19.8)	48(13.4)	0.01
HTN, N (%)	327(70.3)	201 (56.3)	<0.001
Total-C, mmol/L	4.52±1.22	4.73±1.13	0.028
LDL-C, mmol/L	2.73±1.05	2.86±0.88	0.070
HDL-C, mmol/L	1.07±0.34	1.15±0.37	0.005
TG, mmol/L	1.68±1.27	1.54±1.05	0.140
PCSK9, ng/mL	385.0±146.9	340.4±125.2	0.000003

All EmCB samples were from non-diabetic individuals not taking a statin or fibrate at the time of recruitment. Continuous variables presented as mean ± SD and categorical variables as N (%). Abbreviations: BMI, body mass index; HTN, anithypertensive medication; Total-C, total-cholesterol; LDL-C, Low density lipoprotein-cholesterol; HDL-C, high density lipoprotein-cholesterol; TG, triglycerides.

Table 6. Linear regression analysis of the relationships between explanatory variables and the level of PCSK9 in the EmCB sub-study.

Variable	β	P-value
Age, (years)	−0.077	0.054
Male sex	−0.010	0.775
BMI, kg/m^2	−0.015	0.686
Smoking	−0.034	0.348
HTN	−0.058	0.103
CAD	0.199	<0.001

Abbreviations: BMI, body mass index; HTN, anithypertensive medication. N = 822.

not in the EmCB study. In contrast to the increased levels of PCSK9 we observed in acute MI patients (measured 1 to 2 days after MI), plasma levels of LDL-C have been reported to fall transiently following MI [28–30]. Thus, PCSK9 levels are uncoupled from LDL-C, at least at the time of MI. One possibility is that PCSK9 levels increase transiently after the trauma of an MI, as an acute phase reactant. However, a recent study reported that plasma PCSK9 levels were not elevated at the time of admission for severe trauma, but only eight days after a traumatic injury and correlated with the severity of the trauma [31], arguing that PCSK9 is not an acute phase reactant.

Another intriguing possibility is that PCSK9 levels might be elevated prior to acute MI, and even trigger MI. PCSK9 has been reported to bind to the LDL-R related protein LRP8 [32]. LRP8 activation promotes platelet aggregation [33]. If PCSK9 binding activates LRP8 receptor signaling, it could increase platelet aggregation and augment the risk of MI. Acute coronary events are more frequent in the morning [34], at a time when plasma PCSK9 levels are at their highest [35], and when propensity for platelets to aggregate is also increased [36]. Whether PCSK9 contributes to the risk of MI through platelet activation remains to be tested. In addition, in the OHGS sample, smoking was an independent predictor of circulating PCSK9 levels. This effect has been reported previously in a study of 4 healthy cohorts from Sweden comprising 5,722 middle-aged individuals [37], and although the mechanism underlying this association has not been explored, smoking is the second most important modifiable risk factor for MI after elevated LDL-C [38].

Plasma PCSK9 levels are elevated in patients with periodontitis, independently of LDL-C levels [17]. Periodontitis is a known risk factor for CAD and MI [39]. The risk of MI is elevated fivefold after an acute infection [40]. In mice, endotoxin elevates plasma PCSK9 levels [41] and plasma PCSK9 levels might be similarly elevated in humans after an acute infection and contribute to increased risk of subsequent MI. PCSK9-targeted therapies might lower the risk of events after acute infections. More needs to be learned about the functions of PCSK9 beyond its effect on LDL-R degradation.

One limitation of our study is that plasma samples from the OHGS were not carried forward to control for lot-to-lot variability when the EmCB samples were assayed. Thus, the 20% higher values measured for the EmCB samples could reflect a true difference or more likely reflect a lot-to-lot difference. Another limitation of our study is that both the OHGS and the EmCB are cross-sectional rather than longitudinal studies, having recruited angiographically-defined CAD cases and controls at the time of cardiac catheterization. Thus, it remains to be determined whether plasma PCSK9 levels are elevated as a consequence of acute MI (as an acute phase reactant) or prior to MI. In addition, we do not know why PCSK9 levels were not associated with CAD in those not taking statin in the OHGS, but were in the EmCB study. This may be a reflection of the presence of less coronary atherosclerosis in EmCB angiographic controls, where 20% or less

Table 7. Logistic regression analysis of the association of PCSK9 with CAD in the EmCB sub-study.

Variable	β or OR (95% CI)	p
Age, (years)	−0.005 (−0.034, 0.024)	<2E-16
Male sex	3.408 (2.28, 5.094)	2.24E-09
BMI, kg/m^2	0.034 (−0.019, 0.088)	0.103
Smoking	2.774 (1.654, 4.651)	0.0001
HTN	2.002 (1.368, 2.929)	0.0003
LDL-C, mmol/L	0.003 (−0.003, 0.010)	0.235
HDL-C, mmol/L	−0.018 (−0.044, 0.008)	0.089
TG, mmol/L	−0.438 (−1.716, 0.841)	0.256
PCSK9, ng/mL	0.003 (0.001, 0.005)	5.26E-06

All EmCB samples were from non-diabetic individuals not taking a statin at the time of recruitment. Results given as beta for continuous variables and odds ratio (OR) for categorical variables. Abbreviations: BMI, body mass index; HTN, anithypertensive medication; Total-C, total-cholesterol; LDL-C, Low density lipoprotein-cholesterol; HDL-C, high density lipoprotein-cholesterol; TG, triglycerides. N = 677.

Table 8. Logistic regression analysis of the association of PCSK9 with acute MI in the EmCB sub-study.

Variable	β or OR (95% CI)	p
Age, (years)	−0.005 (−0.034, 0.024)	0.718
Male sex	0.745 (0.402, 1.378)	0.200
BMI, kg/m^2	0.034 (−0.019, 0.088)	0.209
Smoking	1.127 (0.576, 2.207)	0.542
HTN	0.627 (0.358, 1.097)	0.370
LDL, mmol/L	0.003 (−0.003, 0.010)	0.316
HDL, mmol/L	−0.018 (−0.044, 0.008)	0.182
TG, mmol/L	−0.438 (−1.716, 0.841)	0.502
PCSK9, ng/mL	0.003 (0.001, 0.005)	0.0008

Results given as beta for continuous variables and odds ratio (OR) for categorical variables. Abbreviations: BMI, body mass index; HTN, anithypertensive medication; Total-C, total-cholesterol; LDL-C, Low density lipoprotein-cholesterol; HDL-C, high density lipoprotein-cholesterol; TG, triglycerides. N = 296.

stenosis was used as an inclusion criterion compared to 30% or less for the OHGS. Another factor could be the inclusion of individuals with aortic valve disease, who showed minimal coronary stenosis, in the OHGS controls [14]. It is not known whether aortic valve disease elevates plasma PCSK9 levels. A recent study of 243 angiographic cases reported a correlation between the severity of coronary artery disease and plasma PCSK9 levels [42]. However, in two larger cohorts, we did not replicate this finding.

Conclusion

Among non-diabetic individuals with angiographically-defined coronary artery disease who are not taking a lipid-lowering medication, plasma PCSK9 levels are elevated at the time of acute myocardial infarction. Future longitudinal studies will be required to determine whether PCSK9 levels are elevated prior to or as a consequence of acute coronary events.

Acknowledgments

We thank Thomas Lagace for providing LDL-C and reading of the manuscript.

Author Contributions

Conceived and designed the experiments: NAMA AFRS. Performed the experiments: NAMA. Analyzed the data: NAMA ROV HHC NG. Contributed reagents/materials/analysis tools: RR AQ SD AFRS. Contributed to the writing of the manuscript: NAMA HHC NG RR AQ AFRS.

References

1. Horton JD, Cohen JC, Hobbs HH (2007) Molecular biology of PCSK9: its role in LDL metabolism. Trends Biochem Sci 32: 71–77.
2. Cohen JC, Boerwinkle E, Mosley TH Jr, Hobbs HH (2006) Sequence variations in PCSK9, low LDL, and protection against coronary heart disease. N Engl J Med 354: 1264–1272.
3. Kathiresan S (2008) A PCSK9 missense variant associated with a reduced risk of early-onset myocardial infarction. N Engl J Med 358: 2299–2300.
4. Benn M, Nordestgaard BG, Grande P, Schnohr P, Tybjaerg-Hansen A (2010) PCSK9 R46L, low-density lipoprotein cholesterol levels, and risk of ischemic heart disease: 3 independent studies and meta-analyses. J Am Coll Cardiol 55: 2833–2842.
5. Lakoski SG, Lagace TA, Cohen JC, Horton JD, Hobbs HH (2009) Genetic and metabolic determinants of plasma PCSK9 levels. J Clin Endocrinol Metab 94: 2537–2543.
6. Dong B, Wu M, Li H, Kraemer FB, Adeli K, et al. (2010) Strong induction of PCSK9 gene expression through HNF1alpha and SREBP2: mechanism for the resistance to LDL-cholesterol lowering effect of statins in dyslipidemic hamsters. J Lipid Res 51: 1486–1495.
7. Truong QA, Murphy SA, McCabe CH, Armani A, Cannon CP (2011) Benefit of intensive statin therapy in women: results from PROVE IT-TIMI 22. Circ Cardiovasc Qual Outcomes 4: 328–336.
8. Kostis WJ, Cheng JQ, Dobrzynski JM, Cabrera J, Kostis JB (2012) Meta-analysis of statin effects in women versus men. J Am Coll Cardiol 59: 572–582.
9. Stein EA, Mellis S, Yancopoulos GD, Stahl N, Logan D, et al. (2012) Effect of a monoclonal antibody to PCSK9 on LDL cholesterol. N Engl J Med 366: 1108–1118.
10. McKenney JM, Koren MJ, Kereiakes DJ, Hanotin C, Ferrand AC, et al. (2012) Safety and efficacy of a monoclonal antibody to proprotein convertase subtilisin/kexin type 9 serine protease, SAR236553/REGN727, in patients with primary hypercholesterolemia receiving ongoing stable atorvastatin therapy. J Am Coll Cardiol 59: 2344–2353.
11. Norata GD, Tibolla G, Catapano AL (2014) Targeting PCSK9 for hypercholesterolemia. Annu Rev Pharmacol Toxicol 54: 273–293.
12. Fan M, Dandona S, McPherson R, Allayee H, Hazen SL, et al. (2013) Two Chromosome 9p21 Haplotype Blocks Distinguish Between Coronary Artery Disease and Myocardial Infarction Risk. Circ Cardiovasc Genet 6: 372–380.
13. Reilly MP, Li M, He J, Ferguson JF, Stylianou IM, et al. (2011) Identification of ADAMTS7 as a novel locus for coronary atherosclerosis and association of ABO with myocardial infarction in the presence of coronary atherosclerosis: two genome-wide association studies. Lancet 377: 383–392.
14. Stewart AFR, Dandona S, Chen L, Assogba O, Belanger M, et al. (2009) Kinesin family member 6 variant Trp719Arg does not associate with angiographically defined coronary artery disease in the Ottawa Heart Genomics Study. J Am Coll Cardiol 53: 1471–1472.
15. Chan K, Patel RS, Newcombe P, Nelson CP, Qasim A, et al. (2013) Association between the chromosome 9p21 locus and angiographic coronary artery disease burden: a collaborative meta-analysis. J Am Coll Cardiol 61: 957–970.
16. Dandona S, Stewart AFR, Chen L, Williams K, So D, et al. (2010) Gene dosage of the common variant 9p21 predicts severity of coronary artery disease. J Am Coll Cardiol 56: 479–486.
17. Miyazawa H, Honda T, Miyauchi S, Domon H, Okui T, et al. (2012) Increased serum PCSK9 concentrations are associated with periodontal infection but do not correlate with LDL cholesterol concentration. Clin Chim Acta 413: 154–159.
18. Persson L, Henriksson P, Westerlund E, Hovatta O, Angelin B, et al. (2012) Endogenous estrogens lower plasma PCSK9 and LDL cholesterol but not Lp(a) or bile acid synthesis in women. Arterioscler Thromb Vasc Biol 32: 810–814.
19. Kosenko T, Golder M, Leblond G, Weng W, Lagace TA (2013) Low Density Lipoprotein Binds to Proprotein Convertase Subtilisin/Kexin Type-9 (PCSK9) in Human Plasma and Inhibits PCSK9-mediated Low Density Lipoprotein Receptor Degradation. J Biol Chem 288: 8279–8288.
20. Dubuc G, Chamberland A, Wassef H, Davignon J, Seidah NG, et al. (2004) Statins upregulate PCSK9, the gene encoding the proprotein convertase neural apoptosis-regulated convertase-1 implicated in familial hypercholesterolemia. Arterioscler Thromb Vasc Biol 24: 1454–1459.
21. Costet P, Hoffmann MM, Cariou B, Guyomarc'h Delasalle B, Konrad T, et al. (2010) Plasma PCSK9 is increased by fenofibrate and atorvastatin in a non-additive fashion in diabetic patients. Atherosclerosis 212: 246–251.

22. Mayne J, Dewpura T, Raymond A, Cousins M, Chaplin A, et al. (2008) Plasma PCSK9 levels are significantly modified by statins and fibrates in humans. Lipids Health Dis 7: 22.
23. Gu Q, Dillon CF, Burt VL (2010) Prescription drug use continues to increase: U.S. prescription drug data for 2007–2008. NCHS data brief: 1–8.
24. Abd TT, Jacobson TA (2011) Statin-induced myopathy: a review and update. Expert opinion on drug safety 10: 373–387.
25. Cohen J, Pertsemlidis A, Kotowski IK, Graham R, Garcia CK, et al. (2005) Low LDL cholesterol in individuals of African descent resulting from frequent nonsense mutations in PCSK9. Nat Genet 37: 161–165.
26. Roberts R, Stewart AFR (2012) Genes and coronary artery disease: where are we? J Am Coll Cardiol 60: 1715–1721.
27. Voight BF, Peloso GM, Orho-Melander M, Frikke-Schmidt R, Barbalic M, et al. (2012) Plasma HDL cholesterol and risk of myocardial infarction: a mendelian randomisation study. Lancet 380: 572–580.
28. Gaziano JM, Hennekens CH, Satterfield S, Roy C, Sesso HD, et al. (1999) Clinical utility of lipid and lipoprotein levels during hospitalization for acute myocardial infarction. Vasc Med 4: 227–231.
29. Wattanasuwan N, Khan IA, Gowda RM, Vasavada BC, Sacchi TJ (2001) Effect of acute myocardial infarction on cholesterol ratios. Chest 120: 1196–1199.
30. Pfohl M, Schreiber I, Liebich HM, Haring HU, Hoffmeister HM (1999) Upregulation of cholesterol synthesis after acute myocardial infarction-is cholesterol a positive acute phase reactant? Atherosclerosis 142: 389–393.
31. Le Bras M, Roquilly A, Deckert V, Langhi C, Feuillet F, et al. (2013) Plasma PCSK9 Is a late biomarker of severity in patients with severe trauma injury. J Clin Endocrinol Metab 98: E732–736.
32. Poirier S, Mayer G, Benjannet S, Bergeron E, Marcinkiewicz J, et al. (2008) The proprotein convertase PCSK9 induces the degradation of low density lipoprotein receptor (LDLR) and its closest family members VLDLR and ApoER2. J Biol Chem 283: 2363–2372.
33. Quinn KL, Henriques M, Tabuchi A, Han B, Yang H, et al. (2011) Human neutrophil peptides mediate endothelial-monocyte interaction, foam cell formation, and platelet activation. Arterioscler Thromb Vasc Biol 31: 2070–2079.
34. ISIS-2 (Second International Study of Infarct Survival) Collaborative Group (1992) Morning peak in the incidence of myocardial infarction: experience in the ISIS-2 trial. Eur Heart J 13: 594–598.
35. Persson L, Cao G, Stahle L, Sjoberg BG, Troutt JS, et al. (2010) Circulating proprotein convertase subtilisin kexin type 9 has a diurnal rhythm synchronous with cholesterol synthesis and is reduced by fasting in humans. Arterioscler Thromb Vasc Biol 30: 2666–2672.
36. Tofler GH, Brezinski D, Schafer AI, Czeisler CA, Rutherford JD, et al. (1987) Concurrent morning increase in platelet aggregability and the risk of myocardial infarction and sudden cardiac death. N Engl J Med 316: 1514–1518.
37. Chernogubova E, Strawbridge R, Mahdessian H, Malarstig A, Krapivner S, et al. (2012) Common and low-frequency genetic variants in the PCSK9 locus influence circulating PCSK9 levels. Arterioscler Thromb Vasc Biol 32: 1526–1534.
38. Yusuf S, Hawken S, Ounpuu S, Dans T, Avezum A, et al. (2004) Effect of potentially modifiable risk factors associated with myocardial infarction in 52 countries (the INTERHEART study): case-control study. Lancet 364: 937–952.
39. DeStefano F, Anda RF, Kahn HS, Williamson DF, Russell CM (1993) Dental disease and risk of coronary heart disease and mortality. BMJ 306: 688–691.
40. Smeeth L, Thomas SL, Hall AJ, Hubbard R, Farrington P, et al. (2004) Risk of myocardial infarction and stroke after acute infection or vaccination. N Engl J Med 351: 2611–2618.
41. Feingold KR, Moser AH, Shigenaga JK, Patzek SM, Grunfeld C (2008) Inflammation stimulates the expression of PCSK9. Biochem Biophys Res Commun 374: 341–344.
42. Li S, Guo YL, Xu RX, Zhang Y, Zhu CG, et al. (2014) Plasma PCSK9 levels are associated with the severity of coronary stenosis in patients with atherosclerosis. Int J Cardiol 174: 863–864.

12

Effects of Insufficient Physical Activity on Mortality and Life Expectancy in Jiangxi Province of China, 2007-2010

Gang Xu[1], Xuemei Sui[2], Shiwei Liu[3]*, Jie Liu[4], Junxiu Liu[5], Yichong Li[3], Shouqing Huang[6], Zhengzhen Wang[7], Steven N. Blair[2]

1 Department of Preventive Medicine, School of Basic Medicine, Jiangxi University of Traditional Chinese Medicine, Nanchang, Jiangxi, China, **2** Department of Exercise Science, Arnold School of Public Health, University of South Carolina, Columbia, South Carolina, United States of America, **3** National Center for Chronic and Noncommunicable Disease Control and Prevention, Chinese Center for Disease Control and Prevention, Beijing, China, **4** Division of Chronic Disease Control and Prevention, Jiangxi Province Center for Disease Control and Prevention, Nanchang, Jiangxi, China, **5** Department of Epidemiology and Biostatisitcs, Arnold School of Public Health, University of South Carolina, Columbia, South Carolina, United States of America, **6** The Second People's Hospital Affiliated to Fujian University of Traditional Chinese Medicine, Fuzhou, Fujian, China, **7** Division of Exercise Rehabilitation, Beijing Sport University Sport Rehabilitation College, Beijing, China

Abstract

Background: Physical inactivity remains an under-researched field in terms of studying burden of disease at provincial level, and no studies have examined the effects of inactivity on life expectancy (LE) in China. The purpose of this study was to estimate mortality risk and LE effects associated with insufficient levels of physical activity in Jiangxi province.

Methods/Findings: Prevalence of risk factors and mortality counts were extracted from Chronic Diseases and Risk Factors Surveillance Survey (CDRFSS) and Disease Surveillance Points system (DSP), respectively. Insufficient physical activity (IPA) was defined as less than 150 minutes of moderate-intensity physical activity or 60 minutes of vigorous-intensity physical activity per week, accumulated across work, home, transport and discretionary domains. Population-attributable fractions (PAF) were used to calculate the mortality attributable to risk factors, and life table methods were used to estimate the LE gains and LE shifts. Monte Carlo simulation techniques were used for uncertainty analysis. Overall, 5 885 (95% uncertainly interval (UI), 5 047–6 506) and 8 578 (95% UI, 8 227–9 789) deaths in Jiangxi province were attributable to IPA in 2007 and 2010, respectively. The LE gains for elimination of attributable deaths were 0.68 (95% UI, 0.61–076) in 2007, and increased to 0.91 (95% UI, 0.81–1.10) in 2010. If the prevalence of IPA in 2010 had been decreased by 50% or 30%, 3 678 (95% UI, 3 220–4 229) or 2 090 (95% UI, 1 771–2 533) deaths would be avoided, and 0.40 (95% UI, 0.34–0.53) or 0.23 (95% UI, 0.16–0.31) years of LE gained, respectively.

Conclusions: Adults in Jiangxi province of China have a high and increasing prevalence of IPA. Due to the deaths and potential LE gains associated with IPA, there is an urgent need to promote physical activity, one of the most modifiable risk factors, within China's health care reform agenda.

Editor: Rui Medeiros, IPO, Inst Port Oncology, Portugal

Funding: This study was funded by the Humanities and Social Sciences Foundation for Young Scholar, Ministry of Education of China (13YJCZH212), Humanities and Social Sciences Development Foundation for Higher Education of Jiangxi Province, China (JC1357), and Development Foundation for Jiangxi University of Traditional Chinese Medicine. The funders had no role in the study design, data collection and analysis, decision to publish, or preparation of the manuscript.

Competing Interests: The authors have declared that no competing interests exist.

* Email: liusw@chinacdc.cn

Introduction

Physical inactivity has been associated with higher risk of many chronic diseases, including coronary heart disease [1,2], ischemic stroke [3,4], type 2 diabetes [5,6], colon cancer [7] and breast cancer [8]. Physical inactivity also is linked to lower life expectancy (LE) [9–12]. Conversely, higher levels of physical activity are associated with lower risk of mortality and longer LE [13]. The comparative risk assessment of the Global Burden of Disease Study indicated that insufficient physical activity (IPA) accounted for 3.2 million deaths and 2.8% of disability-adjusted life years in 2010, and ranked tenth among the 20 leading risk factors in attributable burden of disease [14]. The study estimated that approximately 0.5 million deaths and 3.6% of disability-adjusted life years in China were attributable to IPA, and that IPA ranked tenth among the 67 risk factors examined [15]. Non-communicable diseases account for 85% of annual deaths and are the leading cause of death in China [16]. The 2010 Global Burden of Disease Study reported that the most significant behaviors related to non-communicable diseases in China included dietary risks, smoking, alcohol use, and physical inactivity [15]. Little research, however, has examined the role of physical inactivity on the burden of disease in China, especially at the provincial level. In addition, no studies have examined changes in LE attributable to physical inactivity in China.

The five-year plan for national economic and social development of China, developed in 2011[17], proposed to increase LE by

1 year, from 73.5 years in 2010 to 74.5 years in 2015, as one of 28 core indices. Since then, each provincial government has developed and implemented programs to improve LE in local populations by 1 year. In addition, China launched its new health care reform plan in 2009, and is periodically monitoring progress toward achieving the objectives of the plan [18,19]. Quantitative and comparative studies on mortality attributable to risk factors and LE gains attributable to reducing risk factor are good indices to evaluate public health performance and guide health intervention and policy-making.

Average weekly physical activity among adults ages 18–55 in China decreased 32% between 1991 and 2006 [20]. The Chinese Chronic Diseases and Risk Factors Surveillance Survey (CDRFSS) reported in 2010 that only 11.9% of Chinese ages 18 and above participated in physical activity regularly (defined as ≥3 times per week, and ≥10 minutes every time for recreational physical activities) and that 83.8% did not participate in any physical activities [21]. Jiangxi province, located in southeast China, is situated 24°29′14″ – 30°04′41″ north latitude and 113°34′36″ – 118°28′58″ east longitude, and spans from the banks of the Yangtze River in the north into hillier areas in the south and east. In 2010, national census data showed that the population of Jiangxi province was approximately 44.57 million, with 72.06% of the population engaged in agriculture (nationwide: 70.13%). The urbanization rate was 43.75% (nationwide: 50.27%). The proportion of the population <15 years of age and ≥65 years of age was 18.88% and 7.60%, respectively (nationwide: 14.01% and 8.92%, respectively), in 2010. Generally, Jiangxi has a larger labor force population and lower urbanization than the country as a whole.

The purpose of this study was to estimate the mortality due to IPA in Jiangxi province among adults from 2007 to 2010, based on Chinese CDRFSS data and the corresponding years' mortality data from the Chinese Disease Surveillance Points (DSP) system, and to estimate the number of deaths that could have been averted by reducing this risk factor at different counterfactual scenarios. LE gains and LE shift were calculated using life-table methods.

Methods

Data Sources

Exposure data of Insufficient Physical Activity. Self-reported data on the prevalence of IPA among Jiangxi province adults 18 years of age or older were retrieved from Chinese CDRFSS 2007 and 2010, which were independently carried out in the surveillance points (one point corresponds to one county or district) of DSP system [21–26]. All participants were randomly selected by a multi-stage stratified random sampling method; the sampling procedure and sample size at the national level are described elsewhere [21–25]. There were 1 554 and 2 772 participants surveyed in Jiangxi province in 2007 and 2010, respectively. Data on moderate-intensity or vigorous-intensity physical activity, using questions based on the Global Physical Activity Questionnaire [27], were collected across four domains - work, domestic, transport and discretionary time. In order to make the samples more representative of the total province, the sample weighting [28] and age- and sex- specific structure adjustment on the sample population were based on the whole population across the province [29]. Because the Global Physical Activity Questionnaire may not measure physical activity reliably among persons ≥70 years, data from participants in the age groups 70–74, 75–79 and ≥80 were combined with age group 65–69, and the same prevalence values were utilized for them.

Consistent with the methodology of comparative risk assessment in the Global Burden of Disease Study [30], physical activity was treated as a categorical variable: (1) Physical inactivity (level 1): doing no or very little physical activity at work, at home, for transport or during discretionary time. (2) Low physical activity (level 2): doing some physical activity but less than 150 minutes of moderate-intensity physical activity or 60 minutes of vigorous-intensity physical activity per week, accumulated across work, home, transport or discretionary domains. (3) Physical activity (level 3): at least 150 minutes of moderate-intensity physical activity or 60 minutes of vigorous-intensity physical activity per week accumulated across work, home, transport or discretionary domains. Levels 1 and 2 were defined as IPA.

Mortality data. Mortality data for 2007 and 2010 by underlying cause, age, and sex were extracted from the DSP system [26], which includes 5 surveillance points in Jiangxi province. Completeness of reporting and accuracy of cause of death are the main problems for any surveillance system. Therefore, we adjusted all the mortality data using propensity score methods based on the underreporting survey data and the redistribution of garbage code of cause of death. In addition, we adjusted the age- and sex-specific structure of the sample using the whole provincial population [29] to make it representative of the whole province.

Population data. The population of surveillance points in 2010 was obtained directly from 2010 census data. The population data for 2007 was interpolated from the 2000 and 2010 censuses by adjusting for annual variation by assuming a constant growth rate over all years.

Health outcomes and the relative risk (*RR*). In accordance with comparative risk assessment in the Global Burden of Disease Study [30], ischemic heart disease, ischemic stroke, breast cancer, colon cancer and type 2 diabetes were identified as health outcomes etiologically associated with IPA. The *RR* for each health outcome with adjustment for measurement errors was also selected from the comparative risk assessment [30]. Though many studies [31–33] show the relationship of physical activity to weight status, obesity is excluded from the health outcomes in this study, consistent with comparative risk assessment methodology.

All enrolled participants in the CDRFSS gave written and informed consent for participation. The National Health and Family Planning Commission (NHFPC, previously Ministry of Health) of China and the Ethics Committee of the Chinese Center for Disease Prevention and Control approved the implementation of CDRFSS and mortality surveillance through the DSP system. The records/information of participants was de-identified prior to analysis.

Statistical Analysis

Premature mortality attributable to risk factor. In our analysis, population-attributable fractions (PAF) were calculated to estimate the amount of premature deaths attributable to IPA by comparing the current population exposure with the theoretical minimum distribution of 0% IPA. The formula used was:

$$PAF = \frac{\sum_{i=1}^{k} p_i(RR_i - 1)}{\sum_{i=1}^{k} p_i(RR_i - 1) + 1},$$

where p_i is the prevalence of exposure level i, RR_i is the RR of adverse health outcome in exposure level i, and k is the total number of exposure levels. For each disease causally associated with the risk factor, the attributable mortality was calculated by

Table 1. The prevalence of three levels of physical activity in Jiangxi province of China by age-sex, 2007 and 2010.

Year	Age group in years	Level of activity						
		Male			Female			
		Level 1	Level 2	Level 3	Level 1	Level 2		Level 3
2007	**18–24**	32.1	34.5	33.4	27.1	49.4		23.5
	25–29	37.5	26.3	36.2	38.7	38.1		23.2
	30–34	40.9	24.9	34.2	39.1	32.0		28.9
	35–39	39.3	26.2	34.5	56.7	26.9		16.4
	40–44	43.7	19.9	36.4	52.3	31.6		16.1
	45–49	44.1	32.5	23.4	56.2	26.6		17.2
	50–54	39.2	33.6	27.2	57.7	28.6		13.7
	55–59	42.1	25.3	32.6	66.6	16.9		16.5
	60–64	37.3	33.3	29.4	50.1	28.6		21.3
	65–69	37.7	35.8	26.5	45.0	35.4		19.6
	70–74[a]	37.7	35.8	26.5	45.0	35.4		19.6
	75–79[a]	37.7	35.8	26.5	45.0	35.4		19.6
	≥80[a]	37.7	35.8	26.5	45.0	35.4		19.6
2010	**18–24**	38.4	29.2	32.4	31.1	49.7		19.2
	25–29	34.8	33.1	32.1	39.5	42.9		17.6
	30–34	44.9	22.7	32.4	54.5	37.2		8.3
	35–39	47.9	19.0	33.1	53.1	33.0		13.9
	40–44	50.4	25.3	24.3	66.3	23.3		10.4
	45–49	45.1	26.0	28.9	66.9	17.6		15.5
	50–54	47.3	33.5	19.2		69.3	22.0	8.7
	55–59	55.1	28.1	16.8		59.3	21.7	19.0
	60–64	50.8	31.1	18.1		66.2	22.7	11.1
	65–69	50.1	32.0	17.9		55.4	34.2	10.4
	70–74[a]	50.1	32.0	17.9		55.4	34.2	10.4
	75–79[a]	50.1	32.0	17.9		55.4	34.2	10.4
	≥80[a]	50.1	32.0	17.9		55.4	34.2	10.4

[a]Due to the limited participants in these age groups, we combined them with age group 65–69 and the same prevalence values were utilized.

Table 2. *RR* values (95% CI) for selected health outcomes by age.

Risk level	Age group	Health outcomes[a] and the *RR* values (95% CI)				
		Ischemic heart disease	Ischemic stroke	Breast cancer[b]	Colon cancer	Type 2 diabetes
Level 1[c]	18–44	1.71 (1.58–1.85)	1.53 (1.31–1.79)	1.25 (1.20–1.30)	1.68 (1.55–1.82)	1.45 (1.37–1.54)
	45–69	1.71 (1.58–1.85)	1.53 (1.31–1.79)	1.34 (1.29–1.39)	1.68 (1.55–1.82)	1.45 (1.37–1.54)
	70–79	1.50 (1.38–1.61)	1.38 (1.18–1.60)	1.25 (1.21–1.30)	1.48 (1.36–1.60)	1.32 (1.25–1.45)
	≥80	1.30 (1.21–1.41)	1.24 (1.06–1.33)	1.16 (1.11–1.20)	1.30 (1.20–1.40)	1.20 (1.14–1.28)
Level 2[c]	18–44	1.44 (1.28–1.62)	1.10 (0.89–1.37)	1.13 (1.04–1.22)	1.18 (1.05–1.33)	1.24 (1.11–1.39)
	45–69	1.44 (1.28–1.62)	1.10 (0.89–1.37)	1.13 (1.04–1.22)	1.18 (1.05–1.33)	1.24 (1.11–1.39)
	70–79	1.31 (1.17–1.48)	1.08 (0.87–1.33)	1.09 (1.01–1.18)	1.13 (1.01–1.27)	1.18 (1.04–1.32)
	≥80	1.20 (1.07–1.35)	1.05 (0.85–1.30)	1.06 (0.98–1.15)	1.08 (0.97–1.22)	1.11 (0.99–1.25)

RR, relative ration; CI, confidence interval.
[a]The 10th revision of international classification of diseases (ICD-10) codes for each health outcomes: Ischemic heart diseases: I20–I25. Ischemic stroke: I63, I65–I67 (except I67.4), I69.3. Breast cancer: C50. Colon cancer: C18. Type 2 diabetes: E11.
[b]Just for females.
[c]Level 1: Physical inactivity, defined as doing no or very little physical activity at work, at home, for transport or during discretionary time. Level 2: Low physical activity, defined as doing some physical activity but less than 150 minutes of moderate-intensity physical activity or 60 minutes of vigorous-intensity physical activity a week accumulated across work, home, transport or discretionary domains.

multiplying the PAF with the observed deaths by age and sex, then the attributable disease-specific mortality was summed as the whole mortality attributable to the risk factor [12]. If the counterfactual scenarios were not the theoretical minimum distribution of 0% IPA, but an alternative distribution with decreased prevalence of risk factor for interventions, the formula was:

$$PIF = \frac{\sum_{i=1}^{n} p_i RR_i - \sum_{i=1}^{n} p'_i RR_i}{\sum_{i=1}^{k} p_i RR_i},$$

where PIF is potential impact fractions and p_i' is the prevalence of exposure level i in alternative distribution.

Effects of risk factors on LE. We calculated the LE for each year using standard life table methods, based on the observed age-specific mortality (LEyt), as well as the alternative age-specific mortality by removing the deaths attributable to IPA (LEyr). The difference between the two sets of LEs at birth measures the LE gains (LEyr-LEyt). Also, LE shifts for the current distributions of risk factor exposure changed to an alternative scenario can be calculated using the same methods.

Alternative risk factor exposure distributions. We tracked the effects of IPA on mortality and LE in Jiangxi province relative to three different counterfactual exposure distributions, comparing with that in 2010 treated as current distribution: (i) the prevalence of level 1 and level 2 for each sex-age group was decreased to 0, which means 100% physical activity. This is the same as PAF calculation results, (ii) the prevalence of level 1 and level 2 for each sex-age group was decreased by 50%, and (iii) the prevalence of level 1 and level 2 for each sex-age group was decreased by 30%.

Uncertainty analysis. Inevitably, several forms of uncertainty occurred in our estimate, including stochastic variation, systematic biases and errors. It is not reasonable if we just provided a definite point value as the final estimate. Monte Carlo simulation techniques, which consist of assigning probability distributions to model variables that involve risk and then generating random numbers based on those distributions, were used to present uncertainty ranges around point estimates reflecting the main sources of uncertainty. The @RISK software version 6 for Excel [34] allows multiple recalculations of a spreadsheet. We defined the *RR* and risk factor exposure level as the input variables, and the attributable fractions, attributive deaths and LE as the output variables. For the input variables we specified a log-normal distribution for the *RR* and normal distribution for the prevalence of risk factor. For each of the output variables, 95% uncertainty intervals (95% UI) were calculated bounded by the 2.5[th] and 97.5[th] percentiles of the 2000 iteration values generated.

Results

Table 1 shows the prevalence of three levels of physical activity based on the 2007 and 2010 CDRFSS. These data indicate that level 1 (physical inactivity) and level 2 (low physical activity) were higher in 2010 than 2007, higher for females than males, and increased with age.

The *RR*s and 95% confidence intervals (CI) for selected health outcomes by age are presented in **Table 2**. Except for breast cancer, which included only females, the *RR* values for other health outcomes were similar for both males and females.

Between 2007 and 2010, the attributable fractions of ischemic heart disease, ischemic stroke, breast cancer, colon cancer, and type 2 diabetes attributable to IPA increased from 23.3% to 25.3%, 15.3% to 17.0%, 16.1% to 16.6%, 20.9% to 23.8%, and 14.7% to 18.5% respectively, with the same trend for both males and females. In total, the PAF of the five outcomes increased from 20.3% in 2007 to 22.4% in 2010 (**Table 3**). Attributable fractions of ischemic heart disease were higher in males than females, and colon cancer and type 2 diabetes were higher in females than males in 2007 and 2010. Attributable fractions were generally higher in the age group 35-69 years, and peaked in the 45-49-year age group for males and 55-59-year age group for females in 2007, and in the 55-59-year age group for males and 50-54-year age group for females in 2010 (data not presented here). Overall, 5 885 (95% UI, 5 047–6 506) deaths, accounting for 2.7% (95% UI, 2.3%–3.8%) of total deaths in Jiangxi province in 2007, and 8 578

Table 3. PAF (%), deaths attributable to IPA and LE gains attributable to IPA reduction by age and sex, Jiangxi province of China, 2007 and 2010.

Year	Health outcomes	Male			Female			Both sexes		
		PAF (%)	Deaths	LE gains	PAF (%)	Deaths	LE gains	PAF (%)	Deaths	LE gains
2007	Ischemic heart disease	23.5	2 306		23.2	1 779		23.3	4 085	
	Ischemic stroke	14.9	705		15.8	590		15.3	1 295	
	Breast cancer	–	–		16.1	182		16.1	182	
	Colon cancer	19.8	129		22.3	105		20.9	235	
	Type 2 diabetes	13.7	55		16.7	34		14.7	89	
	Total	20.2	3 196	0.27	20.5	2 690	0.41	20.3	5 885	0.68
	95% UI									
	Lower		2 751	0.22		2 183	0.38		5 047	0.61
	Upper		3 378	0.37		2 809	0.52		6 506	0.76
	% of total deaths		2.4			3.3			2.7	
	95% UI									
	Lower		1.8			2.8			2.3	
	Upper		3.3			4.1			3.8	
2010	Ischemic heart disease	25.9	3 201		24.6	2 673		25.3	5 874	
	Ischemic stroke	17.0	977		16.9	839		17.0	1 816	
	Breast cancer	–	–		16.6	174		16.6	174	
	Colon cancer	23.4	324		24.9	139		23.8	463	
	Type 2 diabetes	17.9	157		19.6	94		18.5	251	
	Total	22.8	4 659	0.41	21.9	3 919	0.50	22.4	8 578	0.91
	95% UI									
	Lower		4 426	0.38		3 575	0.44		8 227	0.81
	Upper		5 372	0.47		4 709	0.66		9 789	1.10
	% of total deaths		3.6			4.4			3.9	
	95% UI									
	Lower		3.1			3.8			3.3	
	Upper		4.3			5.5			4.5	

PAF, population-attributable fractions; LE, life expectancy; IPA, insufficient physical activity; UI, uncertainty interval.

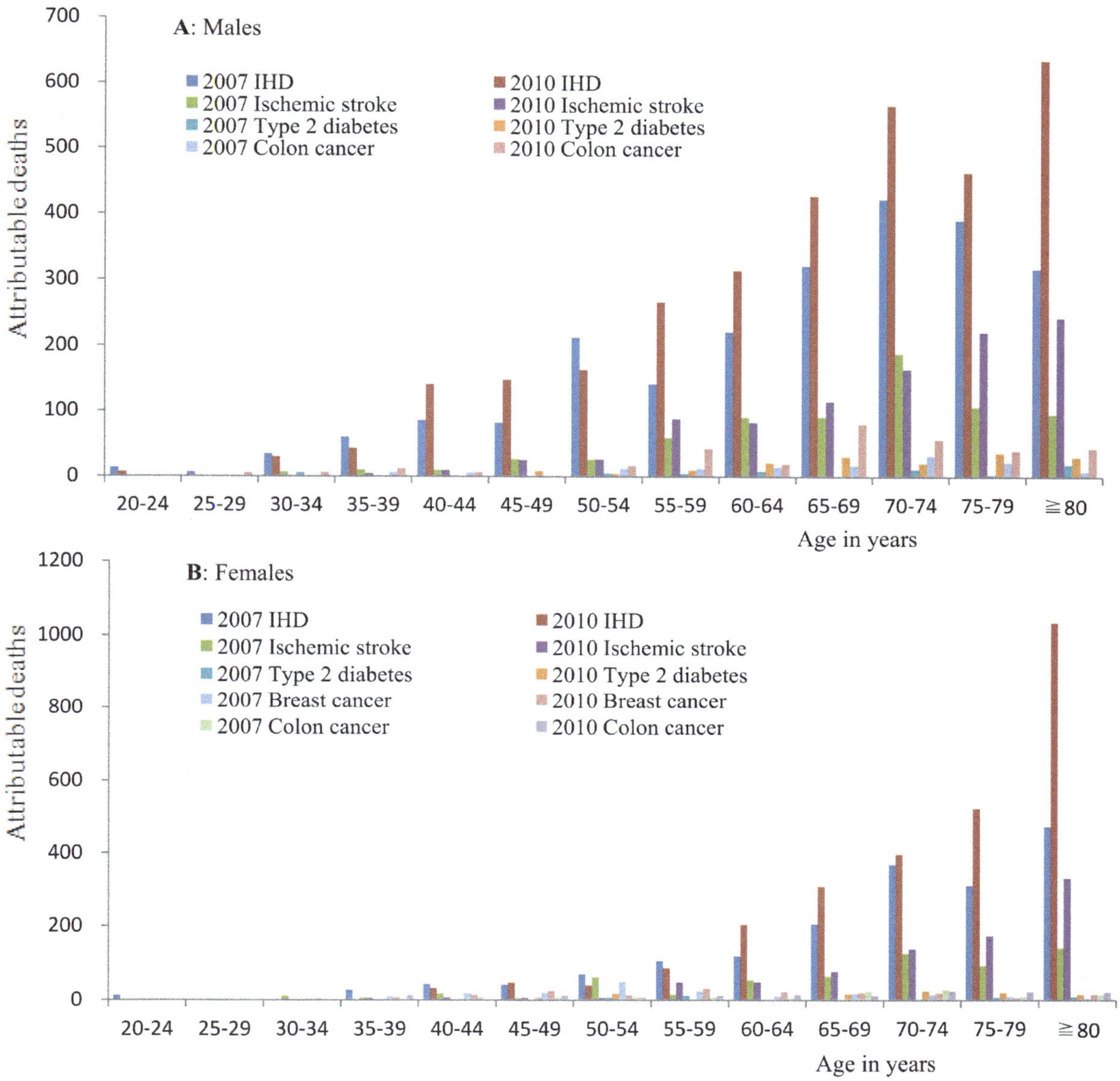

Figure 1. Deaths attributable to insufficient physical activity by age and sex, Jiangxi province of China in 2007 and 2010.

(95% UI, 8 227–9 789) deaths, accounting for 3.9% (95% UI, 3.3%–4.5%) of total deaths in 2010, were attributable to IPA. The majority of the attributable deaths were due to ischemic heart disease. The LE gains for elimination of attributable deaths were 0.68 (95% UI, 0.61–0.76) (0.27 for males and 0.41 for females) in 2007, and increased to 0.91 (95% UI, 0.81–1.10) (0.41 for males and 0.50 for females) in 2010 (**Table 3**).

Figure 1 shows the deaths attributable to IPA across age and sex groups. The overall pattern of deaths for 2010 was different, with a higher proportion at ≥80 years old for females. The total deaths attributable to IPA were higher in older age groups and males and were higher in 2010 than 2007. Most deaths were attributable to ischemic heart disease and ischemic stroke in both 2007 and 2010. A larger proportion of deaths in 2007 occurred in the 50–54 age group, in both males and females, compared to 2010.

Figure 2 shows that the largest proportion of deaths was caused by ischemic heart disease (more than 65%), followed by ischemic stroke (more than 20%). For females, breast cancer accounted for 6.8% of deaths in 2007 and declined to 4.4% in 2010. Colon cancer accounted for 4.0% in 2007 and increased to 6.9% in 2010 for males. The contribution from type 2 diabetes increased for 2010 among both males and females.

Assuming that the prevalence of level 1 and level 2 for all sex-age groups was decreased by 50% in 2010, 3 678 (95% UI, 3 220–4 229) deaths would have been avoided, with 0.40 (95% UI, 0.34–0.53) years of LE gained (**Table 4**). If the prevalence of level 1 and level 2 for all sex-age groups was decreased by 30% in 2010, 2 090 (95% UI, 1 771–2 533) deaths would have been avoided, with 0.23 (95% UI, 0.16–0.31) years of LE gained (**Table 4**).

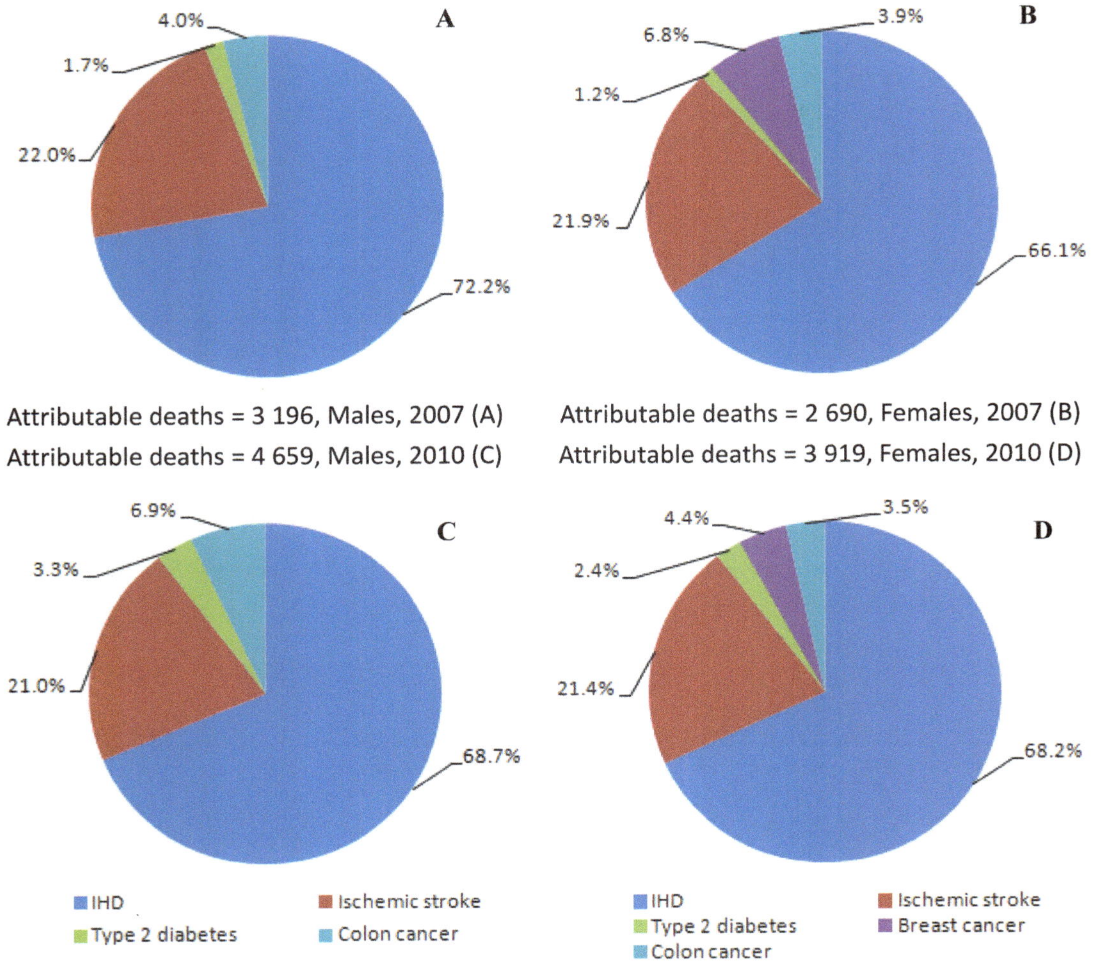

Figure 2. Deaths attributable to insufficient physical activity by sex and conditions, Jiangxi province of China, 2007 and 2010.

Table 4. LE shifts at different counterfactual scenarios of IPA by sex comparing with current distribution in 2010, Jiangxi province of China.

Exposure scenarios	Male		Female		Both sexes	
	Deaths	LE gains	Deaths	LE gains	Deaths	LE gains
Current distribution (i)	4 659	0.41	3 919	0.50	8 578	0.91
Decreased by 50% (ii)	2 668	0.23	2 232	0.28	4 900	0.51
Decreased by 30% (iii)	3 529	0.31	2 959	0.37	6 488	0.68
Burden shifts						
(i)–(ii)	1 991	0.18	1 687	0.22	3 678	0.40
95% UI						
Lower	1 639	0.11	1 400	0.15	3 220	0.34
Upper	2 548	0.24	2 277	0.31	4 229	0.53
(i)–(iii)	1 130	0.10	960	0.13	2 090	0.23
95% UI						
Lower	926	0.05	857	0.08	1 771	0.16
Upper	1 417	0.14	1 266	0.17	2 533	0.31

LE, life expectancy; IPA, insufficient physical activity; UI, uncertainty interval.

Discussion

This study showed an upward trend for the prevalence of IPA, which was associated with higher attributable fractions of deaths from ischemic heart disease, ischemic stroke, breast cancer, colon cancer, and type 2 diabetes from 2007 to 2010 in Jiangxi province of China. Ischemic heart disease and colon cancer accounted for more than 20% of deaths. Although the mortality rate across the country declined from 2007 to 2010, the number of deaths attributable to IPA in 2010 was higher than in 2007. The prevalence of IPA for females was higher than for males. However, the number of attributable deaths for males was greater than for females.

These trends and population distributions of prevalence of IPA in Jiangxi province mirrored the national data [21,22]. The Global Burden of Disease Study [30] and a 51-country survey [35] also showed that females in most regions of the world were slightly more inactive than males and younger adults were less inactive than older adults. The prevalence of physical inactivity (level 1) in Jiangxi province of China was higher than the global average of 17%, and the prevalence of low physical activity (level 2) was lower than the global average of 40.6% [30]. The findings from the current study suggest that lower levels of physical activity are becoming a global concern.

PAFs for IPA were slightly higher in Jiangxi province than in the global study, in which they accounted for 21.5% of ischemic heart disease, 11% of ischemic stroke, 14% of diabetes, 16% of colon cancer and 10% of breast cancer [30], but lower than those found in other emerging market economies and developed countries [2,36]. Another study from China that also was based on the 2007 NCDRFSS showed generally lower PAF of ischemic heart disease and type 2 diabetes than our study, but its exposure measure focused only on physical inactivity, with low physical activity excluded [32]. For some important limitations, the global estimates of the 2000 Global Burden of Disease Study were likely to be an underestimate of the true burden attributable to inactive lifestyles [30]. Although the *RR* values used in our study were directly obtained from comparative risk assessment of the Global Burden of Disease Study, it is reasonable to assume that they are valid and robust since the health benefits of physical activity have been demonstrated in a variety of settings and in many developing countries [36]. Physically inactive lifestyles in Jiangxi province were estimated to cause 5 881 and 8 582 deaths, which accounted for 2.7% and 3.9% of total deaths in 2007 and 2010, respectively. Globally, 3.3% of total deaths were due to physical inactivity in 2000 [30] and the same proportion found in South Africa [36]. In summary, our estimates of the morbidity and mortality burden due to physical inactivity in Jiangxi province are plausible and comparable to previous studies. Our findings further support the effort to promote physical activity and reduce inactivity in China.

In this study, we calculated for the first time the LE gains attributable to reducing physical inactivity in China, which showed that elimination of IPA in 2010 would have increased the LE by nearly a year. Any physical activity-related intervention that decreased the prevalence of IPA by 50% and 30% would increase LE by 0.40 years and 0.23 years, respectively. A recent global study in 2008 [37] estimated that elimination of physical inactivity would increase the LE of the world's population by 0.68 years, and in the Chinese population by 0.61 years, which is similar to our study for 2007 (0.68 years).

In addition, we tracked the effects of IPA on mortality and LE in Jiangxi province for different counterfactual exposure distributions, compared with the distribution in 2010. If the prevalence of level 1 and level 2 in each sex-age group was decreased by 50%, 3 678 deaths would have been avoided and 0.40 years of LE gained. If the prevalence declined by 30%, 2 091 deaths would have been avoided and 0.23 years of LE gained. These estimates are expected to be applied to health policy making and evaluation.

To the best of our knowledge, this is the first study to estimate the burden of disease attributable to insufficient physical activity at the provincial level and track the effects on LE in China. However, there were some limitations to our approach. First, the participants were identified using multi-stage stratified random cluster sampling method across the country in each CDRFSS; therefore, the study population might not be provincially representative. Also, the calculation of LE gains was based on two CDRFSSs with cross-sectional designs, which would impact the comparability between 2010 and 2007. The relatively small sample size involved in the 2007 and 2010 surveys [21,22] might produce unstable prevalence estimates of IPA in Jiangxi province. The same problem exists for the mortality from DSP, which only included 5 points. Fortunately, each field site in CDRFSS is consistent with DSP, which might minimize the impact for the calculation of excess deaths in this study. Lastly, physical activity data were self-reported in CDRFSS, and recall bias and social desirability might influence the exposure estimation [38,39].

China is going through a rapid demographic change, and unhealthful lifestyles associated with socioeconomic improvement have resulted in a greater burden of non-communicable diseases. Although the Movement of National Healthy Lifestyles initiated by the Ministry of Health and the Nationwide Body-building Plan promoted by the State General Administration of Sport have been implemented for many years [40], sedentary lifestyles in China are still very common. There is an increasing need for the Chinese government to take responsibility for expanding prevention strategies, such as taking action to encourage regular physical activity from childhood to older age, promoting a healthier environment, and motivating non-governmental organizations. Even small reductions in behavioral risk factors could generate substantial health benefits. Preventing or reducing IPA behaviors should be a priority within China's health care reform agenda.

Acknowledgments

We appreciate Gaye Christmus for her editorial contribution to the manuscript.

Author Contributions

Conceived and designed the experiments: SL GX XS JL JXL YL SH ZW. Performed the experiments: SL GX XS JL JXL YL SH ZW. Analyzed the data: GX SL JL YL. Contributed reagents/materials/analysis tools: SL GX XS JL JXL YL SH ZW. Wrote the paper: GX SL. Helped revise the manuscript: SL GX XS JL JXL YL SH ZW SB.

References

1. Sattelmair J, Pertman J, Ding EL, Kohl HW, Haskell W, et al. (2011) Dose Response Between Physical Activity and Risk of Coronary Heart Disease: A Meta-Analysis. Circulation 124: 789–795.
2. Rastogi T, Vaz M, Spiegelman D, Reddy KS, Bharathi AV, et al. (2004) Physical activity and risk of coronary heart disease in India. Int J Epidemiol 33: 759–767.
3. Kiely DK, Wolf PA, Cupples LA, Beiser AS, Kannel WB (1994) Physical activity and stroke risk-the Framingham study. Am J Epidemionl 140: 608–620.
4. Kohl HW (2001) Physical activity and cardiovascular disease: evidence for a dose response. Med Sci Sport Exer 33: S472–483.
5. Jeon CY, Lokken RP, Hu FB, Dam RM Van (2007) Physical Activity of Moderate Intensity and Risk of Type 2 Diabetes. Diabetes Care 30: 744–752.

6. Ivy JL, Zderic TW, Fogt DL (1999) Prevention and treatment of non-insulin-dependent diabetes mellitus. Exerc sport Sci Rev 27: 1–35.
7. Wolin KY, Yan Y, Colditz GA, Lee IM (2009) Physical activity and colon cancer prevention: a meta-analysis. Brit J Cancer 100: 611–616.
8. Monninkhof EM, Elias SG, Vlems FA, Van der Tweel I, Schuit AJ (2007) Physical Activity and Breast Cancer: A Systematic Review. Epidemiology 18: 137–157.
9. Franco OH, Laet C, Peeters A, Jonker J, Mackenbach J, et al. (2005) Effects of Physical Activity on Life Expectancy with Cardiovascular Disease. Arch Intern Med 165: 2355–2360.
10. Katzmarzyk PT, Lee IM (2012) Sedentary behaviour and life expectancy in the USA: a cause-deleted life table analysis. BMJ Open 2: e000828. Doi: 10.1136/bmjopen-2012-000828
11. Veerman JL, Healy GN, Cobiac LJ, Vos T, Winkler EAH, et al. (2012) Television viewing time and reduced life expectancy: a life table analysis. Br J Sports Med 46: 927–930. doi: 10.1136/bjsports-2011-085662
12. Danaei G, Rimm EB, Oza S, Kulkarni SC, Murray CJL, et al. (2010) The Promise of Prevention: The Effects of Four Preventable Risk Factors on National Life Expectancy and Life Expectancy Disparities by Race and County in the United States. PLoS Med 7: e1000248. doi: 10.1371/journal.pmed.1000248
13. Wen CP, Wai JPM, Tsai MK, Yang YC, Cheng TYD, et al. (2011) Minimum amount of physical activity for reduced mortality and extended life expectancy. Lancet 378: 1244–1253.
14. Slim S, Vos T, Flaxman AD, Danaei G, Shibuya K, et al. (2012) A comparative risk assessment of burden of disease and injury attributable to 67 risk factors and risk factor clusters in 21 regions, 1990–2010: a systematic analysis for the Global Burden of Disease Study 2010. Lancet 380: 2224–2260.
15. Yang G, Wang Y, Zeng Y, Gao GF, Liang X, et al. (2013) Rapid health transition in China, 1990–2010: findings from the Global Burden of Disease Study 2010. Lancet 381: 1987–2015.
16. Ministry of Health and Chinese Center for Disease Control and Prevention (2011) China Non-communicable Diseases Report. Beijing.
17. The Sate Council of the People's Republic of China (2011) The twelfth five-year plan outline of national economic and social development. Available: http://www.gov.cn/2011lh/content_1825838.htm. Accessed 30 November 2013.
18. The Sate Council of the People's Republic of China (2009) The guiding opinions on deepening the reform of medical care system. http://www.nhfpc.gov.cn/fzs/s9660/200904/5c15883cf95f416792b485514711f2f9.shtml. Accessed 1 December 2013.
19. National Health and Family Planning Commission of the People's Republic of China (2009) Monitoring and evaluation plan of health care reform.
20. Ng SW, Norton EC, Popkin BM (2009) Why have physical activity levels declined among Chinese adults? Findings from the 1991–2006 China health and nutrition surveys. Soc Sci Med 68: 1305–1314.
21. National Center for Chronic and Non-communicable Disease Control and Prevention of Chinese Center for Disease Control and Prevention (2011) The report of 2010 Behavioral Risk Factors Surveillance of China. Beijing: Military Medical Science Press.
22. National Center for Chronic and Non-communicable Disease Control and Prevention of Chinese Center for Disease Control and Prevention (2010) The report of 2007 Behavioral Risk Factors Surveillance of China. Beijing: People's Medical Publishing House.
23. Y Li, Y Jiang, M Zhang, P Yin, F Wu, et al. (2011) Drinking behaviour among men and women in China: the 2007 China Chronic Disease and Risk Factor Surveillance. Addiction 106: 1946–1956.
24. Y Li, M Zhang, Y Jiang, F Wu (2012) Co-variations and clustering of chronic disease behavioral risk factors in China: China Chronic Disease and Risk Factor Surveillance, 2007. PLoS ONE 7: e33881. doi: http://dx.doi.org/10.1371/journal. pone.0033881 PMID:22439010
25. Y Li, L Wang, Y Jiang, M Zhang, L Wang (2013) Risk factors for noncommunicable chronic diseases in women in China: surveillance efforts. Bull World Health Organ 91: 650–660.
26. Zhou M, Jiang Y, Huang Z, Wu F (2010) Adjustment and representativeness evaluation of national disease surveillance points system. Disease Surveillance 25: 239–244.
27. Armstrong T, Bull F (2006) Development of the World Health Organization Global Physical Activity Questionniare (GPAQ). J Public Health 14: 66–70.
28. Hu N, Jiang Y, Li Y, Chen Y (2012) Weighting method for Chinese chronic disease surveillance in 2010. Chinese Journal of Health Statistics 29: 424–426.
29. Wan X, Zhou M, Wang C, Yang G (2007) The application of direct standardization method of rate to the sample rate weighting. Health research 36: 285–286.
30. Bull FC, Armstrong TP, Dixon T, Ham S, Neiman A, et al. (2004) Physical inactivity. In: Ezzati M, Lopez AD, Rodgers A, Murray CJL, editors. Comparative Quantification of Health Risks: Global and Regional Burden of Disease Attributable to Selected Major Risk Fators. Vol.1. Geneva: WHO. pp.729–881.
31. Grundy SM, Blackburn G, Higgins M, Lauer R, Perri MG, et al. (1999) Physical activity in the prevention and treatment of obesity and its comorbidities: evidence report of independent panel to assess the role of physical activity in the treatment of obesity and its comorbidities. Med Sci Sports Exer 31: 1493–1500.
32. Zhang J, Chaaban J (2013) The economic cost of physical inactivity in China. Prev Med 56: 75–78.
33. Hill J, Melanson E (1999) Overview of the determinants of overweight and obesity: current evidence and research issues. Med Sci Sports Exer 33: S515–521.
34. Palisade Corporation (2013) @RISK software version 6 for Excel. Available: http://www.palisade.com/risk/. Accessed 10 December 2013.
35. Guthold R, Ono T, Strong KL, Chatterji S, Morabia A (2008) Worldwide variability in physical inactivity: A 51-country survey. Am J Prev Med 34: 486–494.
36. Joubert J, Norman R, Lambert EV, Groenewald P, Schneider M, et al. (2007) Estimating the burden of disease attributable to physical inactivity in South Africa in 2000. S Afr Med J 97: 725–731.
37. Lee IM, Shiroma EJ, Lobelo F, Puska P, Blair SN, et al. (2012) Effect of physical inactivity on major non-communicable diseases worldwide: an analysis of burden of disease and life expectancy. Lancet 380: 219–229.
38. Podsakoff PM, Organ DW (1986) Self-Reports in Organizational Research: Problems and Prospects. J Manage 12: 531–544.
39. Adams SA, Matthews CE, Ebbeling CB, Moore CG, Cunningham JE, et al. (2005) The Effect of Social Desirability and Social Approval on Self-Reports of Physical Activity. Am J Epidemiol 161: 389–398.
40. Han D, Yang SB (2008) The reflection on the combination between the nationwide body-building plan and the movement of national health lifestyle. J Sport Sci 29: 47–53.

Peak Oxygen Uptake after Cardiac Rehabilitation: A Randomized Controlled Trial of a 12-Month Maintenance Program versus Usual Care

Erik Madssen[1,2], Ingerid Arbo[1], Ingrid Granøien[3], Liv Walderhaug[3], Trine Moholdt[1,4]*

1 K.G. Jebsen Center of Exercise in Medicine, Department of Circulation and Medical Imaging, Faculty of Medicine, Norwegian University of Science and Technology, Trondheim, Norway, **2** Department of Pulmonary Medicine, St. Olavs Hospital, Trondheim, Norway, **3** Ålesund Hospital, Ålesund, Norway, **4** Women's Clinic, St. Olavs Hospital, Trondheim, Norway

Abstract

Background: Exercise capacity is a strong predictor of survival in patients with coronary artery disease (CAD). Exercise capacity improves after cardiac rehabilitation exercise training, but previous studies have demonstrated a decline in peak oxygen uptake after ending a formal rehabilitation program. There is a lack of knowledge on how long-term exercise adherence can be achieved in CAD patients. We therefore assessed if a 12-month maintenance program following cardiac rehabilitation would lead to increased adherence to exercise and increased exercise capacity compared to usual care.

Materials and Methods: Two-centre, open, parallel randomized controlled trial with 12 months follow-up comparing usual care to a maintenance program. The maintenance program consisted of one monthly supervised high intensity interval training session, a written exercise program and exercise diary, and a maximum exercise test every third month during follow-up. Forty-nine patients (15 women) on optimal medical treatment were included following discharge from cardiac rehabilitation. The primary endpoint was change in peak oxygen uptake at follow-up; secondary endpoints were physical activity level, quality of life and blood markers of cardiovascular risk.

Results: There was no change in peak oxygen uptake from baseline to follow-up in either group (intervention group 27.9 (±4.7) to 28.8 (±5.6) mL·kg (-1) min (−1), control group 32.0 (±6.2) to 32.8 (±5.8) mL·kg (−1) min (−1), with no between-group difference, $p = 0.22$). Quality of life and blood biomarkers remained essentially unchanged, and both self-reported and measured physical activity levels were similar between groups after 12 months.

Conclusions: A maintenance exercise program for 12 months did not improve adherence to exercise or peak oxygen uptake in CAD patients after discharge from cardiac rehabilitation compared to usual care. This suggests that infrequent supervised high intensity interval training sessions are inadequate to improve peak oxygen uptake in this patient group.

Trial Registration: ClinicalTrials.gov NCT01246570

Editor: Terence J. Quinn, University of Glasgow, United Kingdom

Funding: Authors were supported by funds from the Liaison Committee for Central Norway Regional Health Authority and the Norwegian University of Science and Technology, Funds for Medical Research at St. Olavs University Hospital, and the Norwegian Fund for Post-Graduate Training in Physiotherapy. The funders had no role in study design, data collection and analysis, decision to publish, or preparation of the manuscript.

Competing Interests: The authors have declared that no competing interests exist.

* Email: trine.moholdt@ntnu.no

Introduction

Exercise-based rehabilitation in patients with coronary artery disease (CAD) reduces mortality [1–4], and cardiorespiratory fitness is a strong, independent predictor of both cardiac- and all-cause mortality in patients with CAD [5,6]. Therefore, it is important to establish effective exercise programs that patients can adhere to in this patient group. Unfortunately, most beneficial effects from physical activity are lost quite rapidly if regular exercise is discontinued. In line with this, peak oxygen uptake (VO_{2peak}) has been found to decline at six months, and more so at 30 months, after discharge from cardiac rehabilitation in patients with CAD [7]. Thus, there is a need for studies to assess interventions that may help patients adhere to regular and effective exercise training after ending a formalized cardiac rehabilitation exercise program [8]. It is known that high intensity interval training (HIIT) is more effective than continuous training with low-to-moderate intensity with respect to increasing VO_{2peak} in patients with CAD [9], but there is a lack of knowledge regarding long-term effects of HIIT interventions.

The primary aim of this study was therefore to assess if a 12-month maintenance program following discharge from formal cardiac rehabilitation would improve adherence to physical activity and peak oxygen uptake We hypothesized that the maintenance program would lead to an attenuated decline in VO_{2peak} 12 months after ending the formal cardiac rehabilitation, compared with patients in usual care. Secondary endpoints were physical activity level, quality of life and blood markers of cardiovascular risk.

Materials and Methods

Design

The protocol for this trial and supporting CONSORT checklist are available as supporting information; see Checklist S1 and Protocol S1. This was a two-centre, open, parallel randomized controlled trial. The study was approved by the Regional Committee for Medical and Health Research Ethics in Middle-Norway (REK-Midt 2010/86), and registered at clinicaltrials.gov (NCT01246570). Patients gave their informed, written consent before entering the study, and we performed the study according to the Helsinki declaration for medical research. After acquisition of all baseline data, patients were randomized stratified by centre the same day, using a web-based randomization tool, developed and administered by Unit of Applied Clinical Research, Department of Cancer Research and Molecular Medicine, Norwegian University of Science and Technology, Trondheim. Stratified for study centre, patients were randomized either to a maintenance exercise program or to usual care for 12 months with a 1:1 allocation ratio (Figure 1).

Participants

We recruited optimal medically treated patients above 18 years of age from the cardiac rehabilitation centres at St. Olav's University Hospital in Trondheim, and Ålesund Hospital, both in central Norway. Inclusion criteria were completion of a 12-week organized in-hospital cardiac rehabilitation program, consisting of 2 exercise sessions per week, including both HIIT and moderate continuous exercise. Patients were included in the current study 1–2 weeks after ending the formal cardiac rehabilitation program. Patients were excluded if they fulfilled one or more of the following criteria; unstable angina pectoris (chest pain at light physical activity), hemodynamic significant valvular disease (valvular disease confirmed by echocardiography and dyspnoea at light physical activity), chronic obstructive pulmonary disease or chronic heart failure with symptoms at rest or in light physical activity, uncontrolled arterial hypertension (hypertension grade 2 despite medical treatment) chronic renal failure (serum creatinine>140 µmol/L), or pregnancy.

Interventions

Maintenance program group. Patients in the maintenance program group received a written exercise program with the aim of three sessions of high intensity interval training (HIIT) per week, and were invited to attend a monthly supervised exercise session at

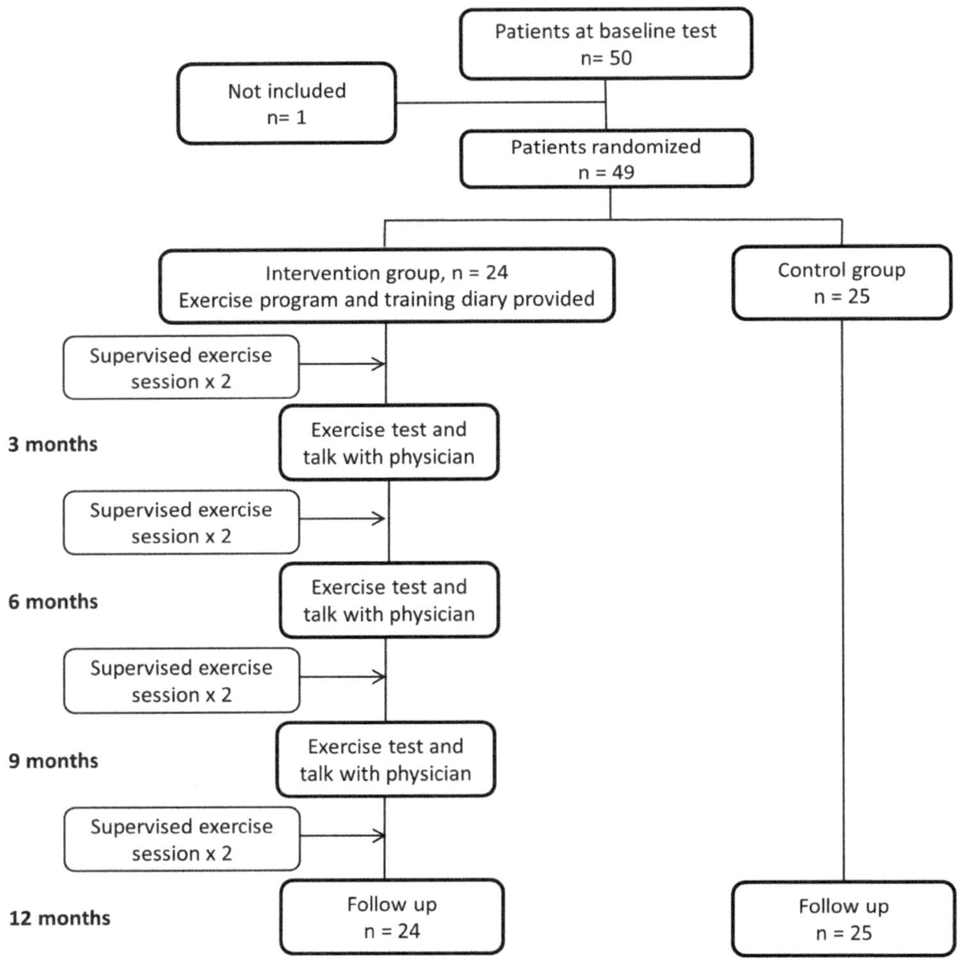

Figure 1. Flow chart of participants throughout the study.

the hospital. The HIIT program was based on protocols from previous studies [10–14], and consisted of 8–10 minutes of warm-up, followed by four times four minutes intervals, with an active pause of three minutes in-between intervals and at the end. The target heart rate was 85–95% of the maximum heart rate as measured at the initial exercise test in intervals, and 70% of maximum heart rate in the active pauses.

During the supervised exercise sessions once per month, patients walked or ran on treadmills (Woodway PPS55, Weil am Rhein, Germany), wearing heart rate monitors (Polar Electro, Kempele, Finland) to ensure that they reached target heart rate. An experienced physiotherapist and/or exercise physiologist instructed and motivated the patients on how to perform HIIT, and patients were asked about their home exercise training and encouraged to maintain a high level of activity. Such instructions have previously been found to be enough to give an acceptable adherence to exercise training during 6 months [10]. The written exercise program also explained in detail how to perform the HIIT, and patients were instructed to perform HIIT as home-based exercise training, as activities which engaged large muscle groups, i.e. walking uphill, running, cross-country skiing, or bicycling. Patients were told to either use a heart rate monitor to ensure that the intensity was adequate, or to exercise with an intensity making them breathe heavily during home exercise training. We gave no advice regarding diet or other lifestyle factors during the follow-up period.

Every third month, patients in the maintenance group did a maximum exercise test as described below. These tests were done to monitor their exercise capacity; to give patients individualized feedback on their VO_{2peak} level, and to ensure them that maximal effort was well tolerated.

Control group. Patients in the control group received no instructions in how to exercise apart from what was given by the rehabilitation staff at the hospitals as usual care. In the two participating hospitals, CAD patients are encouraged to be physically active but are not given any concise exercise prescription. The control group attended baseline and 12 months follow-up tests as described below, without any other contact with the study or hospital personnel.

Outcomes and follow-up

The primary outcome measure was change in VO_{2peak} between baseline and 12 months follow-up. Secondary outcome measures were physical activity level, resting blood pressure, health-related quality of life, cardiometabolic blood markers and anthropometric measurements. In the original study protocol, endothelial function measurements (flow mediated dilatation of the brachial artery) were described. Due to technical issues at one of the participating hospitals, endothelial function could not be included in the study. Physical activity registration was not pre-specified in the original protocol, but during the preparation phase of the study it became clear that such data would be needed and thus physical activity questionnaires and activity monitors were included into the protocol.

Peak oxygen uptake. All patients performed a treadmill cardiopulmonary maximum exercise test at baseline and at follow-up after 12 months, without discontinuation of prescribed medication. Gas exchange data was analysed (Oxycon Pro, Jaeger, Hoechberg, Germany) continuously using mixing chamber, and patients were monitored with a 12-lead electrocardiogram during maximum exercise tests. After 10 minutes of warm-up, we individually adjusted a ramp protocol, by increasing the incline and speed of the treadmill, for the test to last 8–12 minutes as recommended [15]. The test was terminated when the patients reported to be exhausted, or if clinical symptoms occurred. Peak oxygen uptake (VO_{2peak}) was calculated as the mean of the three highest VO_2 measurements during the test, each obtained over a 10-sec average. Peak heart rate was recorded at the end of the test and was not compared to age predicted values as the patients were taking betablockers. We did not use a threshold value of respiratory exchange ratio (RER) as a criterion for reaching VO_{2peak}, but average RER-values obtained during the tests are outlined in the results. Heart rate recovery was defined as the change in heart rate from the peak heart rate to the heart rate after one minute of rest standing on the treadmill.

Physical activity level. All patients reported physical activity level by questionnaires. They were asked how often they exercised (≤ 1, 2–3, ≥ 4 sessions per week), the mean duration of each exercise session (<30, 30–45, 45–60,>60 minutes per session), and the mean intensity-level during sessions (light, medium or hard intensity). In a subgroup of patients (n = 18, 37%), everyday physical activity level was measured with an on-body activity monitoring system (Sensewear, Bodymedia Inc., Pittsburgh, PA, USA) worn for 3–7 days during the first 1–3 weeks and repeated during the last 1–3 weeks in the follow-up period. We measured the numbers of steps taken per day, and the time spent in different activity level zones defined by metabolic equivalents (METs). Sedentary time was defined as activity <3 METs, moderate physical activity was defined as activity ≥ 3 and <6 METs, and vigorous physical activity was defined as ≥ 6 METs.

Resting blood pressure and resting heart rate. Resting systolic and diastolic blood pressure was measured sitting after 10 minutes of rest with a calibrated automated blood pressure monitor (Welch Allyn, Germany). Blood pressure was automatically measured three times by the monitor, and the average value of the two last measurements was used. Resting heart rate was measured, after 10 minutes of rest in supine position, using electrocardiogram. Height was measured to the nearest centimetre and body weight was measured to the nearest 0.1 kg using a Seca 877 scale (Seca Corp, Germany). Body mass index was calculated as body weight in kilograms divided by the square of height in meter. Waist circumference was measured to the nearest half centimetre, using a measuring tape at the height of the umbilicus.

Blood markers. Venous blood samples were drawn after 12 hours of fasting, and analysed using accredited in-hospital procedures for serum glucose, total cholesterol, low-density lipoprotein cholesterol, high-density lipoprotein cholesterol, triglycerides, and high-sensitive C-reactive protein (all using standard commercial kits on a Roche Modular P, Roche, Basel, Switzerland), and glycosylated haemoglobin (Roche Cobas Integra 400).

Health related quality of life. Health related quality of life was measured by MacNew Heart Disease Health-Related Quality of Life Questionnaire [16]. This is a disease-specific questionnaire with a validated Norwegian translation [17]. The questionnaire assesses social, emotional, and physical quality of life using a 1–7 scale. Higher scores indicated better quality of life and a change of 0.5 is found to be clinically significant [16].

Sample size and statistics

A decline in VO_{2peak} of 2.0 $mL \cdot kg^{-1} \cdot min^{-1}$ (SD 4.0) could be expected after 12 months without formal rehabilitation [18]. We anticipated that the intervention program would give an increase of 2.0 $mL \cdot kg^{-1} \cdot min^{-1}$after 12 months, giving a difference of 4.0 $mL \cdot kg^{-1} \cdot min^{-1}$ compared to usual care. This yields a standardised difference of $4/4 = 1$. With a two-tailed t-test for independent samples at a power (1-β) of 0.9 and $\alpha = 0.05$, a total of 44 subjects had to be enrolled [19]. To allow for an expected 10% drop out, we aimed at including 48 patients. The actual statistical analysis performed takes within-person correlation into account and thereby improves power.

Observed data are given as frequencies with percentages in parenthesis, or means ± standard deviation (SD). Baseline characteristics were compared using the chi square test, Mann-Whitney U-test or student t-test where appropriate. Changes from baseline to follow-up are reported with 95% confidence intervals (CI) using a univariate general linear model in the analyses. To test for differences between groups, we used a univariate general linear model analysis of covariance (ANCOVA) with Bonferroni adjustments. In the model, the change in the outcome variable (Δ-values) was the dependent variable, with group as fixed factor and baseline values of the outcome variable as covariates [20]. Between-group differences are reported with 95% CIs and p-values. Within- and between-group differences were considered significant if the 95% CI did not include zero [21]. Physical activity data are only presented as descriptive statistics. All statistical analyses were performed using SPSS (version 20.0, IBM, Chicago, IL, USA).

Results

Forty-nine patients (15 women) were recruited from January 2011 to March 2012 at St.Olav's Hospital and from November 2011 to June 2012 at Ålesund Hospital. Patient characteristics at baseline can be found in Table 1. All registered variables at baseline were comparable between groups except for age, which was lower in the control group ($p<0.05$, Table 1), and VO_{2peak}, which was higher in the control group ($p<0.01$, Table 2).

We experienced no adverse events during maximum exercise testing or training sessions. All participants completed scheduled tests, and the mean attendance at training sessions was 7.8 out of 8 sessions in the intervention group. None of the patients changed their medication use during the study period. During follow-up, two patients in each group were hospitalized. In the intervention group, one patient was diagnosed with a duodenal ulcer and atrial fibrillation, and one patient was diagnosed with chronic lymphatic leukaemia. In the control group, one patient experienced a tibia fracture and one patient underwent surgical treatment for breast carcinoma.

We found no within-group changes in VO_{2peak} from baseline to follow-up, and no between-group difference ($p = 0.22$, Table 2). In the intervention group, VO_{2peak} was at its highest at the third maximum exercise test, and declined slightly at test number four and five (Figure 2). We found no changes in resting heart rate, heart rate recovery, blood pressure, neither within- or between-groups from baseline to follow-up. Blood markers did not change during follow-up in any group (Table 2). Quality of life (social domain) was increased in the control group, but there was no between-group difference ($p = 0.39$).

Self-reported physical activity level is summarized in Table 3. In the intervention group, all patients reported some regular physical activity both at baseline and follow-up, whereas 5 patients in the control group reported no regular physical activity at follow-up. The majority of patients in both groups reported that they had been physically active 2–3 times per week, with duration of 45–60 minutes and with a medium intensity. Physical activity level was adequately monitored in 18 patients (37%). The mean number of steps taken per day was 7024 in the intervention group (10 patients), and 9338 in the control group (8 patients). The mean time spent in sedentary, moderate and vigorous activity level zones per day was 1333 minutes, 58 minutes and 3 minutes in the intervention group. The corresponding numbers in the control

Table 1. Patient characteristics and medication use at baseline.

	Intervention group (n = 24)	Control group (n = 25)
Sex, male/female	18/6	18/7
Age, years (range)	64.4 (47–78)	58.5 (42–71)*
Treatment qualifying for referral to rehabilitation		
PCI	15 (63)	15 (60)
CABG	7 (29)	7 (28)
Valve replacement	2 (8)	1 (4)
Cardiomyopathy	0 (0)	2 (8)
Co-morbidity		
Heart failure	3 (13)	4 (16)
PAD	0 (0)	1 (4)
Hypertension	11 (46)	13 (52)
Diabetes	4 (17)	3 (12)
Medication at baseline		
Aspirin	24 (100)	25 (100)
Clopidogrel	18 (75)	16 (64)
Warfarin	1 (4)	1 (4)
Betablockers	19 (79)	19 (76)
Statins	23 (96)	25 (100)
ACE/ARA	9 (38)	11 (44)

Data are given as numbers with percentages in parenthesis when not otherwise specified. PCI; percutaneous coronary intervention, CABG; coronary artery bypass grafting, PAD; peripheral artery disease, ACE; angiotensin converting enzyme inhibitors, ARA; angiotensin II receptor antagonists. * Between group difference at baseline ($p = 0.02$).

Table 2. Outcome measures at baseline and after 12 months follow-up.

	Intervention group (n = 24)			Control group (n = 25)			ANCOVA	
	Baseline	12 months	Change scores (95% CI)	Baseline	12 months	Change scores (95% CI)	Between-group difference (95% CI)	P value
Exercise test								
VO_{2peak}, ml·kg^{-1}·min^{-1}	27.9±4.7	28.8±5.6	0.9 (−0.6, 2.4)	32.0±6.2	32.8±5.8	0.8 (−0.5, 2.2)	0.6 (−1.5, 2.7)	0.58
VO_{2peak}, ml·min^{-1}	2405±517	2533±576	129 (−18, 275)	2535±760	2614±734	79 (−45, 203)	−0.04 (−0.2, 0.2)	0.70
RER_{peak}	1.09±0.07	1.09±0.09	0.004 (−0.03, 0.04)	1.10±0.07	1.09±0.06	−0.01 (−0.04, 0.01)	−0.01 (−0.05, 0.03)	0.71
HR_{peak}, beats	154.7±13.1	155.8±15.9	1.1 (−5.1, 7.3)	160.6±11.3	161.6±13.1	1.0 (−2.3, 4.2)	1.4 (−5.5, 8.3)	0.68
HR recovery, beats	27.7±11.2	31.2±14.6	3.5 (−1.9, 8.9)	28.9±10.0	30.1±10.2	1.2 (−2.9, 5.4)	−1.7 (−8.3, 4.9)	0.60
Resting measurements								
HR, beats/min	64.0±10.2	65.7±11.6	1.6 (−1.5, 4.8)	61.2±11.5	63.2±11.1	2.0 (−1.4, 5.4)	−0.2 (−4.8, 4.4)	0.92
Systolic BP, mmHg	132.8±14.7	133.7±16.4	0.9 (−4.4, 6.2)	131.3±14.5	134.3±14.0	3.0 (−2.3, 8.2)	1.4 (−5.9, 8.8)	0.69
Diastolic BP, mmHG	78.8±7.2	79.3±7.5	0.5 (−2.1, 3.1)	75.1±10.7	77.5±10.0	2.4 (−1.5, 6.2)	−0.08 (−4.8, 4.6)	0.97
Anthropometric measurements								
Weight, kg	86.8±15.6	89.0±16.5	2.1 (0.8, 3.5)*	79.2±17.8	79.9±17.3	0.7 (−0.8, 2.2)	−1.5 (−3.6, 0.5)	0.14
BMI, kg/m^2	28.0±3.9	28.7±4.1	0.7 (0.2, 1.1)*	25.8±3.3	26.1±3.2	0.3 (−0.2, 0.7)	−0.5 (−1.2, 0.2)	0.16
Waist, cm	101.4±12.1	103.2±11.7	1.8 (0.1, 3.5)*	92.6±9.8	93.0±9.4	0.3 (−0.8, 1.5)	−2.2 (−4.2, −0.1)‡	0.04
Quality of life								
Emotional domain	6.0±0.8	6.0±0.6	0.1 (−0.2, 0.3)	5.7±0.8	6.1±0.8	0.4 (−0.2, 0.7)	0.1 (−0.4, 0.6)	0.69
Physical domain	6.2±0.7	6.3±0.6	0.1 (−0.2, 0.4)	6.3±0.6	6.4±0.5	0.1 (−0.1, 0.3)	0.1 (−0.2, 0.5)	0.40
Social domain	6.4±0.6	6.5±0.4	0.1 (−0.1, 0.3)	6.4±0.6	6.7±0.4	0.3 (0.1, 0.5)*	0.1 (−0.1, 0.4)	0.37
Blood markers								
hsCPR, mg/L	1.09±0.9	1.07±0.6	−0.02 (−0.3, 0.3)	1.2±0.9	1.5±2.5	0.3 (−0.7, 1.3)	0.4 (−0.7, 1.4)	0.51
Cholesterol, mmol/L	4.3±1.0	4.3±0.8	−0.08 (−0.4, 0.2)	3.9±0.6	3.9±0.8	−0.02 (−0.2, 0.2)	−0.1 (−0.5, 0.3)	0.57
LDL, mmol/L	2.2±0.9	2.2±0.7	−0.03 (−0.3, 0.2)	2.0±0.5	2.0±0.6	0.01 (−0.2, 0.2)	−0.0 (−0.4, 0.2)	0.70
HDL, mmol/L	1.5±0.4	1.5±0.4	0.05 (−0.02, 0.13)	1.3±0.4	1.3±0.4	0.004 (−0.05, 0.05)	−0.04 (−0.1, 0.04)	0.34
TG, mmol/L	1.4±0.8	1.2±0.7	−0.19 (−0.4, 0.01)	1.2±0.6	1.3±1.1	0.07 (−0.3, 0.4)	0.2 (−0.2, 0.6)	0.24
Glucose, mmol/L	6.7±3.7	6.4±2.2	−0.3 (−0.6, 0.1)	6.0±1.8	6.2±2.4	0.2 (−0.2, 0.6)	0.3 (−0.4, 1.0)	0.43
HbA1c, %	6.1±1.2	6.0±1.0	−0.1 (−0.2, −0.01)*	6.1±0.7	6.2±1.4	0.1 (−0.1, 0.4)	0.2 (−0.1, 0.6)	0.21

VO_{2peak}; peak oxygen uptake, RER_{peak}; respiratory exchange ratio at peak oxygen uptake, HR_{peak}; peak heart rate, HRR, 1 min; heart rate recovery the first minute after ending an exercise test, HR; resting heart rate, SBP; systolic blood pressure, DBP; diastolic blood pressure, BMI; body mass index, hsCRP; high-sensitive C-reactive protein, LDLc; low-density lipoprotein cholesterol, HDLc; high-density lipoprotein cholesterol, TG; triglycerides, HbA1c; glycosylated haemoglobin.

* indicates within-group changes from baseline to 12 months,

‡ indicates between groups changes in mean difference.

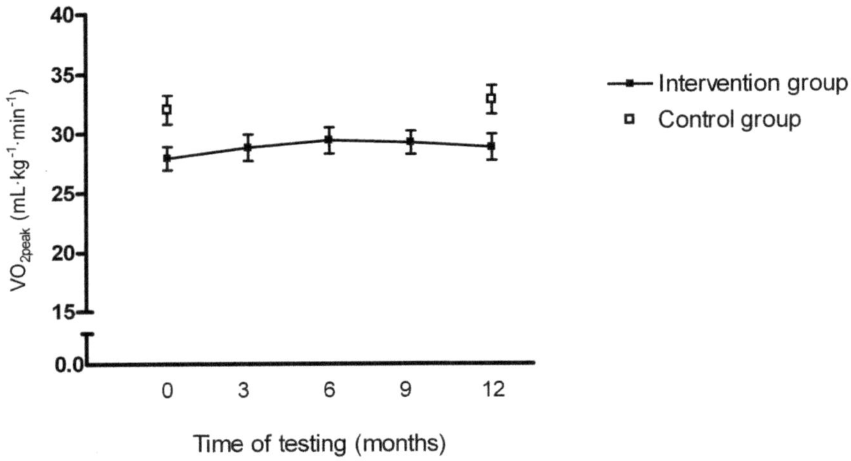

Figure 2. Peak oxygen uptake in the intervention group at baseline, after 3, 6 and 9 months, and at follow-up, and peak oxygen uptake in the control group at baseline and follow-up. The bars represent ± standard error of mean.

group were 1288 minutes, 111 minutes, and 7 minutes, respectively.

Discussion

In this randomized trial we assessed whether patients with CAD discharged from cardiac rehabilitation would benefit with respect to VO_{2peak} by attending a maintenance exercise program for 12 months compared to usual care of no formal follow-up. Our main finding was that the maintenance program did not improve VO_{2peak} compared to usual care. However, neither group deteriorated with respect to exercise capacity during follow-up. This was to us unexpected as exercise capacity has been found to decrease in CAD patients after discharge from formal rehabilitation when the patients were not aware of the last follow-up test [18].

We can only suggest some potential explanations for our findings. Participants enrolled in clinical exercise studies may be highly motivated to perform exercise, especially when they are aware of future follow-up tests. This was illustrated by Gupta et al. [22] who found an increased level of physical activity and 6-minute walking distance at 12 months after discharge from cardiac rehabilitation. Also Izawa et al. [23] demonstrated high exercise maintenance in patients with myocardial infarction 18 months

Table 3. Self-reported physical activity.

	Intervention group (n = 24)		Control group (n = 25)	
	Baseline	**Follow-up**	**Baseline**	**Follow-up**
Self-reported	**n = 19***	**n = 21***	**n = 22***	**n = 22***
Frequency				
No exercise	0 (0)	0 (0)	1 (5)	5 (23)
<1/week	1 (5)	0 (0)	0 (0)	0 (0)
1/week	0 (0)	1 (5)	0 (0)	2 (9)
2–3/week	12 (63)	16 (76)	17 (77)	14 (64)
≥4/week	6 (32)	4 (19)	4 (18)	1 (4)
Duration				
<30 min	0 (0)	1 (5)	1 (5)	0 (0)
30–45 min	6 (31.5)	6 (28.5)	2 (9)	5 (29.5)
45–60 min	10 (52.5)	8 (38)	11 (50)	5 (29.5)
>60 min	3 (16)	6 (28.5)	7 (36)	7 (41)
Intensity				
Low	1 (5)	1 (5)	1 (5)	1 (6)
Medium	16 (84)	11 (52)	13 (62)	10 (59)
High	2 (11)	9 (43)	7 (33)	6 (35)

Data are given as numbers with percentages in parenthesis.
* Valid questionnaires for 19 patients at baseline and 21 patients at follow-up in the intervention group, and 22 patients at baseline and follow-up in the control group.

after cardiac rehabilitation. Both these studies had an observational design without strategies to improve exercise adherence after ending formal rehabilitation, and with patients being aware of future follow-ups. We argue that the knowledge of future follow-up tests by cardiac rehabilitation units may act as a motivation for increased levels of physical activity. This may have also been the case in our study. In fact, the objectively measured physical activity indicated that patients in the control group spent more time in the moderate activity level zone and had a higher daily step count than the patients in the intervention group. Patients randomized to the intervention group were on average 6 years older than in the control group, possibly explaining the tendency for lower level of physical activity in the intervention group. Previous studies have found adherence to physical activity to decline with age [24,25]. However, a previous study found no significant effect of age on improvement in VO_{2peak} after HIIT in patients with CAD [26]. We therefore think that the potential effect of age was on the adherence to exercise rather than on the physiological adaptations to HIIT. Of note, all included patients had some knowledge of HIIT, as this was included in the cardiac rehabilitation program prior to study inclusion.

Several studies have demonstrated that HIIT is superior to moderate continuous exercise in improving VO_{2peak} in patients with CAD [12,27,28] without compromising safety [29]. In the current study, patients in the intervention group were invited to attend a monthly supervised HIIT session at the hospital. However, one monthly session of HIIT is obviously not enough to improve or maintain exercise capacity, and therefore patients also received a training program with the aim of three sessions of HIIT per week. A previous study [10] of home-based HIIT after coronary artery bypass grafting has shown good adherence to such exercise prescription. According to the self-reported physical activity data in the current study, however, only about one third of patients in the intervention group reported that they exercised with high-intensity 2–3 times a week. Thus, a lack of adherence to prescribed exercise at home in the maintenance group is probably the single most important explanation to the lack of VO_{2peak} improvement at 12 months.

Our study may have implications for clinical rehabilitation units. We argue that all patients with CAD enrolled in a rehabilitation program should be offered one or several follow-up sessions, and that a maximum exercise testing should preferably be a part of this follow-up. Our data implies that this type of follow-up may be sufficient to prevent deterioration with respect to VO_{2peak}. However, follow-up programs of infrequent supervised exercise sessions seemed not to be effective. It is possible that a maintenance program with more frequent supervised exercise could have resulted in improvements in VO_{2peak}. In a study of patients with congestive heart failure, Prescott et al. [30] found a small beneficial effect in patients that followed a low-cost maintenance training program with group training sessions every two weeks, indicating that supervised sessions must be more frequent than in our study to result in increased work capacity.

The complete follow-up testing of patients and the high adherence to the supervised exercise are regarded as strengths of our study. Our study is however limited by the fact that the study group consisted of relatively young patients, who probably were quite motivated to exercise without formal follow-up during 12 months. Thus, our results may not be valid for older and less motivated patients with established CAD. Also, neither investigators nor participants were blinded for the study endpoints, which could raise concerns regarding objectivity of testing. However, all patients were told to exercise to complete exhaustion at every exercise test. Further, there was no difference in peak heart rate or peak RER achieved during the baseline and the follow-up test. We also chose to inform the patients in the intervention group about their VO_{2peak} at intermediate tests as we considered it to act motivating for sustained or increase levels of exercise training.

Conclusions

A 12-month maintenance exercise program consisting of infrequent supervised HIIT sessions, a home-based HIIT program and regular exercise testing did not result in improved adherence to exercise or increased VO_{2peak} in CAD patients compared to usual care. However, both the intervention and the control group sustained their VO_{2peak} 12 months after discharge from formal cardiac rehabilitation.

Supporting Information

Checklist S1 CONSORT checklist.

Protocol S1 Study protocol.

Author Contributions

Conceived and designed the experiments: TM EM IA. Performed the experiments: TM EM IA LW IG. Analyzed the data: TM EM. Contributed reagents/materials/analysis tools: IG LW IA TM EM. Wrote the paper: EM TM. Collected all data at Åelsund Hospital: IG LW.

References

1. Jolliffe JA, Rees K, Taylor RS, Thompson D, Oldridge N, et al. (2001) Exercise-based rehabilitation for coronary heart disease. Cochrane Database Syst Rev: CD001800.
2. Taylor RS, Brown A, Ebrahim S, Jolliffe J, Noorani H, et al. (2004) Exercise-based rehabilitation for patients with coronary heart disease: systematic review and meta-analysis of randomized controlled trials. American Journal of Medicine 116: 682–692.
3. Clark AM, Hartling L, Vandermeer B, McAlister FA (2005) Meta-analysis: secondary prevention programs for patients with coronary artery disease. Annals of Internal Medicine 143: 659–672.
4. O'Connor GT, Buring JE, Yusuf S, Goldhaber SZ, Olmstead EM, et al. (1989) An overview of randomized trials of rehabilitation with exercise after myocardial infarction. Circulation 80: 234–244.
5. Myers J, Prakash M, Froelicher V, Do D, Partington S, et al. (2002) Exercise capacity and mortality among men referred for exercise testing. New England Journal of Medicine 346: 793–801.
6. Keteyian SJ, Brawner CA, Savage PD, Ehrman JK, Schairer J, et al. (2008) Peak aerobic capacity predicts prognosis in patients with coronary heart disease. American Heart Journal 156: 292–300.
7. Moholdt T, Aamot IL, Granoien I, Gjerde L, Myklebust G, et al. (2011) Long-term follow-up after cardiac rehabilitation: a randomized study of usual care exercise training versus aerobic interval training after myocardial infarction. International Journal of Cardiology 152: 388–390.
8. Fletcher GF (2007) Cardiac rehabilitation: Something old—something new—more to do. J Cardiopulm Rehabil Prev 27: 21–23.
9. Weston KS, Wisloff U, Coombes JS (2013) High-intensity interval training in patients with lifestyle-induced cardiometabolic disease: a systematic review and meta-analysis. Br J Sports Med. 48: 1227–1234
10. Moholdt T, Bekken Vold M, Grimsmo J, Slordahl SA, Wisloff U (2012) Home-based aerobic interval training improves peak oxygen uptake equal to residential cardiac rehabilitation: a randomized, controlled trial. PLoS One 7: e41199.
11. Moholdt T, Aamot IL, Granoien I, Gjerde L, Myklebust G, et al. (2012) Aerobic interval training increases peak oxygen uptake more than usual care exercise training in myocardial infarction patients: a randomized controlled study. Clin Rehabil 26: 33–44.
12. Rognmo O, Hetland E, Helgerud J, Hoff J, Slordahl SA (2004) High intensity aerobic interval exercise is superior to moderate intensity exercise for increasing aerobic capacity in patients with coronary artery disease. Eur J Cardiovasc Prev Rehabil 11: 216–222.

13. Wisloff U, Stoylen A, Loennechen JP, Bruvold M, Rognmo O, et al. (2007) Superior cardiovascular effect of aerobic interval training versus moderate continuous training in heart failure patients: a randomized study. Circulation 115: 3086–3094.
14. Aamot IL, Forbord SH, Gustad K, Lockra V, Stensen A, et al. (2013) Home-based versus hospital-based high-intensity interval training in cardiac rehabilitation: a randomized study. Eur J Prev Cardiol. doi: 10.1177/2047487313488299
15. Froelicher V, Myers J (2006) Exercise and the heart. 5th edn. Philadelphia: Saunders Elsevier.
16. Hofer S, Lim L, Guyatt G, Oldridge N (2004) The MacNew Heart Disease health-related quality of life instrument: a summary. Health Qual Life Outcomes 2: 3.
17. Hiller A, Helvik AS, Kaasa S, Slordahl SA (2010) Psychometric properties of the Norwegian MacNew Heart Disease health-related quality of life inventory. Eur J Cardiovasc Nurs 9: 146–152.
18. Moholdt T, Aamot IL, Granoien I, Gjerde L, Myklebust G, et al. (2011) Long-term follow-up after cardiac rehabilitation A randomized study of usual care exercise training versus aerobic interval training after myocardial infarction. Int J Cardiol 152: 388–390.
19. Machin D (1997) Sample size tables for clinical studies. 2nd edn. Oxford: Blackwell Science.
20. Vickers AJ, Altman DG (2001) Statistics notes: Analysing controlled trials with baseline and follow up measurements. BMJ 323: 1123–1124.
21. Gardner MJ, Altman DG (1986) Confidence intervals rather than P values: estimation rather than hypothesis testing. Br Med J (Clin Res Ed) 292: 746–750.
22. Gupta R, Sanderson BK, Bittner V (2007) Outcomes at one-year follow-up of women and men with coronary artery disease discharged from cardiac rehabilitation: what benefits are maintained? J Cardiopulm Rehabil Prev 27: 11–18.
23. Izawa KP, Yamada S, Oka K, Watanabe S, Omiya K, et al. (2004) Long-term exercise maintenance, physical activity, and health-related quality of life after cardiac rehabilitation. American Journal of Physical Medicine and Rehabilitation 83: 884–892.
24. Jefferis BJ, Sartini C, Lee IM, Choi M, Amuzu A, et al. (2014) Adherence to physical activity guidelines in older adults, using objectively measured physical activity in a population-based study. BMC Public Health 14: 382.
25. Lohne-Seiler H, Hansen BH, Kolle E, Anderssen SA (2014) Accelerometer-determined physical activity and self-reported health in a population of older adults (65-85 years): a cross-sectional study. BMC Public Health 14: 284.
26. Moholdt T, Madssen E, Rognmo O, Aamot IL (2013) The higher the better? Interval training intensity in coronary heart disease. J Sci Med Sport. doi: 10.1016/j.jsams.2013.07.007
27. Moholdt TT, Amundsen BH, Rustad LA, Wahba A, Lovo KT, et al. (2009) Aerobic interval training versus continuous moderate exercise after coronary artery bypass surgery: a randomized study of cardiovascular effects and quality of life. American Heart Journal 158: 1031–1037.
28. Moholdt T, Aamot IL, Granoien I, Gjerde L, Myklebust G, et al. (2012) Aerobic interval training increases peak oxygen uptake more than usual care exercise training in myocardial infarction patients: a randomized controlled study. Clinical Rehabilitation 26: 33–44.
29. Rognmo O, Moholdt T, Bakken H, Hole T, Molstad P, et al. (2012) Cardiovascular risk of high- versus moderate-intensity aerobic exercise in coronary heart disease patients. Circulation 126: 1436–1440.
30. Prescott E, Hjardem-Hansen R, Dela F, Orkild B, Teisner AS, et al. (2009) Effects of a 14-month low-cost maintenance training program in patients with chronic systolic heart failure: a randomized study. Eur J Cardiovasc Prev Rehabil 16: 430–437.

14

Association between B Vitamins Supplementation and Risk of Cardiovascular Outcomes: A Cumulative Meta-Analysis of Randomized Controlled Trials

Chi Zhang[1], Zhi-Yong Wang[2], Ying-Yi Qin[3], Fei-Fei Yu[3], Yu-Hao Zhou[4]*

1 Department of Neurosurgery, Shanghai Seventh People's Hospital, Shanghai, China, **2** Department of Information, Changhai Hospital, Second Military Medical University, Shanghai, China, **3** Department of Health Statistics, Second Military Medical University, Shanghai, China, **4** Department of Rehabilitation Institute, Shanghai Seventh People's Hospital, Shanghai, China

Abstract

Background: Observational studies suggest that B vitamin supplementation reduces cardiovascular risk in adults, but this association remains controversial. This study aimed to summarize the evidence from randomized controlled trials (RCTs) investigating B vitamin supplementation for the primary or secondary prevention of major adverse cardiovascular outcomes and to perform a cumulative meta-analysis to determine the evidence base.

Methodology and Principal Findings: In April 2013, we searched PubMed, Embase, and the Cochrane Library to identify relevant RCTs. We included RCTs investigating the effect of B vitamin supplementation on cardiovascular outcome. Relative risk (RR) was used to measure the effect using a random-effect model. Statistical heterogeneity scores were assessed using the Q statistic. We included data on 57,952 individuals from 24 RCTs: 12 primary prevention trials and 12 secondary prevention trials. In 23 of these trials, 10,917 major adverse cardiovascular events (MACE) occurred; in 20 trials, 7,203 deaths occurred; in 15 trials, 3,422 cardiac deaths occurred; in 19 trials, 3,623 myocardial infarctions (MI) occurred; and in 18 trials, 2,465 strokes occurred. B vitamin supplementation had little or no effect on the incidence of MACE (RR, 0.98; 95% confidence interval [CI]: 0.93–1.03; $P = 0.37$), total mortality (RR, 1.01; 95% CI: 0.97–1.05; $P = 0.77$), cardiac death (RR, 0.96; 95% CI: 0.90–1.02; $P = 0.21$), MI (RR, 0.99; 95% CI: 0.93–1.06; $P = 0.82$), or stroke (RR, 0.94; 95% CI: 0.85–1.03; $P = 0.18$).

Conclusion/Significance: B vitamin supplementation, when used for primary or secondary prevention, is not associated with a reduction in MACE, total mortality, cardiac death, MI, or stroke.

Editor: Vincenzo Lionetti, Scuola Superiore Sant'Anna, Italy

Funding: This study was funded by Disciplines Group Construction Project of Pudong Health Bureau of Shanghai (PWZxkq2011-01) and Shanghai key speciality of traditional Chinese medicine (ZYXK2012010). The funders had no role in study design, data collection and analysis, decision to publish, or preparation of the manuscript.

Competing Interests: The authors have declared that no competing interests exist.

* Email: zhou_ly@126.com

These authors contributed equally to this work.

Introduction

The potential role of B vitamins (folate, B6, and B12) in reducing cardiovascular risk has been supported by observational studies [1–5]. Although the mechanism of action is unclear, B vitamins may affect cardiovascular outcome by lowering homocysteine concentrations, which correlate strongly with the risk of coronary disease [1–5] and stroke [6–8]. A meta-analysis [9] of observational studies suggested that lowering the plasma homocysteine level by 25% reduced the risk of coronary heart disease by 11% and the risk of stroke by 19%. Daily supplementation with folic acid has been shown to lower the plasma homocysteine level by approximately 25% and adding vitamin B12 further lowers the level by approximately 7%, indicating that B vitamins supplements lower homocysteine levels significantly [10–11]. Despite its ability to lower homocysteine levels, meta-analyses of randomized controlled trials (RCTs) [12–19] indicate that, although folic acid supplementation may reduce the risk of stroke in specific subsets of patients, it is not associated with a reduction in a composite of all-cause death, nonfatal acute myocardial infarction (MI), acute hospitalization for unstable angina pectoris, and nonfatal thromboembolic stroke (MACE), MI, cardiac death, or total mortality. The association between B vitamin supplementation and reduction of cardiovascular risk has not been confirmed by a RCT [20–31]. Furthermore, previous meta-analyses have not investigated the potential interaction of supplementation with both vitamin B6 and B12 on cardiovascular risk [12–17,19].

The effect of B vitamin supplementation on primary and secondary prevention of adverse cardiovascular outcomes has been studied in numerous RCTs [20–43]. In this study, we performed a meta-analysis of these RCTs to evaluate the effect of

Table 1. Design and characteristic of trials included in our meta-analysis*.

Source	Publication year	No. of patients	Mean age, y	Percentage male (%)	Background fortification	Disease status	Primary/ Secondary prevention	Baseline folate status (nmol/L)	Baseline homocysteine (μmol/L)	Net decrease in homocysteine (μmol/L)	Intervention	Follow-up (year)	Jadad score
Baker F(20)	2002	1882	NG	NG	No	CHD	Secondary	NG	11.2	−1.5	5.0 mg folic acid; placebo	1.7	1
The Swiss Heart Study (21)	2002	553	63	80	No	Coronary angioplasty	Secondary	NG	11.2	−2.9	1.0 mg folic acid, 10 mg vitamin B6, and 0.4 mg vitamin B12; Placebo	1.0	3
M Righetti (32)	2003	81	64	56	No	ESRD	Primary	6.06	50.3	−26.0	25 mg folic acid; 5 mg folic acid; untreated	1.0	1
VISP Trial Investigators (22)	2004	3680	66	63	Yes	Ischemic stroke	Secondary	NG	12.3	−2.1	25 mg of vitamin B6, 0.4 mg of vitamin B12, and 2.5 mg of folic acid; 200 μg of vitamin B6, 6 μg of vitamin B12, and 20 μg of folic acid	2.0	5
A Liem(23)	2004	283	59	69	No	CHD	Secondary	NG	NG	NG	5 mg folic acid; placebo	1.0	2
EM Wrone (33)	2004	510	60	50	Yes	ESRD	Primary	47.07	32.9	−3.6	15 mg folic acid, 12.5 mg vitamin B6, 6 μg vitamin B12; 5 mg folic acid, 12.5 mg vitamin B6, 6 μg vitamin B12; 1 mg folic acid, 12.5 mg vitamin B6, 6 μg vitamin B12	2.0	4
H Lange(24)	2004	636	61	77	No	Coronary Stenting	Secondary	NG	12.6	−3.6	1.2 mg of folic acid, 48 mg of vitamin B6,and 60 μg of vitamin B12; placebo	0.7	3
A Liem(25)	2005	593	65	78	No	CHD	Secondary	16	12.1	−1.3	0.5 mg folic acid; usual care	3.2	3
NORVIT Trial Investigators (26)	2006	3749	63	74	No	MI	Secondary	10.95	13.1	−2.3	0.8 mg of folic acid, 0.4 mg of vitamin B12, and 40 mg of vitamin B6; placebo	3.3	5

Table 1. Cont.

Source	Publication year	No. of patients	Mean age, y	Percentage male (%)	Background fortification	Disease status	Primary/ Secondary prevention	Baseline folate status (nmol/L)	Baseline homocysteine (μmol/L)	Net decrease in homocysteine (μmol/L)	Intervention	Follow-up (year)	Jadad score
(HOPE) 2 Investigators (27)	2006	5522	69	72	Parial	DM or vascular disease	Secondary	28.0	12.2	−3.3	2.5 mg of folic acid, 50 mg of vitamin B6, and 1 mg of vitamin B12; placebo	5.0	4
ASFAST Study Group(34)	2006	315	56	68	Yes	ESRD	Primary	NG	27.0	−4.7	15 mg folic acid; placebo	3.6	4
M Righetti(35)	2006	114	64	55	No	Hemodialysis	Primary	22.32	31.7	−15.1	5 mg folic acid plus vitamin B1 250 mg, vitamin B6 250 mg, vitamin B12 500 μg; untreated	2.4	2
ACA Vianna (36)	2007	186	48	59	No	ESRD	Primary	9.99	24.6	−10.5	Folic acid 10 mg 3 times a week; placebo	2.0	2
Polyp Prevention Study Group (37)	2007	1021	57	64	Yes	Colorectal adenomas	Primary	23.70	9.8	NG	1 mg/d of folic acid daily; placebo	7.0	4
Veterans Affairs Site Investigators (38)	2007	2056	66	98	Yes	CKD or ESRD and high tHcy	Primary	35.34	22.4	−5.1	40 mg of folic acid, 100 mg of vitamin B6, and 2 mg of vitamin B12; placebo	3.2	4
WAFACS Study Group(39)	2008	5442	63	0	No	Health professionals	Primary	NG	NG	NG	2.5 mg of folic acid, 50 mg of vitamin B6, and 1 mg of vitamin B12; placebo	7.3	3
WENBIT Study Group(28)	2008	3096	62	80	No	Coronary angiography	Secondary	NG	11.1	−2.8	Folic acid, 0.8 mg, plus vitamin B12, 0.4 mg, plus vitamin B6, 40 mg; folic acid plus vitamin B12; vitaminB6 alone; placebo	3.1	4
BVAIT Research Group(40)	2009	506	61	61	Yes	Initial tHcy>8.5 umol/L	Primary	21.41	9.6	−2.1	5 mg folic acid, 0.4 mg vitamin B12 plus 50 mg vitamin B6; placebo	3.1	3

Table 1. Cont.

Source	Publication year	No. of patients	Mean age, y	Percentage male (%)	Background fortification	Disease status	Primary/ Secondary prevention	Baseline folate status (nmol/L)	Baseline homocysteine (μmol/L)	Net decrease in homocysteine (μmol/L)	Intervention	Follow-up (year)	Jadad score
DIVINe Study Group(41)	2010	238	60	75	Yes	Diabetic nephropathy	Primary	35.12	15.6	−4.8	2.5 mg folic acid, 25 mg vitamin B6, and 1 mg vitamin B12; placebo	3.0	4
J Heinz(42)	2010	650	61	58	No	ESRD	Primary	14.1	29.0	−8.6	2.5 mg folic acid, 25 μg vitamin B12, and 10 mg vitamin B6; 0.1 mg folic acid, 2 μg vitamin B12, and 0.5 mg vitamin B6	2.1	5
SEARCH Collaborative Group(29)	2010	12064	64	83	No	MI	Secondary	16.76	13.5	−3.8	2 mg folic acid plus 1 mg vitamin B12 daily; placebo	6.7	4
SU.FOL.OM3 Collaborative Group(30)	2010	2501	61	79	No	MI, angina, or ischaemic stroke	Secondary	15.29	12.8	−2.7	5-methyltetrah-ydrofolate (560 μg), vitamin B-6 (3 mg), and vitamin B-12 (20 μg); placebo	4.7	5
FAVORIT Study Group(43)	2011	4110	52	63	Yes	Kidney transplant recipients	Primary	NG	16.4	−4.1	5.0 mg folic acid, 50 mg vitamin B6, and 1.0 mg vitamin B12; 1.4 mg vitamin B6 and 0.002 mg vitamin B12	4.0	4
VITATOPS Study Group(31)	2012	8164	63	64	Partial	TIA or stroke	Secondary	NG	14.3	−3.8	2 mg folic acid, 25 mg vitamin B6, and 0·5 mg vitamin B12; placebo	3.4	5

*CHD: coronary heart disease; ESRD: End-stage renal disease; MI: myocardial infarction; DM: diabetes mellitus; CKD: chronic kidney disease; TIA: transient ischaemic attack; NG: not give.

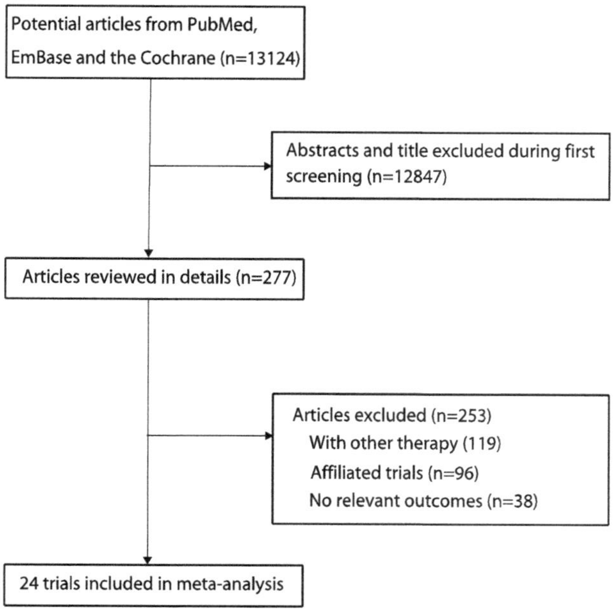

Figure 1. Flow diagram of the literature search and trials selection process.

B vitamin supplementation on cardiovascular risk in specific subpopulations and attempt to determine the role of folic acid supplementation interaction with vitamin B6 and B12 in reducing cardiovascular risk. Furthermore, we used cumulative meta-analysis to determine the evidence base for routine B vitamin supplementation in clinical practice.

Methods

Data Sources, Search Strategy, and Selection Criteria

This review was conducted and reported according to the Preferred Reporting Items for Systematic Reviews and Meta-Analysis Statement, 2009 (Checklist S1) [44]. RCTs evaluating the effect of B vitamin supplementation on cardiovascular risk written in the English language were included in our study, regardless of the publication status (published, in press, or in progress) and the effect of B vitamin supplementation on MACE, total mortality, cardiac death, MI, and stroke were examined. Relevant trials were identified using the following procedure:

(1) Electronic searches: we searched PubMed, Embase, and the Cochrane Central Register of Controlled Trials electronic databases for articles published through April 2013, using "B vitamins" AND "randomized controlled trials" AND "clinical trials" AND "human" AND "English" as the search terms.

(2) Other sources: we searched ongoing RCTs in the metaRegister of Controlled Trials, which lists trials that are registered as completed but not yet published. Furthermore, we reviewed bibliographies of publications for potentially relevant

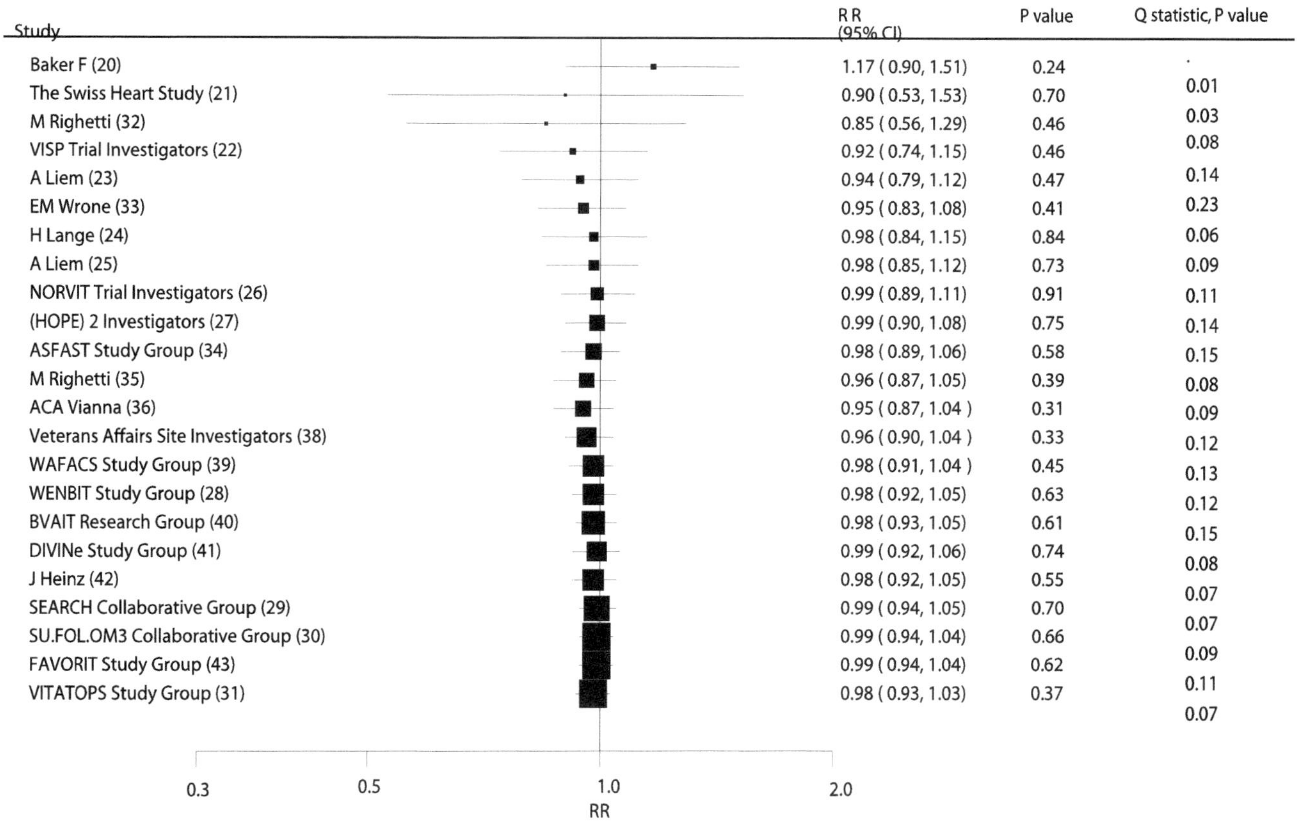

Figure 2. Cumulative meta-analysis of the B vitamins supplementation for major adverse cardiovascular event. RR, relative risk; CI, confidence interval.

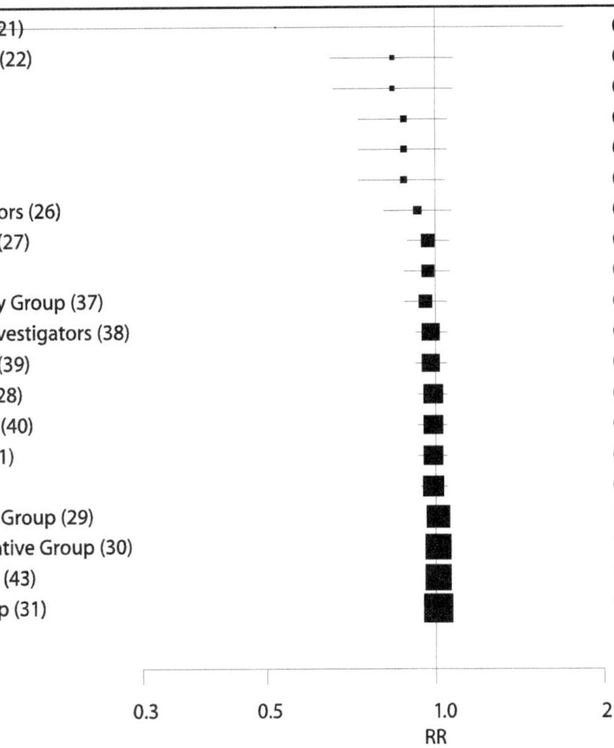

Study	RR (95% CI)	P value	Q statistic, P value
The Swiss Heart Study (21)	0.52 (0.16, 1.70)	0.28	.
VISP Trial Investigators (22)	0.84 (0.65, 1.08)	0.17	0.41
A Liem (23)	0.84 (0.66, 1.08)	0.17	0.71
EM Wrone (33)	0.88 (0.73, 1.05)	0.15	0.82
H Lange (24)	0.88 (0.73, 1.05)	0.16	0.92
A Liem (25)	0.88 (0.73, 1.04)	0.14	0.97
NORVIT Trial Investigators (26)	0.93 (0.81, 1.07)	0.34	0.88
(HOPE) 2 Investigators (27)	0.97 (0.89, 1.06)	0.47	0.90
M Righetti (35)	0.97 (0.88, 1.06)	0.44	0.94
Polyp Prevention Study Group (37)	0.96 (0.88, 1.05)	0.34	0.79
Veterans Affairs Site Investigators (38)	0.98 (0.92, 1.05)	0.64	0.78
WAFACS Study Group (39)	0.98 (0.92, 1.05)	0.59	0.85
WENBIT Study Group (28)	0.99 (0.93, 1.05)	0.66	0.87
BVAIT Research Group (40)	0.99 (0.93, 1.05)	0.65	0.85
DIVINe Study Group (41)	0.99 (0.93, 1.05)	0.66	0.89
J Heinz (42)	0.99 (0.94, 1.05)	0.81	0.89
SEARCH Collaborative Group (29)	1.01 (0.96, 1.06)	0.79	0.90
SU.FOL.OM3 Collaborative Group (30)	1.01 (0.97, 1.06)	0.55	0.54
FAVORIT Study Group (43)	1.01 (0.97, 1.06)	0.54	0.61
VITATOPS Study Group (31)	1.01 (0.97, 1.05)	0.77	0.62

Figure 3. Cumulative meta-analysis of the B vitamins supplementation for total mortality. RR, relative risk; CI, confidence interval.

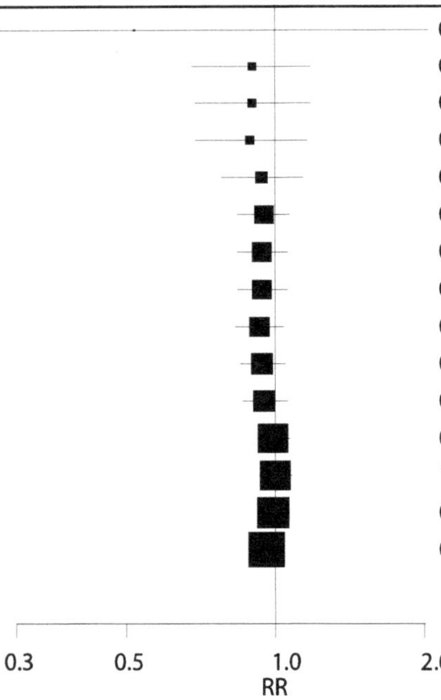

Study	RR (95% CI)	P value	Q statistic, P value
The Swiss Heart Study (21)	0.52 (0.13, 2.04)	0.35	.
VISP Trial Investigators (22)	0.90 (0.68, 1.18)	0.45	0.42
A Liem (23)	0.90 (0.69, 1.18)	0.46	0.72
A Liem (25)	0.89 (0.69, 1.16)	0.39	0.85
NORVIT Trial Investigators (26)	0.94 (0.78, 1.14)	0.53	0.89
(HOPE) 2 Investigators (27)	0.95 (0.84, 1.07)	0.37	0.95
ASFAST Study Group (34)	0.94 (0.84, 1.06)	0.34	0.98
M Righetti (35)	0.94 (0.84, 1.06)	0.30	0.98
ACA Vianna (36)	0.93 (0.83, 1.04)	0.22	0.97
WAFACS Study Group (39)	0.94 (0.85, 1.05)	0.28	0.98
J Heinz (42)	0.95 (0.86, 1.06)	0.36	0.97
SEARCH Collaborative Group (29)	0.99 (0.92, 1.07)	0.79	0.96
SU.FOL.OM3 Collaborative Group (30)	1.00 (0.93, 1.08)	0.97	0.77
FAVORIT Study Group (43)	0.99 (0.92, 1.06)	0.73	0.72
VITATOPS Study Group (31)	0.96 (0.90, 1.02)	0.21	0.56

Figure 4. Cumulative meta-analysis of the B vitamins supplementation for cardiac death. RR, relative risk; CI, confidence interval.

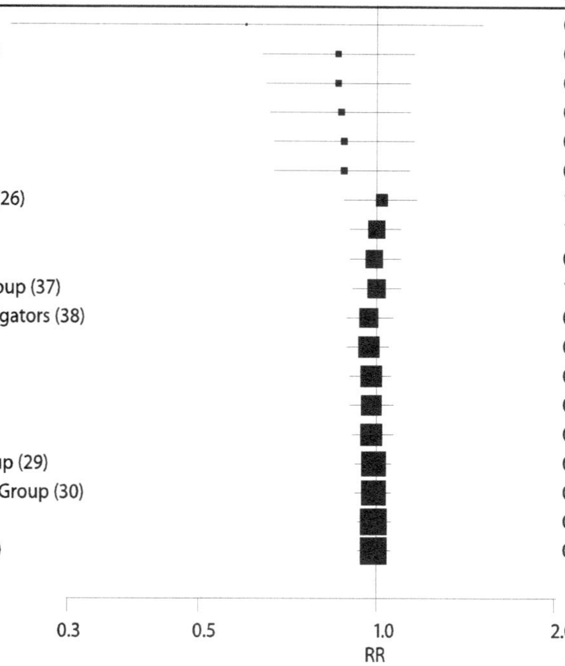

Study	RR (95% CI)	P value	Q statistic, P value
The Swiss Heart Study (21)	0.60 (0.24, 1.51)	0.28	.
VISP Trial Investigators (22)	0.86 (0.64, 1.16)	0.33	0.41
A Liem (23)	0.86 (0.65, 1.14)	0.29	0.71
EM Wrone (33)	0.87 (0.66, 1.14)	0.32	0.84
H Lange (24)	0.88 (0.67, 1.16)	0.36	0.88
A Liem (25)	0.88 (0.67, 1.14)	0.33	0.94
NORVIT Trial Investigators (26)	1.02 (0.88, 1.17)	0.82	0.82
(HOPE) 2 Investigators (27)	1.00 (0.90, 1.10)	0.96	0.88
M Righetti (35)	0.99 (0.90, 1.10)	0.90	0.85
Polyp Prevention Study Group (37)	1.00 (0.91, 1.10)	0.99	0.78
Veterans Affairs Site Investigators (38)	0.97 (0.89, 1.07)	0.57	0.70
WAFACS Study Group (39)	0.97 (0.89, 1.05)	0.45	0.74
WENBIT Study Group (28)	0.98 (0.90, 1.06)	0.61	0.75
DIVINe Study Group (41)	0.98 (0.90, 1.07)	0.67	0.71
J Heinz (42)	0.98 (0.91, 1.07)	0.68	0.77
SEARCH Collaborative Group (29)	0.99 (0.92, 1.06)	0.75	0.82
SU.FOL.OM3 Collaborative Group (30)	0.99 (0.92, 1.06)	0.71	0.86
FAVORIT Study Group (43)	0.99 (0.93, 1.06)	0.77	0.89
VITATOPS Study Group (31)	0.99 (0.93, 1.06)	0.82	0.92

Figure 5. Cumulative meta-analysis of the B vitamins supplementation for myocardial infarction. RR, relative risk; CI, confidence interval.

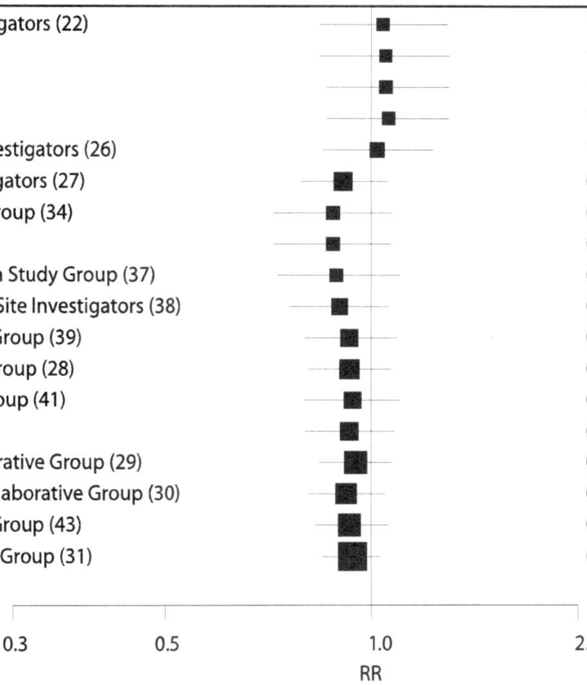

Study	RR (95% CI)	P value	Q statistic, P value
VISP Trial Investigators (22)	1.04 (0.84, 1.29)	0.71	.
A Liem (23)	1.05 (0.84, 1.30)	0.68	0.51
EM Wrone (33)	1.05 (0.86, 1.30)	0.62	0.78
A Liem (25)	1.06 (0.86, 1.30)	0.59	0.90
NORVIT Trial Investigators (26)	1.02 (0.85, 1.23)	0.80	0.89
(HOPE) 2 Investigators (27)	0.91 (0.79, 1.06)	0.23	0.43
ASFAST Study Group (34)	0.88 (0.72, 1.07)	0.21	0.26
M Righetti (35)	0.88 (0.72, 1.07)	0.19	0.25
Polyp Prevention Study Group (37)	0.89 (0.73, 1.10)	0.29	0.23
Veterans Affairs Site Investigators (38)	0.90 (0.76, 1.06)	0.20	0.31
WAFACS Study Group (39)	0.93 (0.80, 1.09)	0.40	0.26
WENBIT Study Group (28)	0.93 (0.81, 1.07)	0.30	0.33
DIVINe Study Group (41)	0.94 (0.80, 1.10)	0.43	0.22
J Heinz (42)	0.93 (0.80, 1.08)	0.33	0.26
SEARCH Collaborative Group (29)	0.95 (0.84, 1.07)	0.40	0.28
SU.FOL.OM3 Collaborative Group (30)	0.92 (0.81, 1.05)	0.24	0.19
FAVORIT Study Group (43)	0.93 (0.83, 1.06)	0.28	0.22
VITATOPS Study Group (31)	0.94 (0.85, 1.03)	0.18	0.27

Figure 6. Cumulative meta-analysis of the B vitamins supplementation for stroke. RR, relative risk; CI, confidence interval.

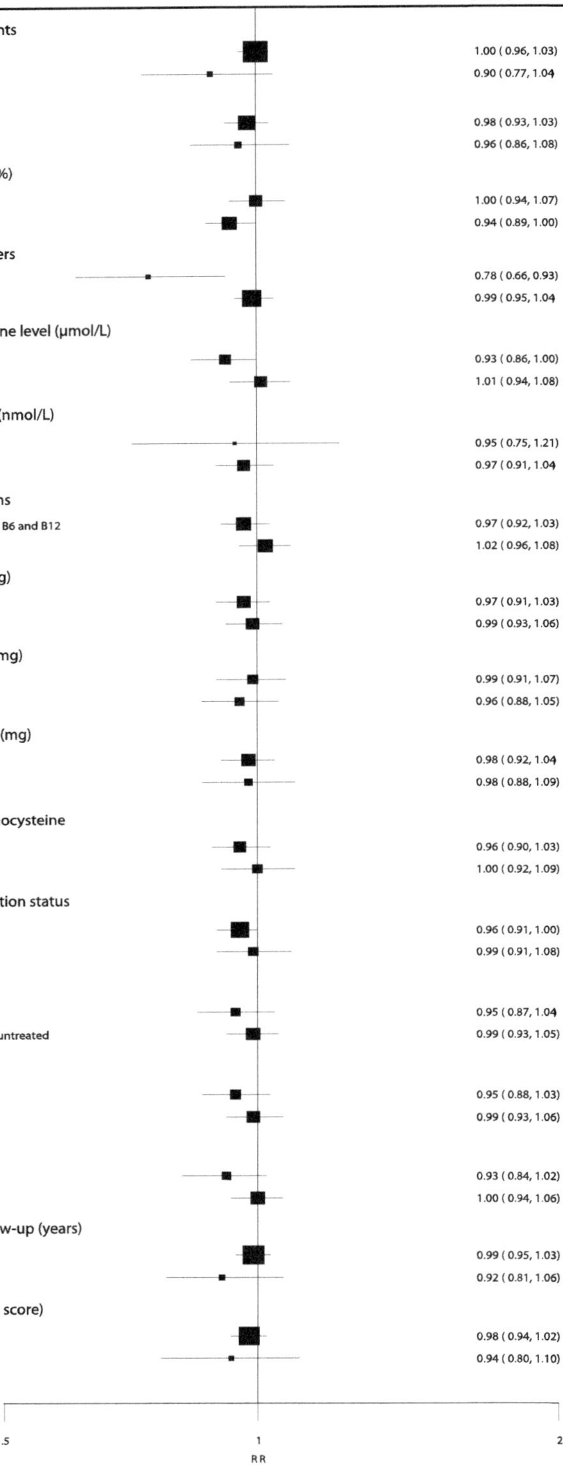

Study	RR (95% CI)	P value	Q statistic, P value	P value for interaction test
Number of participants				
1000 or more	1.00 (0.96, 1.03)	0.899	0.470	0.181
<1000	0.90 (0.77, 1.04	0.149	0.064	
Mean age (years)				
62 or more	0.98 (0.93, 1.03)	0.424	0.085	0.746
<62	0.96 (0.86, 1.08)	0.528	0.196	
Percentage of men (%)				
65 or more	1.00 (0.94, 1.07)	0.914	0.078	0.164
<65	0.94 (0.89, 1.00)	0.034	0.466	
Number of trial centers				
single–center	0.78 (0.66, 0.93)	0.005	0.613	0.008
multi–cencer	0.99 (0.95, 1.04	0.806	0.162	
Baseline homocysteine level (μmol/L)				
>14	0.93 (0.86, 1.00)	0.051	0.196	0.115
14 or less	1.01 (0.94, 1.08)	0.739	0.147	
Baseline folate level (nmol/L)				
Low (<11 nmol/L)	0.95 (0.75, 1.21)	0.720	0.265	0.869
Normal (11–54 nmol/L)	0.97 (0.91, 1.04	0.390	0.186	
Intervention regimens				
Folic acid plus vitamins B6 and B12	0.97 (0.92, 1.03)	0.381	0.049	0.227
Folic acid	1.02 (0.96, 1.08)	0.552	0..481	
Dose of folic acid (mg)				
>2.5	0.97 (0.91, 1.03)	0.302	0.487	0.657
2.5 or less	0.99 (0.93, 1.06)	0.772	0.026	
Dose of vitamin B6 (mg)				
>40	0.99 (0.91, 1.07)	0.772	0.124	0.615
40 or less	0.96 (0.88, 1.05)	0.398	0.070	
Dose of vitamin B12 (mg)				
>0.4	0.98 (0.92, 1.04	0.513	0.060	1.000
0.4 or less	0.98 (0.88, 1.09)	0.739	0.086	
Net decrease in homocysteine				
20% or more	0.96 (0.90, 1.03)	0.267	0.017	0.460
<20%	1.00 (0.92, 1.09)	0.978	0.553	
Background fortification status				
Yes or partial	0.96 (0.91, 1.00)	0.061	0.545	0.537
No	0.99 (0.91, 1.08)	0.856	0.058	
Control				
Low dose B vitamins	0.95 (0.87, 1.04	0.230	0.763	0.454
Usual care, placebo or untreated	0.99 (0.93, 1.05)	0.653	0.037	
Disease prevention				
Primary	0.95 (0.88, 1.03)	0.235	0.216	0.430
Secondary	0.99 (0.93, 1.06)	0.858	0.070	
Renal status				
Yes	0.93 (0.84, 1.02)	0.131	0.172	0.213
No	1.00 (0.94, 1.06)	0.937	0.117	
The duration of follow-up (years)				
3 or more	0.99 (0.95, 1.03)	0.729	0.327	0.306
<3	0.92 (0.81, 1.06)	0.251	0.043	
Study quality (Jadad score)				
4 or 5	0.98 (0.94, 1.02)	0.397	0.267	0.619
<4	0.94 (0.80, 1.10)	0.425	0.039	

Figure 7. Subgroup analysis for the effect of B vitamins supplementation on major cardiovascular events. RR, relative risk; CI, confidence interval.

trials. Medical subject headings, methods, patient population, interventions, and outcome variables of these studies were used to identify relevant trials.

The literature search, data extraction, and quality assessment were undertaken by 2 investigators (CZ and PJM) independently with a standardized approach. Any inconsistencies between these investigators were identified by the primary investigator (YHZ) and resolved by consensus. We restricted our study to RCTs, which are less likely than observational studies to be subject to confounding variables or bias. A study was eligible for inclusion in our meta-analysis if the following criteria were met: (1) the study was a RCT; (2) the trial evaluated the effects of B vitamin supplementation compared with placebo; (3) the study's follow-up continued for at least 6 months; and (4) the trial reported at least 1 of the following outcomes: MACE, total mortality, cardiac death, MI, or stroke.

Data Collection and Quality Assessment

All data from included trials was extracted independently by 2 investigators (CZ and PJM) using a standardized protocol. Each data set was reviewed by a third investigator (YHZ), and any discrepancies between the 2 investigator's data were resolved by discussion. The data collected from each study included first author or study group name, publication year, study design, type of blinding, number of patients, percentage of men, mean age, background fortification, current disease status, baseline total homocysteine level, baseline folate level, intervention regimens, controls, and the duration of follow-up. The outcomes investigated included MACE, total mortality, cardiac death, MI, and stroke. Study quality was assessed using the Jadad score [45], which is based on the 5 following subscales: randomization (1 or 0), concealment of the treatment allocation (1 or 0), blinding (1 or 0), completeness of follow-up (1 or 0), and the use of intention-to-treat analysis (1 or 0). A score system ranging from 1 to 5 has been developed for quality assessment.

Statistical Analysis

We assigned the results of each RCT as dichotomous frequency data. Individual study relative risks (RR) and 95% confidence intervals (CI) were calculated from event numbers extracted from each trial before data pooling. The overall RR and 95% CI of MACE, total mortality, cardiac death, MI, and stroke were also calculated. Both fixed-effect and random-effect models were used to evaluate the pooled RR for B vitamin supplementation compared with placebo. Although both models yielded similar findings, results from the random-effect model, which assume that the true underlying effect varies among included trials, are presented here [46–47]. Heterogeneity of the treatment effect between studies was evaluated using the Q statistic, and P values <0.10 were considered statistically significant [48–49]. In the cumulative meta-analysis, outcome data for MACE, total mortality, cardiac death, MI, and stroke from all available trials were included sequentially according to the year in which they first became available.

We explored potential sources of heterogeneity in estimates of the treatment effect on MACE with univariate meta-regression [50] (for number of participants, mean age, percentage of men, baseline homocysteine level, baseline folate level, dose of folic acid, dose of vitamin B6, dose of vitamin B12, net decrease in homocysteine level, and duration of follow-up). Subsequently, subgroup analyses were conducted for MACE on the basis of number of participants, mean age, percentage of men, number of trial centers, baseline homocysteine level, baseline folate level, intervention regimens, dose of folic acid, dose of vitamin B6, dose of vitamin B12, net decrease in homocysteine level, background fortification, control, disease prevention, renal status, duration of follow-up, and Jadad score [45]. Interaction tests [51] were performed to compare differences between estimates of the 2 subsets, which were based on Student *t* distribution rather than on normal distribution because the number of included studies was small. We also performed a sensitivity analysis by removing each individual trial from the meta-analysis [52]. Several methods were used to check for potential publication bias. Visual inspection of funnel plots for MACE, total mortality, cardiac death, MI, and stroke were conducted. The Egger (53) and Begg test (54) were used to statistically assess publication bias for MACE, total mortality, cardiac death, MI, and stroke. All reported P values were two-sided, and P values of <0.05 were considered statistically significant for all included studies. Statistical analyses were performed using STATA software (version 10.0 StataCorp, Texas, USA).

Results

Search of the Published Literature

We identified 13,124 articles during our initial electronic search, of which 12,847 were excluded during an initial review of the titles and abstracts. We retrieved the full text for the remaining 277 articles, and 24 RCTs [20–43] met the inclusion criteria of our meta-analysis (**Figure 1**). B vitamin supplementation for primary prevention of major cardiovascular outcome was studied in 12 trials [32–43], and the remaining 12 trials studied its use for secondary prevention [20–31].

Characteristics of the Included Studies

Tables 1 and S1 summarizes the baseline characteristics of the 57,952 individuals included in the trials investigated. The follow-up period for participants ranged from 0.7 to 7.3 years, the number of individuals included in each trial ranged from 81 to 12064, and the net change in total homocysteine level ranged from 1.3 to 26.0 μmol/L. In the intervention groups, the dose of folic acid ranged from 0.5 to 40 mg/day, the dose of vitamin B6 ranged from 3 to 250 mg/day, and the dose of vitamin B12 ranged from 6 to 2000 μg/day. In the meta-analysis, the trial outcome was MACE in 23 trials [20–36,38–43], total mortality in 20 trials [21–31,33,35,37–43], cardiac death in 15 trials [21–23,25–27,29–31,34–36,39,42,43], MI in 19 trials [21–31,33,35,37–39,41–43], and stroke in 18 trials [22,23,25–31,33–35,37–39,41–43]. We restricted the inclusion criteria to RCTs with a minimum follow-up of 6 months to ensure a reliable conclusion.

Risk of Bias in Individual Trials

The quality of the trials was assessed using the Jadad score (45) and are summarized in **Table 1**. We considered a score ≥4 to indicate a high-quality study. Five trials [22,26,30,31,42] had a Jadad score of 5, 9 trials [27–29,33,34,37,38,41,43] scored 4, 5 trials [21,24,35,39,40] scored 3, 3 trials [23,35,36] scored 2, and the remaining 2 trials [20,32] scored 1.

Effects of B Vitamins on Major Cardiovascular Outcomes

Data from 56,925 individuals was used to assess the effect of B vitamin supplementation on MACE and included 10,917 MACE. Overall, B vitamin supplementation reduced the risk of MACE by 2%, but this was not statistically significant (RR, 0.98; 95% CI: 0.93–1.03; P = 0.37, **Figure 2** and **Figure S1**). Heterogeneity was observed in the magnitude of the effect across the trials (P = 0.07). However, after sequential exclusion of each trial from all pooled analysis, the conclusion was not affected by the exclusion of any specific trial.

Data from 55,482 individuals was used to assess the effect of B vitamin supplementation on total mortality and included 7,203 deaths. No significant difference in the number of deaths was observed between participants receiving B vitamins compared with those receiving placebo (RR, 1.01; 95% CI: 0.97–1.05; P = 0.77, without evidence of heterogeneity; **Figure 3** and **Figure S2**).

Data from 47,926 individuals was used to assess the effect of B vitamin supplementation on cardiac death and included 3,422 cardiac deaths. B vitamin supplementation caused a 4% reduction in cardiac death; however, this was not a significant change (RR, 0.96; 95% CI: 0.90–1.02; P = 0.21, without evidence of heterogeneity; **Figure 4** and **Figure S3**).

Data from 54,976 individuals was used to assess the effect of B vitamin supplementation on MI, and included 3,623 MIs. There were no significant differences between participants receiving B vitamins compared with placebo for MI (RR, 0.99; 95% CI: 0.93–1.06; P = 0.82, without evidence of heterogeneity, **Figure 5** and **Figure S4**).

Data from 54,102 individuals and 2,465 stroke events was used to assess the effect of B vitamin supplementation on stroke. B vitamin supplementation reduced incident stroke by 6%, but this was not a significant reduction (RR, 0.94; 95% CI: 0.85–1.03; P = 0.18; with no statistical heterogeneity, **Figure 6** and **Figure S5**). Sensitivity analysis was conducted for the incidence of stroke. However, after sequential exclusion of each trial from all pooled analysis, the conclusion was not affected by the exclusion of any specific trial.

Cumulative Meta-Analysis

On cumulative meta-analysis for MACE (**Figure 2**), the original nonsignificant result for a B vitamin effect persisted, and the effect was slight and borderline nonsignificant. Similarly, the nonsignificant result persisted when cumulative meta-analyses for total mortality (**Figure 3**), cardiac death (**Figure 4**), MI (**Figure 5**), and stroke (**Figure 6**) were conducted.

Meta-Regression and Subgroup Analyses

Heterogeneity testing for the analysis showed a P<0.10 for MACE. We concluded that heterogeneity was statistically significant in the overall analysis. We, therefore, conducted a meta-regression analysis [50] for MACE that included the number of participants, mean age, percentage of men, baseline homocysteine level, baseline folate level, dose of folic acid, dose of vitamin B6, dose of vitamin B12, net decrease in homocysteine level, and duration of follow-up. Overall, we detected a net decrease in homocysteine (P = 0.043) that contributed to the association between B vitamin supplementation and MACE (**Figure S6**). However, the number of participants (P = 0.435), mean age (P = 0.763), percentage of men (P = 0.866), baseline homocysteine level (P = 0.094), baseline folate level (P = 0.797), dose of folic acid (P = 0.840), dose of vitamin B6 (P = 0.933), dose of vitamin B12 (P = 0.614), and duration of follow-up (P = 0.186) were not significant factors contributing to the association between B vitamin supplementation and MACE (**Figure S6**).

Subgroup analyses were conducted for MACE to minimize heterogeneity among the included trials and to evaluate the effect of B vitamin supplementation in specific subpopulations. B vitamin supplementation significantly reduced the risk of MACE if the percentage of men in the study was <65% (RR, 0.94; 95% CI: 0.89–1.00; P = 0.034; **Figure 7**) and the study was a single-center trial (RR, 0.78; 95% CI: 0.66–0.93; P = 0.005; **Figure 7**). Furthermore, we noted that B vitamin supplementation was associated with a nonsignificant reduction in MACE when the baseline homocysteine level was>14 μmol/L (RR, 0.93; 95% CI: 0.86–1.00; P = 0.051; **Figure 7**) or dietary grain fortification had been taken to boost the folate level (RR, 0.96; 95% CI: 0.91–1.00; P = 0.061; **Figure 7**). No other significant differences were identified in the predefined factors between those who took B vitamin supplements and those who took placebo (**Figure 7**). Furthermore, there was no significant difference in the effect of B vitamins on MACE between the 2 subgroups by factors that could affect the treatment effect except center of trials (P = 0.008; **Figure 7**).

Publication Bias

Review of funnel plots did not rule out the potential for publication bias for MACE, total mortality, cardiac death, MI, and stroke (**Figure S7**). However, the Egger [53] and Begg tests [54] showed no evidence of publication bias for MACE (P value for Egger, 0.342; P value for Begg, 0.267), total mortality (P value for Egger, 0.312; P value for Begg, 0.183), cardiac death (P value for Egger, 0.631; P value for Begg, 0.621), MI (P value for Egger, 0.816; P value for Begg, 0.944), and stroke (P value for Egger, 0.992; P value for Begg, 1.000).

Discussion

Several observational studies [1–5] have suggested that B vitamin supplementation may improve major cardiovascular outcomes. However, this effect has not been confirmed to date. In the present study, we included RCTs and explored all possible correlations between B vitamin supplementation and the outcomes of MACE, total mortality, cardiac death, MI, and stroke. Furthermore, we conducted a cumulative meta-analysis to explore the value of routine B vitamin supplementation in clinical practice. This large quantitative study included 57,952 individuals from 24 trials with a broad range of baseline characteristics. Our results suggest that B vitamin supplementation has no significant effect on MACE, total mortality, cardiac death, MI, or stroke. Furthermore, in a cumulative meta-analysis, this B vitamin effect persisted and remained nonsignificant.

We reviewed previous meta-analyses and found that the hypothesized protective effect of B vitamins comes from observational studies [9], which, we suggest, may overestimate the effect on major cardiovascular outcomes. Several systematic reviews and meta-analyses of RCTs [12–17] have evaluated the impact of folic acid supplementation on major cardiovascular outcomes and have found no evidence to support a significant association. In a meta-analysis, Wang et al. [19] indicated that B vitamins significantly reduced the risk of stroke, but subgroup analysis showed that this effect was based on trials that included only participants without a previous stroke history. Lee et al. [55] suggested that folic acid supplementation administered as primary prevention significantly reduced the risk of stroke at>3 years of follow-up and that the homocysteine-lowering effect was>20%. However, this meta-analysis included trials with a male: female ratio of >2. Gao et al. [56] found that B vitamin supplementation given to reduce homocysteine levels influenced the risk of stroke events, especially in subgroups with a follow-up of>3 years (RR, 0.92; 95% CI: 0.84–1.00), without a history of grain fortification (RR, 0.91; 95% CI: 0.83–1.00), or without chronic kidney disease (RR, 0.93; 95% CI: 0.86–1.01), but these differences were not significant. In the present study, all pooled RR estimate points for stroke were <1 (evidence accumulated up to 2006) with a potential trend toward moving leftward in the cumulative meta-analysis of B vitamin supplementation. We suggest a potential protective effect of B vitamins on stroke events. However, this trend is not obvious and requires validation.

There was no significant difference between B vitamin supplementation and placebo for the RR of major cardiovascular outcomes. However, several trials included in our study reported inconsistent results. Schnyder et al. [21] indicated that homocysteine-lowering therapy with B complex vitamins reduced the risk of MACE in patients after percutaneous coronary intervention. However, Lange et al. [24] indicated that B vitamin complex supplementation after coronary stenting increases the risk of in-stent restenosis and the need for target-vessel revascularization. The possible reasons for these inconsistencies are as follows: (1) a history of B vitamin supplementation may mask treatment effect; (2) patients in our meta-analysis had variable disease status, which also affects major cardiovascular outcomes; (3) elevated homocysteine levels impair vascular function, but the effect of homocysteine on cardiovascular outcomes may not be directly related to coronary disease pathogenesis, which is largely attributable to plaque formation and rupture [57]; and (4) high doses of B vitamin may adversely affect vascular remodeling and myocardial repair and may increase complications and death in patients with cardiovascular disease [58]. Therefore, although B vitamin supplementation may have direct effects on major cardiovascular outcomes, these effects may be counterbalanced by other effects.

Cumulative meta-analyses suggest that a nonsignificant response persisted for MACE, total mortality, cardiac death, MI, and stroke. However, the proposed nonsignificant protective effect of B vitamin supplementation for MI has been refuted by the NORVIT Trial Investigators [26], who specifically included individuals with MI, which may have contributed to higher recurrence and suggests a nonsignificant harmful effect for B vitamin supplementation. However, the proposed nonsignificant harmful effect of B vitamin supplementation for stroke was refuted by the HOPE 2 Trial [27]. This trial suggested that B vitamin supplementation reduced the risk of stroke by 25% (95% CI: 0.59–0.97), but this may be due to a considerably lower number of stroke events than coronary events. In addition, the CIs of the estimated risk reduction were wide. Furthermore, the results were not adjusted for the multiplicity of potential outcomes.

In our study, subgroup analysis suggested that B vitamin supplementation reduced the risk of MACE in specific subgroups. The main findings were as follows. First, although no significant difference was observed in MACE for the B vitamin supplementation group compared with the placebo group, in populations with a baseline total homocysteine level >14 μmol/L and those with a net decrease in homocysteine level of >20% there seemed to be a slight, but nonsignificant, benefit. In this study, baseline homocysteine levels were only available for whole populations, not individuals. Second, folate fortification of the grain supply may influence the risk of MACE, because it reduces the prevalence of low folate levels and high total homocysteine levels, so the mean difference in total homocysteine levels between groups narrows. Fortification reduces the number of participants with a high total homocysteine level, which is the population most likely to benefit from supplementation [59]. In this study, we found that B vitamin supplementation reduced the risk of MACE if participants had a background of grain fortification. Those with background fortification received higher doses of vitamin B12, which may be more effective at preventing MACE. Third, the protective effect of B vitamins was more evident if the percentage of men in the study was <65%. Among men, there is a higher rate of smoking and drinking, both of which increase the risk of MACE. Therefore, the effect of B vitamins on the risk of MACE in studies with a higher percentage of male subjects may be reduced or balanced by a higher rate of smoking and drinking. Fourth, there was a significant difference between single-center and multi-center trials in the risk for MACE. This difference could be due to chance because only 6 trials were single-center, and they had a low sample size and low rate of cardiovascular disease occurrence. Fifth, no significant differences were observed in MACE between participants with a low folate level and those with a normal folate level. Folate level data were not available for several trials, so this conclusion was similar to those of a previous meta-analysis [60]. Sixth, the B vitamin dose showed no significant effect because all doses investigated were in the mega-dose range, and there may have been differences in the control groups in different studies. Seventh, B vitamin supplementation seems to offer a benefit for primary prevention of MACE but not for secondary prevention. Participants with pre-existing cardiovascular disease have higher recurrence and mortality rates. Finally, B vitamins seem to benefit participants with kidney disease but not those without kidney disease; patients with kidney disease may have higher homocysteine concentrations and a higher rate of cardiovascular disease.

The limitations of our study are as follows: (1) different types and doses of supplements might result in bias; (2) the use of background B vitamin supplementation might have impaired our ability to identify a treatment effect; (3) differences in diagnosis and reporting may have contributed to the differences in major cardiovascular outcomes in some trials; (4) stratified analyses based on background therapy in patients with previous disease were unavailable; (5) data on hemoglobin levels were not available, so we could not evaluate the potential confounding role of hemoglobin when evaluating the effect of vitamins B on the risk of major cardiovascular outcomes; (6) several trials with low Jadad score were included in our study, which could bias the results; and (7) since inherent assumptions are made for any meta-analysis, the analysis used pooled data, and individual patient data were unavailable; this restricted us from performing a more detailed analysis and obtaining more comprehensive results.

In conclusion, we found that B vitamin supplementation has little or no effect on major cardiovascular outcomes across various patient populations. We believe the use of B vitamin supplementation as a structured intervention in everyday clinical practice is not justified. A meta-analysis of individual patient data might be more appropriate to determine how the duration and dose of supplementation influence treatment outcomes.

Supporting Information

Figure S1 Effect of B vitamins supplementation on the risk of major cardiovascular events.

Figure S2 Effect of B vitamins supplementation on the risk of total mortality.

Figure S3 Effect of B vitamins supplementation on the risk of cardiac death.

Figure S4 Effect of B vitamins supplementation on the risk of myocardial infarction.

Figure S5 Effect of B vitamins supplementation on the risk of stroke.

Figure S6 Meta-regression of number of participants, mean age, percentage male, baseline homocyteine, baseline folate status, dose of folic acid, dose of vitamin B6, dose of vitamin B12, net decrease in homocysteine, and the duration of the follow-up periods.

Figure S7 Funnel plots for major cardiovascular events, total mortality, cardiac death, myocardial infarction, and stroke.

Table S1 Additional characteristic of trials included in our meta-analysis.

Checklist S1 PRISMA Checklist.

Author Contributions

Conceived and designed the experiments: YHZ. Performed the experiments: YHZ CZ YYQ FFY ZYW. Analyzed the data: YHZ YYQ FFY. Contributed reagents/materials/analysis tools: YHZ. Wrote the paper: YHZ.

References

1. Folsom AR, Nieto FJ, McGovern PG, Tsai MY, Malinow MR, et al. (1998) Prospective study of coronary heart disease incidence in relation to fasting total homocysteine, related geneitic polymorphisms, and B vitamins: the Atherosclerosis Risk in Communities (ARIC) study. Circulation 98: 204–210.
2. Verhoef P, Kok FJ, Kruyssen DA, Schouten EG, Witteman JC, et al. (1997) Plasma total homocysteine, B vitamins, and risk of atherosclerosis. Arterioscler Thromb Vasc Biol 17: 985–995.
3. Schwartz SM, Siscovick DS, Malinow MR, Rosendaal FR, Beverly RK, et al. (1997) Myocardial infarction in young women in relation to plasma total homocysteine, folate, and a common variant in the methylenetetrahydrofolate reductase gene. Circulation 96: 412–7.
4. Chambers JC, Obeid OA, Refsum H, Ueland P, Hackett D, et al. (2000) Plasma homocysteine concentrations and risk of coronary heart disease in UK Indian, Asian and European men. Lancet 355: 523–527.
5. Robinson K, Mayer EL, Miller DP, Green R, van Lente F, et al. (1995) Hyperhomocysteinemia and low pyridoxal phosphate. Common and independent reversible risk factors for coronary artery disease. Circulation 92: 2825–2830.
6. Perry IJ, Refsum H, Morris RW, Ebrahim SB, Ueland PM, et al. (1995) Prospective study of serum total homocysteine concentration and risk of stroke in middle-aged British men. Lancet 346: 1395–1398.
7. Bots ML, Launer LJ, Lindemans J, Hoes AW, Hofman A, et al. (1999) Homocysteine and short-term risk of myocardial infarction and stroke in the elderly: the Rotterdam Study. Arch Intern Med 159: 38–44.
8. Evers S, Koch HG, Grotemeyer KH, Lange B, Deufel T, et al. (1997) Features, symptoms, and neurophysiological findings in stroke associated with hyperhomocysteinemia. Arch Neurol 54: 1276–1282.
9. The Homocysteine Studies Collaboration (2002) Homocysteine and risk of ischemic heart disease and stroke: a meta-analysis. JAMA 288: 2015–2022.
10. Homocysteine Lowering Trialists' Collaboration (1998) Lowering blood homocysteine with folic acid based supplements: meta-analysis of randomised trials. BMJ 316: 894–898.
11. Homocysteine Lowering Trialists' Collaboration (2005) Dose-dependent effects of folic acid on blood concentrations of homocysteine: a meta-analysis of the randomized trials. Am J Clin Nutr 82: 806–812.
12. Bazzano LA, Reynolds K, Holder KN, He J (2006) Effect of folic acid supplementation on risk of cardiovascular diseases a meta-analysis of randomized controlled trials. JAMA 296: 2720–2726.
13. Zhou Y-H, Tang J-Y, Wu M-J, Lu J, Wei X, et al. (2011) Effect of folic acid supplementation on cardiovascular outcomes: a systematic review and meta-analysis. PLoS ONE 6: e25142.
14. Jardine MJ, Kang A, Zoungas S, Navaneethan SD, Ninomiya T, et al. (2012) The effect of folic acid based homocysteine lowering on cardiovascular events in people with kidney disease: systematic review and meta-analysis. BMJ 344: e3533.
15. Pan Y, Guo LL, Cai LL, Zhu XJ, Shu JL, et al. (2012) Homocysteine-lowering therapy does not lead to reduction in cardiovascular outcomes in chronic kidney disease patients: a meta-analysis of randomised, controlled trials. Br J Nutr 108: 400–7.
16. Clarke R, Halsey J, Lewington S, Lonn E, Armitage J, et al. (2010) Effects of lowering homocysteine levels with B vitamins on cardiovascular disease, cancer, and cause-specific mortality: Meta-analysis of 8 randomized trials involving 37 485 individuals. Arch Intern Med 170: 1622–31.
17. Miller ER, Juraschek S, Pastor-Barriuso R, Bazzano LA, Appel LJ, et al. (2010) Meta-analysis of folic acid supplementation trials on risk of cardiovasculardisease and risk interaction with baseline homocysteine levels. Am J Cardiol 106: 517–27.
18. C Zhang, FL Chi, TH Xie, YH Zhou (2013) Effect of B-vitamin Supplementation on Stroke: a Meta-Analysis of Randomized Controlled Trials. PLoS One 8: e81577.
19. Wang X, Qin X, Demirtas H, Li J, Mao G, et al. (2007) Efficacy of folic acid supplementation in stroke prevention: a meta-analysis. Lancet 369: 1876–82.
20. Baker F, Picton D, Blackwood S, Hunt J, Erskine M, et al. (2002) Blinded comparison of folic acid and placebo in patients with ischemic heart disease: an outcome trial [abstract]. Circulation (suppl 2): 741S.
21. Schnyder G, Roffi M, Flammer Y, Pin R, Hess OM (2002) Effect of homocysteine-lowering therapy with folic acid, vitamin B12, and vitamin B6 on clinical outcome after percutaneous coronary intervention: the Swiss Heart Study: a randomized controlled trial. JAMA 288: 973–979.
22. Toole JF, Malinow MR, Chambless LE, Spence JD, Pettigrew LC, et al. (2004) Lowering Homocysteine in Patients With Ischemic Stroke to Prevent Recurrent Stroke, Myocardial Infarction, and Death The Vitamin Intervention for Stroke Prevention (VISP) Randomized Controlled Trial. JAMA 291: 565–575.
23. Liem AH, van Boven AJ, Veeger NJ, Withagen AJ, Robles de Medina RM, et al. (2004) Folic Acid on Risk Diminishment After Acute Myocarial Infarction Study Group. Efficacy of folic acid when added to statin therapy in patients with hypercholesterolemia following acute myocardial infarction: a randomised pilot trial. Int J Cardiol 93: 175–179.
24. Lange H, Suryapranata H, De Luca G, Börner C, Dille J, et al. (2004) Folate therapy and in-stent restenosis after coronary stenting. N Engl J Med 350: 2673–2681.
25. Liem A, Reynierse-Buitenwerf GH, Zwinderman AH, Jukema JW, van Veldhuisen DJ (2005) Secondary prevention with folic acid: results of the Goes extension study. Heart 91: 1213–1214.
26. The NORVIT Trial Investigators (2006) Homocysteine Lowering and Cardiovascular Events after Acute Myocardial Infarction. N Engl J Med 354: 1578–88.
27. The Heart Outcomes Prevention Evaluation (HOPE) 2 Investigators (2006) Homocysteine Lowering with Folic Acid and B Vitamins in Vascular Disease. N Engl J Med 354: 1567–77.
28. Ebbing M, Bleie Ø, Ueland PM, Nordrehaug JE, Nilsen DW, et al. (2008) Mortality and Cardiovascular Events in Patients Treated With Homocysteine-Lowering B Vitamins After Coronary Angiography A Randomized Controlled Trial. JAMA 300: 795–804.
29. Study of the Effectiveness of Additional Reductions in Cholesterol and Homocysteine (SEARCH) Collaborative Group (2010) Effects of Homocysteine-Lowering With Folic Acid Plus Vitamin B12 vs Placebo on Mortality and Major Morbidity in Myocardial Infarction Survivors A Randomized Trial. JAMA 303: 2486–2494.
30. The SU.FOL.OM3 Collaborative Group (2010) Effects of B vitamins and omega 3 fatty acids on cardiovascular diseases: a randomised placebo controlled Trial. BMJ 341: c6273.
31. The VITATOPS Trial Study Group (2010) B vitamins in patients with recent transient ischaemic attack or stroke in the VITAmins TO Prevent Stroke (VITATOPS) trial: a randomised, double-blind, parallel, placebo-controlled trial. Lancet Neurol 9: 855–65.
32. Righetti M, Ferrario GM, Milani S, Serbelloni P, La Rosa L, et al. (2003) Effects of folic acid treatment on homocysteine levels and vascular disease in hemodialysis patients. Med Sci Monit 9: PI19–PI24.
33. Wrone EM, Hornberger JM, Zehnder JL, McCann LM, Coplon NS, et al. (2004) Randomized trial of folic acid for prevention of cardiovascular events in endstage renal disease. J AmSoc Nephrol 15: 420–426.
34. Zoungas S, McGrath BP, Branley P, Kerr PG, Muske C, et al. (2006) Cardiovascular morbidity and mortality in the Atherosclerosis and Folic Acid Supplementation Trial (ASFAST) in chronic renal failure: a multicenter, randomized, controlled trial. J Am Coll Cardiol 47: 1108–1116.
35. Righetti M, Serbelloni P, Milani S, Ferrario G (2006) Homocysteine- lowering vitamin B treatment decreases cardiovascular events in hemodialysis patients. Blood Purif 24: 379–386.
36. Vianna ACA, Mocelin AJ, Matsuo T, Morais-Filho D, Largura A, et al. (2007) Uremic hyperhomocysteinemia: A randomized trial of folate treatment for the prevention of cardiovascular events. Hemodialysis International 11: 210–216.
37. The Polyp Prevention Study Group (2007) Folic Acid for the Prevention of Colorectal Adenomas A Randomized Clinical Trial. JAMA 297: 2351–2359.
38. The Veterans Affairs Site Investigators (2007) Effect of Homocysteine Lowering on Mortality and Vascular Disease in Advanced Chronic Kidney Disease and End-stage Renal Disease A Randomized Controlled Trial. JAMA 298: 1163–1170.
39. Albert CM, Cook NR, Gaziano JM, Zaharris E, MacFadyen J, et al. (2008) Effect of Folic Acid and B-Vitamins on Risk of Cardiovascular Events and Total

Mortality among Women at High Risk for Cardiovascular Disease: A Randomized Trial. JAMA 299: 2027–2036.
40. The BVAIT Research Group (2009) High-Dose B Vitamin Supplementation and Progression of Subclinical Atherosclerosis A Randomized Controlled Trial. Stroke 40: 730–736.
41. House AA, Eliasziw M, Cattran DC, Churchill DN, Oliver MJ, et al. (2010) Effect of B-Vitamin Therapy on Progression of Diabetic Nephropathy A Randomized Controlled Trial. JAMA 303: 1603–1609.
42. Heinz J, Kropf S, Domröse U, Westphal S, Borucki K, et al. (2010) B Vitamins and the Risk of Total Mortality and Cardiovascular Disease in End-Stage Renal Disease: Results of a Randomized Controlled Trial. Circulation 121: 1432–1438.
43. The FAVORIT Study Group (2011) Homocysteine-Lowering and Cardiovascular Disease Outcomes in Kidney Transplant Recipients Primary Results From the Folic Acid for Vascular Outcome Reduction in Transplantation Trial. Circulation 123: 1763–1770.
44. Moher D, Liberati A, Tetzlaff J, Altman DG, PRISMA Group (2009) Preferred Reporting Items for Systematic Reviews and Meta-Analyses: The PRISMA Statement. Plos Medicine 6: e1000097.
45. Jadad AR, Moore RA, Carroll D (1996) Assessing the quality of reports of randomized clinical trials: is blinding necessary? Control Clin Trials 17: 1–12.
46. DerSimonian R, Laird N (1986) Meta-analysis in clinical trials. Control Clin Trials 7: 177–88.
47. Ades AE, Lu G, Higgins JP (2005) The interpretation of random-effects metaanalysis in decision models. Med Decis Making 25: 646–54.
48. Deeks JJ, Higgins JPT, Altman DG (2008) Analyzing data and undertaking meta-analyses. In: Higgins J, Green S, eds.Cochrane Handbook for Systematic Reviews of Interventions 5.0.1. Oxford, UK: The Cochrane Collaboration: chap 9.
49. Higgins JPT, Thompson SG, Deeks JJ, Altman DG (2003) Measuring inconsistency in meta-analyses. BMJ 327: 557–60.
50. Thompson SG, Higgins JP (2002) How should meta-regression analyses be undertaken and interpreted? Stat Med 21: 1559–73.
51. Altman DG, Bland JM (2003) Interaction revisited: the difference between two estimates. BMJ 326: 219.
52. Tobias A (1999) Assessing the influence of a single study in meta-analysis. Stata Tech Bull 47: 15–17.
53. Egger M, Davey Smith G, Schneider M, Minder C (1997) Bias in meta-analysis detected by a simple, graphical test. BMJ 315: 629–34.
54. Begg CB, Mazumdar M (1994) Operating characteristics of a rank correlation test for publication bias. Biometrics 50: 1088–1101.
55. Lee M, Hong KS, Chang SC, Saver JL (2010) Efficacy of Homocysteine-Lowering Therapy With Folic Acid in Stroke Prevention: A Meta-Analysis. Stroke 41: 1205–1212.
56. Ji Y, Tan S, Xu Y, Chandra A, Shi C, et al. (2013) Vitamin B supplementation, homocysteine levels, and the risk of cerebrovascular disease: A meta-analysis. Neurology 81: 1–10.
57. Eikelboom JW, Lonn E, Genest J Jr, Hankey G, Yusuf S (1999) Homocysteine and cardiovascular disease: a critical review of the epidemiologic evidence. Ann Intern Med 131: 363–375.
58. Loscalzo J (2006) Homocysteine trials: clear outcomes for complex reasons. N Engl J Med 354: 1629–1632.
59. Stampfer MJ, Malinow MR, Willett WC, Newcomer LM, Upson B, et al. (1992) A prospective study of plasma homocyst(e)ine and risk of myocardial infarction in US physicians. JAMA 268: 877–81.
60. Holmes MV, Newcombe P, Hubacek JA, Sofat R, Ricketts SL, et al. (2011) Effect modification by population dietary folate on the association between MTHFR genotype, homocysteine, and stroke risk: a meta-analysis of genetic studies and randomised trials. Lancet 378: 584–94.

15

Relationship of Dickkopf1 (DKK1) with Cardiovascular Disease and Bone Metabolism in Caucasian Type 2 Diabetes Mellitus

Antonia Garcia-Martín[1,2], Rebeca Reyes-Garcia[1,3], Beatriz García-Fontana[1], Sonia Morales-Santana[1,4], Ana Coto-Montes[5], Manuel Muñoz-Garach[6], Pedro Rozas-Moreno[7], Manuel Muñoz-Torres[1]*

1 Bone Metabolic Unit (RETICEF), Endocrinology Division, Hospital Universitario San Cecilio, Instituto de Investigación Biosanitaria de Granada, Granada, Spain, **2** Endocrinology, Hospital Comarcal del Noroeste, Caravaca de la Cruz, Murcia, Spain, **3** Endocrinology Unit, Hospital General Universitario Rafael Mendez, Lorca, Murcia, Spain, **4** Proteomic Research Service, Fundación para la Investigación Biosanitaria de Andalucía Oriental -Alejandro Otero- (FIBAO), Granada, Spain, **5** Department of Morphology and Cellular Biology (RETICEF), Faculty of Medicine, University of Oviedo, Oviedo, Spain, **6** Critical Care and Emergencies Unit, Hospital Universitario San Cecilio, Granada, Spain, **7** Endocrinology Division, Hospital General de Ciudad Real, Ciudad Real, Spain

Abstract

Objectives: Dickkopf-1 (DKK1) is a potent inhibitor of Wnt signalling, which exerts anabolic effects on bone and also takes part in the regulation of vascular cells. Our aims were to evaluate serum DKK1 in type 2 diabetes (T2DM) patients and to analyze its relationships with cardiovascular disease (CVD). We also evaluated the relationship between DKK1 and bone metabolism.

Design: We conducted a cross-sectional study in which we measured serum DKK1 (ELISA, Biomedica) in 126 subjects: 72 patients with T2DM and 54 non-diabetic subjects. We analysed its relationship with clinical CVD, preclinical CVD expressed as carotid intima media thickness (IMT), and bone metabolism.

Results: T2DM patients with CVD ($P = 0{,}026$) and abnormal carotid IMT ($P = 0{,}038$) had higher DKK1 concentrations. DKK1 was related to the presence of CVD in T2DM, independently of the presence of risk factors for atherosclerosis. Therefore, for each increase of 28 pg/ml of serum DKK1 there was a 6,2% increase in the risk of CVD in T2DM patients. The ROC curve analysis to evaluate the usefulness of DKK1 as a marker for high risk of CVD showed an area under the curve of 0,667 (95% CI: 0,538–0,795; $P = 0{,}016$). In addition, there was a positive correlation between serum DKK1 and spine bone mineral density in the total sample ($r = 0{,}183$; $P = 0{,}048$).

Conclusion: In summary, circulating DKK1 levels are higher in T2DM with CVD and are associated with an abnormal carotid IMT in this cross-sectional study. DKK1 may be involved in vascular disease of T2DM patients.

Editor: Rudolf Kirchmair, Medical University Innsbruck, Austria

Funding: This work was supported in part by Consejería de Salud y Bienestar Social, Junta de Andalucia (PI-0514-2012) and Red de Investigación Colaborativa en Envejecimiento y Fragilidad (RETICEF) (RD06/0013/1014-RD12/0043/0014). The funders had no role in study design, data collection and analysis, decision to publish, or preparation of the manuscript.

Competing Interests: The authors have declared that no competing interests exist.

* Email: mmt@mamuto.es

Introduction

Patients with type 2 diabetes mellitus (T2DM) have a higher risk of cardiovascular disease (CVD). This association has serious consequences on the morbidity and the mortality in this population. Atherosclerosis is the main pathological mechanism in macrovascular disease in T2DM, which causes the development of atheroma plaques and the major life-threatening events in atherosclerosis, including myocardial infarction and stroke [1].

Patients with osteoporosis have a higher prevalence of cardiovascular disease, and it has been proposed that both pathologies share common pathophysiologic pathways [2]. In T2DM there is an increased risk of fractures at any skeletal site even with greater bone mineral density (BMD) [3,4], and there are data from epidemiological studies supporting a relationship between low bone mineral density (BMD) and atherosclerosis in T2DM [5,6]. Thus, a better characterization of the pathways that could be involved in both processes is of interest, and may help in the development of new therapeutic tools.

The Wnt signalling pathways are involved in several developmental and physiological processes, including the cell differentiation and tissue/organ morphogenesis [7]. The discovery of the Wnt signaling pathway and its relevance in bone homeostasis has contributed to a better knowledge of the cellular and molecular mechanisms of bone biology [8]. The activation of this pathway results in an expansion of osteoprogenitor cells and also determines a reduction in the apoptosis of osteoblasts, which leads to anabolic effects on bone [8]. The canonical Wnt pathway is regulated by several families of secreted antagonists, such as the soluble frizzled-related receptors, dickkopf-1 (DKK1) and sclerostin. DKK1 regulates the Wnt signaling by binding to the Wnt co-receptor, the low-density lipoprotein-related receptor (LRP) 5/6. In addition to its binding to LRP 5/6, DKK1 binds to other trans-membrane molecules as proteins Kremen, which increases their inhibitory activity on the Wnt signaling pathway [9].

The role of Wnt signaling pathways in atherosclerosis it is a matter of growing interest. In preclinical studies the Wnt signaling pathways are involved in atherosclerosis-related processes as vascular calcification [10], inflammation [11], and the monocyte adhesion and its trans-endothelial migration [12]. In a recent study conducted in bovine aortic endothelial cells (ECs) [13], the authors found that Msx2 and Wnt7 family members stabilize the aortic ECs phenotype, whereas DKK1 promotes an endothelial–mesenchymal transition in cultured bovine aortic ECs, a process associated to the pathogenesis of myocardial fibrosis with ischemia [14] and valve calcification [15]. In addition, in animal models of CKD-MBD (chronic kidney disease-mineral bone disease) [16] there is an increased renal production of Wnt inhibitor family members and higher levels of circulating DKK1, sclerostin, and secreted klotho. In this model, the neutralization of DKK1 by administration of a monoclonal antibody after renal injury stimulated bone formation rates, corrected the osteodystrophy, and prevented CKD-stimulated vascular calcification. Besides, the neutralization of DKK1 suppressed aortic expression of the osteoblastic transcription factor Runx2, increased expression of vascular smooth muscle protein 22-α, and restored aortic expression of klotho"

There is also recent data showing a relationship between serum DKK1 and atherosclerosis in humans [17,18]. In a previous study from Register and colleagues, DKK1 concentrations were inversely related to coronary artery disease and aortic calcification. However, as the authors point, this study has been conducted in Afro-Americans (AAs) with T2DM, which has a different prevalence of atherosclerotic disease and osteoporosis compared to European populations. These differences make it interesting to explore this relationship in Caucasian type 2 diabetes. Besides, the relationship between DKK1 concentrations and bone mass has been explored with conflicting data [19–21], so its evaluation in a population with a high risk of bone fragility such as T2DM is of interest.

In this context, the objectives of our study were to evaluate serum DKK1 levels in a cohort of T2DM patients and to analyze its relationships with CVD and bone metabolism. In addition, we compared serum DKK1 concentrations between T2DM and non-diabetic subjects. Thus, our hypothesis was that DKK1 concentrations may be related to CVD and bone metabolism in T2DM patients.

Materials and Methods

Study population

Our study was a cross-sectional one that included 126 subjects. The estimated size of the sample considering an error of 5% and a statistical power of 80% was 84 subjects. The T2DM group included 72 patients with a diagnosis of diabetes according to the American Diabetes Association criteria (ADA, 2005). From January 2006 to December 2007 we consecutively recruited patients who had been referred to our outpatient clinic from community clinics for treatment of diabetes. The control group included 54 non-diabetic subjects who were consecutively recruited from the general community in the same period of time.

All participants were recruited according to the following criteria: Caucasian, free-living, aged 35 to 65 years and normal values for blood count, renal creatinine, hepatic function, calcium and phosphorus. We considered as exclusion criteria the presence of chronic diseases apart from T2DM in the non-diabetic group, the presence of diseases affecting bone (Paget's disease, rheumatoid arthritis, hyperparathyroidism, hypercortisolism, malignant tumors, renal bone disease, chronic liver disease and post-transplantation bone disease) and also previous or current treatment with drugs affecting bone metabolism (calcium supplements, vitamin D preparations, selective estrogen receptor modulators, calcitonin, estrogens therapy, antiresorptive therapy, thiazides, steroids, glucocorticoids or anticonvulsants). Patients treated with thiazolidinediones were also excluded.

The presence of cardiovascular disease was recorded by the medical history and after that it was checked in medical records. T2DM patients were classified into two groups according to the presence of clinical CVD: CVD group and non-CVD group. Inclusion criteria for patients with CVD were cerebrovascular disease (ischemic stroke or transient ischemic attack); coronary heart disease (previous myocardial infarction, diagnosed stable or unstable angina, or coronary revascularization surgery) or ischemic peripheral arterial disease (diagnosed by a positive Doppler ultrasound or arteriogram, or by a previous revascularization surgery).

The study was approved by the ethical review board of the Hospital Universitario San Cecilio and it was done conformed to the ethical guidelines for research in humans. All the participants in the study provided written informed consent after a full explanation of the purpose of the study and the nature of all the procedures that will be used in the study. Written informed consent was approved for the ethical review board of our hospital, and after that it was filed in the medical record of each patient.

Clinical evaluation

Height, weight, and waist circumference were measured at baseline according to standard procedures. Weight was measured to the nearest 100 grams using digital electronic scales. Height and waist circumference were measured to the nearest 1 mm using a stadiometer and a metal anthropometric tape, respectively. Body mass index (BMI) in Kg/m^2 was calculated as weight divided by the square of height in meters.

Blood pressure was measured in a standardized manner. The subjects remained at rest for at least 5 minutes, and after that blood pressure was measured twice using a standard mercury sphygmomanometer (12 centimeters long, 35 cm wide). The mean of the two values was used for analysis. We defined hypertension when blood pressure values were higher than 140/90 mmHg and/or where subjects were on antihypertensive treatment.

The participants reported their alcohol use, smoking status and their level of physical activity with a specific health questionnaire. Patients were classified as having a significant alcohol intake if it was higher than 40 grams/day in males and 24 grams/day in women; smoking status was categorized as no tobacco use or current tobacco use. Physical activity was collected through a specific questionnaire in which study subjects scored their physical activity on a scale from 0 (none) to 10 (sport more than one hour four times per week). Based on the results, the study sample was divided into two groups: sedentary (<5 on the scale) and no sedentary (≥5 on the scale).

Serum measurements

Samples of venous blood were taken in the morning after a fasting overnight. The sera were stored at −80°C until examina-

Table 1. Characteristics of the study population.

	Total Group (n = 126)	T2DM Group (n = 72)	Non-diabetic Group (n = 54)	P Value
Age (years)	57±6	58±6	55±7	0,018
Male/female (n)	62/64	39/33	25/29	0,472
Medical history				
Duration of diabetes (years)	-	13,7±7,6	-	
Hypertension (%)	53,2	80,6	46,3	<0,001
Dyslipidaemia (%)	65,9	94,4	70,4	<0,001
Albuminuria (%)	20,5	35,0	4,0	0,006
Chronic kidney disease (KDOQI stages) (%)				
Stage 1	51	52	52	0,938
Stage 2	46	44	48	0,815
Stage 3	3	4	0	0,155
Smoker or ex-smoker (%)	15,1	16,7	13	0,623
Alcohol (%)	8,7	6,9	11,1	0,104
Sedentarism (%)	47,6	55,6	37,0	0,048
Clinical evaluation:				
BMI (kg/m^2)	102,6±12,4	31,4±5,7	29,3±5,9	0,043
Waist circumference (cm)	130±20	106,4±11,4	97,4±11,9	<0,001
SBP (mm Hg)	80±13	134±97	124±17	0,002
DBP (mm Hg)	30,5±5,9	80±12	79±15	0,705
Serum parameters:				
FPG (mg/dL)	137,2±61,9	173±60,1	89,4±10,4	<0,001
HbA1$_c$ (%)	6,7±2,2	8±1,9	4,8±0,4	<0,001
GFR (MDR/CKD-EPI)(ml/min/1,73 m^2)	92±23	92±23	93±22	0,745
Calcium (mg/dL)	9,5±0,5	9,6±0,5	9,3±0,4	0,001
Phosphorus (mg/dL)	3,6±0,5	3,7±0,5	3,5±0,5	0,01
PTH (pg/mL)	43,6±19,5	38,5±18,4	50,4±19,1	<0,001
25(OH) D (ng/mL)	19,5±11,3	17,8±11,5	21,6±10,9	0,06
Triglyceride (mg/dl)	142±121	169,9±149,8	104,9±47,7	<0,001
HDL-c (mg/dl)	53,5±15,5	49±16	59,5±12,5	<0,001
LDL-c (mg/dl)	111,7±35,5	96,9±34,1	130,8±27,4	<0,001
DKK1 (pg/ml)	629±374	669±395	575±340	0,163
DXA parameters and VF:				
BMD LS (g/cm^2)	0,977±0,148	0,954±0,146	1±0,148	0,068
BMD FN (g/cm^2)	0,820±0,124	0,817±0,132	0,823±0,117	0,792
BMD TH (g/cm^2)	0,906±0,135	0,903±0,145	0,911±0,125	0,772
T-score LS	−1,08±1,36	−1,3±1,3	0,82±1,3	0,058
T-score FN	−0,55±1,01	−0,6±1,04	−0,49±0,99	0,565
T-score TH	−0,55±0,98	−0,62±1	−0,51±0,92	0,557
Osteoporosis (%)	15,9	24,6	9,4	0,047
Morphometric VF (%)	23,0	30,3	20,0	0,274
Cardiovascular disease:	35,7	58,3	5,6	<0,001
Cerebrovascular disease (%)	11,9	19,4	1,9	0,002
Coronary heart disease (%)	23,8	38,9	3,7	<0,001
Peripheral artery disease (%)	7,9	13,9	0	0,005
Abnormal intima-media thickness (%)	35,7	54,2	11,1	<0,001
Carotid plaques (%)	15,9	29,4	0	<0,001

Data for continuous variables are presented as mean ±SD. Data for categorical variables are presented as numbers and/or percentages. The comparison between groups was done by Student's t test (continuous variables) or Chi-square test (categorical variables).
T2DM: type 2 diabetes mellitus; BMI: body mass index; SBP: sistolic blood pressure; DBP: diastolic blood pressure; FPG: fasting plasma glucose; HbA1c: glycated hemoglobin; GFR: glomerular filtration rate; MDR/CKD-EPI: Chronic Kidney Disease Epidemiology Collaboration; PTH: parathormone; 25(OH) D: 25-hydroxyvitamin D; HDL-c: High-density lipoprotein; LDL-c: Low-density lipoprotein; BMD: bone mineral density; LS: lumbar spine; FN: femoral neck; TH: total hip; VF: vertebral fractures.

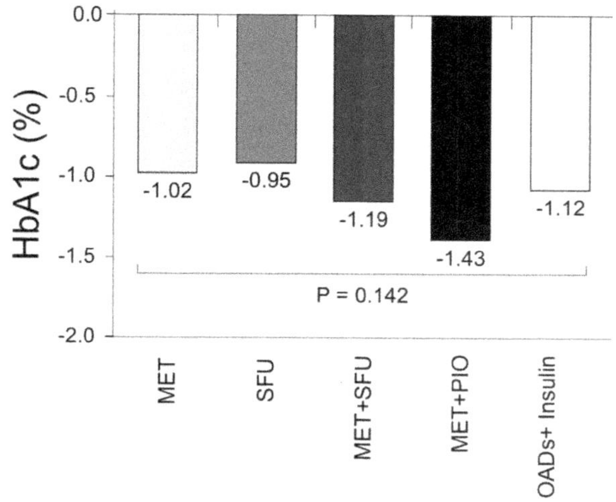

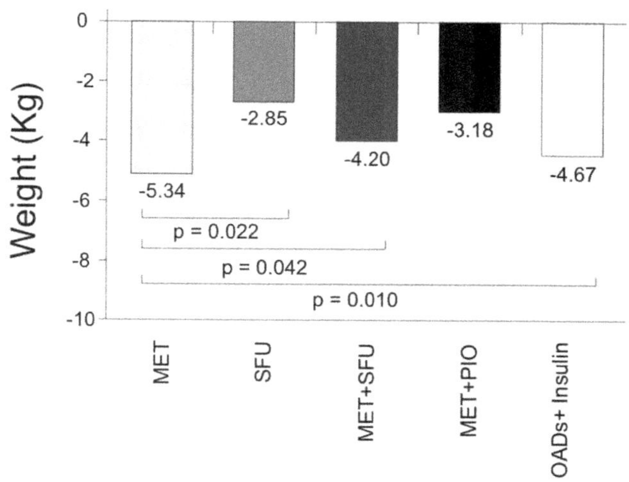

Figure 1. DKK1 serum levels in T2DM patients according to the presence of cardiovascular disease and abnormal intima-media thickness. Between groups differences are indicated through a bar with the P-value given above.

tion. Fasting plasma glucose (FPG), glycated hemoglobin (HbA1c), calcium, phosphorus and creatinine were measured using standard automated laboratory techniques. Glomerular filtration rate (GFR) was calculated by MDRD/CKD-EPI formula [22]. High-density lipoprotein (HDL), low-density lipoprotein (LDL) cholesterol and triglycerides (TGs) were measured by standard biochemical methods. Dyslipidemia was defined according to third report of the expert panel on detection, evaluation, and treatment of high blood cholesterol in adults (ATP-III) criteria or current treatment with statins.

Calciotropic hormones measurement included serum intact parathormone (Two-site immunoassay for iPTH, Roche Diagnostics SL, Barcelona, Spain; intra and interassay variability of 3%) and 25-hydroxyvitamin D (25-OH-D, radioimmunoassay, Dia-Sorin, Stillwater, Minnesota USA. Serum DKK1 was measured using quantitative sandwich enzyme-linked immunosorbent assay (ELISA) developed by Biomedica (Biomedica Medizinprodukte GmbH and Co. KG, Wien, Austria) according to the manufacturer's instructions. The Biomedica DKK-1 ELISA (BI-20412) detects free DKK-1. Intra-assay and interassay variability were of 7% and 9%, respectively. DKK1 measurements are reported throughout in pg/ml after conversion from pMol/L. 1 pMol/l is equivalent to 28,68 pg/ml.

Bone density measurement and vertebral fractures assessment

Bone mineral density at lumbar spine (LS) L2–L4, femoral neck (FN) and total hip (TH) was performed in all patients by dual-energy X-ray absorptiometry (DXA) using Hologic QDR 4500 densitometer (Whatman, MA; variation coefficient <1%). All the BMD measurements were done by the same experienced operator. We used the World Health Organization criteria for osteoporosis (Kanis JA, 1994).

Standardized spinal X-rays were taken for morphometric analysis of all participants of the study and they were interpreted according to the algorithm developed by McCloskey and colleagues [23].

Carotid intima-media thickness Ultrasonographic examination of the carotid arteries was performed with patients in supine position using Doppler ultrasonography (Toshiba Power-Vision 6000). The maximum intima-media thickness (IMT) at the carotid bifurcation (BIF) was determined between the near and far walls of the carotid bifurcation on the right and left sides. Each part was measured from views of both longitudinal and vertical sections at the bifurcation. If a discrepancy was observed in the measured values between longitudinal and vertical sections, the smaller value was selected to avoid overestimation. BIF–IMT was defined as the mean of the measurements from the right and left sides. The value for each side was obtained from the mean of 10 wall measurements. The BIF–IMT, measured in millimeters (mm), was considered pathological if it was ≥0.9 mm, and was considered to be carotid atherosclerosis if the BIF–IMT was ≥ 1.2 mm or 50% greater than the BIF–IMT in the adjacent area [24]. Plaques were identified as calcified by findings of bright white echoes on sonography. A single trained sonographer performed the study in all subjects.

Statistical analysis

Data for continuous variables are presented as mean ± standard deviation (SD). Data for categorical variables are presented as numbers and/or percentages. Kolmogorov–Smirnov test was used to test the normality of distribution of continuous variables. The association between continuous variables was described by Pearson's or Spearman's correlation coefficients. The comparison of categorical variables among groups was performed using Chi-square test or Fisher test. The comparison of continuous variables among groups was performed using unpaired Student's t test or Mann-Whitney test. To determine the independent variables which correlated with DKK1 (dependent variable), the parameters that correlate significantly in univariate analysis and other which are biologically linked to DKK1 were tested in multiple backward model linear regression analysis. Multiple backward model of logistic regression analysis was performed to identify DKK1 as independent predictor for CVD (dependent variable) in T2DM patients. The model included established atherosclerotic risk factors (age, gender, body mass index, hypertension, dislipidaemia, smoking, sedentarism, HbA1c, GFR and intima-media thickness). CVD-defining parameters (cerebrovascular disease, coronary heart disease or ischemic peripheral arterial disease) were not included in the multiple logistic regression model. The usefulness of serum DKK1 as a marker of high risk of atherosclerotic disease in T2DM was

Table 2. DKK1 concentrations according to the presence of cardiovascular disease in the T2DM group.

	Yes	No	P value
Cardiovascular disease	757±416	547±333	0,026
Cerebrovascular disease	854±480	625±363	0,045
Coronary heart disease	694±379	654±408	0,677
Peripheral artery disease	634±247	675±415	0,762
Abnormal intima-media thickness	756±433	567±322	0,042
Carotid plaque	730±422	661±395	0,522

The comparison between groups was done by Student's t test.

analyzed using a receiver operating characteristic curve (ROC Curve). A p value of less than 0,05 was considered to be significant (two-tailed). Data were recorded and analyzed using SPSS version 18.0 software (SPSS Inc, Chicago, IL, USA).

Results

The clinical characteristics of the study population are summarized in Table 1. Serum DKK1 was significantly higher ($P=0{,}026$) in T2DM patients with CVD (757±416 pg/ml) compared with those without CVD (547±333 pg/ml). (Figure 1 and Table 2). T2DM patients with abnormal IMT (756±433 pg/ml *vs* 563±322 pg/ml; $P=0{,}042$) and cerebrovascular disease (854±480 pg/ml *vs* 625±363; $P=0{,}045$) had higher DKK1 concentrations. (Figure 1 and Table 2). However, we did not find differences in DKK1 concentrations according to the presence of carotid plaque ($P=0{,}522$), coronary heart disease ($P=0{,}677$) or ischemic peripheral artery disease ($P=0{,}762$).

A model of logistic regression analysis was performed using the presence of CVD as a dependent variable. Independent variables were serum DKK1 levels and risk factors for atherosclerosis (age, gender, body mass index, hypertension, dislipidaemia, smoking, sedentarism, HbA1c, GFR, and IMT). DKK1 levels were independently associated with the presence of CVD in T2DM (odds ratio: 1,062, 95% confidence interval: 1,003–1,125; $P=0{,}04$). Therefore, for each increase of 28 pg/ml of serum DKK1 there was a 6,2% increased risk of CVD in T2DM patients.

In the ROC curve analysis to evaluate the usefulness of DKK1 as a marker for high risk of CVD, the area under the curve was 0,667 (95% confidence interval: 0,538–0,795; $P=0{,}016$) (Figure 2). A concentration of 494 pg/ml or higher showed a sensitivity of 71,4% and a specificity of 60% to identify an increased risk of CVD.

We found no differences in DKK1 between study groups: T2DM 669±395 vs non-diabetic 575±340 pg/ml, $P=0{,}163$. Serum DKK1 concentrations were significantly higher in females than in males in total sample (697±434 vs 563±293 pg/ml, $P=0{,}046$) and in T2DM group (788±493 vs 569±255 pg/ml, $P=0{,}025$) but were not significantly increased in control females (593±335 vs 553±349 pg/ml, $P=0{,}682$).

Linear regression analysis was performed to determine the influence of independent factors identified in univariate correlation analysis, including group, gender, age, HbA1c, CVD and IMT as independent variables that explain serum DKK1 levels. The analysis demonstrated that gender ($\beta=-0{,}299$, $P=0{,}002$) and CVD ($\beta=0{,}292$, $P=0{,}007$) were positively associated with serum DKK1.

Regarding bone metabolism, lumbar spine BMD was positively related to serum DKK1 in total sample ($r=0{,}183$, $P=0{,}048$). In contrast, we did not found a significant relationship with bone remodelling markers osteoporosis diagnosis or morphometric vertebral fractures (data not shown), in the total sample or in the study groups separately.

Discussion

To our knowledge, there is no previous study evaluating DKK1 concentrations and its relationship with CVD in Caucasian T2DM patients. There is also scarce data concerning the relationship between DKK1 and bone metabolism in T2DM. Our results show that higher levels of DKK1 are associated with clinical CVD and abnormal IMT in T2DM patients. These findings suggest that serum DKK1 are related to the presence of CVD in this population. However, our data showed no differences in serum DKK1 between T2DM patients and non-diabetic patients. Regarding bone metabolism, we found a significant relationship with bone mineral density.

In our study, higher DKK1 levels were positively related to cardiovascular disease in T2DM patients independently of the presence of others risk factors for atherosclerosis, and high concentrations of DKK1 were related to abnormal IMT in these patients. Our results are in accordance with previous reports showing the relationship between vascular disease and DKK1 in other populations. Patients with cerebrovascular disease have higher serum DKK1 levels compared with control subjects [25], and serum DKK1 correlated with coronary artery calcification and atherosclerotic plaques evaluated by coronary computed tomography and coronary artery calcium scoring [17]. Previously, Ueland and colleagues [26] demonstrated that DKK1 expression is enhanced in advanced carotid plaques and that DKK1 is a novel mediator in platelet-mediated endothelial cell activation, which could occur within the atherosclerotic lesions. Moreover, current data clearly demonstrate a novel role for Wnt proteins in the proliferation, migration, and survival of smooth muscle cells (SMCs) [27]. Regarding this, higher levels of DKK1 are present in advanced carotid plaques and DKK1 promotes platelet-mediated activation of endothelial cells. Thus, it has been proposed that this could lead to enhanced inflammation in the atherosclerotic lesion; however, it may also lead to a reduced survival, proliferation, and migration of SMCs, thereby reinforcing the potential complexity of the participation of Wnt proteins in atherosclerosis [27].

In contrast to our findings, DKK1 concentrations were negatively associated with atherosclerotic calcified plaque in African-Americans (AAs) patients with T2DM [18]. There are several reasons that might contribute to this discrepancy. As the authors point, AAs have lower rates of vascular calcification. It has

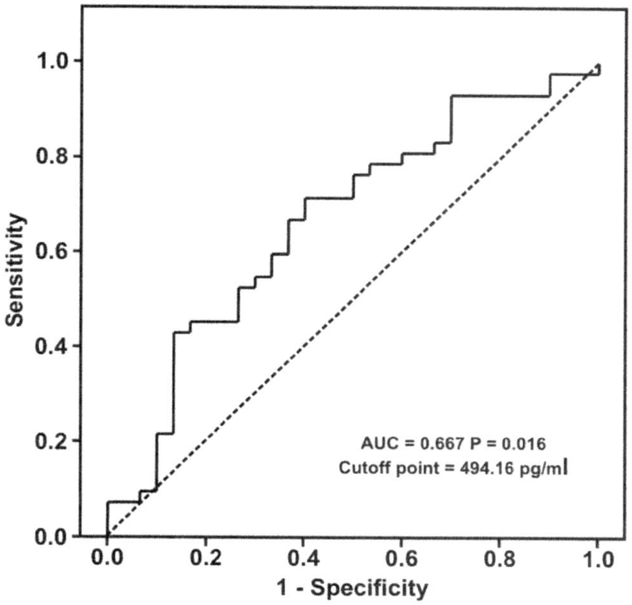

Figure 2. DKK1 ROC curve for cardiovascular disease.

been reported lower levels of coronary artery calcified plaque relative to European Americans (EAs) despite similar or more detrimental cardiovascular risk factor profiles [28,29]. This observation is consistent both in T2DM and subjects without diabetes [30,31], and suggests a differential impact of CV risk factors on atherosclerosis based on ethnicity although the underlying causes of ethnic differences in vascular calcification are not well established [32]. Reinforcing these ethnic differences, AAs are at lower risk for myocardial infarction based on less coronary artery calcification, and they have significantly lower rates of myocardial infarction than EAs, provided equal access to healthcare [33,34]. It has been suggested that AAs may be less susceptible than whites to hyperglycaemia–induced macrovascular disease [35]. Thus, these findings may explain the differences observed in the relationship between vascular disease and DKK1 between our study and the data from Register and colleagues.

Recent data suggest that the association between vascular calcification and osteoporosis is not simply a consequence of age, stressing that the co-incidence of vascular calcification with low bone activity and osteoporosis could be biologically linked. During the development of vascular calcification, there is a transition of vascular SMCs towards an osteoblast- like phenotype, which promotes the mineralization within these structures. In this process there are several players, including those related to mineral metabolism, like phosphorus, calcium or parathyroid hormone, which influences the expression of osteogenic factors [36]. There is emerging evidence suggesting that some inhibitors of the Wnt pathway, such as secreted frizzled Proteins 2 and 4 and DKK-1, may play a role linking vascular calcification and bone loss [26,27]. AAs manifest a skeletal resistance to the effects of parathyroid hormone [37,38] and exhibit opposite relationships between arterial calcification and serum vitamin D concentrations compared with Europeans [39]. In our opinion, these ethnic differences in the effects of calciotropic hormones on bone and vessels may indicate that differences in other pathways, as Wnt pathway, may be expected according to race. However, this hypothesis must be confirmed.

There are other differences between the study from Register and colleagues and ours, which may explain the discrepancy of results. First, the prevalence of cardiovascular disease is lower, 27%, compared to our study where a 58% of patients had previous cardiovascular disease. Second, in the study from Register and colleagues 28,3% of subjects were taking hormonal therapy while no women were on hormonal therapy in our study. Estradiol and progesterone has shown to regulate Wnt pathways in endometrial tissue [40] and brain [41], so an influence of hormonal therapy in DKK1 concentrations can not be excluded. Finally, despite the low expected incidence of arterial calcification in AAs, in the study from Register and colleagues there is a high prevalence of aortic calcification. Thus, differences between study populations apart from the ethnicity may influence the discrepancy of results.

There are no previous studies evaluating differences in serum DKK1 concentrations according to the presence of diabetes. We did not find differences in DKK1 between T2DM patients and subjects without diabetes. These results contrast with our previous data showing higher sclerostin concentrations in the same group of type 2 diabetes patients [42]. However, serum DKK1 and sclerostin have shown to be barely correlated [43], as we found in our sample (data not shown). In addition, the effects of DKK1 and sclerostin may differ due to differences in Kremen binding. While DKK1 is always an inhibitor of Wnt signaling, the effect of sclerostin is variable depending on context [44]. Unlike our previous results about sclerostin, women had higher DKK1 concentrations both in the total sample and in the T2DM group. Estradiol and progesterone have shown to take part in the regulation of the Wnt pathways in endometrial tissue [40] and brain [41], so a sex steroid-induced effect may explain gender differences in DKK1 although this hypothesis must be confirmed.

Regarding the relationship between bone metabolism and DKK1 we only found a weak correlation with BMD at lumbar spine in the total sample, and no relationship with bone turnover markers, osteoporosis or morphometric vertebral fractures (data not shown). In addition, lumbar spine BMD may be affected by aortic calcification. Our findings confirm previous data showing no relationship between DKK1 and bone turnover markers in postmenopausal osteoporosis [20]. The relationship between DKK1 and BMD is not totally established. It has been reported no relationship with volumetric BMD in Afro-American T2DM patients [18]. However, is also been described and inverse relationship between DKK1 and BMD, and higher DKK1 concentrations in patients with osteoporosis [19]. Therefore, in our opinion the data about serum DKK1 and bone metabolism are controversial and thus no clear conclusions can be drawn.

Our study has some limitations. First, the cross-sectional design does not allow to establishing a cause-effect relationship. Second, the sample size is relatively small and might affect the statistic power. Our study has also several strengths, as the evaluation of circulating serum DKK1 in Caucasian patients with T2DM for the first time, the comparison to non-diabetic subjects and the evaluation both of bone metabolism and atherosclerotic disease.

In summary, serum levels of DKK1 are elevated in Caucasian patients with T2DM presenting CVD. These findings suggest that Wnt signaling pathway is involved in vascular disease in diabetic subjects. However, the relations of DKK1 with bone metabolism are inconsistent.

Author Contributions

None. Conceived and designed the experiments: AGM PRM RRG MMT. Performed the experiments: BGF SMS. Analyzed the data: AGM RRG MMT. Contributed reagents/materials/analysis tools: BGF SMS. Wrote the paper: AGM RRG MMT PRM ACM MMG.

References

1. Madonna R, De Caterina R (2011) Cellular and molecular mechanisms of vascular injury in diabetes–part I: Pathways of vascular disease in diabetes. Vascular Pharmacology 54: 68–74.
2. Magnus JH, Brussard DL (2005) Relationship between bone mineral density and myocardial infarction in US adults. Osteoporosis International 16: 2053–2062.
3. Hofbauer LC, Brueck CC, Singh SK, Dognig H (2007) Osteoporosis in patients with diabetes mellitus. Journal of Bone and Mineral Research 22: 1317–1328.
4. Epstein S, Leroith D (2008) Diabetes and fragility fractures — A burgeoning epidemic? Bone 43: 3–6.
5. Carr JJ, Register TC, Hsu FC, Lohman K, Lenchik L, et al. (2008) Calcified atherosclerotic plaque and bone mineral density in type 2 diabetes: the diabetes heart study. Bone 42: 43–52.
6. Divers J, Register TC, Langefeld CD, Wagenknecht LE, Bowden DW, et al. (2011) Relationships between calcified atherosclerotic plaque and bone mineral density in AAs with type 2 diabetes. Journal of Bone and Mineral Research 26: 1554–1560.
7. Gordon MD, Nusse R (2006) Wnt signalling: multiple pathways, multiple receptors and multiple transcription factors. Journal of Biology and Chemistry 281: 22429–22433.
8. Huang H, He X (2008) Wnt/beta-catenin signaling: new (and old) players and new insight. Current Opinion in Cell Biology 20: 119–125.
9. Mao B, Wu W, Davidson G, Marhold J, Li M, et al. (2002) Kremen proteins are Dickkopf receptors that regulate Wnt/-catenin signalling. Nature 417: 664–667.
10. Shao JS, Cheng SL, Pingsterhaus JM, Charlton-Kachigian N, Loewy AP, et al. (2005) Msx2 promotes cardiovascular calcification by activating paracrine Wnt signals. Journal of Clinical Investigation 115: 1210–1220.
11. Sen M, Ghosh G (2008) Transcriptional outcome of Wnt-Frizzled signal transduction in inflammation: evolving concepts. Journal of Immunology 181: 4441–4445.
12. Christman MA 2nd, Goetz DJ, Dickerson E, McCall KD, Lewis CJ, et al. (2008) Wnt5a is expressed in murine and human atherosclerotic lesions. American Journal of Physiology and Heart Circulation and Physiology 294: H2864–2870.
13. Cheng SL, Shao JS, Behrmann A, Krchma K, Towler DA (2013) Dkk1 and MSX2-Wnt7b signaling reciprocally regulate the endothelial-mesenchymal transition in aortic endothelial cells. Arterioscler Thromb Vasc Biol 33: 1679–89.
14. Krenning G, Zeisberg EM, Kalluri R (2010) The origin of fibroblasts and mechanism of cardiac fibrosis. J Cell Physiol 225: 631–637.
15. Wylie-Sears J, Aikawa E, Levine RA, Yang JH, Bischoff J (2011) Mitral valve endothelial cells with osteogenic differentiation potential. Arterioscler Thromb Vasc Biol 31: 598–607.
16. Fang Y, Ginsberg C, Seifert M, Agapova O, Sugatani T, et al. (2014) CKD-Induced Wingless/Integration1 Inhibitors and Phosphorus Cause the CKD-Mineral and Bone Disorder. J Am Soc Nephrol 25: 1760–73.
17. Kim KI, Park KU, Chun EJ, Choi SI, Cho YS, et al. (2011) A novel biomarker of coronary atheroesclerosis: serum DKK1 concentration correlates with coronary artery calcification and atherosclerotic plaques. Journal of Korean Medical Science 26: 1178–1184.
18. Register TC, Hruska KA, Divers J, Bowden DW, Palmer ND, et al. (2013) Plasma Dickkopf (DKK1) concentrations negatively associate with atherosclerotic calcified plaque in african-americans with type 2 diabetes. Journal of Clinical Endocrinology and Metabolism 98: 60–65.
19. Butler JS, Murray DW, Hurson CJ, O'Brien J, Doran PP, et al. (2011) The role of Dkk1 in bone mass regulation: correlating serum Dkk1 expression with bone mineral density. Journal of Orthopaedic Research 29: 414–418.
20. Polyzos SA, Anastasilakis AD, Bratengeier C, Woloszczuk W, Papatheodorou A, et al. (2012) Serum sclerostin levels positively correlate with lumbar spinal bone mineral density in postmenopausal women-the six-month effect of risedronate and teriparatide. Osteoporosis International 23: 1171–1176.
21. Cejka D, Jäger-Lansky A, Kieweg H, Weber M, Bieglmayer C, et al. (2012) Sclerostin serum levels correlate positively with bone mineral density and microarchitecture in haemodialysis patients. Nephrology Dialysis Transplantion 27: 226–230.
22. Levey AS, Stevens LA, Schmid CH, Zhang YL, Castro AF 3rd, et al. (2009) CKD-EPI (Chronic Kidney Disease Epidemiology Collaboration). A new equation to estimate glomerular filtration rate. Ann Intern Med 150: 604–612.
23. McCloskey EV, Spector TD, Eyres KS, Fern ED, O'Rourke N, et al. (1993) The assessment of vertebral deformity: a method for use in population studies and clinical trials. Osteoporosis International 3: 138–147.
24. Junyent M, Gilabert R, Nuñez I, Corbella E, Vela M, et al. (2005) Carotid ultrasound in the assessment of preclinical atherosclerosis. Distribution of intima-media thickness values and plaque frequency in a Spanish community cohort. Medicina Clinica 125: 770–774.
25. Seifert-Held T, Pekar T, Gattringer T, Simmet NE, Scharnagl H, et al. (2011) Circulating Dickkopf-1 in acute ischemic stroke and clinically stable cerebrovascular disease. Atherosclerosis 218: 233–237.
26. Ueland T, Otterdal K, Lekva T, Halvorsen B, Gabrielsen A, et al. (2009) Dickkopf-1 enhances inflammatory interaction between platelets and endothelial cells and shows increased expression in atherosclerosis. Arteriosclerosis Thrombosis and Vascular Biology 29: 1228–1234.
27. Mill C, George SJ (2012) Wnt signalling in smooth muscle cells and its role in cardiovascular disorders. Cardiovascular Research 95: 233–40.
28. Bild DE, Detrano R, Peterson D, Guerci A, Liu K, et al. (2005) Ethnic differences in coronary calcification: the Multi-Ethnic Study of Atherosclerosis (MESA). Circulation 111: 1313–20.
29. Lee TC, O'Malley PG, Feuerstein I, Taylor AJ (2003) The prevalence and severity of coronary artery calcification on coronary artery computed tomography in black and white subjects. J Am Coll Cardiol 41: 39–44.
30. Freedman BI, Hsu FC, Langefeld CD, Rich SS, Herrington DM, et al. (2005) The impact of ethnicity and sex on subclinical cardiovascular disease: the Diabetes Heart Study. Diabetologia 48: 2511–8.
31. Wade AN, Fedyna S, Mehta NN, St. Clair C, Ginwala N, et al. (2011) Type 2 diabetes does not attenuate racial differences in coronary calcification. Diabetes Res Clin Pract 91: 101–7.
32. Divers J, Palmer ND, Lu L, Register TC, Carr JJ, et al. (2013) Admixture mapping of coronary artery calcified plaque in African Americans with type 2 diabetes mellitus. Circ Cardiovasc Genet; 6: 97–105.
33. Karter AJ, Ferrara A, Liu JY, Moffet HH, Ackerson LM, et al. (2002) Ethnic disparities in diabetic complications in an insured population. JAMA 287: 2519–27.
34. Young BA, Maynard C, Boyko EJ (2003) Racial differences in diabetic nephropathy, cardiovascular disease, and mortality in a national population of veterans. Diabetes Care 26: 2392–9.
35. Freedman BI, Hsu FC, Langefeld CD, Rich SS, Herrington DM, et al. (2005) The impact of ethnicity and sex on subclinical cardiovascular disease: the Diabetes Heart Study. Diabetologia 48: 2511–8.
36. Cannata-Andia JB, Roman-Garcia P, Hruska K (2011) The connections between vascular calcification and bone health. Nephrol Dial Transplant 26: 3429–36.
37. Bell NH, Williamson B, Hollis B, Riggs BL (2001) Effects of race on diurnal patterns of renal conservation of calcium and bone resorption in premenopausal women. Osteoporos Int 12: 43–8.
38. Aloia J, Vaswani A, Yeh J, Flaster E (1996) Risk for osteoporosis in black women. Calcif Tissue Int 59: 415–23.
39. Freedman BI, Register TC (2012) Effect of race and genetics on vitamin D metabolism, bone and vascular health. Nature Review Nephrology 8: 459–466.
40. Wang Y, Hanifi-Moghaddam P, Hanekamp EE, Kloosterboer HJ, Franken P, et al. (2009) Progesterone inhibition of Wnt/beta-catenin signaling in normal endometrium and endometrial cancer. Clinical Cancer Research 15: 5784–5793.
41. Scott EL, Brann DW (2012) Estrogen regulation of Dkk1 and Wnt/β-Catenin signaling in neurodegenerative disease. Brain Research 1514: 63–74.
42. García-Martín A, Rozas-Moreno P, Reyes-García R, Morales-Santana S, García-Fontana B, et al. (2012) Circulating levels of sclerostin are increased in patients with type 2 diabetes mellitus. Journal of Clinical Endocrinology and Metabolism 97: 234–241.
43. Thambiah S, Roplekar R, Manghat P, Fogelman I, Fraser WD, et al. (2012) Circulating sclerostin and Dickkopf-1 (DKK1) in predialysis chronic kidney disease (CKD): relationship with bone density and arterial stiffness. Calcified Tissue International 90: 473–480.
44. Kawano Y, Kypta R (2003) Secreted antagonists of the Wnt signalling pathway. J Cell Sci 116: 2627–34.

16

Impact of Age and Gender on the Prevalence and Prognostic Importance of the Metabolic Syndrome and Its Components in Europeans. The MORGAM Prospective Cohort Project

Julie K. K. Vishram[1,2]*, Anders Borglykke[2], Anne H. Andreasen[2], Jørgen Jeppesen[1], Hans Ibsen[3], Torben Jørgensen[2], Luigi Palmieri[4], Simona Giampaoli[4], Chiara Donfrancesco[4], Frank Kee[5], Giuseppe Mancia[6], Giancarlo Cesana[7], Kari Kuulasmaa[8], Veikko Salomaa[8], Susana Sans[9], Jean Ferrieres[10], Jean Dallongeville[11], Stefan Söderberg[12], Dominique Arveiler[13], Aline Wagner[13], Hugh Tunstall-Pedoe[14], Wojciech Drygas[15], Michael H. Olsen[16], on behalf of the MORGAM Project¶

1 Department of Internal Medicine, Glostrup Hospital, University of Copenhagen, Glostrup, Denmark, **2** Research Centre for Prevention and Health, Glostrup Hospital, University of Copenhagen, Glostrup, Denmark, **3** Division of Cardiology, Holbæk University Hospital, Holbæk, Denmark, **4** Cerebro and Cardiovascular Epidemiology Unit, National Centre of Epidemiology Surveillance and Health Promotion, National Institute of Health, Rome, Italy, **5** UKCRC Centre of Excellence for Public Health Research (NI), The Queen's University of Belfast, Belfast, Northern Ireland, **6** Clinica Medica e Istituto Auxologico Italiano, Monza, Milano, Italy, **7** Research Centre on Public Health, University of Milano Bicocca, Monza, Italy, **8** National Institute for Health and Welfare (THL), Helsinki, Finland, **9** Department of Health, Barcelona, Spain, **10** Department of Cardiology, Toulouse University School of Medicine, Rangueil Hospital, Toulouse, France, **11** Institut Pasteur de Lille, Lille, France, **12** Department of Public Health and Clinical Medicine, Cardiology and Heart Centre, Umeå University, Umeå, Sweden, **13** Department of Epidemiology and Public Health, University of Strasbourg, Faculty of Medicine, Strasbourg, France, **14** Cardiovascular Epidemiology Unit, University of Dundee, Ninewells Hospital and Medical School, Dundee, United Kingdom, **15** Department of Epidemiology, CVD Prevention and Health Promotion, National Institute of Cardiology, Warsaw, Poland, **16** Department of Endocrinology, Center of Individualized Medicine in Arterial Diseases (CIMA), Odense University Hospital, Odense, Denmark, and Hypertension in Africa Research Team (HART), North-West University, Potchefstroom, South Africa

Abstract

Objective: To investigate the influence of age and gender on the prevalence and cardiovascular disease (CVD) risk in Europeans presenting with the Metabolic Syndrome (MetS).

Methods: Using 36 cohorts from the MORGAM-Project with baseline between 1982–1997, 69094 men and women aged 19–78 years, without known CVD, were included. During 12.2 years of follow-up, 3.7%/2.1% of men/women died due to CVD. The corresponding percentages for fatal and nonfatal coronary heart disease (CHD) and stroke were 8.3/3.8 and 3.1/2.5.

Results: The prevalence of MetS, according to modified definitions of the International Diabetes Federation (IDF) and the revised National Cholesterol Education Program-Adult Treatment Panel III (NCEP-ATPIII), increased across age groups for both genders ($P<0.0001$); with a 5-fold increase in women from ages 19–39 years to 60–78 years (7.4%/7.6% to 35.4%/37.6% for IDF/NCEP-ATPIII) and a 2-fold increase in men (5.3%/10.5% to 11.5%/21.8%). Using multivariate-adjusted Cox regressions, the associations between MetS and all three CVD events were significant ($P<0.0001$). For IDF/NCEP-ATPIII in men and women, hazard ratio (HR) for CHD was 1.60/1.62 and 1.93/2.03, for CVD mortality 1.73/1.65 and 1.77/2.06, and for stroke 1.51/1.53 and 1.58/1.77. Whereas in men the HRs for CVD events were independent of age (MetS*age, $P>0.05$), in women the HRs for CHD declined with age (HRs 3.23/3.98 to 1.55/1.56; MetS*age, $P=0.01$/$P=0.001$ for IDF/NCEP-ATPIII) while the HRs for stroke tended to increase (HRs 1.31/1.25 to 1.55/1.83; MetS*age, $P>0.05$).

Conclusion: In Europeans, both age and gender influenced the prevalence of MetS and its prognostic significance. The present results emphasise the importance of being critical of MetS in its current form as a marker of CVD especially in women, and advocate for a redefinition of MetS taking into account age especially in women.

Editor: Chiara Lazzeri, Azienda Ospedaliero-Universitaria Careggi, Italy

Funding: The authors did not receive any funding for this study, but overall this work has been sustained by the MORGAM Project's current funding: European Community FP 7 projects ENGAGE (HEALTH-F4-2007-201413), and CHANCES (HEALTH-F3-2010-242244). This has supported central coordination, workshops and part of the activities of the MORGAM Data Centre, at THL in Helsinki, Finland. MORGAM Participating Centres are funded by regional and national governments, research councils, charities, and other local sources. Salary for JKV was partly covered by Interreg IVA. The funders had no role in study design, data collection and analysis, decision to publish, or preparation of the manuscript.

Competing Interests: The authors have declared that no competing interests exist.

* Email: julievishram@hotmail.com

¶ Membership of the MORGAM Project is provided in Text S1.

Introduction

Since Reaven in 1988 [1] established the clinical importance of the clustering of the metabolic disorders dysglycemia, central adiposity, hypertension and dyslipidemia (low levels of high density lipoprotein cholesterol (HDL-C) and high levels of triglycerides), known as the metabolic syndrome (MetS), many studies [2–22] have shown a higher risk of cardiovascular disease (CVD) in the presence of MetS. However, in recent years the clinical relevance of MetS in assessing risk for developing CVD has been questioned since studies [15,23–26] have stated that MetS is no single disease entity and no better than its individual components in identifying individuals at high risk of CVD. This critical appraisal of MetS as a prognostic marker of CVD risk comes at a time when the prevalence of MetS has increased dramatically, with approximately one-fourth of the adult population in Europe carrying this syndrome [27]. Therefore, it is important to clarify whether the utility of MetS can be optimized as a screening tool for identifying individuals at high risk of CVD.

From previous European work there is some indication of age and gender interactions on the association between MetS and CVD risk since the risk of CVD in the presence of MetS was more strongly related to women than men [17–22] and to older individuals [28]. However, despite this well described influence of gender and age on MetS, only few national studies have investigated age and gender specific MetS prevalence [5,8–9,11], and none of the studies looked at the impact of age and gender on the prognostic significance of MetS. Furthermore, if the purpose of MetS is to shift emphasis to earlier intervention with for example lifestyle changes, it is crucial to get a better understanding of the impact of age and gender on its prevalence and prognostic significance in a more representative sample, and therefore, studies incorporating a broader range of study participants are needed.

Using the MORGAM Project, which consists of large European population-based cohorts of men and women aged 19–78 years, with uniform standardized data collection, we aimed to investigate the influence of age and gender on the prevalence and prognostic significance of MetS in regard to fatal and nonfatal CHD, fatal and nonfatal stroke, and CVD mortality, defined by the National Cholesterol Education Program – Adult Treatment Panel (NCEP-ATP III) criteria [29] and the International Diabetes Federation (IDF) criteria [30].

Methods

Cohorts

The present study used baseline (1982–1997) and follow-up data on subsequent cardiovascular events from 36 cohorts in 10 European countries from the MOnica, Risk, Genetics, Archiving and Monograph (MORGAM)-Project [31] (table S1; see supporting information). As seen in table S1, age at baseline, gender composition as well as the follow-up time differed among the countries.

The cohorts in the MORGAM Project had either been a part of the World Health Organization's MONICA Project or had used the same standardized MONICA survey procedures for data collection as described in the MORGAM-manual [32]. Exclusion criteria at baseline included a history of stroke (ischemic or hemorrhagic; n = 969) or CHD (myocardial infarction, angina pectoris, coronary artery by-pass graft, or coronary angioplasty; n = 2899), and missing values on (1) any of the MetS components: blood pressure (BP), use of antihypertensive drugs, serum high density lipoproteins cholesterol (HDL-C), body mass index (BMI), diabetes (n = 4057) and serum triglycerides (n = 1586); and (2) potential confounders such as smoking and total serum cholesterol (n = 167), leaving a total of 69094 participants for analyses.

The use of antihypertensive drugs, daily smoking, and diabetes at baseline were self-reported. BMI was calculated as weight (kg) divided by the square of the height (m^2). Weight was measured with weight balance scales, and height with a stadiometer. Waist circumference (WC) was reported in cm. BP was measured twice in the right arm in the sitting position using a standard or random zero mercury sphygmomanometer after a 5-minute rest [33] except in five cohorts where BP was measured only once. The mean of the first and second systolic BP (SBP) and diastolic BP (DBP) was used when possible. Total cholesterol, HDL-C, and triglycerides were measured in serum samples by local laboratories [33]. Since fasting levels differed between cohorts, a categorized fasting variable was used as adjustment in the Cox model: (1) full fasting: overnight/at least 8 hours of fasting before blood sampling; (2) semi-fasting: between 4–8 hours of fasting; and (3) non-fasting: less than 4 hours of fasting.

As endpoints we chose fatal and nonfatal CHD and stroke, respectively, in order to have statistical power to identify possible endpoint related differences. Furthermore, we chose CVD mortality due to the greater validity of fatal events, as well as to include other clinical manifestations of CVD, besides CHD and stroke, that are also of atherosclerotic origin. Observations continued until death or the end of a fixed follow-up period (December 31st 1998- December 31st 2007 depending on the cohort). The mean follow-up time was 12.2 years. Fatal cases were identified by national or regional health information systems. In most cohorts, nonfatal cases were identified by hospital discharge registers. Most MORGAM centres used the WHO MONICA diagnostic criteria [33] to validate the events occurring during follow-up. Details including quality assessments of MORGAM endpoints and baseline data have been described previously [34–35].

Classification of Metabolic Status

We used modified versions of MetS according to both the IDF criteria [30] and the 2004 revised NCEP-ATP III criteria [29]. In order to maximize sample size, BMI was used in the main analyses; analyses were also replicated using WC. A scatter plot was drawn to find the BMI cut-offs which corresponded to WC with specific reference to a European population. Furthermore, since data on plasma glucose was not available, the self-reported presence of diabetes or use of anti-diabetic drugs was used instead. According to the IDF criteria, MetS was based on the presence of a BMI$\geq$30 kg/m^2 in men and $\geq$25 kg/m^2 in women and 2 or more of the following components: (1) BP$\geq$130 mmHg (systolic) or $\geq$85 mmHg (diastolic) or use of antihypertensive drugs; (2) triglyceride $\geq$1.7 mmol/l; (3) HDL-C $<$1.03 mmol/l in men and $<$1.29 mmol/l in women; and (4) the presence of diabetes or use of anti-diabetic drugs. According to the NCEP-ATP III criteria, MetS was based on the presence of 3 or more of the 5 criteria which are identical to those provided by IDF. With specific reference to a European population, the cut-offs for WC was ≥ 94 cm in men and ≥80 cm in women according to the IDF criteria, and >102 cm in men and >88 cm in women according to the NCEP-ATP III criteria.

Statistical Analyses

Statistical Analysis Software (SAS Institute Inc, Cary, NC) version 9.2 was used for all analyses. Baseline characteristics were presented as median and the 5th and 95th percentiles or as percent. Discrete variables were compared using the Chi-square test, while continuous variables were compared using Student's t-test or non-parametric Mann-Whitney test, according to the normality of variables. Differences in continuous variables between groups were tested using one-way ANOVA. Due to differences in cohort follow-up time, the incidence rates of cardiovascular events per 1000 person years were reported instead of absolute risk for MetS and its individual components.

Since age distribution varied among the populations, the prevalence of MetS at baseline was presented for a fixed age-interval of 50–59 years, allowing for a meaningful comparison between the populations since this age range was covered by all the populations. Furthermore, due to significant interactions between age and gender for the baseline prevalence of MetS and its components using logistic regression models adjusted for country, total cholesterol, smoking- and fasting status (all $P<$ 0.0001, table 1), separate analyses were carried out for men and women in various baseline age groups: 19–39 years, 40–49 years, 50–59 years, and 60–78 years. Although interactions between country and age as well as country and gender were also significant for the prevalence of MetS and most of its components, regression analyses were not carried out separately for men and women within each country due to lack of statistical power. Instead, the Cox proportional hazard model was stratified by country allowing for the baseline hazard to vary between countries. In addition, we adjusted for age, total cholesterol, smoking and fasting status, and used time from baseline as the time scale. Hazard ratios (HRs) and 95% confidence intervals (95% CIs) for CHD, stroke, and CVD mortality in relation to the different definitions of MetS were estimated separately for men and women of various age groups. Only the interaction between MetS and age for women with regards to CHD risk was significant (table 2). In the outcome analysis, for participants who experienced multiple events we only considered the first.

All explanatory variables met the proportional hazards assumption of the Cox regression model, assessed by Schoenfeld residuals. The linearity of the continuous variables was assessed using quadratic and cubic effects as well as cubic splines (a piecewise fitting of polynomial equations).

Analyses were replicated in subsets using WC instead of BMI, and using a reduced dataset excluding participants in antihypertensive treatment and non-fasting or semi-fasting participants.

For all analyses a 2-tailed $P<0.05$ was considered statistically significant.

Results

Risk Factors

For both genders, the median values of the baseline metabolic risk factors as well as the prevalence of the individual components of MetS, except HDL-C, and triglycerides in men, increased across age groups (all $P<0.0001$; table 3 and figure 1, respective-

Table 1. Significance of age, gender, country, and their interactions, for risk of having the metabolic syndrome or its individual components in adjusted logistic regression models.

Influence of:	age	gender	country	age* gender	country* gender	country* age	country* gender* age
P-values:							
MetS ATP	<0.0001	<0.0001	<0.0001	<0.0001	<0.0001	<0.0001	0.41
MetS IDF	<0.0001	<0.0001	<0.0001	<0.0001	<0.0001	<0.0001	0.74
Individual MetS Components (dichotomized):							
Blood Pressure	<0.0001	<0.0001	<0.0001	<0.0001	<0.0001	<0.0001	0.88
Body Mass Index	<0.0001	<0.0001	<0.0001	<0.0001	<0.0001	<0.0001	0.009
Triglycerides	<0.0001	<0.0001	<0.0001	<0.0001	<0.0001	0.0005	0.004
HDL-Cholesterol	<0.0001	<0.0001	<0.0001	<0.0001	<0.0001	<0.0001	<0.0001
Diabetes	<0.0001	0.09	0.45	<0.0001	0.10	0.002	0.15

$P<0.05$ indicates a significant interaction term in the logistic regression model.
Adjusted for age, sex, country, total cholesterol, smoking- and fasting status.
MetS ATP indicates the metabolic syndrome defined by the National Cholesterol Education Program - Adult Treatment Panel III; and MetS IDF, the metabolic syndrome defined by the International Diabetes Federation.

Table 2. Significance of interactions between age, gender, and the metabolic syndrome for subsequent CVD risk in adjusted Cox regression models.

	Fatal and nonfatal		
	CHD	**Stroke**	**CVD mortality**
Interactions:	***P*-values:**	***P*-values:**	***P*-values:**
sex*MetS IDF	0.07	0.97	0.90
sex*MetS ATP	0.005	0.32	0.05
age*MetS IDF	0.004	0.19	0.02
age*MetS ATP	0.0003	0.56	0.01
Men			
age*MetS IDF	0.30	0.91	0.10
age*MetS ATP	0.53	0.13	0.16
Women			
age*MetS IDF	0.01	0.86	0.18
age*MetS ATP	0.001	0.56	0.05

$P<0.05$ indicates a significant interaction term in the Cox regression model.
CHD indicates coronary heart disease; CVD, cardiovascular disease; MetS ATP, the metabolic syndrome defined by the National Cholesterol Education Program - Adult Treatment Panel III; and MetS IDF, the metabolic syndrome defined by the International Diabetes Federation.
Cox model adjusted for smoking (yes/no), cholesterol (continuous), and fasting (full/semi/no fasting).

ly). Age influenced the pattern of the MetS components in men and women, such that young women had a higher prevalence of obesity and low HDL-C, while younger men had a higher prevalence of elevated BP and elevated triglycerides. In older men and women, high BP was the most prevalent component of MetS.

Metabolic Syndrome

Despite comparing men and women separately, and using a fixed age interval of 50–59 years covered by all the populations, baseline MetS prevalence, defined by IDF/NCEP-ATP III, still varied greatly among populations (5.0–18.1%/10.8–34.5% in men and 11.3–45.0%/12.6–46.1% in women; table S1, see supporting information) leading to country interactions independently of differences in age and gender (table 1).

In the total population, there was a higher prevalence of MetS when using the NCEP-ATP III criteria compared to the IDF. This difference between IDF and NCEP-ATP III was more pronounced in men (9.7%/19.9%) than in women (29.5%/32.1%). MetS was slightly more prevalent in women compared to men, but this difference became smaller when using a BMI cut-off of 30 kg/m^2 in both genders (table S1, see supporting information).

Participants who had MetS defined by IDF also had MetS defined by NCEP-ATP III. However, of those participants who had MetS defined by NCEP-ATP III, 30% (4048/13833; 447 women and 3601 men) did not have MetS defined by IDF (data not shown) supporting the conclusion that the IDF definition is more restrictive than NCEP-ATP III, especially in men (figure 2).

Taking into account age group, the prevalence of MetS defined by both IDF and NCEP-ATP III significantly increased across ages for both genders ($P<0.0001$; figure 2). The increase in MetS prevalence from age group 19–39 years to 60–78 years was almost 5-fold (7.4%/7.6% to 35.4%/37.6%, for IDF/NCEP-ATP III, respectively) in women and 2-fold (5.3%/10.5% to 11.5%/21.8%) in men reflecting less increase in men older than 49 years. Within each age group, there was a significantly higher prevalence of MetS in women compared to men when using IDF, while for NCEP-ATP III this was only the case for women aged 50 years or above (all $P<0.0001$; figure 2).

Outcome

During the average of 12.2 years of follow-up, the number of CHD, stroke, and CVD mortality in men/women were 3222/1146, 1189/768, and 1412/638, respectively (table S1, see supporting information). The incidence rates per 1000 person years for the 3 CVD events generally increased with rising number of components of MetS ($P<0.0001$) and age categories ($P<0.0001$) at baseline, with the strongest relations to CHD incidence rates and the weakest relationship with stroke and those below 40 years of age (figure 3). In women three or more elements, resembling MetS, had to be present to identify a significant risk increase (figure 3).

A comparison of men and women within each age group confirmed higher incidence rates in men for CHD in participants older than 39 years with 0–4 risk factors present, for CVD mortality in participants older than 49 years with 1–4 risk factors present, and for stroke in participants older than 49 years with 2–3 risk factors present (figure 3).

Even after adjusting for the known higher incidence rates with aging and male gender ($P<0.0001$; figure 4), MetS at baseline was associated with higher incidence rates especially for CHD and when MetS was defined by NCEP-ATP III. For stroke, the incidence rates were very low for those younger than 50 years with MetS, indicating that MetS was not strongly associated with stroke in younger participants.

The gender-specific HRs for CHD, stroke, and CVD mortality when baseline MetS was defined by either IDF or NCEP-ATP III (table 4) were significantly associated with all three CVD events (all $P<0.0001$), independent of age, total cholesterol, and smoking as well as fasting status, and comparable HRs were observed for both definitions of MetS. However, in women compared to men MetS defined by especially NCEP-ATPIII was closer associated with CHD risk (HRs 1.93/2.03 vs. 1.60/1.62 for IDF/NCEP-ATP III), with CVD mortality risk (HRs 1.77/2.06 vs. 1.73/1.65),

Table 3. Distribution of risk factors in men (a) and women (B) according to age group.

(A) Men	Age				
Risk Factors	19–78 Years	19–39 Years	40–49 Years	50–59 Years	60–78 Years
Number of subjects	38639	8143 (21.1)	8409 (21.8)	17714 (45.8)	4373 (11.3)
Smoker	13463 (34.8)	3559 (43.7)[b]	3475 (41.3)[b]	5051 (28.5)	1378 (31.5)
Diabetes mellitus	1240 (3.2)	73 (0.9)	165 (2.0)	730 (4.1)	272 (6.2)
Antihypertensive treatment	3346 (8.7)	87 (1.1)	419 (5.0)	2053 (11.6)	787 (18.0)
BMI, kg/m^2	26.0 (20.9–32.7)	24.8 (20.3–31.6)	26.0 (21.0–32.7)	26.3 (21.3–32.8)[b]	26.6 (21.1–33.4)[b]
Waist circumference[a], cm	93 (77.5–111)	87 (74–107)	92.5 (77.5–111)	94 (79–112)	96 (79–114)
Total cholesterol, mmol/L	5.61 (4.01–7.53)	5.20 (3.70–7.20)	5.70 (4.10–7.70)[d]	5.74 (4.20–7.58)[d]	5.80 (4.20–7.70)
Triglycerides, mmol/L	1.42 (0.66–3.86)	1.21 (0.58–3.46)	1.54 (0.67–4.31)	1.47 (0.71–3.85)[b]	1.43 (0.70–3.66)[b]
HDL cholesterol, mmol/L	1.19 (0.77–1.85)	1.21 (0.81–1.81)[c]	1.16 (0.73–1.83)	1.19 (0.76–1.86)[c]	1.24 (0.81–1.94)[c]
Systolic blood pressure, mmHg	131 (107–170)	124 (105–150)	128 (106–161)	133 (108–172)	144 (112–188)
Diastolic blood pressure, mmHg	83 (65–104)	79 (61–98)	83 (66–104)	84 (67–105)	85 (67–106)
(B) Women	**Age**				
Risk Factors	**19–78 Years**	**19–39 Years**	**40–49 Years**	**50–59 Years**	**60–78 Years**
Number of subjects	30455	8799 (28.9)	8818 (29.0)	8560 (28.1)	4278 (14.1)
Smoker	8171 (26.8)	2780 (31.6)[b]	2630 (29.8)[b]	2032 (23.7)	729 (17.0)
Diabetes mellitus	810 (2.7)	87 (1.0)	154 (1.8)	303 (3.5)	266 (6.2)
Antihypertensive treatment	2903 (9.5)	104 (1.2)	525 (6.0)	1256 (14.7)	1018 (23.8)
BMI, kg/m^2	25.1 (19.6–35.5)	23.2 (18.9–32.3)	25.0 (35.0–19.9)	26.4 (20.4–36.5)	27.4 (20.5–37.3)
Waist circumference[a], cm	78.5 (65–103)	74 (63.5–96)	78.5 (66–102.5)	82 (68–107)	84.5 (68.5–107)
Total cholesterol, mmol/L	5.59 (4.00–7.73)	4.90 (3.70–6.70)	5.40 (4.00–7.30)	6.10 (4.50–8.20)	6.30 (4.60–8.30)
Triglycerides, mmol/L	1.11 (0.56–2.84)	0.90 (0.50–2.14)	1.06 (0.55–2.71)	1.32 (0.66–3.20)	1.40 (0.72–3.28)
HDL cholesterol, mmol/L	1.44 (0.93–2.14)	1.46 (0.98–2.12)[d]	1.41 (0.90–2.10)	1.43 (0.91–2.16)	1.47 (0.93–2.23)[d]
Systolic blood pressure, mmHg	126 (101–170)	116 (98–140)	124 (101–160)	135 (107–178)	145 (113–185)
Diastolic blood pressure, mmHg	79 (61–100)	73 (58–91)	79 (63–100)	83 (65–104)[c]	83 (66–104)[c]

Values are expressed as numbers (percentages) or median (5% to 95% percentiles).
[a]Number of subjects = 39106 (Men/Women = 23817/15289) since not all cohorts registered waist circumference.
Comparison of risk factor values between age groups (i.e., 19–39 years versus 40–49 years, 40–49 years versus 50–59 years, and so on) for men and women separately, all $P<0.0001$, except. [b]$P<0.01$, [c]$P<0.05$, and [d]$P>0.05$.
Comparison of risk factor values between men and women within each age group, all $P<0.0001$, except for SBP levels in ages 60–78 years, and % of diabetics in ages 19–49 years and ages 60–78 years, where all $P>0.05$.

and with stroke risk (HRs 1.58/1.77 vs. 1.51/1.53). Furthermore, whereas in men the HRs for a CVD event were independent of age (MetS*age, $P>0.05$; table 2), in women the HRs for CHD declined with age (from HRs 3.23/3.98 to 1.55/1.56; MetS*age, $P=0.01/P=0.001$ for IDF/NCEP-ATPIII) while the HRs for stroke tended to increase (from HRs 1.31/1.25 to 1.55/1.83; MetS*age, $P>0.05$).

Sensitivity Analyses

Replicating the above analyses in subsets using WC instead of BMI, and using a reduced dataset excluding participants in antihypertensive treatment and non-fasting or semi-fasting participants, generally showed similar trends. Worth noting is that the mean values of triglycerides, SBP, and DBP, as well as the prevalence/incidence rates of MetS and its components were attenuated. Furthermore, using WC instead of BMI showed a higher prevalence of MetS defined by IDF in men compared to women.

Discussion

Using modified versions of the IDF- and the revised NCEP-ATP III criteria of MetS, the main findings of the present study were that the prevalence and prognostic significance of MetS at baseline showed great variations among countries and were influenced by both age and gender. With older age, the prevalence of MetS increased 5-fold in women and 2-fold in men (figure 2) and the pattern of the individual MetS components changed in women (obesity was surpassed by high SBP) but not in men in whom SBP was dominating in all ages (figure 1). Independently of age the prevalence of MetS based on the NCEP-ATP III criteria almost doubled that of IDF criteria in men whereas it was equal in women (figure 2). Incidence rates for all three CVD events increased with more components of MetS present independently of the type of CVD event, age and gender (figure 3), whereas the risk of a CVD event associated with MetS was (1) higher in women than in men especially when using the NCEP-ATP III criteria

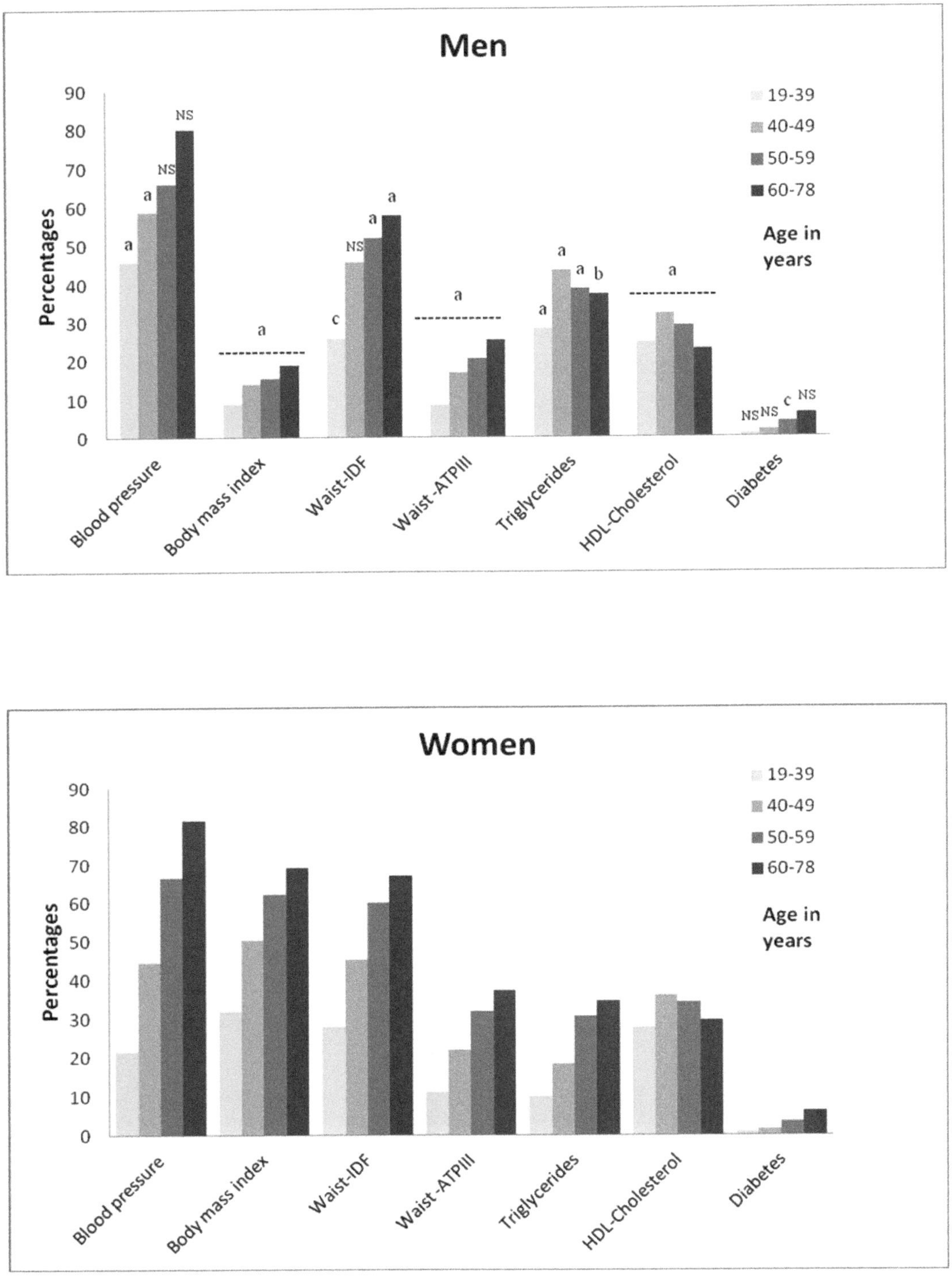

Figure 1. Frequency of each MetS component according to gender and age group. MetS indicates the metabolic syndrome; IDF, the International Diabetes Federation; and ATPIII, Adult Treatment Panel III. The men/women ratio is 38639/30455 for all components except for waist circumference (men/women =23817/152899) since not all cohorts registered waist circumference. $P<0.0001$ for each MetS component across age groups in men and women separately. Gender differences within each age group, with $P<0.0001^{a}$, $P<0.01^{b}$, $P<0.05^{c}$, NS indicates non-significance, $P>0.05$, and the dashed line indicates the same level of significance across the age groups.

(table 4), and (2) independently of age in men whereas in women CHD risk decreased and stroke risk tended to increase with older age (table 4).

These results were reproducible in all sensitivity analyses, although attenuated. To the best of our knowledge this is the first study to examine the age and gender specific prevalence and

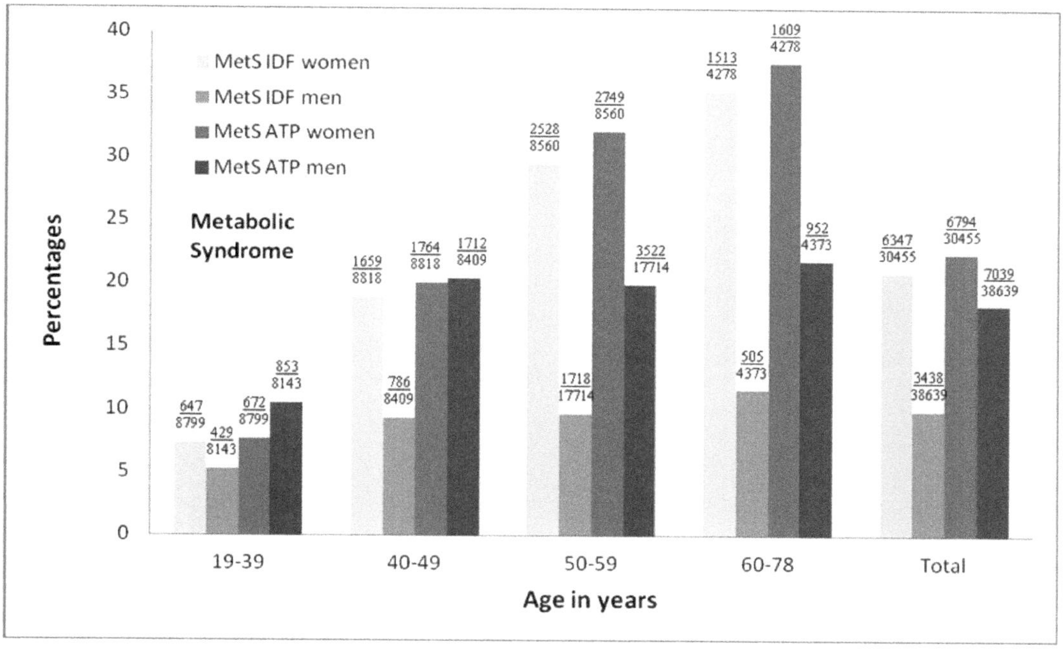

Figure 2. Frequency of MetS according to gender and age group. MetS indicates the metabolic syndrome; IDF, the International Diabetes Federation (MetS IDF) criteria and the National Cholesterol Education Program–Adult Treatment Panel III (MetS ATP) criteria. Numbers above each bar indicate total number of persons with MetS/total number of persons in the given age group; All $P<0.0001$ for each of the 4 MetS/gender combination across age groups. Within each age group, $P<0.0001$ between genders, except for MetS ATP in ages 40–49 years ($P=0.57$).

prognostic significance of MetS using the IDF and the revised NCEP-ATP III criteria in a large European prospective cohorts study.

Prevalence of MetS and its components

Our finding, that MetS prevalence increased with age, is consistent with previous work [3,5,8–9,11,28,36]. Furthermore, the steeper age-related increase in MetS prevalence in women compared to men, has also been shown previously [5,8], and may be attributable to the steep increase in BP in women after menopause which initiates a more rapid decrease in endothelial function. Consistently, we found a shift in the dominance of the individual MetS components with age, from obesity in younger women to elevated BP in older women. Similarly, Lawlor et al [12] found that the most prevalent component of MetS in postmenopausal women was elevated BP. The less steep increase in prevalence of MetS with older age in men, found in the present study, could partly be due to the dominance of the BP component in all age groups. The relative difference between the genders in components of MetS with older age has been shown previously [9].

Country variations in prevalence of MetS have also been found in other studies [5,8,9,11,17–20,27]. For instance, comparing studies from Germany [5], Norway [8], and Greece [11] show variations in MetS prevalence from 9–16% in men below age 40 years to 34–45% in men between ages 60–69 years, and the corresponding prevalence in women was 5–8% and 35–46%. These age differences were slightly accentuated when using the IDF criteria. The country variation in the present study could not be explained by variations in age and gender indicating that it was due to some country specific differences in either genes, lifestyle and/or population selection.

Incidence rates and prognostic importance of MetS and its components

Previously, it has been shown that incidence rates for CVD increase with more components of MetS present [36,37], as well as with the presence of MetS [3,5,22]. Furthermore, some [17–22] but not all [2,12] previous studies have shown a higher CVD event risk conferred by MetS in women compared to men. We confirmed and extended these findings by showing (1) that it was true for the risk of CHD, stroke, and CVD mortality, (2) that the risk associated with MetS was higher in women especially when using the NCEP-ATP III criteria, and (3) that the CVD event risk associated with MetS was independently of age in men whereas in women CHD risk decreased and stroke risk tended to increase with older age.

The CVD event risk associated with MetS can be explained by the fact that MetS includes both metabolic risk factors promoting atherosclerosis and CHD and hemodynamic risk factors promoting arteriosclerosis and stroke [38,39]. In women the revised NCEP-ATP III criteria was more closely associated with outcome than MetS defined by the IDF criteria which might be explained by the fact that elevated BMI, which is mandatory for the IDF definition and very prevalent in women with MetS, is only weakly related to CVD outcome.

Furthermore, the weaker associations between CVD event risk and MetS defined by the IDF as well as NCEP-ATP III criteria found previously in women [2,12] could be due to the lack of age-stratification as well as the lack of inclusion of younger women. The increased relative risk for CHD among young women with MetS might be explained by the low absolute risk of CHD in these young women. Indeed, we showed very low incidence rates per 1000 person years for CHD in women aged 19–39 years without MetS (figure 4A). Consistently, Gami et al [18] showed in a meta-analysis that the association between MetS and incident CVD

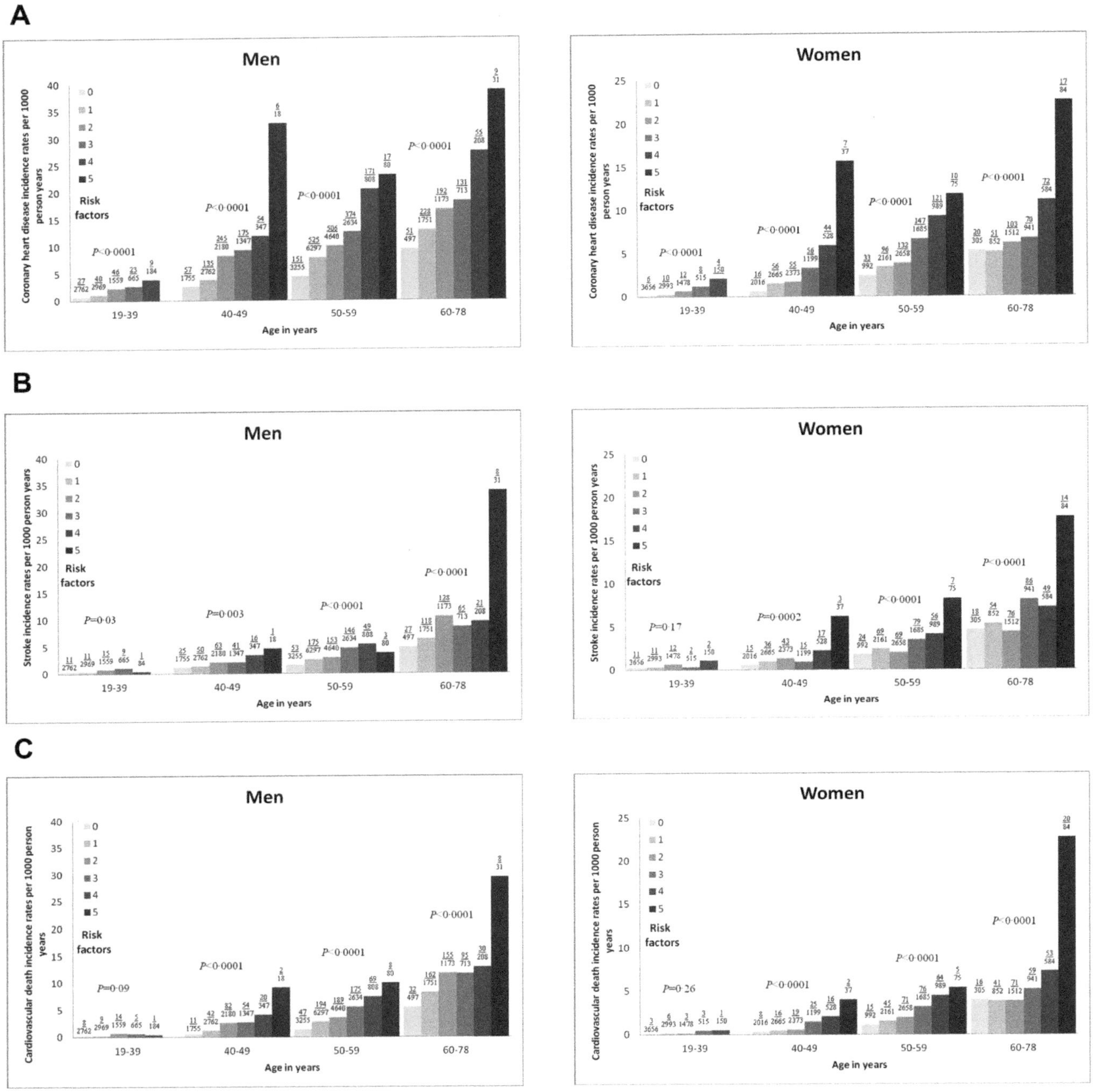

Figure 3. Age- and gender-specific incidence rates per 1000 person years for CVD with increasing number of risk factors. Risk factors refer to the components of the metabolic syndrome (MetS); and CVD, cardiovascular disease: (A) fatal and nonfatal CHD, (B) fatal and nonfatal stroke, and (C) cardiovascular death. Numbers above each bar indicate event/person. Overall trend with $P<0.0001$ for incidence rates with increasing number of MetS risk factors and age categories at baseline. Within each age group, the reported P values indicate significant differences in incidence rates with rising number of MetS risk factors, except in men (for CVD) and women (for stroke and CVD) below age 40 years.

events and death was stronger in studies enrolling lower risk individuals. The apparent age independency of MetS associated CVD event risk in men, can be explained by lower relative risk in younger men with MetS due to higher absolute risk in younger men without MetS, by higher relative risk in middle-aged men due to sufficient exposure time, and finally by a lower relative risk in older men due to selection bias. Alternatively, the reduction of HRs with aging for CHD and to some degree of CVD mortality in women with MetS might be due to increasing competing risk (i.e. cancer) [40], but that would not explain the gender difference. In contrast, the stroke risk associated with MetS seemed to increase with age in women. This age-related increase in HRs for stroke in women with MetS might reflect the increased contribution of SBP to the definition of MetS. As seen in figure 1, we showed that the frequency of the BP component of MetS increased from 20% in women aged 19–39 years to 80% in women aged 60–78 years as

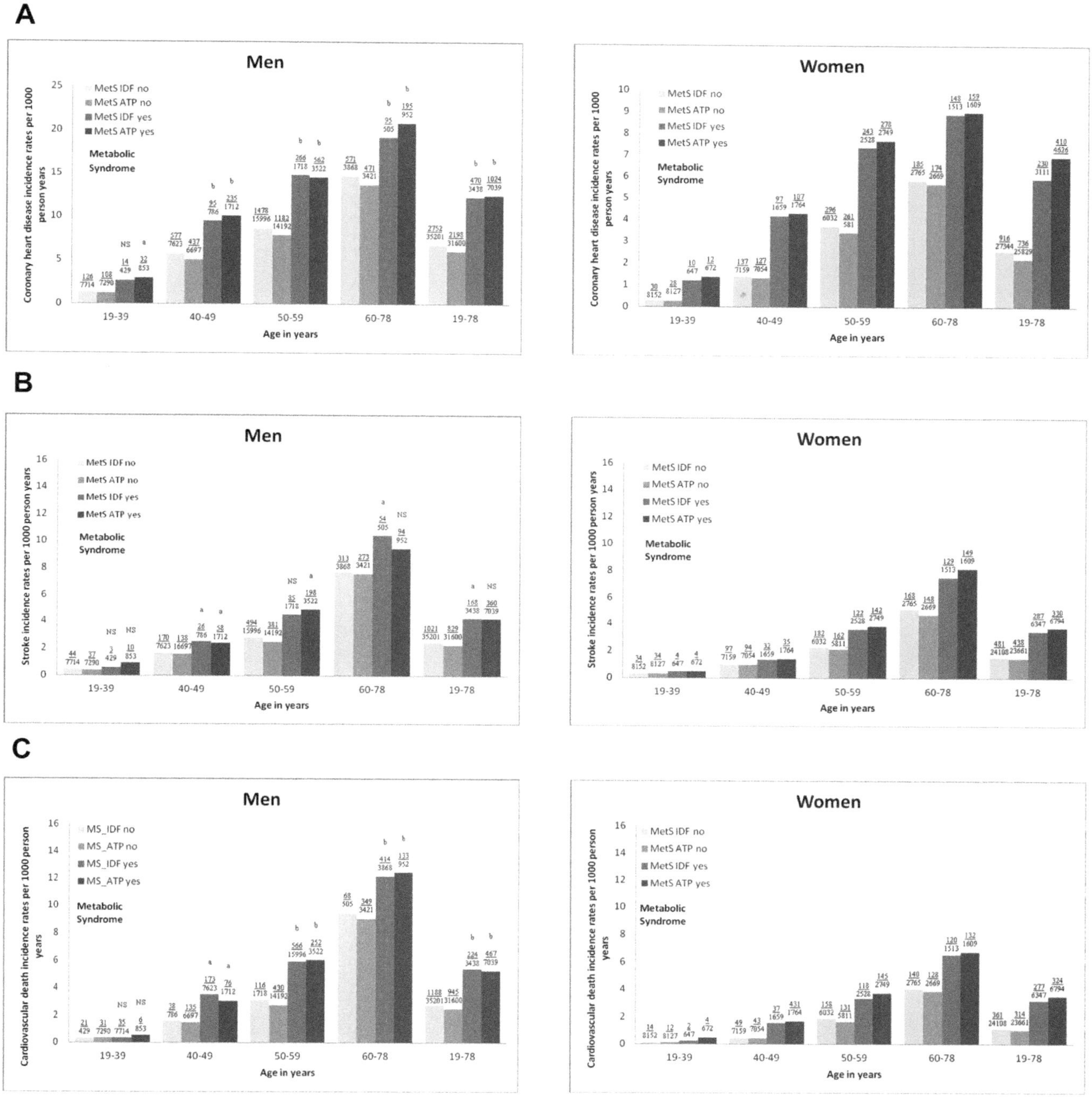

Figure 4. Age- and gender-specific incidence rates per 1000 person years for CVD with or without the presence of MetS. MetS IDF indicates the metabolic syndrome defined according to the International Diabetes Federation criteria; MetS ATP, the metabolic syndrome defined according to the National Cholesterol Eduation Program-Adult Treatment Panel III; and CVD, cardiovascular disease: (A) fatal and nonfatal CHD, (B) fatal and nonfatal stroke, and (C) cardiovascular death. Numbers above each bar indicate events/persons. Comparison of incidence rates between men and women with MetS within each age group using Pearson Chi^2-test, $P<0.05^a$, $P<0.0001^b$, and NS indicates non-significance, $P>0.05$.

compared to 45% and 80% in men. Furthermore, from table 3B it is seen that the median SBP value increased significantly with age. Lastly, in previous work [41] we showed that the HR for SBP does not decrease with age, implying the importance of SBP also in the elderly.

Strengths

The strength of the present investigation was the large sample size of 69 094 individuals, with a mean follow-up time of 12.2 years leading to a relatively large number of CVD events: 4368, 1957, 2050 incident CHD-, stroke- and CVD-events, respectively, which was more than in many previous studies, and which allowed robust sensitivity analyses. Other strengths were the inclusion of a wide age range, an almost equal proportion of men and women,

Table 4. Hazard ratio for different definitions of the metabolic syndrome by age category and event type in men and women.

	Men							Women						
		MetS IDF			MetS ATP				MetS IDF			MetS ATP		
	N	HR	95%CI	*P*-value	HR	95%CI	*P*-value	N	HR	95%CI	*P*-value	HR	95%CI	*P*-value
Coronary heart disease														
19–39 years	140	1.46	0.84–2.55	0.18	1.50	0.99–2.27	0.05	40	3.23	1.51–6.89	0.0025	3.98	1.94–8.20	0.0002
40–49 years	672	1.59	1.28–1.98	<0.0001	1.65	1.40–1.95	<0.0001	234	2.56	1.96–3.35	<0.0001	2.66	2.04–3.48	<0.0001
50–59 years	1744	1.71	1.50–1.95	<0.0001	1.65	1.49–1.83	<0.0001	539	1.88	1.58–2.23	<0.0001	2.02	1.70–2.40	<0.0001
60–78 years	666	1.29	1.03–1.60	0.02	1.46	1.23–1.72	<0.0001	333	1.55	1.24–1.94	0.0001	1.56	1.25–1.94	<0.0001
19–78 years[a]	3222	1.60	1.45–1.77	<0.0001	1.62	1.50–1.75	<0.0001	1146	1.93	1.71–2.18	<0.0001	2.03	1.80–2.29	<0.0001
Stroke														
19–39 years	47	0.98	0.30–3.19	0.97	1.88	0.91–3.89	0.09	38	1.31	0.45–3.78	0.62	1.25	0.43–3.61	0.68
40–49 years	196	1.54	1.01–2.34	0.04	1.37	1.00–1.88	0.05	129	1.33	0.88–2.00	0.17	1.35	0.90–2.01	0.14
50–59 years	579	1.60	1.27–2.02	<0.0001	1.76	1.47–2.09	<0.0001	304	1.74	1.38–2.21	<0.0001	1.95	1.54–2.46	<0.0001
60–78 years	367	1.38	1.03–1.84	0.032	1.25	0.99–1.58	0.066	297	1.55	1.22–1.96	0.0003	1.83	1.44–2.32	<0.0001
19–78 years[a]	1189	1.51	1.28–1.78	<0.0001	1.53	1.35–1.73	<0.0001	768	1.58	1.36–1.84	<0.0001	1.77	1.52–2.05	<0.0001
Cardiovascular death														
19–39 years	37	0.72	0.17–3.03	0.66	1.05	0.42–2.63	0.91	16	1.21	0.26–5.61	0.81	2.90	0.88–9.56	0.08
40–49 years	211	2.17	1.52–3.10	<0.0001	1.70	1.27–2.27	0.0003	86	2.67	1.72–4.15	<0.0001	3.12	2.01–4.84	<0.0001
50–59 years	682	1.91	1.56–2.34	<0.0001	1.84	1.57–2.15	<0.0001	276	1.70	1.33–2.16	<0.0001	2.07	1.62–2.63	<0.0001
60–78 years	482	1.34	1.03–1.73	0.027	1.37	1.12–1.68	0.0022	260	1.60	1.25–2.06	0.0002	1.71	1.33–2.20	<0.0001
19–78 years[a]	1412	1.73	1.50–2.00	<0.0001	1.65	1.47–1.84	<0.0001	638	1.77	1.51–2.09	<0.0001	2.06	1.75–2.42	<0.0001

N indicates the number of events; MetS IDF, metabolic syndrome according to the International Diabetes Federation; and MetS ATP, metabolic syndrome according to the National Cholesterol Education Program – Adult Treatment Panel III.
Cox model adjusted for smoking (yes/no), cholesterol (continuous), and fasting (full/semi/no fasting).
[a]For the total population, the Cox model is adjusted for age, smoking (yes/no), total cholesterol (continuous), and fasting (full/semi/no fasting).

and the standardized baseline and endpoint assessment available from the well-characterized MORGAM cohorts, with individual validation of the diagnosis in the majority of fatal and nonfatal events.

Limitations

Some limitations should also be considered. The baseline age distribution of the various populations differed, and therefore any age difference observed may also reflect differences between the populations. We tried to minimize the influence of the populations by adjusting for country in the Cox model. Furthermore, when comparing MetS prevalence among the populations, we used a fixed age group, which was covered by all populations. However, since most populations are from age 25 years and onwards, our results for the youngest age group should be interpreted with caution due to lack of statistical power to detect associations.

The MetS status of the participants, which is bound to change during the follow-up period, was available only at baseline, causing likely attenuation of the estimates of the hazard ratios.

Since data on plasma glucose was not available, the self-reported presence of diabetes or use of anti-diabetic drugs was used instead. Therefore, we have underestimated the prevalence of diabetes. Although most of the "missed" cases would be defined as having MetS on account of the coexistence of other components of MetS, some might have been "missed" probably leading to an underestimation of the HR associated with MetS because subjects with diabetes generally are at high CVD risk. Therefore, we do not believe that the underestimation of MetS influenced the prognostic interactions between age, gender and the risk of MetS. Although we used BMI instead of WC in order to maximize sample size, this was in line with other studies [6,9,17–20]. In a meta-analysis by Gami et al [18] it was shown that substitution of BMI for WC or waist-to-hip ratio in NCEP-based criteria did not appear to affect the results. Moreover, since fasting levels differed between cohorts, a categorized fasting variable was used as adjustment in the Cox model. In both of these cases, we carried out sensitivity analyses using WC instead of BMI, or including only full-fasting individuals, and showed similar, although slightly attenuated results. For the latter case, Hildrum et al [8] showed no statistically significant difference between the fasting and the non-fasting samples in the prevalence of the IDF- or ATP-proxies of MetS. Finally, our findings may not apply to non-Europeans or patients with CVD because the latter were excluded.

Conclusion

MetS was prevalent and associated with increased incidence of CHD, stroke, and CVD mortality. However, prevalence and prognostic importance were strongly dependent on age and gender, which seemed to account for some of the differences between countries. The CHD risk associated with MetS was higher in women especially when using the NCEP-ATP III criteria and it was independently of age in men whereas in women CHD risk decreased significantly and stroke risk tended to increase with older age. These results emphasise the importance of being critical of MetS in its current form as a marker of CVD especially in women, and advocate for a redefinition of MetS taking into account age especially in women.

Supporting Information

Table S1 Characteristics of the MORGAM cohorts included in the analyses.

Text S1 Appendix.

Author Contributions

Conceived and designed the experiments: JKV AB AHA JJ HI TJ LP SG CD FK GM GC KK VS S. Sans JF JD S. Söderberg DA AW HT WD MHO. Performed the experiments: JKV AB AHA JJ HI TJ LP SG CD FK GM GC KK VS S. Sans JF JD S. Söderberg DA AW HT WD MHO. Analyzed the data: JV MHO AB AHA KK JJ TJ. Contributed reagents/materials/analysis tools: JKV AB AHA JJ HI TJ LP SG CD FK GM GC KK VS S. Sans JF JD S. Söderberg DA AW HT WD MHO. Wrote the paper: JKV MHO. Author contributions to manuscript revision: JKV AB AHA JJ HI TJ LP SG CD FK GM GC KK VS S. Sans JF JD S. Söderberg DA AW HT WD MHO.

References

1. Reaven GM (1988) Role of insulin resistance in human disease. Diabetes 37: 1595–1607.
2. Qiao Q, The DECODE Study Group (2006) Comparison of different definitions of the metabolic syndrome in relation to cardiovascular mortality in European men and women. Diabetologia 49: 2837–2846.
3. Ascaso JF, Millán J, Mateo-Gallego R, Ruiz A, Suarez-Tembra M, et al. (2011) Prevalence of metabolic syndrome and cardiovascular disease in a hypertriglyceridemic population. Eur J Intern Med 22: 177–1781.
4. Benetos A, Thomas F, Pannier B, Bean K, Jégo B, et al. (2008) All-cause and cardiovascular mortality using the different definitions of metabolic syndrome. Am J Cardiol 102: 188–191.
5. Assmann G, Guerra R, Fox G, Cullen P, Schulte H, et al. (2007) Harmonizing the definition of the metabolic syndrome: comparison of the criteria of the Adult Treatment Panel III and the International Diabetes Federation in United States of American and European populations. Am J Cardiol 99: 541–548.
6. Dekker JM, Girman C, Rhodes T, Nijpels G, Stehouwer CDA, et al. (2005) Metabolic syndrome and 10-year cardiovascular disease risk in the Hoorn study. Circulation 112: 666–673.
7. Wang J, Ruotsalainen S, Moilanen L, Lepistö P, Laakso M, et al. (2007) The metabolic syndrome predicts cardiovascular mortality: a 13-year follow-up study in elderly non-diabetic Finns. Eur Heart J 28: 857–864.
8. Hildrum B, Mykletun A, Hole T, Midthjell K, Dahl AA (2007) Age-specific prevalence of the metabolic syndrome defined by the International Diabetes Federation and the National Cholesterol Education Program: the Norwegian HUNT 2 study. BMC Public Health 7: 220.
9. Hu G, Qiao Q, Tuomilehto J, Balkau B, Borch-Johnsen K, et al; for the DECODE Study Group (2004) Prevalence of the metabolic syndrome and its relation to all-cause and cardiovascular mortality in nondiabetic European men and women. Arch Intern Med 164: 1066–1076.
10. Lakka HM, Laaksonen DE, Lakka TA, Niskanen LK, Kumpusalo E, et al. (2002) The metabolic syndrome and total and cardiovascular disease mortality in middle-aged men. JAMA 288: 2709–2716.
11. Athyros VG, Bouloukos VI, Pehlivanidis AN, Papageorgiou AA, Dionysopoulou SG, et al. (2005) The prevalence of the metabolic syndrome in Greece: the MetS-Greece Multicentre Study. Diabetes Obes Metab 7: 397–405.
12. Lawlor DA, Smith GD, Ebrahim S (2006) Does the new International Diabetes Federation definition of the metabolic syndrome predict CHD any more strongly than older definitions? Findings from the British Women's Heart and Health Study. Diabetologia 49: 41–48.
13. Mancia G, Bombelli M, Corrao G, Facchetti R, Madotto F, et al. (2007) Metabolic syndrome in the Pressioni Arteriose Monitorate E Loro Associazioni (PAMELA) study: daily life blood pressure, cardiac damage, and prognosis. Hypertension 49: 40–47.
14. Mancia G, Bombelli M, Facchetti R, Madotto F, Corrao G, et al. (2008) Long-term risk of diabetes, hypertension and left ventricular hypertrophy associated with the metabolic syndrome in a general population. J Hypertens 26: 1602–1611.
15. Giampaoli S, Stamler J, Donfrancesco C, Panico S, Vanuzzo D, et al, for the Progetto CUORE Research Group (2009) The metabolic syndrome: a critical appraisal based on the CUORE epidemiologic study. Preventive Medicine 48(6): 525–531.
16. Woodward M, Tunstall-Pedoe H (2009) The metabolic syndrome is not a sensible tool for predicting the risk of coronary heart disease. Eur J Prev Cardiol 16: 210–214.
17. Galassi A, Reynolds K, He J (2006) Metabolic syndrome and risk of cardiovascular disease. A meta-analysis. Am J Med 119: 812–819.
18. Gami AS, Witt BJ, Howard DE, Erwin PJ, Gami LA, et al. (2007) Metabolic syndrome and risk of incident cardiovascular events and death. A systematic

review and meta-analysis of longitudinal studies. J Am Coll Cardiol 49: 403–414.

19. Mottillo S, Filion KB, Genest J, Joseph L, Pilote L, et al. (2010) The metabolic syndrome and cardiovascular risk. A systematic review and meta-analysis. J Am Coll Cardiol 56: 1113–1132.
20. Ford ES (2005) Risks for all-cause mortality, cardiovascular disease, and diabetes associated with the metabolic syndrome. Diabetes Care 28: 1769–1778.
21. Hunt KJ, Resendez RG, Williams K, Haffner SM, Stern MP (2004) National Cholesterol Education Program versus World Health Organization metabolic syndrome in relation to all-cause and cardiovascular mortality in the San Antonio Heart Study. Circulation 110: 1251–1257.
22. McNeill AM, Rosamond WD, Girman CJ, Golden SH, Schmidt MI, et al. (2005) The metabolic syndrome and 11-year risk of incident cardiovascular disease in the Atherosclerosis Risk in Communities Study. Diabetes Care 28: 385–390.
23. Kahn R, Buse J, Ferrannini E, Steen M (2005) The metabolic syndrome: time for a critical appraisal: joint statement from the American Diabetes Association and the European Association for the Study of Diabetes. Diabetes Care 28(9): 2289–2304.
24. Sundström J, Vallhagen E, Risèrus U, Byberg L, Zethelius B, et al. (2006) Risk associated with the metabolic syndrome versus the sum of its individual components. Diabetes Care 29(7): 1673–1674.
25. Bayturan O, Tuzcu M, Lavoie A, Hu T, Wolski K, et al. (2010) The metabolic syndrome, its component risk factors, and progression of coronary atherosclerosis. Arch Intern Med 170(5): 478–484.
26. Sattar N, McConnachie A, Shaper AG, Blauw GJ, Buckley BM, et al. (2008) Can metabolic syndrome usefully predict cardiovascular disease and diabetes? Outcome data from two prospective studies. Lancet 371(9628): 1927–1935.
27. Grundy SM (2008) Metabolic syndrome pandemic. Arterioscler Thromb Vasc Biol 28: 629–636.
28. Ford ES, Giles WH, Dietz WH (2003) Prevalence of the metabolic syndrome among US adults: Findings from the Third National Health and Nutrition Examination Survey. JAMA 287: 356–359.
29. Grundy SM, Cleeman JI, Daniels SR, Donato KA, Eckel RH, et al. (2005) Diagnosis and management of the metabolic syndrome: an American Heart Association/National Heart, Lung, and Blood Institute scientific statement. Circulation 112: 2735–2752.
30. Alberti KGGM, Zimmet P, Shaw J, for the IDF Epidemiology Task Force Consensus Group (2005) The metabolic syndrome – a new worldwide definition. Lancet 366: 1059–1062.
31. Evans A, Salomaa V, Kulathinal S, Asplund K, Cambien F, et al. (2005) MORGAM (an international pooling of cardiovascular cohorts). Int J Epidemiol 34: 21–27.
32. MORGAM Manual (2001) MORGAM Project e-publications [Internet].URN:NBN:fi-fe20041529. Available: http://www.thl.fi/publications/morgam/manual/contents.htm. Accessed 2010 Aug 27.
33. Tuntall-Pedoe H (2003) Monica Monograph and Multimedia Sourcebook. World Health Organization, Geneva; 2003.
34. Niemelä M, Kulathinal S and Kuulasmaa K, editors, for the MORGAM Project (2007) Description and quality assessment of MORGAM data. MORGAM Project e-publications [Internet]. URN:NBN:fi-fe20071495. Available: http://www.thl.fi/publications/morgam/qa/contents.htm. Accessed 2010 Aug 27.
35. Asplund K, Tuomilehto J, Stemayr B, Wester PO, Tunstall-Pedoe H (1988) Diagnostic criteria and quality control of the registration of stroke events in the MONICA project. Acta Med Scand Suppl 728: 26–39.
36. Ho JS, Cannaday JJ, Barlow CE, Mitchell TL, Cooper KH, et al. (2008) Relation of the number of metabolic syndrome risk factors with all-cause and cardiovascular mortality. AM J Cardiol 102: 689–692.
37. Wilson PW, Kannel WB, Silbershatz H, D'Agostino RB (1999) Clustering of metabolic factors and coronary heart disease. Arch Intern Med 159: 1104–1109.
38. Sarwar N, Sandhu MS, Ricketts SL, Butterworth AS, Di Angelantonio E, et al; Triglyceride Coronary Disease Genetics Consortium and Emerging Risk Factors Collaboration. (2010) Triglyceride-mediated pathways and coronary disease: collaborative analysis of 101 studies. Lancet 375(9726): 1634–1639.
39. Blood Pressure Lowering Treatment Trialists' Collaboration (2003) Effects of different blood-pressure-lowering regimens on major cardiovascular events: results of prospectively designed overview of randomized trials. Lancet 362: 1527–1535.
40. Esposito K, Chiodini P, Colao A, Lenzi A, Giugliano D (2012) Metabolic syndrome and risk of cancer: a systematic review and meta-analysis. Diabetes Care 35(11): 2402–2411.
41. Vishram JK, Borglykke A, Andreasen AH, Jeppesen J, Ibsen H, et al. (2012) Impact of age on the importance of systolic and diastolic blood pressures for stroke risk: the . MOnica, Risk, Genetics, Archiving, and Monograph (MORGAM) Project. Hypertension 60(5): 1117–1123.

17

Elevated C-Reactive Protein Levels and Enhanced High Frequency Vasomotion in Patients with Ischemic Heart Disease during Brachial Flow-Mediated Dilation

Shogo Watanabe[1,2], Eisuke Amiya[1]*, Masafumi Watanabe[1], Munenori Takata[1], Atsuko Ozeki[1], Aya Watanabe[1], Shuichi Kawarasaki[1], Tomoko Nakao[1], Yumiko Hosoya[1], Kohzo Nagata[2], Ryozo Nagai[3], Issei Komuro[1]

1 Department of Cardiovascular Medicine, Graduate School of Medicine, The University of Tokyo, Tokyo, Japan, **2** Department of Pathophysiological Laboratory Sciences, Nagoya University Graduate School of Medicine, Aichi, Japan, **3** Jichi Medical School, Tochigi, Japan

Abstract

Purpose: The physiological role of vasomotion, rhythmic oscillations in vascular tone or diameter, and its underlying mechanisms are unknown. We investigated the characteristics of brachial artery vasomotion in patients with ischemic heart disease (IHD).

Methods: We performed a retrospective study of 37 patients with IHD. Endothelial function was assessed using flow-mediated dilation (FMD), and power spectral analysis of brachial artery diameter oscillations during FMD was performed. Frequency-domain components were calculated by integrating the power spectrums in three frequency bands (in ms^2) using the MemCalc (GMS, Tokyo, Japan): very-low frequency (VLF), 0.003–0.04 Hz; low frequency (LF), 0.04–0.15 Hz; and high frequency (HF), 0.15–0.4 Hz. Total spectral power (TP) was calculated as the sum of all frequency bands, and each spectral component was normalized against TP.

Results: Data revealed that HF/TP closely correlated with FMD ($r = -0.33$, $p = 0.04$), whereas VLF/TP and LF/TP did not. We also explored the relationship between elevated C-reactive protein (CRP) levels and vasomotion. HF/TP was significantly increased in subjects with high CRP levels (CRP;>0.08 mg/dL) compared with subjects with low CRP levels (0.052 ± 0.026 versus 0.035 ± 0.022, $p < 0.05$). The HF/TP value closely correlated with CRP ($r = 0.24$, $p = 0.04$), whereas the value of FMD did not ($r = 0.023$, $p = 0.84$). In addition, elevated CRP levels significantly increased the value of HF/TP after adjustment for FMD and blood pressure ($\beta = 0.33$, $p < 0.05$).

Conclusion: The HF component of brachial artery diameter oscillation during FMD measurement correlated well with FMD and increased in the presence of elevated CRP levels in subjects with IHD.

Editor: Thiruma V. Arumugam, National University of Singapore, Singapore

Funding: This research was supported by the Japan Society for the Promotion of Science through the Funding Program for World-Leading Innovative R&D on Science and Technology program, research grants from the Fukuda Foundation for Medical Technology (to E.A.), and Ministry of Education, Culture, Sports, Science, and Technology of Japan Grant-in-aid 23790837 (to E. A.). The funders had no role in study design, data collection and analysis, decision to publish, or preparation of the manuscript.

Competing Interests: The authors have declared that no competing interests exist.

* Email: amiyae-tky@umin.ac.jp

Introduction

Vasomotion is oscillations in vascular tone or diameter that can be observed in many, if not all, vascular segments. Vasomotion is suggested to play a role in tissue oxygenation and other physiological responses. For example, changes in the pattern or amplitude of vasomotion can set the vascular resistance and conductance to the desired level [1]. However, the precise physiological role of vasomotion and its underlying mechanisms remain unclear. Mechanistic studies have suggested that vasomotion is generated by synchronous oscillations due to the release of calcium via gap junctions between adjacent smooth muscle cells [2]. Vasomotion is also regulated by various extra-myogenic factors including autonomic nervous system activity, hormonal factors, and endothelium-derived factors [2–5].

Rhythmic oscillations during microcirculation can be recorded in various ways depending on the site of observation. Oscillations in the resistance vessels can be recorded using photoplethysmography or near-infrared spectroscopy, whereas those in the skin nutritive and thermoregulatory vessels can be detected using laser Doppler flowmetry (LDF). Although vasomotion predominantly occurs during microcirculation [6], it can also occur in large muscular arteries [7].

Table 1. Basic characteristics of the 37 IHD subjects.

Male/Female	25/12
Age (years)	67.7±7.5
Body mass index (kg/m^2)	24.2±3.2
Systolic blood pressure (mmHg)	126.8±15.7
Diastolic blood pressure (mmHg)	65.5±11.3
Heart rate (Beat/min)	63.4±9.7
Hemoglobin (g/dl)	12.9±1.8
Hemoglobin A1C (%)	6.2±1.4
eGFR (ml/min/1.73 m^2)	64.6±14.3
Low density lipoprotein (mg/dl)	95.7±29.5
CRP (mg/dl)	0.22±0.43
Brachial artery diameter (mm)	4.1±0.7
FMD (%)	4.2±1.5
SDNN (ms)	26.3±10.9
HRV LF/TP	0.24±0.14
HRV HF/TP	0.24±0.14
Smoker (%)	62.1
Myocardial infarction (%)	16.2
Diabetes mellitus (%)	40.5
Beta blocking agents (%)	43.2

IHD; ischemic heart disease, eGFR; estimated glomerular filtration rate, CRP; C-reactive protein, FMD; flow-mediated dilation; SDNN; standard deviation of normal to normal beats, HRV; heart rate variability, LF; low frequency, HF; high frequency, NS; not significant.

The presence of low-grade chronic vascular inflammation is critical for the pathogenesis of atherosclerotic disease. Proinflammatory cytokines, such as tumor necrosis factor-α (TNF-α) and interleukin-6, have been implicated in the initiation and maintenance of the systemic and vascular inflammation that is associated with atherosclerosis [8]. Among the biomarkers of inflammation, C-reactive protein (CRP) is most potent prognostic factor in cardiovascular clinical application that is independently associated with the risk of incident or recurring cardiovascular events [9,10]. These inflammatory factors also affect vascular function. For example, TNF-α and endotoxin impair endothelium-dependent vasodilation [11]. However, little is known about the relationship between vasomotion and inflammation exemplified by these inflammation parameters.

On the other hand, flow-mediated dilation (FMD), a response of vasodilation produced by increased blood flow shear, is a tool for evaluation of endothelial function. In subjects with ischemic heart disease (IHD), the value of FMD is generally impaired and more detailed vasomotion parameters is warranted for evaluating vascular function more minutely beyond FMD.

In this study, we observed oscillations in the brachial artery diameter during FMD in IHD, and we investigated the relationship between vasomotion of the brachial artery and several clinical variables, including C-reactive protein (CRP).

Methods

Subjects

We conducted a retrospective study of 37 patients with IHD who were hospitalized for cardiac catheterization. Inclusion criteria included coronary artery disease documented by angiography. Coronary artery disease was defined as the presence of at least one of the following:>50% luminal diameter narrowing of at least one epicardial coronary artery as shown by angiography, history of coronary revascularization, or history of myocardial infarction. Exclusion criteria included unstable clinical condition and significant valvular dysfunction. All components of standard informed consent, including the purpose of the study, risks, and benefits were fully explained to each subject, and written informed consent was obtained from all participants. The study protocol conformed to the Declaration of Helsinki and was reviewed and approved by the Institutional Review Board of the University of Tokyo (3003). All raw data was available in Table S1.

Flow-mediated dilation (FMD) measurement and vasomotion analysis

Endothelial function was assessed using FMD, as described by the International Brachial Artery Reactivity Task Force [12]. The subjects were instructed to abstain from eating, smoking, and consuming caffeine for at least 4 h, and were asked to lie down for 20 min prior to the beginning of the study. FMD of the brachial artery was measured by amplitude-mode and brightness-mode ultrasonography using a linear-array 10-MHz transducer (UNEXEF18G, UNEX, Nagoya). After baseline diameter measurements were taken for 30 s, the blood pressure cuff was inflated to 50 mmHg above the patient's systolic blood pressure for 5 min, and then deflated. The diameter of the brachial artery was continuously recorded for 2 min after the cuff was deflated. All diameters were measured in the end-diastolic phase, which was defined as the beginning of R wave in the electrocardiogram. FMD was calculated as the percent change in the diameter from baseline before cuff release to the peak value after cuff release. The reproducibility of FMD was confirmed previously ($n = 14$) [13]. Intra-observer reliability yielded an intra-class correlation coefficient of 0.968, with variation of 3.2%.

We also performed spectral analysis of vascular diameter oscillations during FMD. These oscillations were analyzed using Maximum Entropy Calculation Methodology(MemCalc, GMS, Tokyo, Japan). Fourier Spectral analysis was performed on a brachial artery trace registered during the 2-min FMD measurements. Frequency-domain components were calculated by integrating the power spectrum in three frequency bands (in ms^2): (1) very-low frequency (VLF), 0.003–0.04 Hz; (2) low frequency (LF), 0.04–0.15 Hz; and (3) high frequency (HF), 0.15–0.4 Hz. Total spectral power (TP) was calculated as the sum of all frequency bands.

Heart rate variability (HRV)

Patients' electrocardiograms were also recorded during the FMD measurements using a three-lead electrocardiogram system, and the recorded data was converted to R–R intervals using the A/D converter within UNEXEF18G. HRV was analyzed in both the time and frequency domains of these recordings using the autoregressive method. Standard deviation of normal-to-normal beats (SDNN) was used as an indicator of both parasympathetic and sympathetic nerve activities, as mediated by baroreflex activity. SDNN was calculated from 100 heartbeats after cuff release during the FMD measurements. Frequency-domain components were calculated in a similar manner as vascular diameter oscillations. The power of LF and HF was calculated as the marker of sympathetic and parasympathetic nervous system activities.

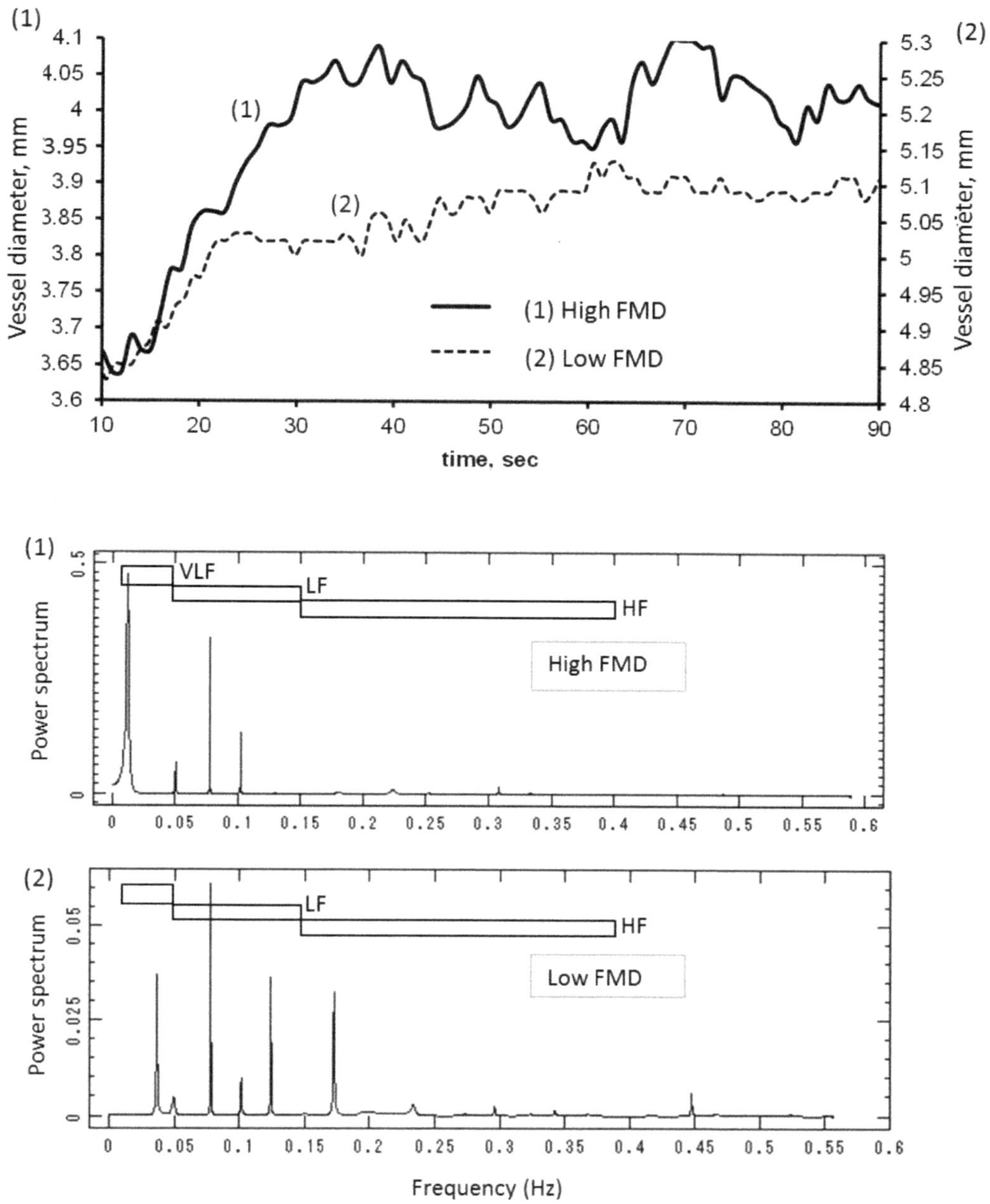

Figure 1. Examples of brachial artery vasomotion of a subject with high FMD (1) and low FMD (2). HF component was enhanced in this subject with low FMD. Brachial artery diameter was continuously measured after cuff release during FMD measurement. FMD, flow-mediated dilation; DM, diabetes; VLF, very-low frequency; LF, low frequency; HF, high frequency.

Table 2. Comparison of HRV and vasomotion in subjects with IHD.

	HRV	Vasomotion
VLF/TP	0.52±0.18	0.74±0.18
LF/TP	0.24±0.14	0.19±0.19
HF/TP	0.24±0.14	0.044±0.025
LF/HF	1.7±1.9	5.1±4.2

HRV; heart rate variability, IHD; ischemic heart disease, VLF; very low frequency, TP; total power, LF; low frequency; HF; high frequency.

Table 3. Correlative relationship between clinical parameters and each frequency in vasomotion.

	HF/TP		LF/TP		VLF/TP		TP	
	r	p value	r	p value	r	p value	r	p value
Age (years)	0.18	0.28	0.16	0.34	−0.15	0.37	−0.12	0.47
Body mass index (kg/m^2)	−0.088	0.60	0.051	0.76	−0.066	0.70	0.23	0.17
Systolic blood pressure (mmHg)	−0.29	0.08	−0.034	0.84	0.068	0.69	0.057	0.74
Diastolic blood pressure (mmHg)	−0.46	0.02*	−0.10	0.55	0.14	0.41	−0.14	0.40
Heart Rate (beat/min)	−0.12	0.55	0.14	0.41	−0.16	0.35	−0.083	0.63
Hemoglobin (g/dl)	−0.31	0.06	−0.082	0.63	0.098	0.56	−0.092	0.59
Hemoglobin A1C (%)	0.090	0.60	0.33	0.04*	−0.35	0.03*	0.098	0.56
eGFR (ml/min/1.73m^2)	−0.40	0.02*	−0.13	0.43	0.22	0.20	0.34	0.04*
Low density lipoprotein (mg/ml)	−0.21	0.22	−0.20	0.25	0.26	0.12	0.14	0.42
CRP (mg/dl)	0.24	0.04*	−0.11	0.35	0.023	0.84	0.04	0.70
Brachial artery diameter (mm)	0.082	0.64	−0.21	0.22	0.16	0.36	0.062	0.71
FMD (%)	−0.33	0.04*	0.12	0.50	−0.080	0.64	−0.11	0.52
SDNN (ms)	−0.020	0.90	−0.12	0.47	0.15	0.37	0.023	0.89
HRV LF/TP	−0.15	0.37	−0.092	0.59	0.12	0.50	−0.034	0.84
HRV HF/TP	0.16	0.35	−0.033	0.85	0.031	0.85	−0.044	0.80
HRV LF/HF	−0.37	0.03*	−0.21	0.22	0.27	0.11	0.33	0.04*

VLF; very low frequency, TP; total power, LF; low frequency; HF; high frequency, Hb; hemoglonin, HbA1c; hemoglobin A1C; eGFR; estimated glomerular filtration rate, CRP; C-reactive protein, BAD; Brachial artery diameter, FMD; flow-mediated dilation; SDNN; standard deviation of normal to normal beats, NS; not significant, *; $p<0.05$.

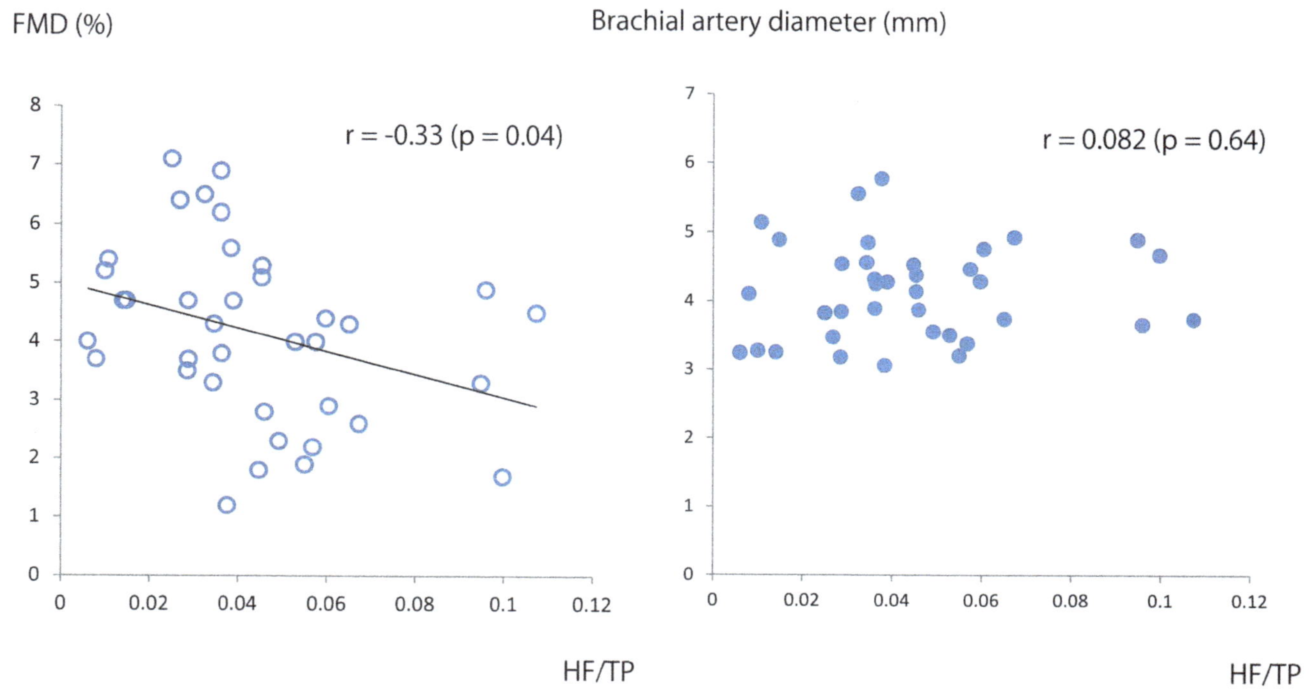

Figure 2. Scatter plot of the relationship between FMD or brachial artery diameter and the HF/TP power ratio of vasomotion in subjects with IHD. FMD, flow-mediated dilation; HF, high frequency; TP, total spectral power; IHD, ischemic heart disease.

Blood samples

Blood samples from fasting subjects were collected for analysis within three days before or after FMD measurement. Hemoglobin and Hemoglobin A1c (HbA1c) levels, estimated glomerular filtration rate (eGFR), and low-density lipoprotein and CRP levels were measured using standard laboratory methods (Tokyo University Hospital).

Statistics

Data are presented as mean±standard deviation. Differences between groups were calculated by Mann–Whitney test, t test and χ2 test. For quantitative variables that were not normally distributed, the Kendall rank correlation was calculated; otherwise, the Person correlation was calculated. A p-value of <0.05 was considered as statistically significant. Data analyses were performed using PASW Statistics 18 (SPSS Inc., Chicago) and JMP Pro 9 (SAS Institute, North Carolina).

Results

Subject characteristics

Table 1 lists the basic characteristics of the 37 subjects with IHD. A history of myocardial infarction was observed in 16.2 % of subjects. It also included 15 patients with diabetes mellitus, and 16 individuals were being treated with beta-blocking agents.

Characteristics of Vasomotion

FMD and the spectral component of vasomotion were both measured as vascular parameters. Figure 1 shows an example of the time course of brachial artery dilation of a subject with high FMD and low FMD. The spectral components of vasomotion were sorted into three frequency bands: VLF, LF, and HF and the amplitude of each component was normalized by TP. The brachial artery generally began to dilate approximately 10–40 s after cuff release, and continued to dilate for 40–120 s. The time required for vasodilation (extended time) ranged from 30 to 80 s. The frequency spectrum of these changes in vascular diameter was estimated to be classified as VLF, whereas LF and HF components were estimated to reflect more minute oscillations. The spectral indices of the LF and HF components were 19±19% and 4.4±2.5% of TP, respectively (Table 2). When compared with the distribution of HRV, vasomotion of the brachial artery was more likely to fluctuate in the lower frequencies than heart rate oscillations. In particular, the HF component of vasomotion was significantly decreased compared with the LF component (Table 2).

Figure 1 also showed that the HF component of vasomotion variously changed among each subject. We investigated the relationships between the spectral components of vasomotion and clinical variables, including FMD, in subjects with IHD. Table 3 shows the correlation between the frequency components of vasomotion and each clinical variable. Data demonstrated that the HF/TP power ratio correlated with diastolic blood pressure ($r = -0.46$; $p = 0.02$), eGFR ($r = -0.40$; $p = 0.02$), CRP ($r = 0.24$; $p = 0.04$) and FMD ($r = -0.33$; $p = 0.04$), and HRV LF/HF ($r = -0.37$; $p = 0.03$) (Figure 2). The correlation between the HF/TP power ratio and these parameters suggested that the HF/TP component of vasomotion was influenced by factors in addition to endothelium-derived factors and autonomic nervous system activity. The lack of correlative relationship between brachial artery diameter and the HF/TP power ratio ($r = 0.082$; $p = 0.64$) suggested the correlation between FMD and the the HF/TP power ratio was independent from vessel diameter.

We also investigated the contribution of the presence of the medication of beta-blocking agents on the behavior of vasomotion that affect the autonomic nervous system and the vascular tone. It unexpectedly revealed that there was no significant difference

Table 4. Characterization of subjects with high CRP and low CRP.

	High CRP	low CRP	
N	19	18	
Male/Female	14/5	11/7	NS
Age (years)	68.0±6.6	67.3±8.4	NS
Body mass index (kg/m^2)	24.0±3.2	24.4±3.3	NS
Systolic blood pressure (mmHg)	127.2±18.0	126.4±13.3	NS
Diastolic blood pressure (mmHg)	64.5±9.7	66.7±12.9	NS
Heart rate (/min)	65.3±10.2	61.4±9.1	NS
Hemoglobin (g/dl)	12.5±1.9	13.3±1.7	NS
Hemoglobin A1C (%)	6.3±1.7	6.1±1.1	NS
eGFR (ml/min/1.73m^2)	60.3±13.6	69.2±13.9	NS
CRP (mg/dl)	0.39±0.56	0.044±0.022	p<0.05
Brachial artery diameter (mm)	4.4±0.6	3.9±0.7	NS
FMD (%)	4.2±1.1	4.1±1.8	NS
SDNN (m)	24.0±8.6	28.6±12.7	NS
HRV LF/TP	0.22±0.13	0.25±0.17	NS
HRV HF/TP	0.27±0.15	0.21±0.12	NS
Smoker (%)	63.2	61.1	NS
Diabetes mellitus (%)	42.1	38.9	NS
Beta-blocker (%)	47.4	38.9	NS

BP; blood pressure, eGFR; estimated glomerular filtration rate, CRP; C-reactive protein, FMD; flow-mediated dilation; HRV; heart rate variability, LF; low frequency, HF; high frequency, NS; not significant.

between subjects with and without beta-blocking agents in each component of oscillation (VLF/TP; 0.78±0.13 vs 0.70±0.21, LF/TP; 0.15±0.13 vs 0.23±0.22, HF/TP; 0.047±0.006 vs 0.041±0.006). Therefore, there was no significant effect of beta-blocking agents on the behavior of vasomotion.

Effect of elevated CRP levels on vasomotion frequency bands

We next explored the effect of elevated CRP levels on vasomotion. Subjects were divided into two groups based on their CRP level (median, 0.08 mg/dL). Each parameter of vasomotion was compared among subjects with high (>0.08 mg/dL) and low CRP (<0.08 mg/dL) levels. Clinical parameters including FMD and brachial artery diameter were not different between groups (Table 4). Blood pressure and heart rate were not also significantly different between these two groups because of the minute difference of CRP. We then investigated the relationship between the spectral component of vasomotion and elevated CRP levels (Figure 3). Of the different components of vasomotion (HF/TP, LF/TP, VLF/TP, and TP), HF/TP was significantly different between patients with high and low CRP levels (0.052±0.026 versus 0.035±0.022, respectively, $p<0.05$) suggesting that this was affected by the presence of elevated CRP levels. Consistent with this, there was a fine correlative relationship between HF/TP and CRP ($r = 0.24$, $p = 0.04$). By contrast, FMD was not correlated with CRP ($r = 0.023$, $p = 0.84$). In addition, elevated CRP levels significantly increased the value of HF/TP after adjustment for FMD and blood pressure ($\beta = 0.33$, $p<0.05$). This result suggests that HF/TP may reflect more minute influence of elevated CRP levels on vasomotion than the value of FMD.

Discussion

To the best of our knowledge, this is the first study to investigate the oscillatory behavior of the brachial artery diameter. It correlated well with FMD and it can also detect the minute change of vasomotion in the presence of elevated CRP. The oscillating movements of the brachial artery have been recently documented [14], however it had not been clearly characterized. Oscillating movements measured in the brachial artery in this study are a direct measurement of vasomotion in blood vessels; therefore, this measurement might more accurately reflect the interaction among myogenic components, vessel diameter oscillations, and other interacting factors compared with vasomotor oscillations measured using other modalities.

Spectral analysis of vasomotion

The mechanism of oscillatory calcium ion release in smooth muscle cells is responsible for vasomotion [15,16]. However, these motions are greatly affected by extrinsic factors other than the smooth muscle cell system. In a study of LDF, VLF vasomotion was related to nitric oxide production by endothelial cells [17]. In contrast, LF vasomotion is considered to be under autonomic control. Decreased vasomotion around the LF spectral band in diabetic patients with sympathetic dysfunction, as demonstrated by Meyer et al., supports this hypothesis. [5]. These findings suggest the behavior of the vasomotion is modified by the extrinsic factors and that the source of oscillation may be predicted by the precise characterization of the oscillation spectrum.

In contrast, in the vasomotion of the brachial artery during FMD, the HF component was associated with several clinical parameters such as FMD, diastolic blood pressure and CRP, whereas the VLF or LF spectral components of vasomotion did not correlate with any clinical parameters except HbA1c. This

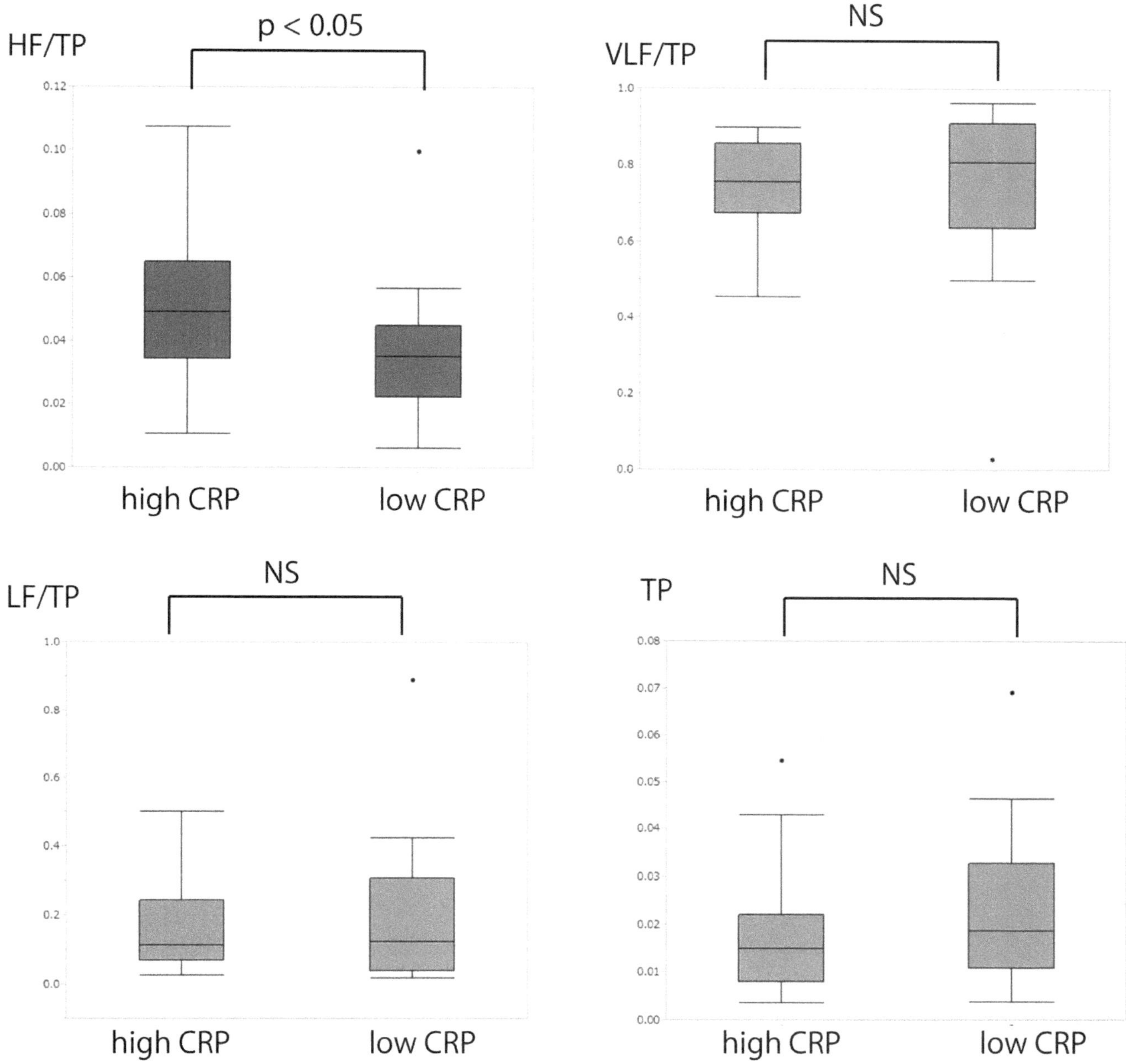

Figure 3. Comparison of each spectral component of vasomotion among subjects with high and low CPR level. HF, high frequency; TP, total spectral power; VLF, very low frequency; LF, low frequency; CRP, C-reactive protein.

character was markedly different from previous studies of vasomotion that were performed using other modalities [18–20]. Among factors that associated with HF component, FMD was a potent parameter; decreased FMD corresponded to an enhanced HF component of vasomotion. This suggests that the increase in the HF component of vasomotion reflects vascular impairment in endothelial function. In contrast, HRV LF/HF, another determining parameter, affected the HF component differently, because enhanced sympathetic nerve activity attenuated the HF component of vasomotion. In this way, the HF component of vasomotion was associated with endothelial function and autonomic nervous system activity.

The correlative relationship between decreased FMD and increased HF component suggests the increased HF component might be a compensatory mechanism that is triggered when tissue perfusion is compromised by vascular damage [15]. Podgoreanu et al. demonstrated that HF vasomotion emerged in the absence of physiological flow oscillation, and was derived from a peripheral origin through a parasympathetic nervous mechanism [21]. Our findings supported this enhancement of the HF component. In addition, the decrease of HF component with enhanced sympathetic nerve activity observed in the present study was compatible with the hypothesis that this compensatory mechanism is mediated through parasympathetic nervous system. However, further investigation is warranted to verify it.

Elevated CRP levels and vasomotion

In this study, vasomotion also correlated with CRP. This correlation was independent of FMD and elevated CRP levels were shown to affect the HF component of vasomotion itself. There have been few reports that demonstrate the relationship between elevated CRP levels and the behavior of vasomotion. Schindler et al. demonstrated a direct association between systemic low-grade inflammation and vasomotor function [22], whereas Verma et al. reported that CRP levels did not correlate with the value of FMD [23]. The current study also failed to demonstrate an association between FMD and CRP. In contrast, the artery diameter oscillation measurement can detect the change derived from the presence of elevated CRP. Elevated CRP levels correlated with an increase in the HF component of vasomotion, suggesting that the inflammatory state, or specific humoral factors such as CRP or other inflammatory cytokines, might enhance the HF component in this subgroup of patients. Indeed, pro-inflammatory cytokines such as TNF-α activate calcium-related vasomotion by enhancing intracellular calcium levels and increasing the availability of calcium to refill the sarcoplasmic reticulum [24]. This enhanced calcium handling might lead to an increased HF component. CRP or other inflammatory cytokines also exert direct effects on the endothelium, which might also change smooth muscle vasomotion through endothelial modification [25–27].

Physiological relevance and future directions

A vessel with an oscillating diameter has a higher conductance (and thus greater flow) than a vessel with a constant diameter of the same mean width [28]. In addition, oscillating contractions might be less costly in terms of energy use than constant contractions. Therefore, the increase of HF component in the presence of vascular injury is a reasonable physiological compensatory response to maintain the blood flow to peripheral tissue. In addition, the correlative relationship of the HF component with several clinical parameters suggested that the evaluation of the HF component could be a good risk parameter of vascular injury, which is difficult to detect using previous methods of vasomotion analysis.

We analyzed oscillating brachial arteries only during FMD. The analysis of vasomotion may disclose another aspect of vascular condition other than FMD. In this manner, the oscillating movements of the brachial artery in other conditions or changes in oscillation movements under different conditions might provide additional useful information regarding the conditions and characteristics of the measured vasculature. Therefore, this method can also be applied to other blood vessels such as the carotid artery. Examining the characteristics of vasomotion might be a promising tool during the diagnostic workup of cardiac patients.

Conclusions

In the present study, we investigated the oscillatory behavior of the brachial artery diameter for the first time. The HF component of oscillation correlated well with FMD and increased in the presence of elevated CRP levels in subjects with IHD. Assessing vessel diameter oscillations in various clinical settings might allow a more accurate evaluation of the interaction between vasomotion and clinical conditions such as inflammation.

Limitations

The primary limitations of this study were the small sample size and the retrospective nature of data collection. Because of the small sample size, there may possibly be some type II errors. For instance, other clinical parameters may be associated with the HF component of the brachial artery diameter oscillation or there may be association between FMD and CRP. In addition, performing multivariate analyses was limited because of small sample size in the current study. However, the relationships between elevated CRP levels and the enhancement of HF component remained significant after adjustment for FMD and blood pressure. The relationship between elevated CRP levels and the enhancement of HF component is sufficiently robust. Ideally, hypotheses should be tested in prospective studies with larger samples. We selected the median (0.08 mg/dl) for dividing subjects into groups with low and high CRP levels. There is no consensus about the threshold level of CRP level for predicting the risk of atherosclerosis. A similar value was applied in previous reports [23,29], suggesting the value in the current study is reasonable. In addition, the interpretation of total autonomic nervous system activity might be limited by the fact that autonomic nervous system activity measurements were made solely during resting short-term HRV. Generally, vasomotion is reported to be a central feature to the microcirculation. However, the relationship between vasomotion observed in this study and that in the microcirculation remained to be unknown and further exploration is needed. Nitroglycerin-mediated dilation measurements were not performed because it was not possible to use nitroglycerin in all IHD subjects owing to the associated risks.

Supporting Information

Table S1 All raw data in this study.

Author Contributions

Conceived and designed the experiments: SW EA. Performed the experiments: SW EA MW MT AO AW SK TN YH. Analyzed the data: SW EA KN RN IK. Contributed reagents/materials/analysis tools: SW EA MW. Wrote the paper: SW EA.

References

1. Diehl R R, Diehl B, Sitzer M, Hennerici M (1991) Spontaneous oscillations in cerebral blood flow velocity in normal humans and in patients with carotid artery disease. Neurosci Lett 127:5–8.
2. Mauban J R, Lamont C, Balke C W, Wier W G (2001) Adrenergic stimulation of rat resistance arteries affects Ca(2+) sparks, Ca(2+) waves, and Ca(2+) oscillations. Am J Physiol Heart Circ Physiol 280:H2399–2405.
3. Lamboley M, Schuster A, Beny J L, Meister J J (2003) Recruitment of smooth muscle cells and arterial vasomotion. Am J Physiol Heart Circ Physiol 285:H562–569.
4. Bernardi L, Rossi M, Leuzzi S, Mevio E, Fornasari G, et al. (1997) Reduction of 0.1 Hz microcirculatory fluctuations as evidence of sympathetic dysfunction in insulin-dependent diabetes. Cardiovasc Res 34:185–191.
5. Meyer M F, Rose C J, Hulsmann J O, Schatz H, Pfohl M (2003) Impaired 0.1-Hz vasomotion assessed by laser Doppler anemometry as an early index of peripheral sympathetic neuropathy in diabetes. Microvasc Res 65:88–95.
6. Funk W, Endrich B, Messmer K, Intaglietta M (1983) Spontaneous arteriolar vasomotion as a determinant of peripheral vascular resistance. Int J Microcirc Clin Exp 2:11–25.
7. Hayoz D, Tardy Y, Rutschmann B, Mignot J P, Achakri H, et al. (1993) Spontaneous diameter oscillations of the radial artery in humans. Am J Physiol 264:H2080–2084.
8. McKellar G E, McCarey D W, Sattar N, McInnes I B (2009) Role for TNF in atherosclerosis? Lessons from autoimmune disease. Nat Rev Cardiol 6:410–417.
9. Ridker P M, Rifai N, Clearfield M, Downs J R, Weis S E, et al. (2001) Measurement of C-reactive protein for the targeting of statin therapy in the primary prevention of acute coronary events. N Engl J Med 344:1959–1965.
10. Ridker P M, Group J S (2003) Rosuvastatin in the primary prevention of cardiovascular disease among patients with low levels of low-density lipoprotein cholesterol and elevated high-sensitivity C-reactive protein: rationale and design of the JUPITER trial. Circulation 108:2292–2297.

11. Bhagat K, Vallance P (1997) Inflammatory cytokines impair endothelium-dependent dilatation in human veins in vivo. Circulation 96:3042–3047.
12. Corretti M C, Anderson T J, Benjamin E J, Celermajer D, Charbonneau F, et al. (2002) Guidelines for the ultrasound assessment of endothelial-dependent flow-mediated vasodilation of the brachial artery: a report of the International Brachial Artery Reactivity Task Force. J Am Coll Cardiol 39:257–265.
13. Watanabe S, Amiya E, Watanabe M, Takata M, Ozeki A, et al. (2013) Simultaneous heart rate variability monitoring enhances the predictive value of flow-mediated dilation in ischemic heart disease. Circ J 77:1018–1025.
14. Cary T W, Reamer C B, Sultan L R, Mohler E R 3rd, Sehgal C M (2014) Brachial artery vasomotion and transducer pressure effect on measurements by active contour segmentation on ultrasound. Med Phys 41:022901.
15. Nilsson H, Aalkjaer C (2003) Vasomotion: mechanisms and physiological importance. Mol Interv 3:79–89, 51.
16. Peng H, Matchkov V, Ivarsen A, Aalkjaer C, Nilsson H (2001) Hypothesis for the initiation of vasomotion. Circ Res 88:810–815.
17. Kvandal P, Stefanovska A, Veber M, Kvernmo H D, Kirkeboen K A (2003) Regulation of human cutaneous circulation evaluated by laser Doppler flowmetry, iontophoresis, and spectral analysis: importance of nitric oxide and prostaglandines. Microvasc Res 65:160–171.
18. Kvernmo H D, Stefanovska A, Kirkeboen K A, Kvernebo K (1999) Oscillations in the human cutaneous blood perfusion signal modified by endothelium-dependent and endothelium-independent vasodilators. Microvasc Res 57:298–309.
19. Kastrup J, Bulow J, Lassen N A (1989) Vasomotion in human skin before and after local heating recorded with laser Doppler flowmetry. A method for induction of vasomotion. Int J Microcirc Clin Exp 8:205–215.
20. Soderstrom T, Stefanovska A, Veber M, Svensson H (2003) Involvement of sympathetic nerve activity in skin blood flow oscillations in humans. Am J Physiol Heart Circ Physiol 284:H1638–1646.
21. Podgoreanu M V, Stout R G, El-Moalem H E, Silverman D G (2002) Synchronous rhythmical vasomotion in the human cutaneous microvasculature during nonpulsatile cardiopulmonary bypass. Anesthesiology 97:1110–1117.
22. Schindler T H, Nitzsche E U, Olschewski M, Magosaki N, Mix M, et al. (2004) Chronic inflammation and impaired coronary vasoreactivity in patients with coronary risk factors. Circulation 110:1069–1075.
23. Verma S, Wang C H, Lonn E, Charbonneau F, Buithieu J, et al. (2004) Cross-sectional evaluation of brachial artery flow-mediated vasodilation and C-reactive protein in healthy individuals. Eur Heart J 25:1754–1760.
24. Sathish V, Delmotte P F, Thompson M A, Pabelick C M, Sieck G C, et al. (2011) Sodium-calcium exchange in intracellular calcium handling of human airway smooth muscle. PLoS One 6:e23662.
25. Pasceri V, Willerson J T, Yeh E T (2000) Direct proinflammatory effect of C-reactive protein on human endothelial cells. Circulation 102:2165–2168.
26. Mohamed F, Monge J C, Gordon A, Cernacek P, Blais D, et al. (1995) Lack of role for nitric oxide (NO) in the selective destabilization of endothelial NO synthase mRNA by tumor necrosis factor-alpha. Arterioscler Thromb Vasc Biol 15:52–57.
27. Yan G, You B, Chen S P, Liao J K, Sun J (2008) Tumor necrosis factor-alpha downregulates endothelial nitric oxide synthase mRNA stability via translation elongation factor 1-alpha 1. Circ Res 103:591–597.
28. Meyer C, de Vries G, Davidge S T, Mayes D C (2002) Reassessing the mathematical modeling of the contribution of vasomotion to vascular resistance. J Appl Physiol 92:888–889.
29. Gupta N K, de Lemos J A, Ayers C R, Abdullah S M, McGuire D K, et al. (2012) The relationship between C-reactive protein and atherosclerosis differs on the basis of body mass index: the Dallas Heart Study. J Am Coll Cardiol 60:1148–1155.

18

Myocardial Metastases on 6-[^{18}F] fluoro-L-DOPA PET/CT: A Retrospective Analysis of 116 Serotonin Producing Neuroendocrine Tumour Patients

Walter Noordzij[1]*, André P. van Beek[2], René A. Tio[3], Anouk N. van der Horst-Schrivers[2], Elisabeth G. de Vries[4], Bram van Ginkel[5], Annemiek M. Walenkamp[4], Andor W. Glaudemans[1], Riemer H. Slart[1], Rudi A. Dierckx[1]

1 Department of Nuclear Medicine and Molecular Imaging, University of Groningen, University Medical Center Groningen, Groningen, The Netherlands, **2** Department of Endocrinology, University of Groningen, University Medical Center Groningen, Groningen, The Netherlands, **3** Department of Cardiology, University of Groningen, University Medical Center Groningen, Groningen, The Netherlands, **4** Department of Medical Oncology, University of Groningen, University Medical Center Groningen, Groningen, The Netherlands, **5** Faculty of Medicine, University of Groningen, University Medical Center Groningen, Groningen, The Netherlands

Abstract

Purpose: This study evaluates the prevalence of cardiac metastases in patients with serotonin producing neuroendocrine tumours (NET), examined with ^{18}F-FDOPA PET/CT, and the relationship of these metastases to the presence of carcinoid heart disease (CHD) based on echocardiography.

Background: CHD occurs in patients with serotonin producing NET. The diagnostic method of choice remains echocardiography. The precise prevalence of cardiac metastases is unknown given the limitations of standard technologies. Nuclear medicine modalities have the potential to visualize metastases of NET.

Methods: All patients who underwent ^{18}F-FDOPA PET/CT because of serotonin producing NET between November 2009 and May 2012 were retrospectively analyzed. The presence of cardiac metastasis was defined as myocardial tracer accumulation higher than the surrounding physiological myocardial uptake. Laboratory tests and transthoracic echocardiography (TTE) results were digitally collected.

Results: 116 patients (62 male) underwent ^{18}F-FDOPA PET/CT, mean age was 61 ± 13 years. TTE was performed in 79 patients. Cardiac metastases were present in 15 patients, of which 10 patients also underwent TTE. One patient had both cardiac metastasis (only on ^{18}F-FDOPA PET/CT) and echocardiographic signs of CHD. There were no differences in echocardiographic parameters for CHD between patients with and without cardiac metastases. TTE in none of the 79 patients showed cardiac metastases.

Conclusion: The prevalence of cardiac metastases detected with ^{18}F-FDOPA PET/CT in this study is 13%. ^{18}F-FDOPA PET/CT can visualize cardiac metastases in serotonin producing NET patients. There appears to be no relationship between the presence of cardiac metastases and TTE parameters of CHD.

Editor: Carmine Pizzi, University of Bologna, Italy

Funding: The authors have no support or funding to report.

Competing Interests: The authors have declared that no competing interests exist.

* Email: w.noordzij@umcg.nl

Introduction

Neuroendocrine tumours (NET) are rare but well-defined neuroendocrine malignancies, with a low worldwide incidence; approximately 1–2 per 100,000 persons [1]. Nuclear medicine modalities and three-phase CT scans are the cornerstones in clinical staging of NET [1]. Indium-111 (^{111}In) labelled pentetreotide scintigraphy (SRS, planar whole body scan with or without additional single photon emission computed tomography and CT (SPECT/CT)) and gallium-68 (^{68}Ga) labelled (DOTA-Phe-Tyr)-octreotide (DOTATOC) positron emission tomography (PET) are both used to visualize somatostatin receptor density. 6-[^{18}F]fluoro-L-DOPA (^{18}F-FDOPA) uptake in NET is analogous to the uptake of amine precursors in these tumours. The overall sensitivity of ^{18}F-FDOPA PET/CT for the detection of (metastatic) NET lesions is higher than that of SRS [2]. All these nuclear medicine modalities have the potential to visualize tracer uptake in myocardial metastases in patient with NET [3,4].

NET of the small bowel frequently produces serotonin which, in case of metastatic disease, may lead to carcinoid syndrome, consisting of diarrhoea, flushing and carcinoid heart disease (CHD). CHD, present in up to 60% of patients with carcinoid syndrome, is characterized by plaque-like endocardial deposits of fibrous tissue on the ventricular aspect of the tricuspid valve leaflets, the arterial side of the pulmonary valve cusps, but also in the right atrium, and right ventricle [5,6]. This plaque formation and subsequent endocardial thickening eventually result in valve dysfunction [7]. Tricuspid valve involvement usually leads to regurgitation, whereas pulmonary valve involvement rather results into stenosis. Despite the indolent character of CHD, it is associated with a worse clinical outcome, especially when developing into heart failure [7].

Echocardiography is the modality of choice for diagnosing CHD [8,9]. Characteristic findings consist of thickening of leaflets/cusps that become retracted and eventually immobile, leading to the combination of valvular regurgitation and stenosis. Myocardial metastases are sometimes considered as a feature of CHD. However, these metastases are not always detected with echocardiography, and do not necessarily lead to typical valve dysfunction [10,11]. The prevalence of cardiac NET metastases is still not well established, partly due to lacking literature. Only few studies report on cardiac metastases, with a prevalence of 4% [12]. This is possibly an underestimation, partly due to low sensitivity of conventional imaging modalities.

The purpose of this retrospective study was to establish the prevalence of cardiac metastases in patients with serotonin producing NET, detected by ^{18}F-FDOPA PET/CT, and its relationship with the presence of echocardiography based CHD.

Patients and Methods

All patients who were referred to the Department of Nuclear Medicine and Molecular Imaging for an ^{18}F-FDOPA PET/CT between November 2009 and May 2012, were retrospectively analyzed. Selected were patients with serotonin producing NET based on elevated urinary 5-hydroxyindole acetic acid (5-HIAA, upper reference limit 3.8 mmol/mol creatinine) and elevated serotonin in platelets (upper reference limit 5.4 nmol/10^9 platelets). Serum creatinine level was used to determine the estimated glomerular filtration rate (eGFR). Presence of chronic kidney disease (CKD) was based on the Kidney Disease Outcomes Quality Initiative CKD classification [13].

Previous medical history was retrieved from the electronic patient chart, especially history of hypertension (defined as either systolic pressure higher than 140 mmHg, diastolic pressure higher than 90 mm Hg, or the use of anti-hypertensive medication), atrial fibrillation (AF) and myocardial infarction. Electrocardiograms (ECG) at the time point of the ^{18}F-FDOPA PET/CT scan (±3 months) were collected from the electronic patient chart, when available. ECGs were re-evaluated regarding rhythm, heart rate, QRS axis, PQ interval, QRS duration, presence of bundle branch block, QTc interval and STT segments. Transthoracic echocardiography (TTE) findings at the same time point were collected from the local digital archive of the Department of Cardiology of our hospital. Patients were followed until May 2013: one year after the ^{18}F-FDOPA PET/CT scan of the last included patient. Information on cardiac events (either myocardial infarction, or sudden cardiac death) or death during follow-up was retrieved from the electronic chart. This study was approved by the Institutional Ethics Review Board (name: 'medisch ethische toetsingscommissie' of the University Medical Center Groningen). According to the Dutch law, no additional informed consent was required. Patient information was anonymized and de-identified before data analysis.

^{18}F-FDOPA PET/CT scanning

All patients fasted for at least 6 hours and were allowed to continue all medication. Whole-body (from top of the skull through midthigh) three-dimensional PET images were acquired 60 minutes after intravenous administration of a standard dose of 200 MBq ^{18}F-FDOPA on a Biograph mCT (Siemens Medical Systems, Knoxville, TN, USA). ^{18}F-FDOPA PET/CT scans were performed with a mean amount of 140±15.5 mg carbidopa premedication, and mean administered activity of 186±39.8 MBq ^{18}F-FDOPA. Acquisition was performed in 7 bed positions of 2 minutes emission scan for patients 60–90 kg. Patient with body weight less than 60 kg and more than 90 kg body weight, were scanned with 1 minute and 3 minutes per bed position, respectively. Low dose transmission CT was used for attenuation correction. For the reduction of tracer decarboxylation and subsequent renal clearance, all patients received 2 mg/kg carbidopa (with a maximum of 150 mg) orally as pre-treatment, 1 hour before the ^{18}F-FDOPA injection, to decrease peripheral uptake and to increase tracer accumulation in tumor cells. Low dose CT and ^{18}F-FDOPA PET scans were automatically fused by use of three-dimensional fusion software (Siemens) with manual fine adjustments. All scans were interpreted by well trained nuclear medicine physicians as part of routine care. For this study, all scans were retrospectively analyzed for the presence of myocardial metastases.

Raw data were reconstructed through ultra high definition (Siemens) and guidelines based standardized algorithms [14,15], for visual assessment and standardized uptake value (SUV) calculations, respectively. Focal left and/or right ventricle ^{18}F-FDOPA uptake higher than the surrounding physiological myocardial uptake was considered abnormal, and thus suspicious for cardiac metastases.

Transthoracic echocardiography

The following variables were measured according to standard recommendations in the M-mode transthoracic echocardiographic examination: left ventricular internal end-diastolic and end-systolic dimensions, inter-ventricular wall thickness and left ventricular posterior wall thickness at end-diastole. An eyeballing left ventricular ejection fraction (LVEF) >55% was considered to be normal, between 55% and 40% mildly disturbed, between 30% and 40% moderately disturbed, and <30% was considered to represent a severely impaired systolic function.

Serotonin induced cardiac involvement was defined as tricuspid or pulmonary valvular dysfunction (i.e. valve leaflet thickening, shortening, retraction, hypomobility, or incomplete coaptation) associated with regurgitation or stenosis [16,17]. Pulmonary valve

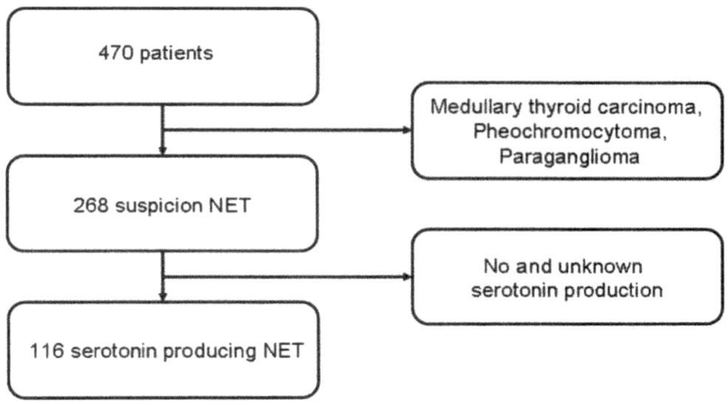

Figure 1. CONSORT diagram.

Table 1. Characteristics of all patients, and patients with and without abnormal cardiac ^{18}F-FDOPA uptake.

Parameter	All patients		No cardiac metastases		Cardiac metastases		*p*-value
	N (%)	Mean ± SD, or median (range)	N (%)	Mean ± SD, or median (range)	N (%)	Mean ± SD, or median (range)	
Age (y)	116 (100)	64±9.3	101 (87)	64±8.5	15 (13)	67±8.1	NS
Male patients	62 (53)		55 (54)		7 (47)		NS
History of							
- Hypertension	48 (41)		39 (39)		9 (60)		NS
- Atrial fibrillation	3 (3)		2 (1)		0		NS
- Myocardial infarction	7 (6)		6 (6)		1 (7)		NS
Cardiac medication							
- β blocker	34 (29)		28 (28)		6 (40)		NS
- Angiotensin converting enzyme inhibitor	18 (16)		16 (16)		2 (13)		NS
- Diuretic	21 (18)		15 (15)		6 (40)		0.021
- Angiotensin II antagonist	9 (8)		8 (8)		1 (7)		NS
- Statin	28 (24)		25 (25)		3 (20)		NS
- Calcium channel blocker	12 (10)		9 (9)		3 (20)		NS
Laboratory tests	116 (100)		101 (87)		15 (13)		
Serum							
- Creatinine (μmol/L)	114 (98)	84±29	99 (98)	84±30	15 (100)	80±6	NS
- Estimated glomerular filtration rate (mL/min/1.73 m^2)	114 (98)	77±20	99 (98)	78±21	15 (100)	72±18	NS
- Chromogranin A (μg/L)	116 (100)	185 (29.0–44.6×10^3)	101 (100)	168 (29.0–44.6×10^3)	15 (100)	320 (48.0–19.1×10^3)	NS
- Platelet serotonin (nmol/10^9)	116 (100)	18 (3.8–58)	101 (100)	17 (3.8–48)	15 (100)	20 (8.2–58)	NS
Urine							
- Serotonin (μmol/mol creatinine)	98 (84)	69 (16–1.2×10^3)	89 (88)	67 (16–1.2×10^3)	9 (60)	96 (36–4.3×10^2)	NS
- 5-Hydroxyindole acetic acid (mmol/mol creatinine)	110 (95)	8.5 (1.8–3.9×10^2)	96 (95)	7.3 (1.8–2.3×10^2)	14 (93)	11 (3.2–3.9×10^2)	NS
Electrocardiography	60 (52)		51 (50)		9 (60)		
- Heart rate (bpm)	60 (100)	68±17	51 (100)	68±17	9 (100)	67±24	NS
- Sinus rhythm	58 (97)		50 (98)		8 (89)		NS
- Atrial fibrillation (n)	2 (3)		1 (1)		1 (11)		NS
- PQ duration (ms)	58 (97)	158±23	50 (98)	157±22.6	8 (89)	162±23.2	NS
- QRS duration (ms)	60 (100)	90±15	51 (100)	90±15	9 (100)	93±10	NS
- QTc duration (ms)	60 (100)	416±28	51 (100)	416±29.0	9 (100)	420±25.0	NS

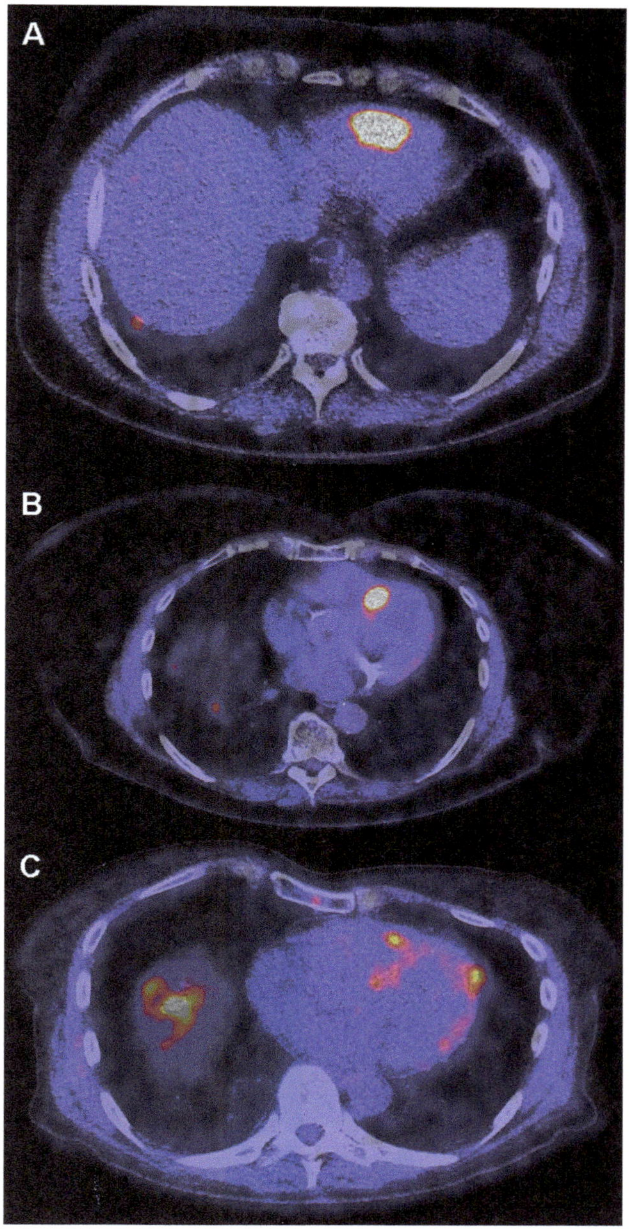

Figure 2. Three fusion images of ^{18}F-FDOPA PET/CT scan in three different patients, indicating cardiac metastases. A: Intense tracer accumulation in the apex of the right ventricle wall. B: Intense uptake in the inter-ventricular septum. C: One lesion in the apex of both the left and right ventricle, with physiological uptake in the rest of the myocardium. The more diffuse and intense uptake projected in the basal part of the right lung is actually located in large liver metastases.

(PV) stenosis (peak gradient across the valve) was graded as mild (<25 mmHg), moderate (25 to 50 mmHg), or severe (>50 mmHg). Tricuspid valve (TV) stenosis (mean gradient across the valve) was graded as mild (0 to 5 mmHg), moderate (5 to 8 mmHg), or severe (>8 mmHg) [18]. Tricuspid annular plane systolic excursion (TAPSE) was measured by M-mode echocardiography at the RV free wall in the apical four-chamber view [19].

Table 2. 6-[fluoride-18]fluoro-L-DOPA (^{18}F-FDOPA PET/CT) results.

	All patients		No cardiac metastases		Cardiac metastases		
Parameter	**N (%)**	**Mean ± SD**	**N (%)**	**Mean ± SD**	**N (%)**	**Mean ± SD**	***p*-value**
^{18}F-FDOPA PET/CT scan	116 (100)		101 (87)		15 (13)		
SUV_{max} right ventricle	116 (100)	2.1±1.6	101 (87)	1.9±0.41	15 (13)	3.9±4.4	<0.001
SUV_{mean} right ventricle	116 (100)	1.4±0.37	101 (87)	1.3±0.32	15 (13)	1.6±0.65	0.015
SUV_{max} left ventricle	116 (100)	2.9±1.6	101 (87)	2.8±1.3	15 (13)	3.7±2.8	0.029
SUV_{mean} left ventricle	116 (100)	1.7±0.36	101 (87)	1.7±0.35	15 (13)	1.7±0.47	NS

SUV denotes Standardized Uptake Value.

Table 3. Echocardiography results of all patients, and patients with and without abnormal cardiac tracer uptake.

	All patients		No cardiac metastases		Cardiac metastases		*p*-value
Parameter	**N (%)**	**Mean ± SD, or median (range)**	**N (%)**	**Mean ± SD, or median (range)**	**N (%)**	**Mean ± SD, or median (range)**	
Heart rate (bpm)	72 (91)	71±18	64 (91)	72±17	8 (89)	68±27	NS
Inter-ventricular septal thickness (mm)	63 (88)	9.4±1.8	54 (77)	9.2±1.7	9 (100)	11±2.1	0.037
Left ventricle posterior wall thickness (mm)	63 (88)	8.5±1.7	54 (77)	8.4±1.6	9 (100)	9.3±2.0	NS
Left ventricle end diastolic volume (mL)	38 (48)	96.8 (41.3–214)	34 (49)	95.2 (41.3–214)	4 (44)	116 (87.2–160)	NS
Left ventricle end systolic volume (mL)	40 (51)	30 (18–95)	36 (51)	30 (18–95)	4 (44)	58 (20–90)	NS
Left ventricle diastolic internal diameter (mm)	63 (88)	46 (34–76)	54 (77)	46 (34–76)	9 (100)	50 (36–58)	NS
Left ventricle systolic internal diameter (mm)	64 (91)	28 (22–46)	55 (79)	28 (22–46)	9 (100)	34 (23–44)	NS
Left ventricle ejection fraction (%)	62 (78)	60±9.8	54 (77)	61±8.6	8 (89)	52±14	0.010
Left atrium diameter (mm)	57 (72)	35±5.6	50 (71)	35±5.6	7 (78)	35±6.3	NS
Right atrium length (mm)	55 (70)	52±5.3	49 (70)	52±5.3	6 (67)	55±5.0	NS
Right atrium wide (mm)	50 (63)	39±6.6	45 (64)	40±6.5	5 (56)	39±8.7	NS
Left atrium length (mm)	53 (67)	54±8.1	47 (67)	54±8.4	6 (67)	55±4.6	NS
Left atrium wide (mm)	53 (67)	40±6.0	47 (67)	39±5.9	6 (67)	45±4.8	0.019
Pulmonary valve peak flow (mmHg)	45 (57)	7.7±6.2	37 (53)	7.9±5.9	8 (89)	6.9±7.7	NS
- Mild pulmonary valve stenosis (<25 mmHg)	45 (100)		37 (100)		8 (100)		NS
Tricuspid valve peak gradient (mmHg)	11 (14)	3.3±3.1	10 (14)	3.4±3.3	1 (11)	2.2	NS
- Mild tricuspid valve stenosis (<5 mmHg)	7 (64)		6 (60)		1 (100)		NS
- Moderate tricuspid valve stenosis (5–8 mmHg)	4 (36)		4 (40)		0		NS
Tricuspid valve regurgitation peak flow (mmHg)	37 (47)	24±7.2	29 (41)	23±7.1	8 (89)	28±6.7	NS
TAPSE (mm)	63 (80)	24±4.4	56 (80)	24±4.3	7 (78)	26±4.7	NS

TAPSE denotes tricuspid annular plane systolic excursion.

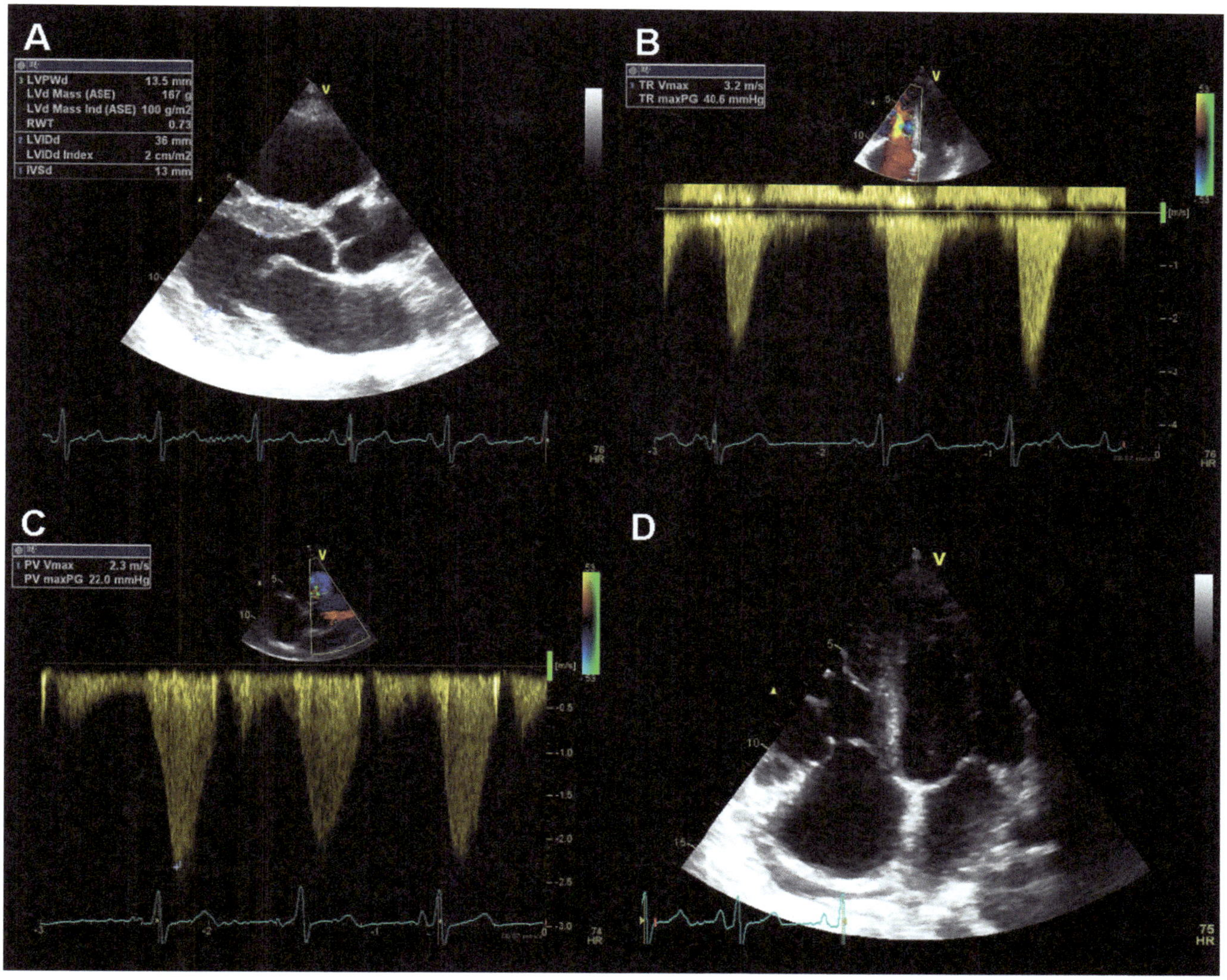

Figure 3. Example of echocardiographic characteristics of a patient with carcinoid heart disease. A: Parasternal long axis view showing thickened LV walls (inter-ventricular septum 13 mm, posterior wall 13 mm). B: Continuous wave Doppler of the tricuspid valve jet. The peak velocity (41 mm Hg) indicates severe tricuspid insufficiency. C: Continuous wave Doppler of the pulmonary valve. The peak gradient (22 mmHg) indicates mild pulmonary valve stenosis. D: 2D four chamber image. On the right in the image normal function of the mitral valve. On the left in the image retraction and immobilisation of the tricuspid valve. The leaflets of the tricuspid valves are also hyperechogenic than normal.

Statistical analysis

Results are expressed as mean value ± standard deviation, or median (range) in the case of an abnormal distribution. The differences between patient categories were evaluated using unpaired Student's *t*-tests (in case of normal distribution), independent sample test (Mann-Whitney U, in case of abnormal distribution), or Chi-square in case of categories. A p value <0.05 was considered significant. Survival was analyzed using log rank test. Statistical analysis was performed using the SPSS package version 20 (IBM Corp., Armonk, NY, USA).

Results

Patient characteristics

Patient selection is shown in Fig. 1.Of the 470 patients who underwent ^{18}F-FDOPA PET/CT, those with medullary thyroid carcinoma, pheochromocytoma and paraganglioma ($n = 202$) were excluded. Of the remaining 268 patients with any form of NET, 116 patients had a serotonin producing NET. Of these patients 103 had a primary location in the small bowel, three a primary in lung, and in 10 patients the exact location of the primary tumour was unknown.

Characteristics of the 116 patients are presented in Table 1. There was a slight male predominance: 62 (53%) vs 54 female. None of the patients had recordings or complaints of ventricular dysrhythmia. During follow up (median 24, range 1–42 months), no cardiac event (either myocardial infarction, or sudden cardiac death) was reported. Eventually 30 patients (26%) died during follow-up. Metastatic disease was the main cause of death. Two patients died from non-disease related causes (one because of a cerebro-vascular accident, the other patient died due to pneumonia during the treatment of her co-existing non-Hodgkin's lymphoma).

In 114 patients (98%), eGFR as a marker for kidney function was determined. Mean eGFR was within normal ranges. In 22 patients, eGFR was moderately decreased (values 30–60 mL/

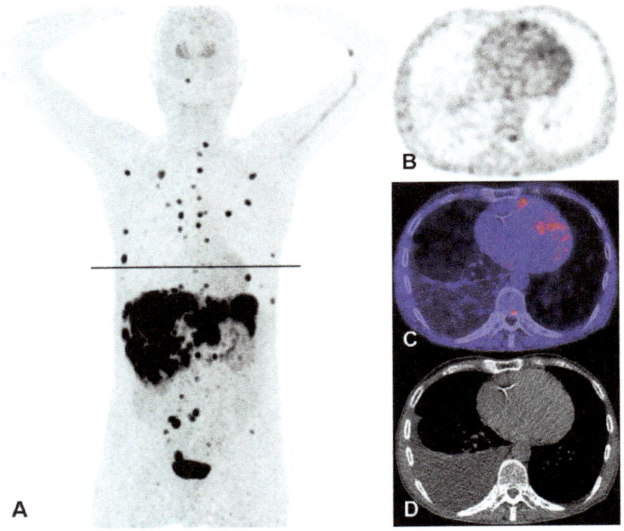

Figure 4. ^{18}F-FDOPA PET/CT scan of the patient illustrated in Fig 2. A: Maximum intensity projection showing multiple metastases of the carcinoid tumour in the mediastinum, thoracic wall, liver, mesentery and skeleton. Physiological uptake in the striatum. Administration artefact in the left elbow and vein in the left upper arm. The black line is the slice position of panels B, C, and D. PET alone (B), fused PET/CT (C) and CT alone (D) images on the slice position indicated in panel A. Physiological uptake in the myocardium with a focus of increased uptake in the right ventricle wall. Also small focal uptake in the posterior part of a thoracic vertebral body, right sided pleural effusion and atherosclerosis of the right coronary artery.

min*1.73 m^2), however, none of the patients had severe impaired kidney function, defined as eGFR <30 mL/min*1.73 m^2.

An ECG in the period of the ^{18}F-FDOPA PET/CT was available in 60 patients (52%). The majority of patients had sinus rhythm at the time of the ECG. In two patients (2%) AF was recorded. One of these patients was newly diagnosed with AF, whereas also one patient with previous reported AF was in sinus rhythm at the time of ECG registration.

^{18}F-FDOPA PET/CT findings

Table 2 shows the results of the ^{18}F-FDOPA PET/CT scans. Fifteen patients (13%) showed abnormal tracer uptake (focal myocardial uptake higher than the surrounding physiological myocardial uptake), suspected of being a result of myocardial metastases of the NET. Of these 15 patients, one patient had a serotonin producing NET originating from the lung. All others had serotonin producing NET originating from the small bowel. Three patients had manifestation of one cardiac metastasis in the left ventricle only, six patients only one metastasis in the right ventricle free wall, and six patients showed lesions in both left and right ventricle walls (Fig. 2).

Of these 15 patients, 4 (27%) died during follow-up after the diagnosis of cardiac metastasis (median 5, range 0–22 months). This was not significantly different from 26 (26%) patients who died with normal cardiac tracer distribution (median 17, range 2–37 months).

Echocardiography

Echocardiography was performed in 79 patients (68%, Table 3). The median time between the ^{18}F-FDOPA PET/CT and echocardiography was 0.80 (range 0.20–1.4) months. Mean LV wall thickness and atrial diameter measurements were within normal ranges. In 10 patients inter-ventricular septum thickness was more than 11 mm, whereas posterior wall was thicker than 11 mm in three patients.

Of these 79 patients, nine patients had abnormal cardiac ^{18}F-FDOPA uptake (Table 3). In six patients with abnormal cardiac uptake, no echocardiography was performed. All of these 15 patients had metastatic disease, based upon the ^{18}F-FDOPA PET/CT. Of the echocardiographic parameters, septum thickness, LVEF, left atrium (wide) measurement and mean peak flow across the aortic valve appeared to be significantly different in the patients with abnormal cardiac tracer distribution. Only one of the nine patients with abnormal ^{18}F-FDOPA uptake had echocardiographic signs of carcinoid heart disease: hypertrophic left ventricle (both septum and posterior wall thickness 13 mm), estimated ejection fraction of 30%, severe tricuspid valve (peak gradient 41 mmHg) and pulmonary valve insufficiency, and a mild pulmonary stenosis (peak gradient 22 mmHg, Figs. 3 and 4). In none of the patients with abnormal ^{18}F-FDOPA uptake in the LV wall who underwent echocardiography a patent foramen ovale could be retrieved on the saved images.

Seven patients with echocardiographic parameters of CHD showed no signs of myocardial metastases on the ^{18}F-FDOPA PET/CT. However, the right ventricle diameter in these patients appeared to be relatively wide (Fig. 5). In two of these patients CHD was based on relatively high maximum peak gradient of TV regurgitation (31 and 37 mm Hg) and peak gradient across the PV (22 and 16 mmHg). In this small group of CHD patients urine level of 5-HIAA was higher than those without echo-based CHD: median 153 (range 4.30–385) vs 5.70 (range 1.70–160) mmol/mol creatinine, $p = 0.001$).

Discussion

This study showed cardiac metastases in 15 out of 116 patients (13%). The presence of cardiac metastases was not related to the occurrence of CHD.

There is slowly growing awareness that cardiac metastases occur rather frequently. However, the early detection of these metastases, especially with echocardiography, remains a challenge. The main limitation is that lesions smaller than 10 mm are non-detectable [20]. The conventional nuclear medicine modality ^{111}In-SRS has the same limitation, especially in whole body imaging. The addition of SPECT/CT of the thorax contributes to a better spatial resolution, with more precise anatomic localization of abnormal tracer accumulation. The introduction of newer imaging modalities with PET tracers ^{68}Ga-DOTATOC and ^{18}F-FDOPA provide an even better spatial resolution (up to 4 mm) and overall more sensitive detection of metastases of NET [4]. This is the largest cohort of patients referred for ^{18}F-FDOPA PET/CT scans, showing that cardiac metastases of NET are more prevalent than previously assumed.

In a review of the reported literature thus far in 2010, a total of 45 patients with cardiac metastases based on imaging, surgery and autopsy findings were retrospectively analyzed [4]. In 21 cases, the presence of cardiac metastasis was based on echocardiographic findings, whereas nuclear medicine modalities were positive in 10 patients. PET scans visualized cardiac metastases in three out of those 10 cases. In all of these cases, the presence of cardiac metastases could be verified with other imaging modalities: echocardiography and MRI. This indicates that both PET tracers are accurately able to visualize cardiac metastases. A recent report on rare metastases of NET further confirms this statement [21]. In this study a total of 4,210 ^{68}Ga-somatostatin-receptor PET/CT

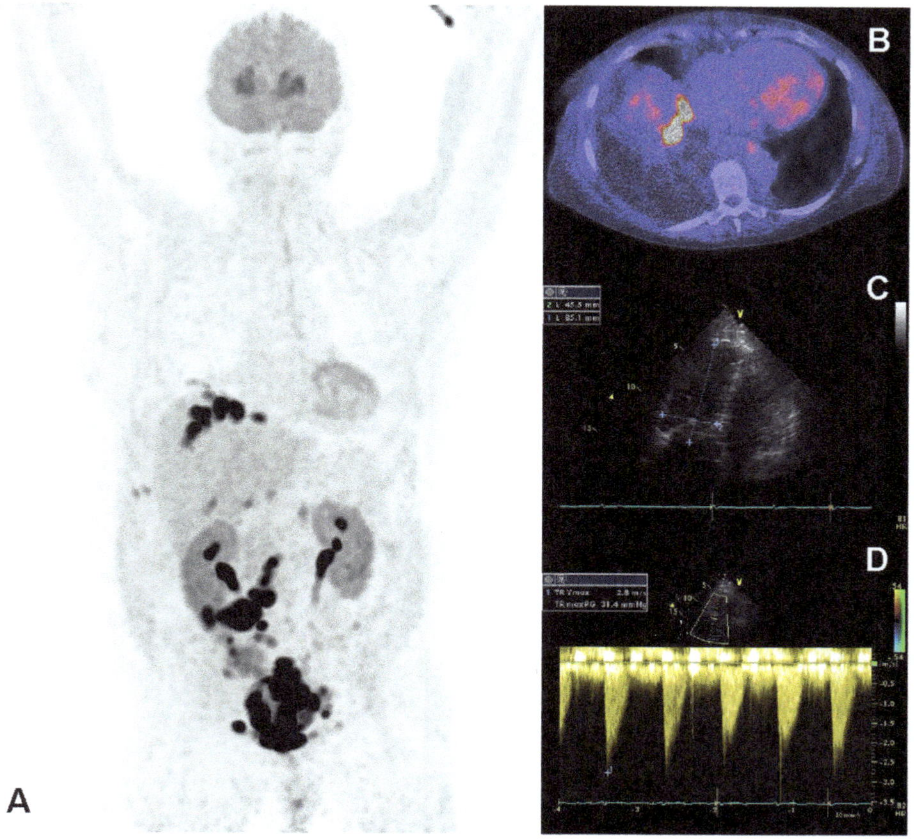

Figure 5. Maximum intensity projection (A) of an ^{18}F-FDOPA PET/CT scan in a patient with echocardiographic signs of carcinoid heart disease, but without myocardial metastases on the ^{18}F-FDOPA PET/CT scan. B: Fused PET/CT image showing only physiological tracer distribution in the myocardium. The intense uptake in liver is due to liver metastases. Ascites surrounding the right liver half. C: Measurements of the right ventricle (85 mm long, 46 mm wide). D: Continuous wave Doppler of the tricuspid valve (peak gradient 31 mmHg), indicating tricuspid insufficiency.

scans performed in a 5-year period were retrospectively analyzed. Cardiac metastases appeared to be rare: in merely 29 of all cases. Both these reports also included non-serotonin producing and non-metastatic NET. Therefore, the prevalence of cardiac metastases in these cohorts is less than 1%. However, this is even less than the low prevalence of 4%, as mentioned previously, and probably a result of selection bias [12]. On the other hand, the most recent study on the presence of cardiac metastases in patients with NET of the small bowel reported that cardiac metastases detected by ^{68}Ga-DOTATOC PET/CT were present in four out of 92 patients with ileal NET [22]. These four patients showed in total seven cardiac metastases, supporting the previously acclaimed prevalence of approximately 4%. As in our study, all patients with myocardial metastases had high tumour burden. Although cardiac metastases are usually detected in patients with widespread metastatic disease, the myocardium can occasionally be the only location of NET metastases [4]. Our study consists of the largest cohort of patients referred for ^{18}F-FDOPA PET/CT scans. We clearly add the novel information that cardiac metastases of NET occur more frequently than previously assumed, and that ^{18}F-FDOPA PET/CT appears to be more sensitive in detecting these metastases than other imaging modalities reported so far.

We showed no relationship between the presence of cardiac metastases and echocardiographic parameters for CHD. This suggests that myocardial metastases and typical CHD are two different entities, which do not seem to affect each other. We could not identify a patent foramen ovale in patients with cardiac metastases, which may support the idea that the presence of cardiac metastases is independent of flow. Lower eyeballing LVEF and wider left atrium measurements were considered to be coincidental findings due to the small group of patients. Urinary excretion of 5-HIAA was higher in patients with echocardiographic signs of CHD, but not in patients with cardiac metastases. Although the duration of the disease was not investigated in this retrospective study, this finding implies that CHD patients probably had long standing disease. Other laboratory tests, as well as ECG findings did not differ. This finding is concordant with the progression of CHD [23].

Conclusions

The prevalence of cardiac metastases found on ^{18}F-FDOPA PET/CT is higher that previously assumed. Cardiac metastases were not related with typical echocardiographic features of CHD, suggesting that these findings are two different entities within the same disease. Of importance, the clinical consequences of this higher incidence of cardiac metastases found on ^{18}F-FDOPA PET/CT may not be of high importance, due to the indolent character of the disease, leading to a comparable survival in patients without cardiac metastases. A large prospective study of serotonin producing NET patients with cardiac metastases should be performed to further establish the clinical role of ^{18}F-FDOPA PET/CT for this indication.

Acknowledgments

We would like to thank Adrienne H. Brouwers, MD PhD, for her expertise in the fields of nuclear medicine and neuroendocrine tumours, and Paul van Snick for reconstructing the raw PET data.

Author Contributions

Conceived and designed the experiments: APB AWG RAD. Performed the experiments: WN BG. Analyzed the data: WN. Contributed reagents/materials/analysis tools: AWG RHS RAD. Wrote the paper: WN APB RAT ANH EGV AMW AWG RHS RAD.

References

1. Pape UF, Perren A, Niederle B, Gross D, Gress T, et al (2012) ENETS Consensus Guidelines for the management of patients with neuroendocrine neoplasms from the jejuno-ileum and the appendix including goblet cell carcinomas. Neuroendocrinology 95: 135–56.
2. Koopmans KP, Neels OC, Kema IP, Elsinga PH, Sluiter WJ, et al (2008) Improved staging of patients with carcinoid and islet cell tumors with ^{18}F-dihydroxy-phenyl-alanine and ^{11}C-5-hydroxy-tryptophan positron emission tomography. J Clin Oncol 26: 1489–1495.
3. Fiebrich HB, Brouwers AH, Links TP, de Vries EGE (2008) Myocardial metastases of carcinoid visualized by F-18-dihydroxy-phenyl-alanine positron emission tomography. Circulation 118: 1602–1604.
4. Jann H, Wertenbruch T, Pape U, Ozcelik C, Denecke T, et al (2010) A matter of the heart: myocardial metastases in neuroendocrine tumors. Horm Metab Res 42: 967–976.
5. Anderson AS, Krauss D, Lang R (1997) Cardiovascular complications of malignant carcinoid disease. Am Heart J 134: 693–702.
6. Roberts WC, Sjoerdsma A (1964) The cardiac disease associated with the carcinoid syndrome (carcinoid heart disease). Am J Med 36: 5–34.
7. Palaniswamy C, Frishman WH, Aronow WS (2012) Carcinoid heart disease. Cardiol Rev 20: 167–176.
8. Bernheim AM, Connolly HM, Hobday TJ, Abel MD, Pellikka PA (2007) Carcinoid heart disease. Prog Cardiovasc Dis 49: 439–451.
9. Rudski LG, Lai WW, Afilalo J, Hua L, Handschumacher MD, et al (2010) Guidelines for the echocardiographic assessment of the right heart in adults: a report from the American Society of Echocardiography endorsed by the European Association of Echocardiography, a registered branch of the European Society of Cardiology, and the Canadian Society of Echocardiography. J Am Soc Echocardiogr 23: 685–713.
10. Møller JE, Pellikka PA, Bernheum AM, Schaff HV, Rubin J, et al (2005) Prognosis of carcinoid heart disease: analysis of 200 cases over two decades. Circulation 112: 3320–3327.
11. Bhattacharyya S, Toumpanakis C, Burke M, Taylor AM, Caplin ME, et al (2010) Features of carcinoid heart disease identified by 2- and 3-dimensional echocardiography and cardiac MRI. Circ Cardiovasc Imaging 3: 103–11.
12. Pellikka PA, Tajik AJ, Khandheria BK, Seward JB, Callahan JA, et al (1993) Carcinoid heart disease. Clinical and echocardiographic spectrum in 74 patients. Circulation 87: 1188–1196.
13. National Kidney Foundation (2002) KDOQI clinical practice guidelines for chronic kidney disease: evaluation, classification, and stratification. Kidney Disease Outcome Quality Initiative. Am J Kidney Dis 39: S1–S266.
14. Boellaard R, Oyen WJ, Hoekstra CJ, Hoekstra OS, Visser EP, et al (2008) The Netherlands protocol for standardisation and quantification of FDG whole body PET studies in multi-centre trials. Eur J Nucl Med Mol Imaging 35: 2320–2333.
15. Boellaard R, O'Doherty MJ, Weber WA, Mottaghy FM, Lonsdale MN, et al (2010) FDG PET and PET/CT: EANM procedure guidelines for tumour PET imaging: version 1.0. Eur J Nucl Med Mol Imaging 37: 181–200.
16. Castillo JG, Silvay G, Solis J (2013) Current concepts in diagnosis and perioperative management of carcinoid heart disease. Semin Cardiothorac Vasc Anesth 2013 17: 212–223.
17. Zoghbi WA, Enriquez-Sarano M, Foster E, Grayburn PA, Kraft CD, et al (2003) Recommendations for evaluation of the severity of native valvular regurgitation with two-dimensional and Doppler echocardiography. J Am Soc Echocardiogr 16: 777–802.
18. Bonow RO, Carabello BA, Chatterjee K, de Leon AC Jr, Faxon DP, et al (2006) ACC/AHA 2006 guidelines for the management of patients with valvular heart disease: a report of the American College of Cardiology/American Heart Association Task Force on Practice Guidelines. J Am Coll Cardiol 48: e1–148.
19. Koestenberger M, Ravekes W, Everett AD, Stueger HP, Heinzl B, et al (2009) Right ventricular function in infants, children and adolescents: reference values of the tricuspid annular plane systolic excursion (TAPSE) in 640 healthy patients and calculation of z score values. J Am Soc Echocardiogr 22: 715–719.
20. Pandya UH, Pellikka PA, Enriquez-Sarano M, Edwards WD, Schaff HV, et al (2002) Metastatic carcinoid tumor to the heart: Echocardiographic-pathologic study of 11 patients. J Am Coll Cardiol 40: 1328–1332.
21. Carreras C, Kulkarni HR, Baum RP (2013) Rare metastases detected by (68)Ga-somatostatin receptor PET/CT in patients with neuroendocrine tumors. Recent Results Cancer Res 194: 379–84.
22. Calissendorff J, Sundin A, Falhammar H (2014). 68Ga-DOTA-TOC-PET/CT detects heart metastases from ileal neuroendocrine tumors. Endocrine 47: 169–76.
23. Denney WD, Kemp WE Jr, Anthony LB, Oates JA, Byrd BF 3rd (1998). Echocardiographic and biochemical evaluation of the development and progression of carcinoid heart disease. J Am Coll Cardiol 32: 1017–22.

19

The Incidence and Prevalence of Diabetes Mellitus and Related Atherosclerotic Complications in Korea: A National Health Insurance Database Study

Bo Kyung Koo[1,2], Chang-Hoon Lee[1], Bo Ram Yang[3,4], Seung-sik Hwang[5], Nam-Kyong Choi[3,6]*

1 Department of Internal Medicine, Seoul National University College of Medicine, Seoul, Republic of Korea, **2** Department of Internal Medicine, Boramae Medical Center, Seoul, Republic of Korea, **3** Division of Clinical Epidemiology, Medical Research Collaborating Center, Seoul National University College of Medicine, Seoul, Republic of Korea, **4** Department of Preventive Medicine, Seoul National University College of Medicine, Seoul, Republic of Korea, **5** Department of Social and Preventive Medicine, Inha University School of Medicine, Incheon, Republic of Korea, **6** Institute of Environmental Medicine, Seoul National University Medical Research Center, Seoul, Republic of Korea

Abstract

Aims/Introduction: The incidence and prevalence of type 2 diabetes mellitus (T2DM) and related macrovascular complications in Korea were estimated using the Health Insurance Review and Assessment (HIRA) database from 2007–2011, which covers the claim data of 97.0% of the Korean population.

Materials and Methods: T2DM, coronary artery disease (CAD), cerebrovascular disease (CVD), and peripheral artery disease (PAD) were defined according to ICD-10 codes. We used the Healthcare Common Procedure Coding System codes provided by HIRA to identify associated procedures or surgeries. When calculating incidence, we excluded cases with preexisting T2DM within two years before the index year. A Poisson distribution was assumed when calculating 95% confidence intervals for prevalence and incidence rates.

Results: The prevalence of T2DM in Korean adults aged 20–89 years was 6.1–6.9% and the annual incidence rates of T2DM ranged from 9.5–9.8/1,000 person-year (PY) during the study period. The incidence rates of T2DM in men and women aged 20–49 years showed decreasing patterns from 2009 to 2011 ($P<0.001$); by contrast, the incidence in subjects aged 70–79 years showed increased patterns from 2009 to 2011 ($P<0.001$). The incidence rates of CAD and CVD in patients newly diagnosed with T2DM were 18.84/1,000 PY and 11.32/1,000 PY, respectively, in the year of diagnosis. Among newly diagnosed individuals with T2DM who were undergoing treatment for PAD, 14.6% underwent angioplasty for CAD during the same period.

Conclusions: Our study measured the national incidences of T2DM, CAD, CVD, and PAD, which are of great concern for public health. We also confirmed the relatively higher risk of CAD and CVD newly detected T2DM patients compared to the general population in Korea.

Editor: Mohammad Ebrahim Khamseh, Institute of Endocrinology and Metabolism, Islamic Republic Of Iran

Funding: This study was supported by a grant from the Korean Diabetes Association (2012-228). The funders had no role in study design, data collection and analysis, decision to publish, or preparation of the manuscript.

Competing Interests: The authors have declared that no competing interests exist.

* Email: likei1@snu.ac.kr

Introduction

The International Diabetes Federation (IDF) estimated the global prevalence of diabetes to be 151 million in 2000 [1] and 285 million in 2010 [2]. The IDF reported that 366 million people had diabetes in 2011, and this prevalence is expected to rise to 552 million by 2030 [3].

From 1970 to 2000, the prevalence of diabetes in South Korea increased about threefold [4], and 9–10% of Korean adults aged ≥30 years were affected by the disease in the early 2000s according to the Korea National Health and Nutritional Examination Survey (KNHANES) [4,5]. The prevalence of diabetes is also increasing in other developing countries in Asia such as China [6–8] and India [9]. A recent meta-analysis reported that the prevalence of diabetes mellitus has significantly increased in China from 2.6% to 9.7% from 2000–2010 [10]. In developed countries such as Canada [11] and the US [12], the prevalence of diabetes has also continued to increase throughout the past decade. However, the prevalence in the Korean population remained stable over the same time period [13]. Furthermore, we recently reported that the prevalence of diabetes among women aged 30–59 years decreased trend from 2001 to

2010 [14]. It is important to investigate the incidence and prevalence of diabetes mellitus in the Korean population considering these trends in the occurrence of diabetes mellitus; however, current data are limited. In one community-based cohort study that included individuals in Korea between the ages of 40 and 79, the annual incidence of type 2 diabetes (T2DM) ranged from 1.33% to 5% [15].

The National Health Insurance (NHI) program in Korea was initiated in 1977 and achieved universal coverage of the population by 1989. The Health Insurance Review and Assessment (HIRA) service covers the claims of 97.0% of the population in Korea; those of the remaining 3% of the population are covered by the Medical Aid Program. Accordingly, the HIRA database contains information on almost the entirety of the insurance claims, including prescribed medications and procedures, for the Korean population of approximately 50 million [16]. The present study was performed to estimate the incidence and prevalence of T2DM and related macrovascular complications in the entire population of South Korea using the NHI claims database from 2007–2011.

Methods

Data collection

We used HIRA data recorded between 1 January 2007 and 31 December 2011. The HIRA database contains information on all insurance claims for about 97.0% of the population in Korea [16]. The HIRA service provided the data after de-identification, and the data included age, gender, diagnosis, date of hospital visits, drug prescriptions received during inpatient and outpatient visits, hospital admissions, medical procedures, and emergency department visits. Drug information included the brand name, generic name, prescription date, and duration and route of administration. Diagnoses were coded according to the International Classification of Disease (10th revision; ICD-10). The study was approved by the Boramae Medical Center Institutional Review Board.

Study population

The prevalence of T2DM patients aged 20–89 years from 2008 to 2010 was defined according to the following eligibility criteria: the presence of (1) at least two claims per year under ICD-10 codes E11–14 or (2) at least one claim per year for the prescription of anti-diabetic medication (under ICD-10 codes E11–14) [17]. Anti-diabetic medications included insulin, sulfonylureas, metformin, thiazolidinediones, α-glucosidase inhibitors, and meglitinides. We excluded patients with type 1 diabetes mellitus, defined as those who (i) were prescribed insulin without oral anti-diabetic agents and (ii) had at least one claim under the ICD-10 code E10, without the code E11, from 2007 to 2011 (**Figure 1**).

The incidence of T2DM from 2009 to 2011 was defined in individuals who met either of the selection criteria, (1) or (2), for estimating the prevalence of T2DM. We subsequently excluded those with preexisting diabetes two or more years before the study period, which included patients who were diagnosed with any type of diabetes mellitus (E10–14) or prescribed any anti-diabetic medications from 1 January 2007 to 31 December 2008 (**Figure 1**). Accordingly, the remaining cases had at least two years and up to five years of disease-free status before the index date and were regarded as the new cases of T2DM. The date of the earliest claim regarding T2DM on or after 1 January 2009 was defined as the index date. The index date was regarded as the incident time, and the patient was counted as a new case in that year.

Case definition of cardiovascular and cerebrovascular disease

To investigate the incidence and prevalence of macrovascular complications in subjects with T2DM, we constructed sub-cohorts of new cases of T2DM and pre-existing cases of T2DM in 2009 (**Figure 1**). The incidence and prevalence, from 2009 to 2011, of macrovascular diabetic complications such as coronary artery disease (CAD), cerebrovascular disease (CVD), and peripheral artery disease (PAD), and amputation were analyzed within the sub-cohorts. CAD and CVD were identified by the following criteria, respectively: (1) medical claim(s) (including all inpatient hospital, outpatient hospital, medical visit, and emergency room claims) with the corresponding disease as the principal diagnosis, or additional diagnosis with an ICD-10 diagnosis code, or procedure code (**Table S1** in File S1) and (2) medical claim(s) regarding any percutaneous intervention or surgery associated with the corresponding disease. We used the Healthcare Common Procedure Coding System codes provided by the HIRA service to identify the associated procedure or surgery (**Table S1** in File S1). Since previous studies showed that the current diagnostic coding system is less sensitive to and less specific for PAD-related illness and treatment than for CAD or CVD [18,19], we did not use ICD-10 diagnosis codes for defining PAD; instead, we defined PAD using claims regarding any percutaneous intervention or surgery associated with PAD (**Table S1** in File S1). Amputation of lower extremities was identified by the medical claim(s) that included an associated procedure or surgery code (**Table S1** in File S1). To detect new cases of CAD, CVD, and PAD in each cohort year, we eliminated all cases with a claim for each corresponding disease that occurred before the cohort year. Hospital admissions for CAD, CVD, and PAD were measured using inpatient claims with the principal diagnosis of the corresponding disease.

Statistical analysis

All data were analyzed using SAS software version 9.3 (SAS Institute, Inc., Cary, NC, USA). Age- and gender-specific annual prevalence rates of T2DM from 2008 to 2010 were calculated by dividing the number of T2DM patients by the Korean population from the 2010 Population and Housing Census (**Table S2** in File S1) [20]. The age- and gender-specific annual incidence rate (number of new cases in each year/number of individuals at risk), and the person-time incidence rate, for 2009–2011, were calculated. The number of individuals at risk in each year was calculated using the following equation [the total population from the 2010 Census – (number of pre-existing cases in the previous year + half of the number of new cases in the year)]; this equation which assumes that new cases developed in the middle of a year. A Poisson distribution was assumed for calculating 95% confidence intervals (CIs) for rates of prevalence and incidence. The annual trends in prevalence and incidence were tested using Poisson regression within age–gender strata. Additionally, Poisson regression was used to analyze the annual trends in prevalence and incidence, with adjustment for age and gender.

Results

Prevalence and incidence of type 2 diabetes mellitus

There were 2,224,876 cases in 2008, 2,368,587 cases in 2009, and 2,516,350 cases in 2010 that fulfilled the study criteria for T2DM and were included in the final analysis. The prevalence of T2DM was 6.1% in 2008, 6.5% in 2009 and 6.9% in 2010 (6.4–7.3% in men and 5.7–6.4% in women from 2008–2010) (**Table 1**). With adjustment for age and gender, annual preva-

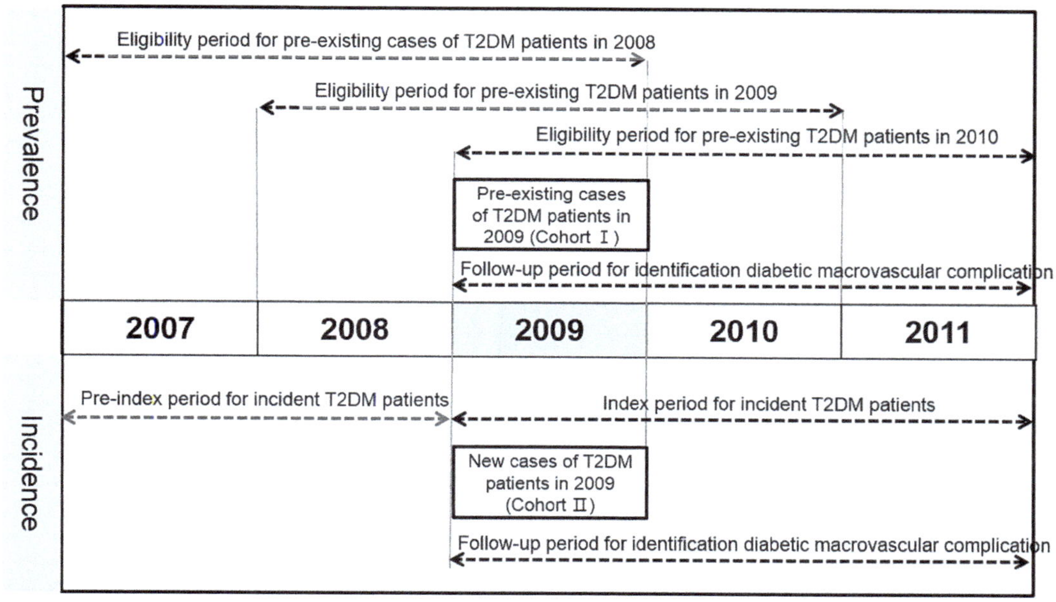

Figure 1. Schematic description of the study period.

lence increased from 2008 to 2010 ($P<0.0001$). In men aged 60–79, the prevalence of T2DM increased each year and reached 19.2–20.0% in 2010 ($P<0.0001$). In women, the prevalence of T2DM was substantially lower than in men of same age in subjects aged <60 years; notably, women aged 30–49 years were shown to have about half the prevalence of T2DM than men of the same age (**Table 1**).

The numbers of newly diagnosed T2DM patients in each year were 336,078, 331,387, and 321,966 in 2009, 2010, and 2011, respectively. The corresponding annual incidence rates of T2DM were 9.8, 9.7, and 9.5 per 1,000 person-years (PY), respectively (**Table 2**). The annual incidence of T2DM decreased after adjusting for age and gender ($P<0.0001$). We subsequently analyzed the annual incidence rate according to gender and age groups. The incidence rates per 1,000 PY were 10.7, 10.6, and 10.4 for men and 9.0, 8.9, and 8.5 for women (**Table 2**). Men and women aged 20–49 years showed a decreasing rate of incidence from 2009 to 2011; the incidence of diabetes in individuals aged 40–49 years decreased from 11.4 to 10.6 (per 1,000 PY) in men and from 6.0 to 5.2 (per 1,000 PY) in women ($P<0.0001$ in both).

Prevalence of macrovascular complication in the 2009 cohort

A total of 1,233,009 men and 1,135,578 women were defined as T2DM patients in 2009 (Cohort I). Among them, 177,999 men and 158,079 women were newly diagnosed as T2DM in that year (Cohort II). In Cohort I, the prevalence of CAD during the three-year period was 16.82%; among these individuals, 11.2% (N = 45,488, 1.92% of Cohort I) and 1.00% (N = 3,984, 0.17% of Cohort I) underwent percutaneous coronary intervention (PCI) and coronary artery bypass graft surgery (CABG), respectively (**Table 3**). As a marker of PAD incidence, 12,282 (0.52% of Cohort I) and 1,162 (0.05% of Cohort I) underwent percutaneous or open revascularization therapy, respectively, which corresponded to about 27% of the number of interventions for CAD during the same period. The amputation of lower extremities was detected in 6,891 (0.29% of Cohort I). CVD was detected in 11.38% of Cohort I from 2009–2011.

In Cohort II, the prevalence of CAD and CVD from 2009–2011 was 14.05% and 8.75%, respectively, which were lower rates than those in Cohort I (**Table 3**). Percutaneous and open revascularization for PAD was performed in 772 (0.23% of Cohort II) and 126 (0.04% of Cohort II) subjects, respectively; and the amputation of lower extremities was detected in 512 (0.15%) subjects in Cohort II from 2009–2011.

Next, we analyzed the incidence of macrovascular complications in Cohort II. Among 336,078 subjects in Cohort II, 21,634 (mean days of follow-up ± standard deviation, 401±283 days) and 13,430 (408±280 days) subjects were newly diagnosed with CAD and CVD, respectively, from 2009–2011 (**Table 4**). Among these individuals, 6,107 and 4,510 were admitted for the management of CAD and CVD, respectively. The annual incidence rates of CAD per 1,000 PY in Cohort II were 18.84 in 2009, 25.71 in 2010, and 21.98 in 2011. About 30% of subjects diagnosed with CAD underwent admission for management of CAD (**Table 4**). The annual incidence rates of PCI for CAD per 1,000 PY in Cohort II were 1.58 in 2009, 2.43 in 2010, and 2.44 in 2011, while the annual incidence rates of percutaneous and open revascularization for PAD were 0.4, 0.6, and 0.7 during the same time period. From 2009–2011, 2,292 and 533 subjects in Cohort II underwent angioplasty for CAD and PAD, respectively. Among them, 78 subjects received angioplasty for both CAD and PAD. The annual incidence rates of admission for CVD per 1,000 PY were 3.83, 5.02, and 4.65 in 2009, 2010, and 2011, respectively.

Discussion

Our retrospective cohort study evaluated the incidence and prevalence of T2DM and associated macrovascular complications in Korea using the NHI HIRA database, which includes information for about 97% of Koreans. The prevalence of T2DM in Korean adults aged 20–89 years ranged from 6.1–6.9% from 2008–2010, and the annual incidence rate of T2DM ranged from 9.5–9.8/1,000 PY from 2009–2011. Women aged <

Table 1. The prevalence of type 2 diabetes mellitus in the Korean population aged 20–89 years.

		Year								*P*-value*
		2008		2009		2010		2008–2010		
		N	Prevalence % (95% CI)	N	Prevalence % (95% CI)	N	Prevalence % (95% CI)	N	Prevalence % (95% CI)	
Total		**2,224,876**	**6.1 (6.1–6.1)**	**2,368,587**	**6.5 (6.4–6.5)**	**2,516,350**	**6.9 (6.9–6.9)**	**3,079,126**	**8.4 (8.4–8.4)**	**<0.0001**
Men	Total	1,152,366	6.4 (6.4–6.4)	1,233,009	6.9 (6.9–6.9)	1,315,234	7.3 (7.3–7.3)	1,605,387	8.9 (8.9–9.0)	<0.0001
	20–29	8,379	0.2 (0.2–0.2)	8,592	0.3 (0.2–0.3)	8,382	0.2 (0.2–0.2)	14,936	0.4 (0.4–0.4)	0.982
	30–39	57,920	1.5 (1.5–1.5)	58,464	1.5 (1.5–1.5)	57,000	1.5 (1.4–1.5)	87,496	2.2 (2.2–2.2)	0.007
	40–49	220,675	5.4 (5.3–5.4)	229,411	5.6 (5.6–5.6)	228,034	5.5 (5.5–5.6)	308,762	7.5 (7.5–7.5)	<0.0001
	50–59	341,748	10.5 (10.5–10.6)	369,824	11.4 (11.3–11.4)	400,527	12.3 (12.3–12.4)	472,318	14.5 (14.5–14.6)	<0.0001
	60–69	321,544	17.0 (17.0–17.1)	341,361	18.1 (18.0–18.1)	363,451	19.2 (19.2–19.3)	429,228	22.7 (22.6–22.8)	<0.0001
	70–79	171,270	15.8 (15.7–15.9)	190,251	17.6 (17.5–17.6)	216,713	20.0 (19.9–20.1)	243,737	22.5 (22.4–22.6)	<0.0001
	80–89	30,830	11.9 (11.7–12.0)	35,106	13.5 (13.4–13.6)	41,127	15.8 (15.7–16.0)	48,910	18.8 (18.6–19.0)	<0.0001
Women	Total	1,072,510	5.7 (5.7–5.7)	1,135,578	6.1 (6.1–6.1)	1,201,116	6.4 (6.4–6.4)	1,473,739	7.9 (7.9–7.9)	<0.0001
	20–29	8,024	0.3 (0.2–0.3)	8,225	0.3 (0.3–0.3)	7,774	0.2 (0.2–0.3)	15,005	0.5 (0.5–0.5)	0.048
	30–39	30,799	0.8 (0.8–0.8)	30,816	0.8 (0.8–0.8)	30,974	0.8 (0.8–0.8)	50,097	1.3 (1.3–1.3)	0.481
	40–49	107,543	2.6 (2.6–2.6)	111,253	2.7 (2.7–2.7)	109,449	2.7 (2.7–2.7)	153,814	3.8 (3.7–3.8)	<0.0001
	50–59	230,093	6.9 (6.9–7.0)	243,840	7.4 (7.3–7.4)	256,632	7.7 (7.7–7.8)	318,061	9.6 (9.6–9.6)	<0.0001
	60–69	343,318	16.3 (16.3–16.4)	354,917	16.9 (16.8–16.9)	365,360	17.4 (17.3–17.4)	443,797	21.1 (21.0–21.2)	<0.0001
	70–79	281,703	18.0 (17.9–18.0)	304,826	19.5 (19.4–19.5)	334,111	21.3 (21.3–21.4)	382,547	24.4 (24.3–24.5)	<0.0001
	80–89	71,030	11.7 (11.6–11.8)	81,701	13.5 (13.4–13.6)	96,816	16.0 (15.9–16.1)	110,418	18.2 (18.1–18.3)	<0.0001

CI = confidence interval.
**P*-values were obtained using Poisson regression.

Table 2. The incidence of type 2 diabetes mellitus in the Korean population aged 20–89 years.

		Year								
		2009		2010		2011		2009–2011		
		N	Incidence per 1,000 PY (95% CI)	N	Incidence per 1,000 PY (95% CI)	N	Incidence per 1,000 PY (95% CI)	N	Incidence per 1,000 PY (95% CI)	*P*-value*
Total		**336,078**	**9.8 (9.8–9.8)**	**331,387**	**9.7 (9.7–9.7)**	**321,966**	**9.5 (9.4–9.5)**	**989,431**	**9.7 (9.6–9.7)**	**<.0001**
Men	Total	177,999	10.7 (10.6–10.7)	175,808	10.6 (10.5–10.6)	172,967	10.4 (10.4–10.5)	526,774	10.6 (10.5–10.6)	<.0001
	20–29	2,931	0.9 (0.8–0.9)	2,748	0.8 (0.8–0.8)	2,622	0.8 (0.7–0.8)	8,301	0.8 (0.8–0.8)	<.0001
	30–39	16,609	4.3 (4.2–4.4)	15,445	4.0 (3.9–4.1)	15,216	3.9 (3.9–4.0)	47,270	4.1 (4.0–4.1)	<.0001
	40–49	44,215	11.4 (11.3–11.5)	41,628	10.8 (10.7–10.9)	40,838	10.6 (10.5–10.7)	126,681	10.9 (10.9–11.0)	<.0001
	50–59	52,070	18.1 (17.9–18.2)	52,952	18.6 (18.4–18.7)	53,702	19.0 (18.9–19.2)	158,724	18.6 (18.5–18.6)	<.0001
	60–69	38,778	25.0 (24.8–25.3)	38,627	25.3 (25.0–25.5)	36,400	24.1 (23.9–24.4)	113,805	24.8 (24.7–25.0)	<.0001
	70–79	19,482	21.6 (21.3–21.9)	20,331	23.0 (22.7–23.3)	20,104	23.5 (23.1–23.8)	59,917	22.7 (22.5–22.9)	0.002
	80–89	3,914	17.2 (16.7–17.8)	4,077	18.3 (17.7–18.8)	4,085	18.8 (18.3–19.4)	12,076	18.1 (17.8–18.4)	0.057
Women	Total	158,079	9.0 (9.0–9.0)	155,579	8.9 (8.8–8.9)	148,999	8.5 (8.5–8.6)	462,657	8.8 (8.8–8.8)	<.0001
	20–29	3,275	1.0 (1.0–1.1)	2,889	0.9 (0.9–0.9)	2,606	0.8 (0.8–0.9)	8,770	0.9 (0.9–0.9)	<.0001
	30–39	9,529	2.5 (2.4–2.5)	9,653	2.5 (2.5–2.6)	8,840	2.3 (2.3–2.4)	28,022	2.4 (2.4–2.5)	<.0001
	40–49	23,621	6.0 (5.9–6.0)	22,463	5.7 (5.6–5.7)	20,762	5.2 (5.2–5.3)	66,846	5.6 (5.6–5.7)	<.0001
	50–59	40,022	13.1 (12.9–13.2)	40,481	13.3 (13.1–13.4)	40,424	13.3 (13.2–13.4)	120,927	13.2 (13.1–13.3)	0.157
	60–69	42,119	24.2 (24.0–24.4)	40,756	23.6 (23.3–23.8)	37,756	22.0 (21.7–22.2)	120,631	23.2 (23.1–23.4)	<.0001
	70–79	30,783	24.2 (24.0–24.5)	30,587	24.5 (24.3–24.8)	29,938	24.6 (24.3–24.9)	91,308	24.5 (24.3–24.6)	0.001
	80–89	8,730	16.4 (16.1–16.8)	8,750	16.8 (16.5–17.2)	8,673	17.2 (16.8–17.5)	26,153	16.8 (16.6–17.0)	0.666

PY = person-years; CI = confidence interval.
* P-values were obtained using Poisson regression.

Table 3. The prevalence of diabetic macrovascular complications in patients with type 2 diabetes mellitus aged 20–89 years.

Year		N (%)							
		Pre-existing cases of T2DM in 2009 (N = 2,368,587, Cohort I)				New cases of T2DM in 2009 (N = 336,078, Cohort II)			
		2009	2010	2011	2009–2011	2009	2010	2011	2009–2011
CAD	Total*	241,924 (10.21)	244,348 (10.32)	244,988 (10.34)	398,389 (16.82)	29,365 (8.74)	26,444 (7.87)	26,067 (7.76)	47,211 (14.05)
	PCI	17,026 (0.72)	15,850 (0.67)	15,973 (0.67)	45,488 (1.92)	2,362 (0.70)	1,377 (0.41)	1,278 (0.38)	4,641 (1.38)
	Coronary bypass	1,583(0.07)	1,253 (0.05)	1,152 (0.05)	3,984 (0.17)	206 (0.06)	77 (0.02)	91 (0.03)	373 (0.11)
CVD	Total*	159,698 (6.74)	158,704 (6.70)	157,526 (6.65)	269,538 (11.38)	18,458 (5.49)	16,876 (5.02)	16,305 (4.85)	29,412 (8.75)
PAD	Percutaneous angioplasty	4,067 (0.17)	3,867 (0.16)	4,348 (0.18)	12,282 (0.52)	300 (0.09)	236 (0.07)	236 (0.07)	772 (0.23)
	Open revascularization	480 (0.02)	404 (0.02)	327 (0.01)	1,162 (0.05)	74 (0.02)	38 (0.01)	26 (0.01)	126 (0.04)
Amputation	Total	2,703 (0.11)	2,418 (0.10)	2,408 (0.10)	6,891 (0.29)	280 (0.08)	147 (0.04)	120 (0.04)	512 (0.15)
	Femur	147 (0.01)	131 (0.01)	118 (0.00)	386 (0.02)	26 (0.01)	15 (0.00)	12 (0.00)	53 (0.02)
	Below knee	729 (0.03)	645 (0.03)	603 (0.03)	1,914 (0.08)	71 (0.02)	39 (0.01)	22 (0.01)	131 (0.04)
	Foot	502 (0.02)	434 (0.02)	479 (0.02)	1,367 (0.06)	43 (0.01)	23 (0.01)	12 (0.00)	77 (0.02)
	Toe	1,722 (0.07)	1,550 (0.07)	1,579 (0.07)	4,529 (0.19)	175 (0.05)	90 (0.03)	84 (0.02)	329 (0.10)

T2DM = type 2 diabetes mellitus; CAD = coronary artery disease; CVD = cardiovascular disease; PAD = peripheral artery disease; PCI = percutaneous coronary intervention.
*Claim with an ICD-10 diagnosis code as the principal or additional diagnosis, or claims involving a procedure related to the corresponding disease.

Table 4. The incidence of diabetic macrovascular complications in Cohort II.

		Incidence, N (/1,000 person-year) (N = 336,078)								
Year		**2009**		**2010**		**2011**		**2009–2011**		**Mean days of follow-up (SD)**
CAD	Total*	6,274	(18.84)	8,373	(25.71)	6,987	(21.98)	21,634	(22.17)	400.8 (283.2)
	PCI	531	(1.58)	816	(2.43)	817	(2.44)	2,164	(2.15)	439.9 (287.6)
	Coronary bypass	37	(0.11)	45	(0.13)	63	(0.19)	145	(0.14)	463.5 (301.1)
	Admission†	1,725	(5.15)	2,293	(6.88)	2,089	(6.31)	6,107	(6.11)	409.4 (291.0)
CVD	Total*	3,782	(11.32)	5,189	(15.74)	4,459	(13.73)	13,430	(13.59)	408.3 (279.7)
	Admission†	1,286	(3.83)	1,677	(5.02)	1,547	(4.65)	4,510	(4.50)	414.9 (285.6)
PAD	Percutaneous angioplasty	108	(0.32)	183	(0.54)	205	(0.61)	496	(0.49)	453.0 (291.7)
	Open revascularization	24	(0.07)	19	(0.06)	14	(0.04)	57	(0.06)	320.1 (243.6)
Amputation	Total	160	(0.48)	126	(0.4)	102	(0.30)	388	(0.39)	340.3 (293.7)
	Femur	18	(0.05)	13	(0.04)	11	(0.03)	42	(0.04)	317.7 (270.1)
	Below knee	39	(0.12)	37	(0.11)	21	(0.06)	97	(0.10)	341.9 (286.2)
	Foot	26	(0.08)	23	(0.07)	11	(0.03)	60	(0.06)	303.8 (277.4)
	Toe	99	(0.29)	78	(0.23)	73	(0.22)	250	(0.25)	353.0 (304.1)

CAD = coronary artery disease; CVD = cardiovascular disease; PAD = peripheral artery disease; PCI = percutaneous coronary intervention; SD = standard deviation.
*Claim with an ICD-10 diagnosis code as the principal or additional diagnosis, or claims involving a procedure related to the corresponding disease.
†Hospital admissions were measured using inpatient claims with the principal diagnosis of the corresponding disease.

60 years showed a lower prevalence of T2DM compared to men of the same age, and women between the ages of 30 and 49 years demonstrated about half the prevalence and incidence rate of men of the same age.

The incidence of T2DM in our study is similar to a previous report in Taiwan, that used diagnosis code-based claim data to show that the incidence was 7.8/1,000 PY in 2004. In Japan, a recent pooled analysis showed that the incidence rate of T2DM was 8.8/1,000 PY, which is also similar to our results [21]. Given that the populations of countries adjacent to Korea such as China and Japan have similar genetic backgrounds related to the risk of developing T2DM [22–24], and that such countries have similar T2DM prevalence [5,6,8,25], our results for the Korean population are reasonable.

However, claim-based diagnoses may underestimate the real prevalence or incidence of T2DM. The mean annual incidence rate of T2DM in a Korean community-based cohort was 21.5/1,000 PY in adults aged 40–69 years [15,26], which is higher than our results. The prevalence of T2DM in adults aged ≥30 years in 2010, according to the KNHANES 2010 was 10.1%, which is also higher than our result [13]. The consideration that only 73.0% of diabetic subjects were aware of their glucose disorder in 2008–2010 according to the KNHANES [13] may explain these differences explained. A previous national survey of diabetes in Korea based on 2003 HIRA data showed an incidence rate of diabetes of 5.7/1,000 PY, which is lower than our results [27]. As the proportion of diabetic subjects with a medical diagnosis of diabetes increased from 43% in 2001 and 66.5% in 2005 [28] to 73.0% in 2008–2010, according to the KNHANES [13], misclassification bias may account for a potential underestimation in the incidence of diabetes based on claims data in 2003 compared with data from 2009–2011.

Interestingly, the incidence of T2DM in men and women aged 20–49 years showed a decrease from 2009 to 2011, despite an increase in the prevalence of T2DM in the overall population. The incidence of diabetes in individuals aged 40–49 years decreased from 11.4 to 10.6/1,000 PY in men and from 6.0 to 5.2/1,000 PY in women, which corresponds to previous data from the KNHANES showing that the prevalence of diabetes among women aged 30–59 years decreased from 2001 to 2010 [14]. Lifestyle improvements such as decreasing total daily energy intake and performing regular exercise along with decreased rates of obesity in young adults in Korea, may be the causes of these trends [14]. In contrast, both the incidence and the prevalence of T2DM in individuals aged ≥70 years increased in our study. Korea is one of most rapidly aging countries, similar to Japan; the proportion of the elderly population aged ≥65 in Korea increased from 7.2% of the total population in 2000 to 11.0% in 2010 [29]. Our study showed that the incidence of T2DM in individuals aged 70–79 years was as high as that in individuals aged 60–69 years; furthermore, in women, individuals aged 70–79 years showed a higher incidence rate than those aged 60–69 years, which is worth noting. In general, the incidence of diabetes increases with age until about 65 years of age, after which both incidence and prevalence seem to decrease [30,31]. We cannot explain the cause of the relatively high incidence of newly detected T2DM in individuals aged ≥70 years; further studies characterizing the elderly population with incident T2DM should be performed because increasing rates of T2DM among these individuals may increase the economic burden in Korea.

The prevalence of CAD and CVD in diabetic subjects in our study ranged from 10.2–10.3% and 6.7%, respectively, which was more than 2 times higher than the general population. In the 2010 KNHANES, the prevalence of CAD and CVD in adults aged ≥30 years was 2.4% and 1.4%, respectively [13]. Previous studies based on the NHI system in the general Korean population also showed a lower prevalence of both CAD and CVD (2.5% and 2.4%, respectively) [32,33]. Comparing the newly diagnosed T2DM patients (Cohort II) with all T2DM patients (Cohort I), the prevalence of CAD and CVD was lower in Cohort II than in Cohort I. However, in Cohort II, up to 8.7% and 5.5% of Cohort II had CAD and CVD, respectively, in the year of T2DM diagnosis, which are still higher rates than those in the general Korean population.

The incidence of CAD and CVD in newly detected T2DM patients (Cohort II) was 18.84/1,000 PY and 11.32/1,000 PY in the year of T2DM diagnosis; these increased in subsequent years. The incidence of CAD was 25.71/1,000 PY in 2010 and 21.98/1,000 PY in 2011, and the incidence of CVD was 15.74/1,000 PY in 2010 and 13.73/1,000 PY in 2011. The incidence of ischemic stroke (resulting from CVD) in the general population of Korea was reported as 1.3/1,000 PY in 2004 [34].

The number of claims for PAD was relatively small compared to CAD and CVD. However, the finding that, among the 533 subjects in Cohort II who underwent angioplasty for PAD during study period, 78 (14.6%) of them experienced angioplasty for CAD during the same period emphasizes the importance of screening for CAD in T2DM patients with PAD considering the morbidity and mortality from CAD [35].

We confirmed the relatively higher risk of CAD and CVD in diabetic subjects compared to the general Korean population using nationwide health insurance claim data from HIRA. However, there are limitations regarding the accuracy of the diagnoses from claim data, since they were not based on clinical data. Furthermore, claims data provide limited information on disease severity, co-morbid conditions, past history, and specific treatment. As previously mentioned, the proportion of the population aware of their disease status may influence the estimation of prevalence or incidence of a disease in a claim study. In addition, three years of follow-up is a relatively short time period to evaluate trends in the incidence of T2DM. However, the usefulness of claim data in the nationwide survey for T2DM has been confirmed previously [36,37]. The accuracy of diagnosis of T2DM from claim data reached a sensitivity of 68–71% and positive predictive value of 85–88% for clinically diagnosed T2DM from health examinations [37]. In addition, we extensively reviewed two years of prior claim data to calculate the incidence of T2DM, which may result in reasonable incidence rates compared to those from adjacent Asian populations and previous reports in Korea.

In summary, in recent years, the prevalence of T2DM in Korean adults aged 20–89 years was 6.1–6.9% and the annual incidence rate of T2DM was 8.8–9.2/1,000 PY. The fact that the incidence of T2DM in the elderly population increased significantly in the opposite direction to that in young men and women in the same period may result in an increasing economic burden in Korea, and necessitates a call for public health planning for the elderly population. Even in newly detected T2DM subjects, the prevalence of CAD and CVD was much higher than that in the general population. Our extensive investigation of epidemiologic data from nationwide claim data should be invaluable for planning national public health strategies.

Supporting Information

File S1 Supporting tables.

Author Contributions

Conceived and designed the experiments: BK CL NC. Performed the experiments: BY NC. Analyzed the data: BK BY SH NC. Contributed reagents/materials/analysis tools: BY NC. Wrote the paper: BK NC.

References

1. International Diabetes Federation (2000) IDF Diabetes Atlas. Brussels: International Diabetes Federation.
2. International Diabetes Federation (2009) IDF Diabetes Atlas. Brussels: International Diabetes Federation.
3. Whiting DR, Guariguata L, Weil C, Shaw J (2011) IDF diabetes atlas: global estimates of the prevalence of diabetes for 2011 and 2030. Diabetes Res Clin Pract 94: 311–321.
4. Kim DJ (2011) The epidemiology of diabetes in Korea. Diabetes Metab J 35: 303–308.
5. Choi YJ, Kim HC, Kim HM, Park SW, Kim J, et al. (2009) Prevalence and management of diabetes in Korean adults: Korea National Health and Nutrition Examination Surveys 1998–2005. Diabetes Care 32: 2016–2020.
6. Ning F, Pang ZC, Dong YH, Gao WG, Nan HR, et al. (2009) Risk factors associated with the dramatic increase in the prevalence of diabetes in the adult Chinese population in Qingdao, China. Diabet Med 26: 855–863.
7. Yang W, Lu J, Weng J, Jia W, Ji L, et al. (2010) Prevalence of diabetes among men and women in China. N Engl J Med 362: 1090–1101.
8. Shen J, Goyal A, Sperling L (2012) The emerging epidemic of obesity, diabetes, and the metabolic syndrome in china. Cardiol Res Pract 2012: 178675.
9. Ramachandran A, Snehalatha C, Vijay V (2002) Temporal changes in prevalence of type 2 diabetes and impaired glucose tolerance in urban southern India. Diabetes Res Clin Pract 58: 55–60.
10. Li H, Oldenburg B, Chamberlain C, O'Neil A, Xue B, et al. (2012) Diabetes prevalence and determinants in adults in China mainland from 2000 to 2010: A systematic review. Diabetes Res Clin Pract.98: 226–235.
11. Lipscombe LL, Hux JE (2007) Trends in diabetes prevalence, incidence, and mortality in Ontario, Canada 1995–2005: a population-based study. Lancet 369: 750–756.
12. Cowie CC, Rust KF, Ford ES, Eberhardt MS, Byrd-Holt DD, et al. (2009) Full accounting of diabetes and pre-diabetes in the U.S. population in 1988–1994 and 2005–2006. Diabetes Care 32: 287–294.
13. Korea Centers for Disease Control and Prevention (2010) The Korean National Health and Nutrition Examination Survey. Chungwon: Ministry of Health and Welfare.
14. Koo BK, Kim EK, Choi H, Park KS, Moon MK (2013) Decreasing trends of the prevalence of diabetes and obesity in korean women aged 30–59 years over the past decade: results from the korean national health and nutrition examination survey, 2001–2010. Diabetes Care 36: e95–96.
15. Cho NH (2010) The epidemiology of diabetes in Korea: from the economics to genetics. Korean Diabetes J 34: 10–15.
16. Choi NK, Chang Y, Choi YK, Hahn S, Park BJ (2010) Signal detection of rosuvastatin compared to other statins: data-mining study using national health insurance claims database. Pharmacoepidemiol Drug Saf 19: 238–246.
17. Sloan FA, Belsky D, Ruiz D, Jr., Lee P (2008) Changes in incidence of diabetes mellitus-related eye disease among US elderly persons, 1994–2005. Arch Ophthalmol 126: 1548–1553.
18. Hirsch AT, Hartman L, Town RJ, Virnig BA (2008) National health care costs of peripheral arterial disease in the Medicare population. Vasc Med 13: 209–215.
19. Margolis J, Barron JJ, Grochulski WD (2005) Health care resources and costs for treating peripheral artery disease in a managed care population: results from analysis of administrative claims data. J Manag Care Pharm 11: 727–734.
20. Statistics Korea (2010) 2010 Population and Housing Census. Daejeon: Statistics Korea.
21. Goto A, Goto M, Noda M, Tsugane S (2013) Incidence of type 2 diabetes in Japan: a systematic review and meta-analysis. PLoS One 8: e74699.
22. Ng MC, Tam CH, Lam VK, So WY, Ma RC, et al. (2007) Replication and identification of novel variants at TCF7L2 associated with type 2 diabetes in Hong Kong Chinese. J Clin Endocrinol Metab 92: 3733–3737.
23. Ng MC, Park KS, Oh B, Tam CH, Cho YM, et al. (2008) Implication of genetic variants near TCF7L2, SLC30A8, HHEX, CDKAL1, CDKN2A/B, IGF2BP2, and FTO in type 2 diabetes and obesity in 6,719 Asians. Diabetes 57: 2226–2233.
24. Miyake K, Horikawa Y, Hara K, Yasuda K, Osawa H, et al. (2008) Association of TCF7L2 polymorphisms with susceptibility to type 2 diabetes in 4,087 Japanese subjects. J Hum Genet 53: 174–180.
25. Ramachandran A, Snehalatha C, Kapur A, Vijay V, Mohan V, et al. (2001) High prevalence of diabetes and impaired glucose tolerance in India: National Urban Diabetes Survey. Diabetologia 44: 1094–1101.
26. Korea Centers for Disease Control and Prevention (2008) Results of the Second Follow-up Survey of Ansung and Ansan Cohort. Chungwon: Korea Centers for Disease Control and Prevention.
27. Task Force Team for Basic Statistical Study of Korean Diabetes Mellitus of Korean Diabetes A, Park Ie B, Kim J, Kim DJ, Chung CH, et al. (2013) Diabetes epidemics in Korea: reappraise nationwide survey of diabetes "diabetes in Korea 2007". Diabetes Metab J 37: 233–239.
28. Korea Centers for Disease Control and Prevention (2005) The Korean National Health and Nutrition Examination Survey. Chungwon: Korea Centers for Disease Control and Prevention
29. Statistics Korea (2011) Population Projections for Korea. Daejeon: Statistics Korea.
30. Selvin E, Coresh J, Brancati FL (2006) The burden and treatment of diabetes in elderly individuals in the u.s. Diabetes Care 29: 2415–2419.
31. Kirkman MS, Briscoe VJ, Clark N, Florez H, Haas LB, et al. (2012) Diabetes in older adults. Diabetes Care 35: 2650–2664.
32. Chang HS, Kim HJ, Nam CM, Lim SJ, Jang YH, et al. (2012) The socioeconomic burden of coronary heart disease in Korea. J Prev Med Public Health 45: 291–300.
33. Lim SJ, Kim HJ, Nam CM, Chang HS, Jang YH, et al. (2009) Socioeconomic costs of stroke in Korea: estimated from the Korea national health insurance claims database. J Prev Med Public Health 42: 251–260.
34. Hong KS, Kim J, Cho YJ, Seo SY, Hwang SI, et al. (2011) Burden of ischemic stroke in Korea: analysis of disability-adjusted life years lost. J Clin Neurol 7: 77–84.
35. Su Kyung Park M-KP, Ji Hye Su, Mi Kyung Kim, Yong Ki Kim, In Ju Kim, Yang Ho Kang, Kwang Jae Lee, Hyun Seung Lee, Chang Won Lee, Bo Hyun Kim, Kyung Il Lee, Mi Kyoung Kim, Duk Kyu Kim (2009) Cause-of-Death Trends for Diabetes Mellitus over 10 Years Korean Diabetes Journal 33: 65–72.
36. Ngo DL, Marshall LM, Howard RN, Woodward JA, Southwick K, et al. (2003) Agreement between self-reported information and medical claims data on diagnosed diabetes in Oregon's Medicaid population. J Public Health Manag Pract 9: 542–544.
37. Southern DA, Roberts B, Edwards A, Dean S, Norton P, et al. (2010) Validity of administrative data claim-based methods for identifying individuals with diabetes at a population level. Can J Public Health 101: 61–64.

Weak Prediction Power of the Framingham Risk Score for Coronary Artery Disease in Nonagenarians

Josef Yayan*

Department of Internal Medicine, Division of Pulmonary, Allergy, and Sleep Medicine, Saarland University Medical Center, Homburg/Saar, Germany

Abstract

Background: Coronary artery disease (CAD) is caused by an acute myocardial infarction and is still feared as a life-threatening heart disease worldwide. In order to identify patients at high risk for CAD, previous studies have proposed various risk assessment scores for the prevention of CAD. The most commonly used risk assessment score for CAD worldwide is the Framingham Risk Score (FRS). The FRS is used for middle-aged people; hence, its appropriateness has not been demonstrated to predict the likelihood of CAD occurrence in very elderly people. This article examines the possible predictive value of FRS for CAD in very elderly people over 90 years of age.

Methods: Data on all patients over 90 years of age who received a cardiac catheter were collected from hospital charts from the Department of Internal Medicine, Saarland University Medical Center, and HELIOS Hospital Wuppertal, Witten/Herdecke University Medical Center, Germany, within a study period from 2004 to 2013. The FRSs and cardiovascular risk profiles of patients over 90 years of age with and without CAD after cardiac catheterization were compared.

Results: One hundred and seventy-five (91.15%, mean age 91.51 $\pm$ 1.80 years, 74 females [42.29%]; 95% confidence interval [CI], 0.87–0.95) of a total 192 of the very elderly patients were found to have CAD. Based on the results of our study, the FRS seems to provide weak predictive ability for CAD in very elderly people ($P = 0.3792$).

Conclusion: We found weak prediction power of FRS for CAD in nonagenarians.

Editor: Ralf Krahe, University of Texas MD Anderson Cancer Center, United States of America

Funding: The author has no funding or support to report.

Competing Interests: The author has declared that no competing interests exist.

* Email: josef.yayan@hotmail.com

Introduction

Coronary artery disease (CAD) is the most common heart disease and hides the high risk for the cause for the development of acute myocardial infarction [1]. Numerous studies and international and national clinical practice guidelines have proven that CAD is caused by the manifestation of atherosclerosis in coronary arteries [2–10]. According to data from epidemiological studies, CAD has an increasingly high mortality rate around the world [11]. For this reason, the prediction of CAD risk has gained significant attention in the medical science community worldwide. The identification of risk factors for CAD is a basic requirement for establishing possible targeted medical therapy for the primary and secondary prevention of CAD. Therefore, several national and international guidelines and recommendations for preventing CAD were previously published after identifying the risk factors for CAD [12–15]. There are still ongoing efforts and attempts to improve the risk assessment methods for the prediction of CAD. To achieve this goal, several risk prediction scores for CAD have been developed in recent years [16]. Five or 10 risk assessments for CAD have been assumed worldwide according to the recommendations of the guidelines [17–18]. Currently available CAD risk prediction scores are mostly based on multivariable regression analysis deduced from the Framingham Heart Study [19] in which the traditional risk factors for CAD are taken into consideration such as age, cholesterol levels, blood pressure, smoking, and body weight [20–21]. The Framingham Risk Score (FRS) provides an estimation of the probability of an individual developing CAD in 10 years to detect high-risk persons and to take preventive actions [22]. Based on data obtained through the FRS calculations, high-risk patients should be treated, according to the guidelines' recommendations, with lipid-lowering medication and aspirin in the primary prevention of CAD [23,24]. FRS and other presently common risk estimation scores are designed for people in middle age [20,25,26]. The mean age in the FRS was 49 years old and people younger than 30 years and older than 74 years of age were not considered [20,27]. Present risk prediction with the FRS might operate less effectively in elderly compared to middle-aged persons, and various traditional risk factors have a weak association with CAD risk in the elderly; for example, hypercholesterolemia is a strong cardiovascular risk factor in middle-aged individuals, but not in the elderly [27,28]. Thus, new questions arise as to whether the FRS could be used to estimate cardiovascular risk for very elderly people over 90 years of age. We conducted the present investigation to better understand the FRS as an eligible prediction system for CAD in very elderly people over 90 years of age. Therefore, we collected data on all patients of this age group with CAD according to the International Classification of Disease from the hospital database at the Department of Internal Medicine, Saarland University Medical Center, and HELIOS Hospital Wuppertal, Witten/Herdecke University Medical Center, Germany. We used a risk assessment tool based on information from the Framingham Heart Study to calculate the FRS after confirming the presence or absence of CAD by performing cardiac catheterization to examine the FRS as an eligible scoring system for very elderly people. The variety of calculated FRS for CAD in people over 90 years of age were age, gender, systolic blood pressure, total cholesterol, high density lipoproteins (HDL), tobacco smoking, and former smoking. CAD diagnosis was made only after cardiac catheterization. The FRS for CAD was compared in patients older than 90 years of age after excluding CAD by performing cardiac catheterization. Only once we have identified the cardiovascular risk factors of CAD can we develop appropriately tailored therapies for all patients to take precautions against CAD.

Materials and Methods

Ethics Statement

All patients' data were anonymized prior to analysis. Due to the retrospective nature of the study protocol, the Medical Association of Saarland's Institutional Review Board approved this study and waived the need for informed consent.

Patients

In this study, the FRS for CAD was retrospectively examined in patients over 90 years of age using hospital chart data at the Department of Internal Medicine, Saarland University Medical Center, and HELIOS Hospital Wuppertal, Witten/Herdecke University Medical Center, during the study period from 2004 to 2013.

The FRS for CAD in the last decade of a patient's life was considered theoretically, assuming that the average life expectancy would be 100 years of age. For the control group, the last highest decade of life was chosen to avoid any distortion in the data analysis due to age. The last highest decade of life refers to patients over 90 years old. Thus, the study population was composed of very elderly patients over 90 years of age diagnosed with CAD, and the control group was composed of elderly patients over 90 years of age without CAD, as determined after cardiac catheterization. All patients older than 90 years who were treated at the internal medicine emergency rooms or in one of the internal departments of the two hospitals were included after receiving a cardiac catheter in this study. Patients over 90 years who were treated in other departments or had no cardiac catheter were excluded from this study.

The FRS assessment tool from the National Heart, Lung, and Blood Institute (NHLBI) in Bethesda, Maryland [12,29] was used to calculate FRSs in very elderly people over 90 years of age after CAD was confirmed to be present or absent by cardiac catheterization. The study population received a point score based on the categorical values of age, total cholesterol, high-density lipoprotein cholesterol (HDL), blood pressure, diabetes, and smoking [30]. Former smokers were considered smokers when calculating the FRS in this study. All patients' 0–5 Risk Scores for CAD were determined, giving one point for existing cardiovascular risk factors. A score of 0 means no risk for CAD, 1 very low risk, 2 moderate risk, 3 increased risk, 4 high risk, and 5 very high risk for CAD. Once CAD was detected or excluded by cardiac catheterization, we calculated FRSs retrospectively using the data from very elderly people over 90 years of age collected from the two hospital charts data, assuming that the examined cardiovascular risk factors in this study existing at the time of detection or exclusion of CAD would also have existed 10 years ago.

CAD has been defined as a chronic disease of the coronary arteries characterized by the manifestation of atherosclerosis with variable coronary artery stenosis, resulting in myocardial ischemia. CAD symptoms are classified as stable angina and ACS. ACS is a collective term for unstable angina, NSTEMI, and STEMI. The main symptom of coronary insufficiency is angina pectoris; it involves localized retrosternal pain triggered by physical and mental stress. Such chest pain may spread to the neck, lower jaw, shoulder, back, left arm to the fingertips, or the upper abdomen. Unstable angina refers to angina pectoris occurring for the first time, as well as a worsening of pain intensity and the duration of episodes.

NSTEMI was described for unstable angina and myocardial infarction with an increase in cardiac enzymes such as high-sensitivity cardiac troponin T without ST-segment elevation on an electrocardiogram. A 12-lead electrocardiogram was used at rest for the temporary recording of the sum of the heart's electrical activity to diagnose STEMI or cardiac arrhythmias in all patients. Typical ST-segmental change in the electrocardiogram for STEMI was considered ST-segment elevation>0.1 mV in at least one derivation. The diagnosis of CAD was made after cardiac catheterization. The quantitative determination of high-sensitivity troponin T in human plasma was measured after sample collection in lithium heparin SARSTEDT Monovette 4.7 ml (orange top) using a standard immunoturbidimetric assay on the COBAS INTEGRA system (the normal value is less than 14 pg/ml) after conservation from cardiac troponin T on September 2, 2010. A second measurement of high-sensitivity troponin T was carried out three hours after the first blood sample.

Prior to this, from January 1, 2004, to September 2, 2010, electrochemiluminescence immunoassay (ECLIA) was performed to determine cardiac troponin T (the normal value is less than 0.01 μg/l) on Elecsys 2010 and cobas e 411 immunoassay analyzers (Roche Diagnostics Ltd., Mannheim, Germany).

The classification of CAD was performed in each case according to the latest edition of the International Classification of Disease (ICD I25.11–I25.13) from 2004 to 2013. Coronary artery disease injuries were categorized as 1-, 2, or 3-vessel. Further, examiners visually estimated the degree of stenosis diameter as a percentage of the cardiac catheter, as per the stenosis morphology classification recommendations of the American College of Cardiology/American Heart Association [31].

We compared the cardiovascular risk factors in accordance with the guidelines of the International Atherosclerosis Society [32], such as arterial hypertension, diabetes mellitus, hypercholesterolemia, hyperlipidemia, obesity, tobacco smoking, and former smoking in very elderly patients over 90 years of age with and without CAD (ICD I25.0–I25.10) after completing cardiac catheterization.

Arterial hypertension was described as a condition in which the blood pressure of the arterial vascular system is chronically elevated. According to the World Health Organization (WHO) [33], hypertension can be diagnosed with a systolic blood pressure of at least 140 mmHg or a diastolic blood pressure of at least 90 mmHg (ICD I10.90). The manifestation of hypertension was described as a known history of hypertension where the patient has been treated with drugs. Blood pressure was measured by the indirect method following Riva-Rocci, 24-hour blood pressure measurement and blood pressure monitors DINAMAP (GE

Medical Systems Information Technologies Ltd., Freiburg, Germany).

Diabetes mellitus (ICD E14.90) was diagnosed as a chronic metabolic disease based on an absolute or relative lack of insulin with elevated blood glucose levels when fasting values were more than 126 mg/dl or when, occasionally, a measured value above 200 mg/dl was detected in the serum of the patients. Blood glucose was determined in the serum of all patients using the SARSTEDT serum Monovette 4.7 ml (brown top) blood collection system with a multifly blood collection needle.

As hypercholesterolemia (ICD E78.0) is considered a lipid metabolic disorder characterized by elevated blood cholesterol levels higher than 200 mg/dl, total cholesterol and HDL (reference range 35–65 mg/dl) were measured after 12 hours of fasting in all patients in the plasma after blood collection in lithium heparin SARSTEDT Monovette 4.7 ml (orange top) with a multifly blood collection needle as an enzymatic colorimetric test using Roche cobas c 701 systems (Roche Diagnostics Ltd., Mannheim, Germany). Hyperlipidemia (ICD E78.2–E78.3) is mainly diagnosed through elevated triglycerides in the blood plasma of patients. The reference range for hypertriglyceridemia has been specified as>200 mg/dl in blood plasma after 12 hours of fasting following blood collection in lithium heparin SARSTEDT Monovette 4.7 ml (orange top) with a multifly blood collection needle as an enzymatic colorimetric test using Roche cobas c 701 systems (Roche Diagnostics Ltd., Mannheim, Germany).

Obesity (ICD E66.99) was defined as the excessive growth of adipose tissue in the body. The transition from overweight to obese was achieved with a body mass index (BMI) of 30. The designation of obese was made by calculating the body weight in kilograms divided by height in meters squared. Nicotine abuse (ICD F17.1) was designated as the abusive consumption of products that contain nicotine, including cigarettes, cigars, and other tobacco products. The study population was categorized into smokers, former smokers, and non-smokers. The quantification of tobacco smoking by measuring packs per year was not considered in this study because the harmful effect of nicotine was not the focus of the research.

We analyzed acute and chronic comorbidities as predisposing factors for the development of CAD in elderly people. In addition, the length of the study and control groups' hospital stays was compared.

Statistical analysis

The data were expressed in proportion, mean, and standard deviation wherever appropriate. We calculated 95% confidence intervals (CIs) for the total number of patients with CAD. Odds ratios were calculated for the presence of cardiovascular risk factors for CAD, sex, and acute and chronic comorbidities. Gender difference was calculated using the chi-square test for two independent standard normal variables of two probabilities. A calculation of the chi-square test for four independent standard normal variables of two probabilities was used to compare the association between cardiovascular risk factors and stable angina, unstable angina, NSTEMI, or STEMI. Fisher's exact test for three variables of two probabilities was calculated for cardiovascular risk factors in different forms of CAD. One-way analysis of variance (ANOVA) for independent samples was performed to compare the duration of hospital stays, BMI, body height, body weight, cholesterol, HDL, and systolic blood pressure between the two groups. The survival rates for both groups were calculated using the Kaplan-Meier method. All tests were expressed as two-tailed, and a P value of <0.05 was considered statistically significant.

Results

In the two hospital databases, we found 126,931 patients who underwent cardiac catheterization at the Department of Internal Medicine, University Hospital of Saarland, and HELIOS Hospital Wuppertal, Witten/Herdecke University Medical Center, Germany, during the study period from 2004 to 2013. A total of 192 (0.15%, mean age 91.45±1.75 years, 97 females [50.52%]; 95% confidence interval [CI], 0.0013–0.0017) patients over 90 years of age with a cardiac catheter met the inclusion criteria for this trial. A total of 175 (91.15%, mean age 91.51±1.80 years, 74 females [42.29%]; 95% confidence interval [CI], 0.87–0.95) patients over 90 years of age had CAD (study group); in 17 patients (8.85%, mean age 90.77±0.88 years, 10 females [58.82%]; 95% CI, 0.05–0.13), CAD was excluded by means of cardiac catheter (control group). We found a higher prevalence of CAD in males, but without increased risk (1.4450 odds ratio; 95% CI, 0.5261–3.9687; P = 0.4752).

FRSs did not differ between very elderly people over 90 years of age compared with and without CAD (P = 0.3792, Table 1). The calculation of Risk Scores 0–5 including one point for each cardiovascular risk factor showed statistical difference only for risk score 3 with statistical difference (P = 0.0244) compared between both study groups (Table 1). A statistical difference was also found in systolic blood pressure with higher levels in the group without CAD with statistical difference (P = 0.465). The levels of cholesterol, HDL, and BMI were statistically no different between the two groups (Table 1). The duration of hospital stays showed no statistical significance between the two groups (Table 1).

Following the results of this study, we identified a five-fold higher cardiovascular risk of developing CAD in patients over 90 years of age with arterial hypertension (P = 0.0035, Table 2). Very elderly diabetics had a three-fold, those with hypercholesterolemia had a one-fold, and very elderly former smokers had a two-fold increased risk of developing CAD, but without a statistically significant difference (Table 2). Neither group was distinguished statistically according to the number of subjects of normal weight, although most of the patients in the study population were not overweight (Table 2).

The largest group in the study group had 3-vessel CAD, followed by 2-vessel CAD, and the small group 1-vessel CAD (Table 3). A comparison of the traditional cardiovascular risk factors with the number of coronary arteries that were afflicted with CAD showed no statistical difference (Table 3).

Only for hypertension did we find a statistically significant difference after comparing the tested traditional cardiovascular risk factors with the clinical manifestation of CAD, such as stable angina or ACS (P<0.0001, Table 4). We also found no statistically significant difference between risk factors and the acute comorbidities in the two groups (Table 5). Cases with a negative outcome were found numerically and exhibited a statistical difference in acute comorbidities such as syncope, falls, and attacks of gout (Table 5). These acute comorbidities showed no increased risk for CAD.

Chronic comorbidities exhibited no increased risk for CAD (Table 6). We found cases with negative outcomes with a statistically significant difference in terms of chronic lumbago and pacemakers. However, chronic lumbago and patients with pacemakers demonstrated no increased risk for CAD (Table 6).

There were six (3.43%, 4 [66.67%] females; 95% CI, 0.0073–0.0613) deaths in the study group and no deaths in the control group (P = 0.4379). Thus, the survival rate was 96.57% (95% CI, 0.94–0.99) in the study group and 100% in the control group.

Table 1. Comparison of demographic data, duration of hospital stay, cholesterol, high sensitivity lipoproteins, systolic blood pressure, Framingham Risk Score, and Risk Score between elderly people over 90 years of age with and without CAD.

	CAD (%)	Without CAD (%)	P value
Number of patients (N = 192)	175 (91.15)	17 (8.85)	
Male	88 (50.29)	7 (41.18)	0.4733
Female	87 (49.71)	10 (58.82)	0.4733
BMI (kg/m^2)	25.59±3.57	25.67±25.65	0.9205
Body height (cm)	166.31±8.85	163.13±8.36	0.1852
Body weight (kg)	70.38±10.61	68.27±11.58	0.4676
Duration of hospital stay (day)	6.02±8.03	6.29±6.21	0.8877
Framingham Score (%)	18.70±9.16	15±8.60	0.3792
Cholesterol (mg/dl)	168.89±42.21	196±27.40	0.1579
HDL (mg/dl)	52.96±20.86	59.6±13.48	0.4854
Systolic blood pressure (mmHg)	140.74±26.08	154.73±23.25	**0.0465**
Risk Score 0	16 (9.14)	3 (17.65)	0.2623
Risk Score 1	40 (22.86)	7 (41.18)	0.0935
Risk Score 2	60 (34.29)	3 (17.65)	0.163
Risk Score 3	41 (23.43)	0	**0.0244**
Risk Score 4	12 (6.86)	1 (5.88)	0.8786
Risk Score 5	6 (3.43)	0	0.4379

Abbreviations: CAD: coronary artery disease; BMI: body mass index; HDL: high sensitivity lipoproteins. **Notes:** Significant *P* values are shown in bold.

Discussion

Past researchers have assumed that the incidence of acute myocardial infarction increases with advancing aging [34,35]. According to the results of this study, after confirmation by cardiac catheterization, the FRS had an insufficient predictive value for CAD in very elderly people over 90 years of age with CAD. In this study, the assessment tool that was used to estimate 10-year risk after having a heart attack considered age, sex, total cholesterol, HDL, systolic blood pressure, smoking status, and whether patients were currently under medication for hypertension. However, age is in and of itself the strongest predictor of CAD.

For this reason, in one study, researchers examined the possibility of the prediction value of a risk factor on the prevalence of CAD to vary over a wide range of ages from middle age to old age [36]. The positive association between hypertension and CAD decreased considerably with age, primarily due to the significantly increased risk of CAD in elderly men without hypertension. The outcomes of total cholesterol on CAD also appeared to decrease with age, although variations were not statistically significant. In contrast, men with diabetes had a dependable two-fold additional risk of CAD transversely across all age groups, while a positive relationship with body mass index in younger men became negative in those who were the oldest. Due to the occasional smoking amongst the elderly, the relationship between smoking and CAD deteriorated with age. The results of this study suggest that changes in risk factor effects on the incidence of CAD with advancing age may require efficient approaches for CAD prevention as people age [35]. The influence of age on the incidence of CAD was not investigated in our study. Overall, the size of the study population in our study over the course of nearly 10 years was small. Therefore, we included the data of two

Table 2. Comparison of traditional risk factors for CAD in very elderly people over 90 years of age with and without CAD.

	Elderly>90 years of age				
Risk factors	**CAD (n = 175) (%)**	**Without CAD (n = 17) (%)**	**Odds ratio**	**95% CI**	**P value**
Hypertension	147 (84)	9 (52.94)	4.6667	1.6584–13.1318	**0.0035**
Diabetes	48 (27.43)	1 (5.88)	6.0472	0.7805–46.8540	0.0849
Hypercholesterolemia	17 (9.71)	1 (5.88)	1.7215	0.2148–13.7984	0.6090
Hyperlipidemia	47 (26.86)	3 (17.65)	1.7135	0.4712–6.2312	0.4136
Obesity	22 (12.57)	3 (17.65)	0.6710	0.1784–2.5236	0.5550
Smoker	6 (3.43)	0	1.3422	0.0725–24.8432	0.8433
Former smoker	14 (8)	0	3.1424	0.1796–54.9851	0.4330

Abbreviations: CAD: coronary artery disease; CI: confidence interval. **Notes:** Significant *P* values are shown in bold.

Table 3. Comparison of traditional cardiovascular risk factors in different forms of coronary artery disease.

	Coronary artery disease			
Risk factors	**1-vessel (n = 26)(%)**	**2-vessel (n = 53)(%)**	**3-vessel (n = 96)(%)**	**P value**
Hypertension	19 (73.08)	45 (84.91)	83 (86.46)	0.2433
Diabetes	4 (15.38)	12 (22.64)	32 (33.33)	0.1320
Hypercholesterolemia	4 (15.38)	5 (9.43)	8 (8.33)	0.5620
Hyperlipidemia	3 (11.54)	14 (26.42)	30 (31.25)	0.1290
Obesity	4 (15.38)	3 (5.66)	15 (15.63)	0.1748
Smoker	1 (3.85)	1 (1.89)	4 (4.17)	0.8601
Former smoker	0	3 (5.66)	11 (11.46)	0.1450

hospitals in this study. This may be due to the patients' biological age, because with increasing age, the population decreases. We found that for patients over 90 years of age, only those with hypertension had a high risk for CAD. Traditional cardiovascular risk factors such as progressing age, diabetes mellitus, hypertension, dyslipidemia, smoking, and obesity are known to have a relationship with CAD [36,37].

Veeranna et al. reported that age and male sex, but not hypertension or dyslipidemia, represented an increased risk for CAD. Only diabetes was an independent predictor of CAD, and smoking was associated with the occlusion of the left main trunk artery of the heart in their study [38]. This was quite different from our outcome, as we found a high risk of CAD in very elderly people with hypertension. Diabetes increased the risk of developing CAD, but without statistical significance, and smoking presented absolutely no increased risk for CAD in our analysis. While the number of male patients with CAD was slightly increased in our study, we could not find a statistically significant difference in sex regarding the risk for CAD.

In one study, researchers examined the influence of advancing age on clinical presentation and hospital reports in a large sample of patients with STEMI [39]. There was a significant converse relationship between age and the probability of presenting with STEMI. For each period of life, the probability of presenting with STEMI decreased. Noticeably fewer elderly patients were frequently treated by cardiologists, they were not examined as thoroughly, and when presenting with STEMI, a smaller number were likely to be treated with cardiac catheterization. Hospital mortality was augmented in the elderly. Fewer elderly patients presented with STEMI but had considerable in-hospital mortality rates; however, they had obviously fewer intensive treatments and investigations [39]. The amount of STEMI was decreased in our study as well. We did not investigate whether the very elderly were treated less often with cardiac catheterization and by cardiologists.

Although several scoring systems have been recommended to compute cardiovascular risk factors, some information has been lacking on significant variables such as family history of CAD or LDL cholesterol. Based on acute coronary events happening within 10 years of follow-up after enrollment into the Prospective Cardiovascular Münster (PROCAM) study [26], the authors of the study developed a Cox proportional hazards model using the following eight independent risk factors for CAD, graded in order of importance: age, LDL cholesterol, smoking, HDL cholesterol, systolic blood pressure, family history of previous myocardial infarction, diabetes mellitus, and triglycerides. They then developed a point scoring system created on the beta-coefficients of this model. The exactness of this point scoring system was similar to coronary event prediction when the continuous variables themselves were used. The scoring system accurately predicted detected coronary events [26]. Similar to this model, we could detect a statistical difference only for risk score 3 in the predictive value of traditional risk factors for CAD for very elderly people in our study

Table 4. Comparison of cardiovascular risk factors with stable angina pectoris and acute coronary syndrome in very elderly people over 90 years of age with CAD.

	Coronary artery disease				
Risk factors	**Stable angina (n = 30)(%)**	**Unstable angina (n = 121)(%)**	**NSTEMI (n = 61)(%)**	**STEMI (n = 47)(%)**	**P value**
Hypertension	30 (100)	99 (81.82)	52 (85.25)	24 (51.06)	**<0.0001**
Diabetes	8 (26.67)	31 (25.62)	17 (27.87)	5 (10.64)	0.1429
Hypercholesterolemia	3(10)	18 (14.88)	9 (14.75)	4 (8.51)	0.6594
Hyperlipidemia	8 (26.67)	30 (24.79)	18 (29.51)	6 (12.77)	0.2186
Obesity	3 (10)	16 (13.22)	9 (14.75)	3 (6.38)	0.5459
Smoker	2 (6.67)	3 (2.48)	2 (3.28)	0	0.3618
Former smoker	3 (10)	10 (8.26)	6 (9.84)	2 (4.26)	0.722

Abbreviations: NSTEMI: non-ST segment elevation myocardial infarction; STEMI: ST segment elevation myocardial infarction. **Notes:** Significant *P* values are shown in bold.

Table 5. Comparison of acute illnesses in patients with and without CAD.

Cardiovascular diseases	**CAD (n = 175) (%)**	**Without CAD (n = 17) (%)**	**Odds ratio**	**95% CI**	**P value**
Acute heart failure	103 (58.86)	9 (52.94)	1.2716	0.4683–3.4526	0.6373
Anemia	8 (4.57)	0	1.7761	0.0983–32.0995	0.6973
Cardiac arrhythmia	62 (35.42)	8 (47.06)	0.6173	0.2267–1.6804	0.3451
Cardiac decompensation	18 (10.29)	3 (17.65)	0.5350	0.1402–2.0412	0.3599
Circulatory collapse	1 (0.57)	0	0.0118	0.0118–7.6681	0.4672
Derailed blood pressure	8 (4.57)	0	1.7761	0.00983–32.0995	0.6973
Shock	4 (2.29)	0	0.9184	0.0475–17.7742	0.9551
Syncope	1 (0.57)	4 (23.53)	0.0187	0.0019–0.1795	**0.0006**
Pulmonary diseases					
Acute respiratory failure	2 (1.14)	1 (5.88)	0.1850	0.0159–2.1532	0.1778
Aspiration pneumonia	1 (0.57)	0	0.3009	0.0118–7.6681	0.4672
Bronchopulmonary infection	3 (1.71)	1 (7.14)	0.2791	0.0274–2.8411	0.2841
Pneumonia	2 (1.14)	0	0.5043	0.0233–10.9290	0.6627
Pulmonary edema	4 (2.89)	0	0.9184	0.0475–17.4442	0.9551
Gastrointestinal diseases					
Duodenal ulcer	1 (0.57)	0	0.3009	0.0118–7.6681	0.4672
Gastritis	2 (1.14)	0	0.5043	0.0233–10.9290	0.6627
Gastrointestinal bleeding	2 (1.14)	0	0.5043	0.0233–10.9290	0.4672
Hyperglycemia	1 (0.57)	0	0.3009	0.0118–7.6681	0.4672
Reflux esophagitis 2 (1.14)	0	0.5043	0.0233–10.9290	0.4672	
Kidney diseases					
Acute kidney injury	3 (1.71)	0	0.7101	0.0352–14.3174	0.8233
Acute urinary tract infection	10 (5.71)	1 (5.88)	0.3009	0.0118–7.6681	0.4672
Macrohematuria	3 (1.71)	0	0.7101	0.0352–14.3174	0.8233
Water-electrolyte imbalance	2 (1.14)	0	0.5043	0.0233–10.9290	0.4672
Thyroid diseases					
Hyperthyroidism	1 (0.57)	0	0.3009	0.0118–7.6681	0.4672
Hypothyroidism	5 (2.86)	0	1.1290	0.0599–21.2845	0.9354
Other conditions					
Acute stroke	1 (0.57)	0	0.3009	0.0118–7.6681	0.4672
Abscess	1 (0.57)	0	0.3009	0.0118–7.6681	0.4672
Dizziness	2 (1.14)	0	0.5043	0.0233–10.9290	0.4672
Fall	0	1 (5.88)	0.0313	0.0012–0.8004	**0.0362**
Attack of gout	0	1 (5.88)	0.0313	0.0012–0.8004	**0.0362**
Delirium	2 (1.14)	1 (5.88)	0.1850	0.0159–2.1532	0.1778

Abbreviations: CAD: coronary artery disease; CI: confidence interval. **Notes:** Significant *P* values are shown in bold.

when we calculated one point for each traditional risk factor, such as hypertension, diabetes, hypercholesterolemia, hyperlipidemia, obesity, and smoking. This risk assessment model was easy to calculate. Apparently, it makes no difference whether the exact numbers of serum lipids or their global viewpoint was used when calculating this risk factor. Because the risk factor of a family history of previous myocardial infarction cannot be influenced, we did not consider this established risk factor of family history for CAD when evaluating the very elderly in our study.

The question of the use of risk assessment for the primary prevention of CAD remains controversial. The validity of the FRS was assessed in a previous study [40]. Comparisons of prediction models and reality in tertiles were performed, and the individual survival functions were calculated. The mean risk for men was increased. Cardiovascular disease events happened in the highest risk tertiles. The negative predictive values in both sexes were noteworthy, and the specificity in women and sensitivity in men were high when their risk for cardiovascular disease was high. This model overestimated the risk in older women and in middle-aged men. The cumulative probability of individual survival by tertiles was significant in both sexes [40]. The results of this study warrant the reclassification of FRS.

Rodondi et al. also reached the conclusion that the FRS miscalculates the risk for CAD in the elderly, mainly in women [27]. They proposed that traditional risk factors best predict CAD. We detected no sex differences in the mean study population in

Table 6. Comparison of chronic comorbidities in elderly people over 90 years of age with and without CAD.

Cardiovascular diseases	CAD (n = 175) (%)	Without CAD (n = 17) (%)	Odds ratio	95% CI	P value
Aneurysm	1 (0.57)	1 (5.88)	0.0920	0.0055–1.5408	0.0970
Cardiomyopathy	4 (2.29)	0	0.9184	0.0475–17.7742	0.9551
Carotid stenosis	3 (1.71)	1 (5.88)	0.2791	0.0274–2.8411	0.2810
Cor pulmonale	9 (5.14)	2 (11.76)	0.4066	0.0804–2.0563	0.2765
Hypertensive heart disease	29 (16.57)	4 (23.53)	0.6455	0.1965–2.1207	0.4708
Pacemaker	20 (11.43)	5 (29.41)	0.3097	0.0988–0.9707	**0.0443**
Peripheral arterial occlusive disease	17 (9.71)	0	3.8644	0.2226–67.0875	0.3533
State after syncope	3 (1.71)	0	0.7101	0.0352–14.3174	0.8233
Cardiac valvular defect	50 (28.57)	8 (47.06)	0.4500	0.1643–1.2322	0.1202
Chronic venous insufficiency	1 (0.57)	0	0.3009	0.0118–7.6681	0.4672
Varicose veins	2 (1.14)	0	0.5043	0.0233–10.9290	0.6627
State after bypass surgery	10 (5.71)	0	2.2205	0.1247–39.5395	0.5871
Pulmonary diseases					
Chronic obstructive pulmonary disease	12 (6.86)	2 (11.76)	0.5521	0.1129–2.7012	0.4639
Emphysema	2 (1.14)	0	0.5043	0.0233–10.9290	0.6627
Obstructive sleep apnea syndrome	1 (0.57)	0	0.3009	0.0118–7.6681	0.4672
State after tuberculosis	2 (1.14)	0	0.5043	0.0233–10.9290	0.6627
Gastrointestinal diseases					
Appendectomy	1 (0.57)	0	0.3009	0.0118–7.6681	0.4672
Cholecystectomy	16 (9.14)	1 (5.88)	1.6101	0.2002–12.9484	0.6543
Colonic diverticula	4 (2.29)	0	0.9184	0.0475–17.7742	0.9551
Gallbladder disease	1 (0.57)	0	0.3009	0.0118–7.6681	0.4672
Gastric carcinoma	6 (3.43)	0	1.3422	0.0725–24.8432	0.8433
Liver cysts	1 (0.57)	0	0.3009	0.0118–7.6681	0.4672
Pancreatic disease	1 (0.57)	0	0.3009	0.0118–7.6681	0.4672
Splenectomy	1 (0.57)	0	0.3009	0.0118–7.6681	0.4672
State after bowel surgery	3 (1.71)	0	0.7101	0.0352–14.3174	0.8233
State after hepatitis	3 (1.71)	0	0.7101	0.0352–14.3174	0.8233
State after hernia operation	4 (2.29)	0	0.9184	0.0475–17.7742	0.9551
State after gastric surgery	4 (2.29)	0	0.9184	0.0475–17.7742	0.9551
Kidney diseases					
Chronic renal failure	45 (25.71)	5 (29.41)	0.8308	0.2774–2.4883	0.7404
Contracted kidney	1 (0.57)	0	0.3009	0.0118–7.6681	0.4672
Diabetic nephropathy	3 (1.71)	0	0.7101	0.0352–14.3174	0.8233
Nephrectomy	3 (1.71)	0	0.7101	0.0352–14.3174	0.8233
Renal adenoma	2 (1.14)	0	0.5043	0.0233–10.9290	0.6627
Renal cysts	5 (2.86)	0	1.1290	0.0599–21.2845	0.9354
State after kidney stones	1 (0.57)	0	0.3009	0.0118–7.6681	0.4672
Diseases of the genitourinary system					
Benign prostate hyperplasia	4 (2.29)	1 (5.88)	0.3743	0.0394–3.5526	0.3920
Hysterectomy	4 (2.29)	0	0.9184	0.0475–17.7742	0.9551
Prostate cancer	3 (1.71)	1 (12.50)	0.2791	0.0274–2.8411	0.2810
Prostatectomy	3 (1.71)	0	0.7101	0.0352–14.3174	0.8233
State after bladder carcinoma	2 (1.14)	0	0.5043	0.0233–10.9290	0.6627
Thyroid diseases					
Struma	2 (1.14)	0	0.5043	0.0233–10.9290	0.6627
Strumectomy	2 (1.14)	1 (5.88)	0.1850	0.0159–2.1532	0.1778
Nervous system disorders					
Chronic lumbago	0	1 (5.88)	0.0313	0.0012–0.8004	**0.0362**

Table 6. Cont.

Cardiovascular diseases	CAD (n = 175) (%)	Without CAD (n = 17) (%)	Odds ratio	95% CI	P value
Disc herniation	2 (1.14)	0	0.5043	0.0233–10.9290	0.6627
Polyneuropathy	4 (2.29)	1 (5.88)	0.3743	0.0394–3.5526	0.3920
Parkinson disease	6 (3.43)	0	1.3422	0.0725–24.8432	0.8433
Restless legs syndrome	3 (1.71)	0	0.7101	0.0352–14.3174	0.8233
Spinal canal stenosis	2 (1.14)	1 (5.88)	0.1850	0.0159–2.1532	0.1778
Status after stroke	12 (6.86)	1 (5.88)	1.1779	0.1437–9.6544	0.8787
Orthopedic disorders					
Osteoarthritis	9 (5.14)	3 (17.65)	0.2530	0.0614–1.0425	0.0571
Osteoporosis	5 (2.86)	1 (5.88)	0.4706	0.0518–4.2786	0.5033
Rheumatism	2 (1.14)	0	0.5043	0.0233–10.9290	0.6627
Psychiatric disorders					
Alzheimer disease	1 (0.57)	0	0.3009	0.0118–7.6681	0.4672
Dementia	4 (2.29)	1 (5.88)	0.3743	0.0394–3.5526	0.3920
Depression	3 (1.71)	0	0.7101	0.0352–14.3174	0.8233
Ear, nose, and throat diseases					
Nasal polypectomy	1 (0.57)	0	0.3009	0.0118–7.6681	0.4672
Tonsillectomy	1 (0.57)	0	0.3009	0.0118–7.6681	0.4672
Skin disorders					
Allergy	1 (0.57)	0	0.3009	0.0118–7.6681	0.4672
Psoriasis	1 (0.57)	0	0.3009	0.0118–7.6681	0.4672
State post-herpes zoster	1 (0.57)	0	0.3009	0.0118–7.6681	0.4672
Ophthalmologic diseases	13 (7.43)	1 (5.88)	1.2840	0.1576–10.4623	0.8154
Gynecological disorders					
Status after breast cancer	3 (1.71)	0	0.7101	0.0352–14.3174	0.8233

Abbreviations: CAD: coronary artery disease; CI: confidence interval. **Notes:** Significant *P* values are shown in bold.

very elderly people over 90 years of age with and without CAD in our study.

In one study, classic risk factors' validity was examined with several new biomarkers in predicting cardiovascular mortality in the very elderly from the general population with no history of CAD [40]. All classic risk factors were comprised in the FRS as well as serum concentrations of the biomarkers homocysteine, folic acid, C reactive protein, and interleukin 6 [40]. Classic risk factors did not forecast cardiovascular mortality when used in the FRS. Of the novel biomarkers investigated, homocysteine had the greatest predictive value. The inclusion of some additional risk factors or a combination of factors into the homocysteine prediction model did not increase its discriminative value. In very elderly people with no history of CAD, only serum levels of homocysteine were able to precisely detect those at high risk of cardiovascular mortality, whereas classic risk factors incorporated into the FRS did not [40]. Further investigations are warranted to confirm these findings.

Other findings have suggested that the FRS and PROCAM should not be carried out to calculate the absolute CAD risk of middle-aged men without any CAD history because of a clear overestimation [41]. In our study, some FRSs overestimated the probability of CAD occurrence, mainly in the very elderly after excluding CAD by cardiac catheterization. In contrast, a small number very elderly people with CAD were underestimated after the calculation of FRSs in our study.

In previous studies, researchers found that risk factors could have supplementary predictive value outside of what the FRS can predict [42]. However, most of the results of the examined studies had mistakes in their design, methods, and descriptions that limit their reliability and validity [42]. While hypertension was treated by medication in the very elderly, our study showed that the risk for CAD was high. While diabetes has been found in nearly over one-quarter of elderly patients with CAD, about one-tenth had hypercholesterolemia in our study, without statistical significance. Neither hyperlipidemia nor obesity was an increased risk factor for CAD in the very elderly patients in our study population. The same result was reported by Kim et al. in relation to the elderly [43]. These results raise questions about the value of weight loss and diet for the prevention of CAD in the elderly.

The effects of smoking on mortality in the elderly population have been studied previously [44]. When comparing the mortality rates for older smokers, ex-smokers, and non-smokers, lower mortality was observed for non-smokers and former smokers than for older smokers [44]. We found more very elderly former smokers and smokers with CAD than non-smokers in our study, but this was not statistically significant.

However, it continues to be difficult to correlate CAD and atherosclerosis. Even when this was evaluated angiographically, the connection has not been well established, and previous studies have reported different and varying outcomes concerning the link between CAD and atherosclerosis [45–47]. The severity of CAD in the elderly seemed to correlate poorly with the prevalence of established traditional cardiovascular risk factors in our study.

There are probably reasons for the different risk profiles for CAD in very elderly people. The assessment and identification of cardiovascular risk factors for CAD in the elderly may be challenging for further investigations.

Study limitations

In this study, the FRS and traditional risk factors for CAD in very elderly people in two departments of internal medicine were examined, but not in very elderly people with CAD in other medical departments. The FRS was calculated after an acute myocardial infarction and preformation of cardiac catheterization to confirm CAD under the assumption that the identified risk factors would have existed 10 years ago. Another limitation was that we were unable to identify very elderly patients with ACS who had not undergone cardiac catheterization for any reason. Moreover, aging itself was considered a risk factor for CAD in previous studies. It is also possible that the risk profiles change over the time among all age groups. The influence of lifestyle and diet in the traditional risk factors were not considered in the very elderly in this study. Therefore, it is difficult to identify the risk profile for CAD in very elderly people. Various causes of the development of CAD have been discussed in the current scientific-medical literature. Most of the very elderly patients had CAD. Therefore, the group of very elderly patients without CAD was small. For this reason, we conducted a two-center study to exclude a statistical error in the limited sample size in the group of very elderly patients without CAD.

Conclusions

We were not able to demonstrate that the FRS has sufficient predictive value in patients over 90 years of age with CAD. In addition, the scoring system with a point for each risk factor for CAD did not have sufficient predictive power for CAD in very elderly people. However, established risk factors such as hypertension, diabetes, hyperlipidemia, obesity, and smoking should be carefully considered in the therapeutic management and prevention of CAD in very elderly people, in addition to treatment for acute and chronic comorbidities.

Author Contributions

Conceived and designed the experiments: YJ. Performed the experiments: YJ. Analyzed the data: YJ. Contributed reagents/materials/analysis tools: YJ. Wrote the paper: YJ.

References

1. Jneid H, Alam M, Virani SS, Bozkurt B (2013) Redefining myocardial infarction: what is new in the ESC/ACCF/AHA/WHF third universal definition of myocardial infarction? Methodist Debakey Cardiovasc J 9: 169–172.
2. Exarchos KP, Exarchos TP, Bourantas CV, Papafaklis MI, Naka KK, et al. (2013) Prediction of coronary atherosclerosis progression using dynamic Bayesian networks. Conf Proc IEEE Eng Med Biol Soc 3889–3892.
3. Schoenhagen P, Tuzcu EM, Apperson-Hansen C, Wang C, Wolski K, et al. (2006) Determinants of arterial wall remodeling during lipid-lowering therapy: serial intravascular ultrasound observations from the Reversal of Atherosclerosis with Aggressive Lipid Lowering Therapy (REVERSAL) trial. Circulation 113: 2826–2834.
4. de Graaf MA, Broersen A, Kitslaar PH, Roos CJ, Dijkstra J, et al. (2013) Automatic quantification and characterization of coronary atherosclerosis with computed tomography coronary angiography: cross-correlation with intravascular ultrasound virtual histology. Int J Cardiovasc Imaging 29: 1177–1190.
5. Priester TC, Litwin SE (2009) Measuring progression of coronary atherosclerosis with computed tomography: searching for clarity among shades of gray. J Cardiovasc Comput Tomogr 3 Suppl 2: S81–90.
6. Martin SS, Abd TT, Jones SR, Michos ED, Blumenthal RS, et al. (2014) American cholesterol treatment guideline: what was done well and what could be done better. J Am Coll Cardio. pii: S0735-1097(14)01579-4.
7. Kavousi M, Leening MJ, Nanchen D, Greenland P, Graham IM, et al. (2014) Comparison of application of the ACC/AHA guidelines, Adult Treatment Panel III guidelines, and European Society of Cardiology guidelines for cardiovascular disease prevention in a European cohort. JAMA 311: 1416–1423.
8. Fihn SD, Gardin JM, Abrams J, Berra K, Blankenship JC, et al. (2012) ACCF/AHA/ACP/AATS/PCNA/SCAI/STS Guideline for the diagnosis and management of patients with stable ischemic heart disease: a report of the American College of Cardiology Foundation/American Heart Association Task Force on Practice Guidelines, and the American College of Physicians, American Association for Thoracic Surgery, Preventive Cardiovascular Nurses Association, Society for Cardiovascular Angiography and Interventions, and Society of Thoracic Surgeons. J AM Coll Cardiol 60: e44–e164.
9. Perk J, De Backer G, Gohlke H, Graham I, Reiner Z, et al. (2012) European guidelines on cardiovascular disease prevention in clinical practice (version 2012). The Fifth Joint Task Force of the European Society of Cardiology and Other Societies on Cardiovascular Disease Prevention in Clinical Practice (constituted by representatives of nine societies and by invited experts). Eur Heart J 33: 1635–1701.
10. Alexander KP, Newby LK, Cannon CP, Armstrong PW, Gibler WB, et al. (2007) Acute coronary care in the elderly, part I: non-ST-segment-elevation acute coronary syndromes: a scientific statement for healthcare professionals from the American Heart Association Council on Clinical Cardiology: in collaboration with the Society of Geriatric Cardiology. Circulation 115: 2549–2569.
11. Lloyd-Jones D, Adams R, Carnethon M, De Simone G, Ferguson TB, et al. (2009) American Heart Association Statistics Committee and Stroke Statistics Subcommittee heart disease and stroke statistics—2009 update. Circulation Jan., 119: 480–486.
12. Third Report of the National Cholesterol Education Program (NCEP) (2002) Expert panel on detection, evaluation, and treatment of high blood cholesterol in adults (Adult Treatment Panel III) final report. Circulation 106: 3143–3421.
13. McPherson R, Frohlich J, Fodor G, Genest J (2006) Canadian Cardiovascular Society position statement: recommendations for the diagnosis and treatment of dyslipidemia and prevention of cardiovascular disease. Can J Cardiol 22: 913–927.
14. Mosca L, Banka CL, Benjamin EJ, Berra K, Bushnell C, et al. (2007) Evidence-based guidelines for cardiovascular disease prevention in women: 2007 update. Circulation 115: 1481–1501.
15. Wood D, De Backer G, Faergeman O, Graham I, Mancia G, et al. (1998) Prevention of coronary heart disease in clinical practice: recommendations of the Second Joint Task Force of European and Other Societies on Coronary Prevention. Atherosclerosis 140: 199–270.
16. Lloyd-Jones DM (2010) Cardiovascular risk prediction, basic concepts, current status, and future directions. Circulation 121: 1768–1777.
17. De Backer G, Ambrosioni E, Borch-Johnsen K, Brotons C, Cifkova R, et al. (2004) European guidelines on cardiovascular disease prevention in clinical practice: Third Joint Task Force of European and Other Societies on Cardiovascular Disease Prevention in Clinical Practice. Atherosclerosis 173: 381–391.
18. Jackson R (2000) Updated New Zealand cardiovascular disease risk-benefit prediction guide. BMJ 320: 709–710.
19. Mahmood SS, Levy D, Vasan RS, Wang TJ (2014) The Framingham Heart Study and the epidemiology of cardiovascular disease: a historical perspective. Lancet 15, 383: 999–1008.
20. Wilson PW, D'Agostino RB, Levy D, Belanger AM, Silbershatz H, et al. (1998) Prediction of coronary heart disease using risk factor categories. Circulation 97: 1837–1847.
21. D'Agostino RB, Grundy SM, Sullivan LM, Wilson P (2001) Validation of the Framingham coronary heart disease prediction scores: results of a multiple ethnic groups investigation. JAMA 286: 180–187.
22. Giampaoli S, Palmieri L, Mattiello A, Panico S (2005) Definition of high risk individuals to optimize strategies for primary prevention of cardiovascular diseases. Nutr Metab Cardiovasc Dis 15: 79–85.
23. NCEP (2001) Executive summary of the third report of the national cholesterol education program (NCEP) expert panel on detection, evaluation, and treatment of high blood cholesterol in adults (Adult Treatment Panel III). JAMA 285: 2486–2497.
24. USPSTF (2008) Aspirin for the prevention of cardiovascular disease: U.S. Preventive Services Task Force recommendation statement. Ann Intern Med 150: 396–404.
25. Conroy RM, Pyorala K, Fitzgerald AP, Sans S, Menotti A, et al. (2003) Estimation of ten-year risk of fatal cardiovascular disease in Europe: the SCORE project. Eur Heart J 24: 987–1003.
26. Assmann G, Cullen P, Schulte H (2002) Simple scoring scheme for calculating the risk of acute coronary events based on the 10-year follow-up of the prospective cardiovascular Munster (PROCAM) study. Circulation 105: 310–315.

27. Rodondi N, Locatelli I, Aujesky D, Bulter J, Vittinghoff E, et al. (2012) Framingham risk score and alternatives for prediction of coronary heart disease in older adults. PLoS One 7: e34287.
28. Psaty BM, Anderson M, Kronmal RA, Tracy RP, Orchard T, et al. (2004) The association between lipid levels and the risks of incident myocardial infarction, stroke, and total mortality: the cardiovascular health study. J Am Geriatr Soc 52: 1639–1647.
29. National Heart, Lung, and Blood Institute (NHLBI) Clinical Practice Guidelines, Cardiovascular Risk Calculator. Available: http://cvdrisk.nhlbi.nih.gov/. Accessed 2014 September 14.
30. National Heart, Lung, and Blood Institute, NHLBI, Estimate of 10-Year for CHD. Available: Nhlbi.nih.gov. Accessed 2014 September 14.
31. Levine GN, Bates ER, Blankenship JC, Bailey SR, Bittl JA, et al. (2011) ACCF/AHA/SCAI guideline for percutaneous coronary intervention: executive summary: a report of the American College of Cardiology Foundation/American Heart Association Task Force on Practice Guidelines and the Society for Cardiovascular Angiography and Interventions. Circulation 124: 2574–2609.
32. Expert Dyslipidemia Panel of the International Atherosclerosis Society Panel member (2014) An international atherosclerosis society position paper: global recommendations for the management of dyslipidemia—full report. J Clin Lipidol 8: 29–60.
33. Whitworth JA (2003) World Health Organization, International Society of Hypertension Writing Group. J Hypertens 21: 1983–1992.
34. Rosengran A, Wallentin L, Gitt AK, Behar S, Battler A, et al. (2004) Sex, age, and clinical presentation of acute coronary syndromes. Eur Heart J 5: 663–670.
35. Abbott RD, Curb JD, Rodriquez BL, Masaki KH, Yano K, et al. (2002) Age-related changes in risk factor effects on the incidence of coronary heart disease. Ann Epidemiol 12: 173–181.
36. Rosamond W, Flegal K, Furie K, Go A, Greenlund K, et al. (2008) Heart disease and stroke statistics—2008 update: a report from the American Heart Association Statistics Committee and Stroke Statistics Subcommittee. Circulation 117: e25–146.
37. Greenland P, Knoll MD, Stamler J, Neaton JD, Dyer AR, et al. (2003) Major risk factors as antecedents of fatal and nonfatal coronary heart disease events. JAMA 290: 891–897.
38. Rosengren A, Wallentin L, Simoons M, Gitt AK, Behar S, et al. (2006) Age, clinical presentation, and outcome of acute coronary syndromes in the Euroheart acute coronary syndrome survey. Eur Heart J 27: 789–795.
39. Artigao-Rodenas LM, Carbayo-Herencia JA, Divisón-Garrote JA, Gil-Guillén VF, Massó-Orozco J, et al. (2013) Framingham risk score for prediction of cardiovascular diseases: a population-based study form southern Europe. PLoS One 8: e73529.
40. de Ruijter W, Westendorp RG, Assendelft WJ, den Elzen WP, de Craen AJ, et al. (2009) Use of Framingham risk score and new biomarkers to predict cardiovascular mortality in older people: population based observational cohort study. BMJ 338: a3083.
41. Empana JP, Ducimetière P, Arveiler D, Ferrières J, Evans A, et al. (2003) Are the Framingham and PROCAM coronary heart disease risk functions applicable to different European populations? The PRIME Study. Eur Heart J 24: 1903–1911.
42. Tzoulaki I, Liberopoulos G, Ioannidis JP (2009) Assessment of claims of improved prediction beyond the Framingham risk score. JAMA 302: 2345–2352.
43. Kim DJ, Bergstrom J, Barrett-Connor E, Laughlin GA (2008) Visceral adiposity and subclinical coronary artery disease in elderly adults: Rancho Bernardo Study. Obesity (Silver Spring) 16: 853–858.
44. Gentleman JF, Brown KS, Forbes WF (1978) Smoking and its effect on mortality of the elderly. Am J Med Sci 276: 173–183.
45. Gehnai AA, al-Mulla AW, Chaikhouni A, Ammar AS, Mahrous F, et al. (2001) Myocardial infarction with normal coronary angiography compared with severe coronary artery disease without myocardial infarction: the crucial role of smoking. J Cardiovasc Risk 8: 1–8.
46. Da Costa A, Isaaz K, Faure E, Mourot S, Cerisier A, et al. (2001) Clinical characteristics, aetiological factors and long-term prognosis of myocardial infarction with an absolutely normal coronary angiogram; a 3-year follow-up study of 91 patients. Eur Heart J 22: 1459–1465.
47. Sun YH, Yang YJ, Pei WD, Wu YJ, Gao RL (2006) Patients with low high-density lipoprotein-cholesterol or smoking are more likely to develop myocardial infarction among subjects with a visible lesion or stenosis in coronary artery. Circ J 70: 1602–1605.

Hyperhomocysteinemia in Patients with Polypoidal Choroidal Vasculopathy

Hui-Chen Cheng[1,2], Jorn-Hon Liu[1,2,3], Shui-Mei Lee[1,2], Po-Kang Lin[1,2,4,5*]

1 Department of Ophthalmology, School of Medicine, National Yang-Ming University, Taipei, Taiwan, **2** Department of Ophthalmology, Taipei Veterans General Hospital, Taipei, Taiwan, **3** Department of Ophthalmology, Cheng Hsin Rehabilitation Medical Center, Taipei, Taiwan, **4** Graduate Institute of Biomedical Electronics and Bioinformatics, National Taiwan University, Taipei, Taiwan, **5** Biomedical Electronics Translational Research Center, National Chiao Tung University, Hsinchu, Taiwan

Abstract

Purpose: To determine whether elevated plasma homocysteine and serum high sensitivity C-reactive protein (hsCRP) levels, two established risk factors of vascular diseases, are associated with polypoidal choroidal vasculopathy (PCV).

Design: Retrospective case-control study.

Methods: One hundred and nineteen consecutive patients with PCV and 119 matched controls were enrolled in a tertiary hospital from September 2008 to June 2013. Plasma homocysteine and serum hsCRP levels were measured. Associations among plasma homocysteine, serum hsCRP levels and PCV were further evaluated using multivariable logistic regression analysis.

Results: The median plasma homocysteine level was significantly higher in patients with PCV than in the controls (12.20 μmol/L vs. 9.80 μmol/L, $p<0.001$). The median serum hsCRP level was slightly higher in the PCV group (0.16 mg/dl vs. 0.11 mg/dl in control group, $p=0.07$). After multivariable logistic regression analysis, each 1 μmol/L increase of plasma homocysteine was associated with a 1.5-fold increase in likelihood of having PCV (OR, 1.54; 95% confidence interval (CI), 1.33–1.79, $p<0.001$).

Conclusions: Hyperhomocysteinemia was associated with PCV and might play a role in the pathogenesis of PCV.

Editor: Alfred S. Lewin, University of Florida, United States of America

Funding: The authors would like to thank the National Science Council of the Republic of China, Taiwan, for supporting this research under Contract No. NSC101-2220-E-010-001. This work was also supported by the "Aim for the Top University Plan" of the National Chiao Tung University and Ministry of Education, Taiwan, R. O. C. The funders had no role in study design, data collection and analysis, decision to publish, or preparation of the manuscript.

Competing Interests: The authors have declared that no competing interests exist.

* Email: pklin123@hotmail.com

Introduction

Polypoidal choroidal vasculopathy (PCV), first proposed by Yannuzzi et al, [1] is characterized by an inner choroidal vascular network ending in an aneurysmal bulge, visible clinically as a reddish orange, polyp-like structure. The affected eye typically presents with multiple recurrent serous or hemorrhagic detachments of the retinal pigment epithelium (RPE) [1,2]. The diagnostic features of PCV are the presence of subretinal nodular hyperfluorescence (the polyps), which may be associated with branching vascular networks in fundus indocyanine green angiography (ICGA) [3]. In earlier reports, PCV accounts for 20–50% of cases manifesting as exudative age-related macular degeneration (AMD) in Asia, compared to approximately 10% in patients of Western descent [2,4–6]. However, PCV has been proposed as a distinct disease entity with its characteristic polypoidal structures and branching vascular networks, which is different from choroidal neovascularization (CNV) of AMD [7]. PCV tends to present at a younger age compared to exudative AMD, with a male preponderance and more frequently in black or Asian patients [1,2,8,9]. Although the pathogenesis of PCV remains largely unknown, there have been several pathological reports that have noted inner choroidal vessel abnormalities with arteriosclerosis in PCV, possibly indicating an association with vascular diseases [10–12].

Homocysteine is a naturally occurring sulfur-containing amino acid that is produced during the metabolism of methionine. High plasma levels of homocysteine have been identified as an independent risk factor of vascular diseases, such as cardiovascular disease and stroke, dementia and Alzheimer's disease [13–15]. Elevated plasma homocysteine levels are also observed in patients with retinal vascular occlusion diseases, pseudoexfoliative glaucoma and diabetic retinopathy [16–19]. Patients with AMD may also present with elevated plasma homocysteine levels but results are inconsistent [20,21].

C-reactive protein (CRP) is a systemic inflammatory biomarker and a risk factor of cardiovascular disease [22]. *Kikuchi et al* [23] found a significant association between elevated high sensitivity

CRP (hsCRP) levels and PCV in the Japanese, and concluded that inflammatory processes were involved in the pathogenesis of PCV. However, further correlations need to be elucidated.

From the clinical manifestations and pathological reports, we propose a hypothesis that PCV is a vascular disorder related to arteriosclerosis, which may be associated with the risk factors of vascular diseases. The purpose of this study is to determine whether elevated plasma homocysteine and serum hsCRP levels, two established risk factors of vascular diseases, are associated with PCV.

Materials and Methods

Study subjects

The authors conducted a case-control study with retrospective recruitment of study subjects from a tertiary hospital between September 2008 and June 2013. The study protocol adhered to the tenets of the Declaration of Helsinki. It was approved by the Institutional Review Board of the Taipei Veterans General Hospital. Though the requirement for informed consent was waived by the approving IRB, verbal informed consent was obtained and recorded on the medical chart.

Patients diagnosed with PCV were recruited consecutively during the study period. The control group included subjects who were undergoing routine physical examinations or follow-up for diseases other than AMD, retinal vascular disease, diabetic retinopathy or glaucoma. Each case was then matched with one control subject on age and gender. All study subjects were of Chinese ethnicity.

Exclusion criteria included subjects without data of plasma homocysteine level, significant comorbidity that could confuse the clinical picture, such as retinal vascular occlusion, uveitis, trauma-related eye disease, other neovascular maculopathies, and media opacities preventing adequate fundus examination. Subjects with renal dysfunction, defined as having a serum creatinine level more than 1.5 mg/dl or having a history of renal failure, and a history of taking vitamin supplements, were also excluded due to their effect on plasma homocysteine [24,25].

All participants received a complete ophthalmic examination consisting of best-corrected visual acuity, slit lamp biomicroscopy and fundoscopy. Fundus photography with fluorescein angiography (FA) taken with a fundus camera (CF-60 UD, Canon Inc., Tokyo, Japan) and ICGA (Heidelberg Retina Angiograph II, Heidelberg Engineering, Heidelberg, Germany) were performed through dilated pupils in all case subjects. The retinal images were all reviewed by two retina specialist (P.K.L. and J.H.L) in a masked fashion. Only subjects with characteristic polyp-like choroidal vessel dilatation (polypoidal lesions or polyps) on ICGA were diagnosed to have PCV [26]. The diagnosis was confirmed when both of them had come to an agreement. Location of PCV was divided into extrafoveal, juxtafoval (within 200 µm of the fovea), subfoveal and peripapillary area (within one disc diameter of the optic disc) [27].

Data including age, gender, lifestyle factors of smoking and alcohol consumption, medication histories, medical histories of hypertension, diabetes mellitus (DM), coronary artery disease, cerebrovascular event and renal dysfunction were obtained from all subjects.

Total plasma homocysteine analysis

Fasting venous blood samples were obtained in the sitting position and collected in test tubes containing heparin. The samples were immediately centrifuged at 4°C, and the plasma homocysteine levels were measured by automated chemiluminescent immunoassay (ADVIA Centaur system, Siemens, East Walpole, MA, USA), with a sensitivity of 0.5 µmol/L and a total coefficient of variation (CV) of 6.8% at 4.9 µmol/L, 3.9% at 61.6 µmol/L. This assay correlates well with other assays, including fluorescent polarization immunoassay and high-performance liquid chromatography (HPLC) [28].

High sensitivity C-reactive protein (hsCRP) analysis

Venous blood samples were obtained and collected in serum-separation tubes. Serum hsCRP was measured by rate nephelometry on an automated nephelometer (Immage 800, Beckman Coulter, Fullerton, CA, USA). This hsCRP assay, with an analytical sensitivity of 0.2 mg/L and a total coefficient of variation (CV) of 5.17% at 0.79 mg/L, and 3.8% at 13.4 mg/L, has been shown to correlate well with other commonly used assays [29].

Hyperhomocysteinemia and elevated hsCRP level were defined as levels above the 95th percentile of the control group.

Statistical analysis

Continuous and categorical variables in demographic and medical characteristics were compared between PCV cases and control subjects using Student's *t*-test and Pearson's chi-square test, respectively. Plasma homocysteine and serum hsCRP levels were presented as median (interquartile range) and compared to controls using the Mann-Whitney U test because homocysteine and hsCRP levels were not normally distributed.

Multivariable logistic regression models were used to evaluate whether or not PCV was associated with plasma homocysteine or serum hsCRP. All odds ratios (ORs) were adjusted for age, gender, lifestyle factors (smoking and alcohol consumption) and medical histories (hypertension, DM, coronary artery disease, cerebrovascular event).

SPSS for Windows version 18 (SPSS Inc, Chicago, Illinois, USA) was used for these calculations. All reported P values were based on 2-sided tests and a P value of less than 0.05 was considered to be statistically significant.

Results

One hundred and twenty-four case subjects were enrolled initially. Three patients were excluded due to renal dysfunction and two were excluded due to revised diagnosis of CNV with AMD. Finally, a total of 119 patients with PCV and 119 matched controls were enrolled in this study.

The mean age was 72.1±13.0 years in the PCV group and 69.3±10.9 years in the control group, with a male preponderance (74.8%) in both groups. There were no statistically significant differences in age, gender, medical histories of hypertension, DM, coronary artery disease, cerebrovascular event and lifestyle factors including smoking and alcohol consumption between case subjects and controls (Table 1).

The median plasma homocysteine level was significantly higher in the PCV group (median, 12.20 µmol/L; interquartile range, 9.67–16.66 µmol/L) than in the control group (median, 9.80 µmol/L; interquartile range, 8.13–11.26 µmol/L; $p<0.001$). The homocysteine evaluation can be further categorized into subgroup with DM and without DM. The plasma homocsyteine level of PCV patients with DM was significantly higher than controls with DM ($p = 0.001$). Also, the plasma homocsyteine level of PCV patients without DM was significantly higher than controls without DM ($p<0.001$). The median serum hsCRP level was slightly higher in the PCV group (median, 0.16 mg/dl; interquartile range, 0.06–0.30 mg/dl) than in the control group

Table 1. Basic characteristics of patients with polypoidal choroidal vasculopathy and the control subjects.

	PCV (n = 119)	Control (n = 119)	P value
Age (years)	72.1±13.0 (36.0–93.0)	69.3±10.9 (36.0–94.0)	0.07
Gender (% male)	89 (74.8%)	89 (74.8%)	1.00
Medical history			
Hypertension	56 (47.1%)	54 (45.4%)	0.80
Diabetes mellitus	26 (21.8%)	28 (23.5%)	0.76
Coronary artery disease	21 (17.6%)	19 (16.0%)	0.73
Cerebrovascular event	5 (4.2%)	3 (2.5%)	0.47
Lifestyle determinants			
Smoking (current/former)	8 (6.7%)	4 (3.4%)	0.24
Alcohol consumption	2 (1.7%)	0 (0%)	0.16

PCV, polypoidal choroidal vasculopathy;
Continuous variables are presented as mean ± standard deviation (range) and compared using Student's *t*-test.
Categorical variables were presented as numbers (percentage) and compared using Pearson's chi-square test.

(median, 0.11 mg/dl; interquartile range, 0.06–0.25 mg/dl, p = 0.07) (Table 2).

The 95th percentile of the homocysteine level in the control group was 13.26 μmol/L. Of the 119 PCV patients, 47 (39.5%) patients exceeded this cutoff value, compared with 5 of 119 (4.2%) patients in the control group (p<0.001). The 95th percentile of the hsCRP level in the control group was 0.70 mg/dl. In the PCV group, 13 of 118 (11.1%) patients exceeded the cutoff value, compared with 6 of 113 (5.4%) patients in the control group (p = 0.12) (Table S1).

After stratified by genders, both males and females of the PCV group had significantly higher plasma homocysteine levels (p< 0.001 in male and p = 0.02 in female) and proportions of hyperhomocysteinemia (p<0.001 in male and p = 0.02 in female), compared to those of the controls. The results of hsCRP levels were generally insignificant except for the higher proportions of elevated hsCRP in female (26.7% vs 3.4% in controls, p = 0.01) (Table 2 and Table S1). If we stratified the homocysteine levels into tertiles, significantly higher proportion of PCV patients had homocysteine levels in the highest tertile, compared to controls (67.2% vs. 32.8% in controls, p<0.001) (Table 3).

In the multivariable logistic regression analysis, after adjusting for age, gender, hypertension, DM, coronary artery disease, cerebrovascular event, smoking and alcohol consumption, it was observed that elevated plasma homocysteine levels were significantly associated with an increasing risk of PCV (OR, 1.54; 95% confidence interval (CI), 1.33–1.79, p<0.001), but not the hsCRP (OR, 1.82; 95% CI 0.61–5.45, p = 0.29). If we defined hyperhomocysteinemia and elevated hsCRP as levels above the 95th percentile of the control group, hyperhomocysteinemia is still significantly associated with PCV (OR, 22.04; 95% CI 7.05–68.92, p<0.001) in the multivariable logistic regression analysis, but not with the elevated hsCRP (OR, 2.45; 95% CI 0.75–7.94, p = 0.14). Moreover, people in the highest tertile of homocysteine had an approximately 9-fold increased risk of PCV (OR, 8.84; 95% CI 3.68–21.21, p<0.001) in the regression model (Table 3).

Of the 119 PCV patients, 17 (14.3%) had bilateral involvement, 49 (41.2%) had right-side involvement and 53 (44.5%) had left-side involvement. Comparing the bilateral involvement with unilateral involvement of PCV, no statistically significant differences in plasma homocysteine levels, serum hsCRP levels, age, gender, lifestyle factors, or medical histories were noted between the two groups.

Of the 136 eyes with PCV, PCV lesions were found in the extrafoveal area in 74 (54.4%) eyes, juxtafoveal in 51 (37.5%) eyes, subfoveal in 9 (6.6%) eyes and peripapillary in 2 (1.5%) eyes. Branching vascular network was noted in 130 (95.6%) eyes. Eighty-one (59.6%) eyes had serous pigment epithelial detachment (PED), 16 (11.8%) eyes had hemorrhagic PED, 51 (37.5%) eyes had subretinal fluid and 20 (14.7%) eyes had subretinal hemorrhage.

Discussion

In our study, total plasma homocysteine levels were significantly higher in the PCV group than in the control group (median, 12.20 μmol/L vs 9.80 μmol/L in controls, p<0.001). On a multivariable logistic regression analysis, each 1 μmol/L increase of plasma homocysteine was associated with a 1.5-fold increase in the likelihood of having PCV (OR, 1.54; 95% CI, 1.33–1.79, p< 0.001). Hyperhomocysteinemia, defined as levels above the 95th percentile of the control group, remained a relevant factor for PCV after regression analysis (OR, 22.04; 95% CI 7.05–68.92, p< 0.001). The increase in risk was also significant for the highest tertile of homocysteine for PCV (OR, 8.84; 95% CI 3.68–21.21, p<0.001). Hyperhomocysteinemia was identified to be associated with PCV in this study. However, whether the plasma homocysteine contributes to direct toxicity on the pathogenesis of PCV or acts as a disease marker needs to be further determined.

The pathogenesis of PCV remains largely unknown. Possible association with systemic cardiovascular risk factors, such as hypertension, has been proposed [30]. The histopathology studies of PCV also showed inner choroidal vessel abnormalities with arteriosclerosis change [10–12,31]. A significant proportion of PCV patients in our study had hypertension or coronary artery disease (47.1% and 17.6%, respectively), provided additional evidence of the association between PCV and arteriosclerosis. Homocysteine is a potent excitatory neurotransmitter that binds to the N-methyl-D-aspartate (NMDA) receptor and leads to oxidative stress, cytoplasmic calcium influx, cellular apoptosis, and endothelial dysfunction, which contributes to atherogenesis [32]. Given the observation that PCV was a choroidal vessel abnormality with arteriosclerosis change, the toxic effect of hyperhomocysteinemia on vessel may contribute to the pathogenesis of PCV.

Table 2. Plasma homocysteine and serum C-reactive protein levels in overall and different genders of patients with polypoidal choroidal vasculopathy and the control subjects.

	Overall			Male			Female		
	PCV (n = 119)	Control (n = 119)	P value	PCV (n = 89)	Control (n = 89)	P value	PCV (n = 30)	Control (n = 30)	P value
Homocysteine (μmol/L)	12.20 (9.67–16.66)	9.80 (8.13–11.26)	<0.001	13.91 (11.43–17.65)	10.48 (8.86–11.91)	<0.001	9.29 (7.70–11.11)	8.18 (7.31–9.00)	0.02
hsCRP (mg/dl)[a]	0.16 (0.06–0.30)	0.11 (0.06–0.25)	0.07	0.17 (0.06–0.30)	0.11 (0.06–0.24)	0.14	0.15 (0.06–0.42)	0.09 (0.06–0.26)	0.22

hsCRP, high sensitivity C-reactive protein; PCV, polypoidal choroidal vasculopathy
Continuous variables are presented as median (interquartile range) and compared using the Mann-Whitney U test.
[a]Only 117 patients of PCV and 112 control subjects received examination of the serum hsCRP level.

Kondo et al [33] identify the elastin gene, a potent and specific regulator of the migration and proliferation of vascular smooth muscle cells, is a susceptible gene for PCV. The dysfunction of this signaling may lead to the development of vascular diseases such as arteriosclerosis [34]. The disruption of vascular elastin has also been proven to lead to aneurysm formation on animal model [35]. We proposed that elastin gene variation, which may be associated with the loss of function of vascular smooth muscle cells and the elastic layer of the vessel walls, together with homocysteine-mediated oxidative stress and endothelial dysfunction, and intraluminal pressure dysregulation, may lead to the final endpoint of choroidal aneurysmal bulging in PCV.

After stratified by gender, the plasma homocysteine level was found to be significantly different between male and female in our study (median, 13.91 umol/L in male with PCV vs. 9.29 umol/L in female with PCV, $p<0.001$). The trend was similar in both case and control subjects. After puberty, males have higher plasma homocysteine levels than females, with a gender difference in plasma homocysteine of approximately 2 μmol/L [24]. The male-female difference has been attributed to sex differences in muscle mass, circulating sex hormones, and it may possibly modify the contribution of the methylenetetrahydrofolate reductase (MTHFR) mutation to homocysteine concentrations [36]. In our study, there were only 30 females in the PCV group, and they had a significantly lower rate of coronary artery disease compared to the males (3.3% in female vs. 22.5% in male $p = 0.02$). This may suggest different contributions to the pathogenesis in females with PCV, but further study is required given the small female sample size in this study.

Kikuchi et al [23] have found a significantly increasing risk for the highest quartile of hsCRP for PCV in Japanese. However, we found no significant difference in serum hsCRP levels between the PCV and control groups in our study. Although a higher proportion of elevated hsCRP seemed to be observed in females with PCV ($p = 0.01$), the small sample size precluded further analysis. From a previous report, focal aggregates of chronic inflammatory cells have been shown in the PCV specimens [37]. The discrepancy in the study results of hsCRP in PCV may suggest the role of chronic inflammation in the pathogenesis of PCV.

There were some limitations in this study. First, it was a retrospective case-control study in a single medical center. Second, MTHFR polymorphism, serum cobalamin and folate levels were not checked, which might influence plasma homocysteine levels [24]. However, the subjects in this study were all well-nourished and people who had history of taking vitamin supplements were excluded to prevent their effect on plasma homocysteine levels. Third, the median plasma homocysteine level (12.20 μmol/L) in the PCV group was within the conventional definition of normal range (<15 μmol/L). However, plasma homocysteine level may be affected by many factors including age, gender, ethnicity, nutritional status, lifestyle, and disease [24]. Reference intervals should be established for different populations or even different laboratories [24]. Considering the relative small sample size and heterogeneous characteristics in this study, the reference upper-limit was calculated as level above the 95th percentile for presumed healthy individuals. If we used conventional definition of hyperhomocysteinemia (>15 μmol/L), 40 (33.6%) PCV patients still had elevated plasma homocysteine level, compared to 1 subject (0.8%) in the control group ($p<0.001$). The association still existed in the male group (43.8% in PCV vs 1.1% in controls, $p<0.001$) but not in the female group (3.3% in PCV vs 0% in controls, $p = 0.31$). After adjusting for age, gender, hypertension, DM, coronary artery disease, cerebrovascular event, smoking and

Table 3. Distribution of polypoidal choroidal vasculopathy cases and controls within tertiles of homocysteine and C-reactive protein levels.

	PCV (n = 119)	Control (n = 119)	Multivariable-adjusted OR (95% CI)[a]	P value
Tertile of homocysteine (μmol/L)				
1 (≤8.62)	16 (13.5%)	40 (33.6%)	1.00 (reference)	
2 (>8.62–10.81)	23 (19.3%)	40 (33.6%)	1.99 (0.83–4.77)	0.12
3 (>10.81)	80 (67.2%)	39 (32.8%)	8.84 (3.68–21.21)	<0.001
Tertile of hsCRP (mg/dl)[b]				
1 (<0.07)	34 (29.1%)	38 (33.9%)	1.00 (reference)	
2 (0.07–<0.17)	26 (22.2%)	36 (32.2%)	0.77 (0.38–1.55)	0.46
3 (≥0.17)	57 (48.7%)	38 (33.9%)	1.72 (0.91–3.24)	0.10

CI, confidence interval; hsCRP, high sensitivity C-reactive protein; OR, odds ratio; PCV, polypoidal choroidal vasculopathy
Categorical variables were presented as numbers (percentage).
[a]Adjusted for age, gender, hypertension, diabetes mellitus, coronary artery disease, cerebrovascular event, smoking and alcohol consumption.
[b]Only 117 patients of PCV and 112 control subjects received examination of the serum hsCRP level.

alcohol consumption, conventional hyperhomocysteinemia (> 15 μmol/L) is still significantly associated with PCV (OR, 64.55; 95% CI 9.79–567.73, p<0.001) in the multivariable logistic regression analysis.

In conclusion, our study showed hyperhomocysteinemia was significantly associated with PCV. The results also supported PCV might be related to arteriosclerosis. Further prospective controlled trials with large sample sizes are needed to improve our understanding of the role of hyperhomocysteinemia in PCV.

Supporting Information

Table S1 Proportions of hyperhomocysteinemia and elevated C-reactive protein levels in overall patients and different genders of patients with polypoidal choroidal vasculopathy and the control subjects.

Acknowledgments

The authors thank Ling-Chen Tai (Biostatistics Task Force and Division of General Surgery, Department of Surgery, Taipei-Veterans General Hospital) for help with statistical analysis.

Author Contributions

Conceived and designed the experiments: HCC JHL SML PKL. Performed the experiments: HCC JHL SML PKL. Analyzed the data: HCC JHL SML PKL. Contributed reagents/materials/analysis tools: HCC JHL SML PKL. Wrote the paper: HCC JHL SML PKL.

References

1. Yannuzzi LA, Sorenson J, Spaide RF, Lipson B (1990) Idiopathic polypoidal choroidal vasculopathy (IPCV). Retina 10: 1–8.
2. Yannuzzi LA, Wong DW, Sforzolini BS, Goldbaum M, Tang KC, et al. (1999) Polypoidal choroidal vasculopathy and neovascularized age-related macular degeneration. Arch Ophthalmol 117: 1503–1510.
3. Spaide RF, Yannuzzi LA, Slakter JS, Sorenson J, Orlach DA (1995) Indocyanine green videoangiography of idiopathic polypoidal choroidal vasculopathy. Retina 15: 100–110.
4. Liu Y, Wen F, Huang S, Luo G, Yan H, et al. (2007) Subtype lesions of neovascular age-related macular degeneration in Chinese patients. Graefes Arch Clin Exp Ophthalmol 245: 1441–1445.
5. Scassellati-Sforzolini B, Mariotti C, Bryan R, Yannuzzi LA, Giuliani M, et al. (2001) Polypoidal choroidal vasculopathy in Italy. Retina 21: 121–125.
6. Maruko I, Iida T, Saito M, Nagayama D, Saito K (2007) Clinical characteristics of exudative age-related macular degeneration in Japanese patients. Am J Ophthalmol 144: 15–22.
7. Ciardella AP, Donsoff IM, Yannuzzi LA (2002) Polypoidal choroidal vasculopathy. Ophthalmol Clin North Am 15: 537–554.
8. Sho K, Takahashi K, Yamada H, Wada M, Nagai Y, et al. (2003) Polypoidal choroidal vasculopathy: incidence, demographic features, and clinical characteristics. Arch Ophthalmol 121: 1392–1396.
9. Laude A, Cackett PD, Vithana EN, Yeo IY, Wong D, et al. (2010) Polypoidal choroidal vasculopathy and neovascular age-related macular degeneration: same or different disease? Prog Retin Eye Res 29: 19–29.
10. Okubo A, Sameshima M, Uemura A, Kanda S, Ohba N (2002) Clinicopathological correlation of polypoidal choroidal vasculopathy revealed by ultrastructural study. Br J Ophthalmol 86: 1093–1098.
11. Kuroiwa S, Tateiwa H, Hisatomi T, Ishibashi T, Yoshimura N (2004) Pathological features of surgically excised polypoidal choroidal vasculopathy membranes. Clin Experiment Ophthalmol 32: 297–302.
12. Nakashizuka H, Mitsumata M, Okisaka S, Shimada H, Kawamura A, et al. (2008) Clinicopathologic findings in polypoidal choroidal vasculopathy. Invest Ophthalmol Vis Sci 49: 4729–4737.
13. Clarke R, Daly L, Robinson K, Naughten E, Cahalane S, et al. (1991) Hyperhomocysteinemia: an independent risk factor for vascular disease. N Engl J Med 324: 1149–1155.
14. (2002) Homocysteine and risk of ischemic heart disease and stroke: a meta-analysis. JAMA 288: 2015–2022.
15. Seshadri S, Beiser A, Selhub J, Jacques PF, Rosenberg IH, et al. (2002) Plasma homocysteine as a risk factor for dementia and Alzheimer's disease. N Engl J Med 346: 476–483.
16. Cahill MT, Stinnett SS, Fekrat S (2003) Meta-analysis of plasma homocysteine, serum folate, serum vitamin B(12), and thermolabile MTHFR genotype as risk factors for retinal vascular occlusive disease. Am J Ophthalmol 136: 1136–1150.
17. Aydemir O, Turkcuoglu P, Guler M, Celiker U, Ustundag B, et al. (2008) Plasma and vitreous homocysteine concentrations in patients with proliferative diabetic retinopathy. Retina 28: 741–743.
18. McGimpsey SJ, Woodside JV, Cardwell C, Cahill M, Chakravarthy U (2009) Homocysteine, methylenetetrahydrofolate reductase C677T polymorphism, and risk of retinal vein occlusion: a meta-analysis. Ophthalmology 116: 1778–1787 e1771.
19. Turgut B, Kaya M, Arslan S, Demir T, Guler M, et al. (2010) Levels of circulating homocysteine, vitamin B6, vitamin B12, and folate in different types of open-angle glaucoma. Clin Interv Aging 5: 133–139.
20. Wu KH, Tan AG, Rochtchina E, Favaloro EJ, Williams A, et al. (2007) Circulating inflammatory markers and hemostatic factors in age-related maculopathy: a population-based case-control study. Invest Ophthalmol Vis Sci 48: 1983–1988.
21. Rochtchina E, Wang JJ, Flood VM, Mitchell P (2007) Elevated serum homocysteine, low serum vitamin B12, folate, and age-related macular degeneration: the Blue Mountains Eye Study. Am J Ophthalmol 143: 344–346.
22. Ridker PM (2001) High-sensitivity C-reactive protein: potential adjunct for global risk assessment in the primary prevention of cardiovascular disease. Circulation 103: 1813–1818.
23. Kikuchi M, Nakamura M, Ishikawa K, Suzuki T, Nishihara H, et al. (2007) Elevated C-reactive protein levels in patients with polypoidal choroidal

vasculopathy and patients with neovascular age-related macular degeneration. Ophthalmology 114: 1722–1727.
24. Refsum H, Smith AD, Ueland PM, Nexo E, Clarke R, et al. (2004) Facts and recommendations about total homocysteine determinations: an expert opinion. Clin Chem 50: 3–32.
25. (2005) Dose-dependent effects of folic acid on blood concentrations of homocysteine: a meta-analysis of the randomized trials. Am J Clin Nutr 82: 806–812.
26. (2005) [Criteria for diagnosis of polypoidal choroidal vasculopathy]. Nippon Ganka Gakkai Zasshi 109: 417–427.
27. Cackett P, Wong D, Yeo I (2009) A classification system for polypoidal choroidal vasculopathy. Retina 29: 187–191.
28. Tewari PC, Zhang B, Bluestein BI (2004) Analytical and clinical evaluation of the Bayer ADVIA Centaur homocysteine assay. Clin Chim Acta 342: 171–178.
29. Ng MK, Liu PY, Williams AJ, Nakhla S, Ly LP, et al. (2002) Prospective study of effect of androgens on serum inflammatory markers in men. Arterioscler Thromb Vasc Biol 22: 1136–1141.
30. Ross RD, Gitter KA, Cohen G, Schomaker KS (1996) Idiopathic polypoidal choroidal vasculopathy associated with retinal arterial macroaneurysm and hypertensive retinopathy. Retina 16: 105–111.
31. Nakajima M, Yuzawa M, Shimada H, Mori R (2004) Correlation between indocyanine green angiographic findings and histopathology of polypoidal choroidal vasculopathy. Jpn J Ophthalmol 48: 249–255.
32. McCully KS (2009) Chemical pathology of homocysteine. IV. Excitotoxicity, oxidative stress, endothelial dysfunction, and inflammation. Ann Clin Lab Sci 39: 219–232.
33. Kondo N, Honda S, Ishibashi K, Tsukahara Y, Negi A (2008) Elastin gene polymorphisms in neovascular age-related macular degeneration and polypoidal choroidal vasculopathy. Invest Ophthalmol Vis Sci 49: 1101–1105.
34. Karnik SK, Brooke BS, Bayes-Genis A, Sorensen L, Wythe JD, et al. (2003) A critical role for elastin signaling in vascular morphogenesis and disease. Development 130: 411–423.
35. Hoh BL, Rabinov JD, Pryor JC, Ogilvy CS (2004) A modified technique for using elastase to create saccular aneurysms in animals that histologically and hemodynamically resemble aneurysms in human. Acta Neurochir (Wien) 146: 705–711.
36. Russo GT, Friso S, Jacques PF, Rogers G, Cucinotta D, et al. (2003) Age and gender affect the relation between methylenetetrahydrofolate reductase C677T genotype and fasting plasma homocysteine concentrations in the Framingham Offspring Study Cohort. J Nutr 133: 3416–3421.
37. Rosa RH, Jr., Davis JL, Eifrig CW (2002) Clinicopathologic reports, case reports, and small case series: clinicopathologic correlation of idiopathic polypoidal choroidal vasculopathy. Arch Ophthalmol 120: 502–508.

Effects of Cytochrome P450 2C19 and Paraoxonase 1 Polymorphisms on Antiplatelet Response to Clopidogrel Therapy in Patients with Coronary Artery Disease

Damrus Tresukosol[1], Bhoom Suktitipat[2,3], Saowalak Hunnangkul[4], Ruttakarn Kamkaew[2], Saiphon Poldee[2], Boonrat Tassaneetrithep[4], Atip Likidlilid[2]*

1 Division of Cardiology, Department of Internal Medicine, Faculty of Medicine, Siriraj Hospital, Mahidol University, Siriraj, Bangkoknoi, Bangkok, Thailand, **2** Department of Biochemistry, Faculty of Medicine, Siriraj Hospital, Mahidol University, Siriraj, Bangkoknoi, Bangkok, Thailand, **3** Integrative Computation BioScience Center (ICBS), Mahidol University, Salaya, Nakhon Prathom, Thailand, **4** Department of Health Research and Development, Faculty of Medicine, Siriraj Hospital, Mahidol University, Siriraj, Bangkoknoi, Bangkok, Thailand

Abstract

Clopidogrel is an antiplatelet prodrug that is recommended to reduce the risk of recurrent thrombosis in coronary artery disease (CAD) patients. Paraoxonase 1 (PON1) is suggested to be a rate-limiting enzyme in the conversion of 2-oxo-clopidogrel to active thiol metabolite with inconsistent results. Here, we sought to determine the associations of *CYP2C19* and *PON1* gene polymorphisms with clopidogrel response and their role in ADP-induced platelet aggregation. Clopidogrel response and platelet aggregation were determined using Multiplate aggregometer in 211 patients with established CAD who received 75 mg clopidogrel and 75–325 mg aspirin daily for at least 14 days. Polymorphisms in *CYP2C19* and *PON1* were genotyped and tested for association with clopidogrel resistance. Linkage disequilibrium (LD) and their epistatic interaction effects on ADP-induced platelet aggregation were analysed. The prevalence of clopidogrel resistance in this population was approximately 33.2% (n = 70). The frequencies of *CYP2C19**2 and *3 were significantly higher in non-responder than those in responders. After adjusting for established risk factors, *CYP2C19**2 and *3 alleles independently increased the risk of clopidogrel resistance with adjusted ORs 2.94 (95%CI, 1.65–5.26; $p<0.001$) and 11.26 (95%CI, 2.47–51.41; $p=0.002$, respectively). Patients with *2 or *3 allele and combined with smoking, diabetes and increased platelet count had markedly increased risk of clopidogrel resistance. No association was observed between *PON1* Q192R and clopidogrel resistance (adjusted OR = 1.13, 95%CI, 0.70–1.82; $p=0.622$). Significantly higher platelet aggregation values were found in *CYP2C19**2 and *3 patients when compared with *1/*1 allele carriers ($p=1.98\times10^{-6}$). For *PON1* Q192R genotypes, aggregation values were similar across all genotype groups ($p=0.359$). There was no evidence of gene-gene interaction or LD between *CYP2C19* and *PON1* polymorphisms on ADP-induced platelet aggregation. Our findings indicated that only *CYP2C19**2 and *3 alleles had an influence on clopidogrel resistance. The risk of clopidogrel resistance increased further with smoking, diabetes, and increased platelet count.

Editor: Carmine Pizzi, University of Bologna, Italy

Funding: This study was partly supported by Graduate Thesis Scholarship grant from Faculty of Medicine Siriraj Hospital, Mahidol University to RK. AL and BS were supported by "Chalermphrakiat" grant, Faculty of Medicine Siriraj Hospital, Mahidol University. The funders had no role in study design, data collection and analysis, decision to publish, or preparation of the manuscript.

Competing Interests: The authors have declared that no competing interests exist.

* Email: atip.lik@mahidol.ac.th

Introduction

Acute coronary syndromes (ACS), the leading cause of sudden death worldwide, including Thailand [1], occurs as a result of platelet aggregation (thrombosis) within the human artery. Clopidogrel and aspirin are dual antiplatelet therapy that inhibit platelet function, preventing ischemic events and improving outcomes following ACS and percutaneous coronary intervention (PCI) with stent implantation [2]. Clopidogrel is a thienopyridine prodrug that requires enzymatic biotransformation into the active thiol metabolite to inhibit platelet ADP P2Y12 receptor. Aspirin (acetylsalicylic acid) is a cyclooxygenase-1 (COX-1) inhibitor, thereby preventing the production of thromboxane A_2, which plays a prominent role in platelet aggregation. Due to the different pathways that clopidogrel and aspirin inhibit platelet aggregation, combined antiplatelet therapy provides additive benefit compared with either agent alone and is considered as a therapy of choice for preventing thrombosis in patients undergoing coronary stenting [3]. However, inter-individual variability in the response to clopidogrel is multifactorial and can be influenced by environmental, clinical, and genetic factors [4–6]. Many investigations have indicated that 4% to 44% of patients fail to attain platelet inhibition after clopidogrel therapy [7–12]. Recent studies have confirmed that *in vivo* bioactivation of clopidogrel is a two-step process which is closely linked to the cytochrome P450 (CYP) 2C19 enzyme [13]. The common genetic variants within the CYP2C19 gene, the loss-of-function hepatic CYP2C19*2 (rs4244285) and *3 (rs4986893) polymorphisms were found to be dominantly associated with a lower clopidogrel responsiveness [14–16] and a higher risk of adverse cardiac events such as the occurrence of stent thrombosis and recurrent myocardial infarction [17–19].

Recently, Bouman et al [20] reported that clopidogrel metabolism involved in two steps of bioactivation. First, clopidogrel undergoes oxidation to 2-oxo-clopidogrel by hepatic CYP450 enzyme. Then, in the second step, PON1 and PON3, the paraoxonases synthesized in the liver associated with HDL, play a crucial role in clopidogrel biotransformation to convert clopidogrel to its thiol active metabolite. Contrary to the prior observations, Bouman identified PON1 Q192R (rs662) as a single key factor for the bioactivation and clinical response of clopidogrel, and found no evidence for CYP2C19 involvement in this step of clopidogrel activation. Specifically, carriers of the QQ genotype were found to have a significantly higher risk of stent thrombosis after PCI as compared with individual with QR or RR genotype with an odds ratio (OR) of 3.3 (95% CI, 1.6–7.9; $p = 0.003$). However, other investigators had found no association between PON1 Q192R genotype and platelet response to clopidogrel in either Caucasian populations or populations with mixed racial background [21–23]. This may be due to the lower enzymatic activity of Q allele in a dose dependent manner (QQ<QR<RR) [24,25]. Additionally, PON1 also contains the antioxidant property by breaking down biologically active oxidized phospholipids and oxidized cholesteryl esters [26], thereby preventing oxidation of HDL and LDL. Therefore, PON1 has been proposed as an atherosclerotic susceptibility gene. Many studies have reported the association between PON1 Q192R polymorphism and coronary artery disease (CAD) with mixed results. A meta-analysis of 39 studies (10,738 cases and 17,068 controls) reported a pooled OR of 1.10 (95%CI, 1.06–1.13; $p<0.001$) per R allele for CAD [27]. The prospective REGRESS study in 739 secondary prevention patients reported a hazard ratio (HR) of 1.71 (95%CI, 1.0–2.8; $p = 0.03$) per Q allele for death due to ischemic disease [28]. The GeneBank study in 1,399 sequential patients undergoing diagnostic coronary angiography reported that the Q allele was associated with an increased risk of major adverse cardiovascular events (HR, 1.48; 95%CI, 1.09–2.03; $p = 0.01$) [25]. This discrepancy may be due to the *PON1* allele frequency which vary greatly across human populations; a relatively high frequency of the *PON1* R192 allele is reported in Blacks, Japanese, Chinese and Thai ranging from 58% to 65% [29–31] as compared with Caucasians (25% to 30%) [32]. The frequency of *CYP2C19* alleles associated with poor metabolizer phenotype also showed high variability from 2–6% in Caucasians to 13–23% in Asians [33]. Since most studies were in Caucasians, there was a paucity of data in Asian populations who have different genetic background. Therefore, the aim of this study was to investigate the impact and interaction of *PON1* Q192R, *CYP2C19**2 and *CYP2C19**3 genotypes on clopidogrel platelet inhibition using multiple electrode platelet aggregometry (MEA) in Thai population.

Methods

Study population

211 patients who resided in Bangkok with aged-range from 39–94 years were recruited if they had established CAD and were on dual antiplatelet therapy with clopidogrel 75 mg and aspirin 75–325 mg daily at least 14 days prior to enrollment for secondary prevention. Subjects were excluded if they had a history of drug or alcohol abuse, bleeding disorder, current warfarin use, myelodysplastic or myeloproliferative disorders, chronic liver disease or any contraindication against aspirin or clopidogrel. Subjects were also excluded if they were pregnant, if the platelet count was less than 10^5 cell/mm^3 (thrombocytopenia), or if there was prior usage of glycoprotein IIb/IIIa antagonist. Questionnaires and medical records were used to collect family and medical history, smoking habit, platelet count, diabetic status, and physical activities. The study protocols were approved by Siriraj Institutional Review Board, Faculty of Medicine Siriraj Hospital, Mahidol University. Informed consent was signed by all subjects after explanation on aims and benefits of this research project.

Platelet aggregation assays

After 14 days of taking 75 mg clopidogrel combined with 75–325 mg aspirin daily, peripheral venous blood samples were obtained from subjects in a catheterization laboratory prior to the next dose of clopidogrel and aspirin. Platelet aggregation was measured using MEA on the Multiplate analyser (Dynabyte, Munich Germany). Blood was placed in 4.5 ml plastic tubes containing hirudin with a final concentration of 25 µg/ml. The final concentration of ADP (6.5 µM) -induced platelet aggregation was assessed as previously reported [34]. Platelet aggregation measured with MEA was quantified as area under the curve (AUC = AU×min) of aggregation unit (AU). A 10 AU×min corresponds to 1 unit (U). The cut off point for this clopidogrel resistance was 50 U as previously reported [35]. All material used for platelet aggregation study was obtained from the manufacturer.

Genotyping

Genomic DNA was isolated from whole blood by guanidine-HCl methods. Subjects were genotyped for *CYP2C19**2 (681 G>A), *CYP2C19**3 (636 G>A), and *PON1* Q192R (575 A>G) using PCR-RFLP as previously described [36–38]. Sequence specific primers were used to amplify the alleles of interest. Primers 5′ AATTACAACCAGAGCTTGGC 3′ and 5′ TATCACTTTCCATAAAAGCAAG 3′ were used to amplified the sequence of the *CYP2C19**2 in exon 5 of the gene. Primers 5′ AAATTGTTTCCAATCATTTAGCT 3′ and 5′ ACTTCAGGGCTTGGTCAATA 3′ were used to amplified the sequence of the *CYP2C19**3 in exon 4. Primers 5′ TATTGTTGCTGTGGGACCTGAG 3′ and 5′ CCTGAGAATCTGAGTAAATCCACT 3′ were used to amplify the sequence of the *PON1* gene containing the Q192R polymorphism in exon 6. PCR cycles for denaturation, annealing and extension were 35 cycles for all polymorphism with initial denaturation at 94°C for 5 min and final extension at 72°C for 5 min. PCR profile of *CYP2C19**2 polymorphism was denatured at 94°C for 30 sec, annealing at 60°C for 30 sec and extension at 72°C for 30 sec. PCR profile for *CYP2C19**3 polymorphism was denatured at 94°C for 30 sec, annealing at 58°C for 30 sec and extension at 72°C for 30 sec. For *PON1* polymorphism, denaturation was at 94°C for 1 min, annealing at 60°C for 1 min, and extension at 72°C for 30 sec. The PCR product for *CYP2C19**2, *CYP2C19**3 and *PON1* were 169, 271 and 238 bp, and were cut by 10 units of *SmaI*, *BamHI*, and *BspPI* restriction enzymes, respectively. Products from *SmaI* enzyme were 120 and 49 bp for G allele and 169 bp for A allele. For *BamHI*, the products were 175 and 96 bp for G allele and 271 bp for A allele and the products from *BspPI* were 175 and 63 bp for R192 allele and 238 bp for Q192 allele. The restriction site cut products were detected by 3.5% agarose gel electrophoresis.

Table 1. Baseline characteristics of study participants.

Parameters	Total (n=211)	Non-responders (n=70)	Responders (n=141)	p-value*
Age	66.25±11.15	64.47±10.51	67.13±11.39	0.102
BMI (kg/m^2)	25.54±4.08	25.59±4.13	25.57±4.08	0.970
Female (%)	68 (32.3)	21 (30.0)	47 (33.3)	0.626
Type of CAD				
- Single vessel disease (%)	51 (24.1)	19 (27.1)	32 (22.7)	0.477
- Multi vessel disease (%)	143 (67.8)	46 (65.7)	97 (68.8)	0.757
- Others (%)	17 (8.1)	5 (7.1)	12 (8.5)	0.731
Cardiomyophaty (%)	7 (3.3)	3 (4.3)	4 (2.8)	0.580
Diabetes (%)	97 (46.0)	43 (61.4)	54 (38.3)	0.002*
Hypertension (%)	184 (87.8)	61 (87.1)	123 (87.2)	0.985
Dyslipidemia (%)	149 (70.6)	52 (74.3)	97 (68.8)	0.410
Stroke (%)	14 (6.6)	6 (8.6)	8 (5.7)	0.426
Renal impairment (%)	23 (10.9)	6 (8.6)	17 (12.1)	0.444
Peripheral arterial disorder (%)	13 (6.2)	4 (5.7)	9 (6.4)	0.849
Smoking (%)	85 (40.3)	35 (50.0)	50 (35.5)	0.043*
Medication				
- Proton pump inhibitors (%)	83 (39.3)	30 (42.9)	53 (37.6)	0.461
- Calcium channel blockers (%)	67 (31.8)	22 (31.4)	45 (31.9)	0.943
- Statin (%)	183 (86.7)	65 (92.9)	118 (83.7)	0.065
Platelet count (×10^5/mm^3)	2.55±0.76	2.73±0.84	2.47±0.72	0.033*
ADP platelet aggregation (U)	43.98±26.19	73.33±18.26	28.95±10.42	<0.001

* Variable is significant difference between responders and non-responders at p-value<0.05.

Statistical analyses

Variables were presented as mean ± standard deviation (SD). Chi-square goodness-of-fit test or Fisher's exact test was used to test for a possible deviation of genotype distribution from Hardy-Weinberg equilibrium (HWE) proportions. Normally distributed continuous variables were compared across two groups with the two-sided student's t-test and for genotype group comparisons with the one-way ANOVA test. The differences in allele and genotype frequencies between groups were compared using Chi-square test. A nominal p value <0.05 was considered statistically significant.

Univariable and multivariable logistic regression analyses were applied to examine whether *PON1* Q192R, *CYP2C19**2 and *3 genotypes were associated with clopidogrel resistance after adjusting for age, sex, diabetes, smoking status and platelet count, assuming an additive genetic model coded as the number of mutated allele. Bonferroni's method was used for multiple testing correction considering three genetic loci tests. Statistical significant level was set at $p \leq 0.017$.

Interaction between *PON1* variants and *CYP2C19**2 and *3 was performed using Cordell's test for epistatic interactions [39], using models containing two genetic markers with and without interaction term and covariates (age, sex, diabetic status, smoking status, and platelet count). Likelihood ratio test was performed with 10,000 permutations to calculate the empirical significance of the interaction term, and empirical statistically significant level was set to $p<0.05$. All analyses were performed using SPSS 13 (SPSS Inc. Chicago, IL, USA) and R version 2.14.2. Cordell's test was performed using *scrime* package in R [40,41]. To determine the extent of linkage disequilibrium (LD) in our samples, standardized LD coefficient (D′) and correlation coefficient (r) were calculated for all pairs of polymorphism.

Results

Baseline characteristics of study participants

Based on the result from platelet function test using MEA, the CAD patients were categorized into responders and non-responders to clopidogrel. Among 211 patients included in this study, 70 patients (33.2%) were classified as non-responders and 141 patients (66.8%) as responders. There was no significance between the two groups regarding differences in age, BMI, sex, number of vessel diseases, underlying diseases (cardiomyopathy, hypertension, dyslipidemia, stroke, renal impairment, and peripheral disorder), and concurrent medications ($p>0.05$). However, clopidogrel non-responders had a significantly higher proportion of diabetes ($p=0.002$), smokers ($p=0.043$), and higher platelet counts ($p=0.033$) as shown in Table 1.

Distribution and allele frequencies of *CYP2C19**2, *3 and *PON1* Q192R genotypes

The distribution of *CYP2C19**2, *3 and *PON1* Q192R genotypes in the clopidogrel responsive and non-responsive groups were summarized in Table 2, which indicates consistency with the Hardy-Weinberg equilibrium ($p>0.05$). There was no homozygous *CYP2C19**3 genotype detected in the study population, which is consistent with its very rare frequency in Caucasians, Africans, Americans, Japanese and Koreans. Moreover, the high frequency of *PON1* R192 in this study was consistent with the

Table 2. Distribution of CYP2C19*2, *3 and PON1 genotypes in clopidogrel responders and non-responders.

CYP2C19*2 (rs4244285)				
Genotype	**Non-responders (n = 70)**	**Responders (n = 141)**	**Total (n = 211)**	**p-value***
GG (*1/*1)	27 (38.6%)	85 (60.3%)	112 (53.1%)	2.9×10^{-3}†
GA (*1/*2)	31 (44.3%)	53 (37.6%)	84 (35.8%)	0.349
AA (*2/*2)	12 (17.1%)	3 (2.1%)	15 (7.1%)	1.6×10^{-4}†
HWE p-value‡	0.549	0.106	0.889	-
Allele frequency				
Allele*2 (95%CI)	0.39 (0.32–0.48)	0.21 (0.16–0.26)	0.27 (0.23–0.31)	6.3×10^{-5}†
CYP2C19*3 (rs4986893)				
Genotype	**Non-responders (n = 70)**	**Responders (n = 141)**	**Total (n = 211)**	**p-value***
GG (*1/*1)	60 (85.7%)	137 (97.2%)	197 (93.4%)	2.9×10^{-3}†
GA (*1/*3)	10 (14.3%)	4 (2.8%)	14 (6.6%)	2.9×10^{-3}†
AA (*3/*3)	0 (0)	0 (0)	0	-
HWE p-value‡	0.520	0.864	0.618	-
Allele frequency				
Allele*3 (95%CI)	0.07 (0.03–0.11)	0.01 (0.0003–0.03)	0.03 (0.02–0.05)	3.4×10^{-3}†
CYP2C19*2 and *3 Combination				
Genotype	**Non-responders (n = 70)**	**Responders (n = 141)**	**Total (n = 211)**	**p-value***
*1/*1	24 (34.3%)	82 (58.2%)	106 (50.2%)	1.1×10^{-3}†
*1/*2	24 (34.3%)	52 (36.9%)	76 (36.0%)	0.712
*1/*3	3 (4.3%)	3 (2.1%)	6 (2.9%)	0.401
*2/*2	12 (17.1%)	3 (2.1%)	15 (7.1%)	1.6×10^{-4}†
*2/*3	7 (10.0%)	1 (0.7%)	8 (1.8%)	2.1×10^{-3}†
*3/*3	0 (0)	0 (0)	0	-
HWE p-value‡	0.127	0.451	0.083	-
Allele frequency				
Allele*1 (95%CI)	0.54 (0.45–0.62)	0.78 (0.72–0.83)	0.70 (0.65–0.74)	4.0×10^{-7}†
Allele*2 (95%CI)	0.39 (0.31–0.47)	0.21 (0.16–0.26)	0.27 (0.23–0.31)	6.5×10^{-5}†
Allele*3 (95%CI)	0.07 (0.04–0.10)	0.01 (0.0003–0.02)	0.03 (0.02–0.05)	3.6×10^{-4}†
PON1 (Q192R; rs662)				
Genotype	**Non-responders (n = 70)**	**Responders (n = 141)**	**Total (n = 211)**	**p-value***
GG (RR)	34 (48.6%)	71 (50.4%)	105 (49.8%)	0.807
AG (QR)	29 (41.4%)	55 (39.0%)	84 (39.8%)	0.735
AA (QQ)	7 (10.0%)	15 (10.6%)	22 (10.4%)	0.886
HWE p-value‡	0.824	0.381	0.399	0.886
Allele frequency				
Allele Q (95%CI)	0.31 (0.24–0.38)	0.30 (0.25–0.35)	0.30 (0.26–0.34)	0.904

* Comparison of genotype and allele frequencies between non-responders and responders.
†Statistically significant difference at $p<0.05$.
‡p-value of Hardy-Weinberg equilibrium.

other reports in Asian populations. The frequencies of both *2/*2 and *2/*3 genotypes (17.10, 10.00 vs 2.10, 0.70%) and *2 and *3 alleles (39.29, 7.14 vs 20.92, 1.42%) were significantly higher in clopidogrel non-responders than those in responders ($p = 1.6 \times 10^{-4}$, $p = 2.1 \times 10^{-3}$ and $p = 6.5 \times 10^{-5}$, $p = 3.6 \times 10^{-4}$, respectively). Similarly, the frequencies of *CYP2C19*1* genotype

Table 3. Association between CYP2C19*2, *3, PON1 Q192R and clopidogrel resistance.

Genotype	Crude OR (95%CI)	p-value	Adjusted OR (95%CI)†	p-value
***CYP2C19*2* (rs4244285)**				
GG (*1/*1)	1	-	1	-
GA (*1/*2)	1.84 (0.99–3.42)	0.053	2.30 (1.14–4.66)	0.021
AA (*2/*2)	12.59 (3.31–47.96)	<0.001*	13.23 (2.87–60.88)	0.001*
Allele A (*2)	2.57 (1.59–4.14)	<0.001*	2.86 (1.63–5.03)	<0.001*
***CYP2C19*3* (rs4986893)**				
GG (*1/*1)	1	-	1	-
GA (*1/*3)	5.71 (1.72–18.93)	0.004*	10.59 (2.39–46.85)	0.002*
AA (*3/*3)	-	-	-	-
Allele A (*3)	5.71 (1.72–18.93)	0.004*	10.59 (2.39–46.85)	0.002*
***CYP2C19*2* and *3 combination**				
***1/*1**	1	-	1	-
***1/*2**	1.58 (0.81–3.06)	0.179	2.01 (0.95–4.29)	0.070
***1/*3**	3.42 (0.65–18.04)	0.148	3.70 (0.46–30.01)	0.221
***2/*2**	13.67 (3.56–52.43)	<0.001*	13.09 (2.83–60.57)	0.001*
***2/*3**	23.92 (2.80–204.11)	0.004*	84.06 (6.89–1026.24)	0.001*
Allele *2 ‡	2.63 (1.62–4.27)	<0.001*	2.94 (1.65–5.26)	<0.001*
Allele *3 ‡	6.18 (1.80–21.17)	0.004*	11.26 (2.47–51.40)	0.002 *
***PON1* (Q192R; rs662)**				
GG (RR)	1	-	1	-
AG (QR)	1.10 (0.60–2.02)	0.756	1.36 (0.68–2.72)	0.381
AA (QQ)	0.98 (0.36–2.61)	0.959	1.05 (0.35–3.16)	0.925
Allele A (Q)	1.03 (0.67–1.57)	0.907	1.13 (0.70–1.82)	0.622

* Risk is statistical significant when compared to the reference genotype at p-value<0.017.
†Adjusted for diabetes, age, sex, history of smoking and platelet count.
‡Adjusted for concurrent *2 or *3 allele and covariates (diabetes, age, sex, history of smoking, and platelet count).

and allele (34.30, 53.57 vs 58.20, 77.66%) were significantly lower in non-responders than those in responders ($p = 1.1 \times 10^{-3}$ and 4.0×10^{-7}, respectively). There were no significant differences of *PON1* Q192R genotypes and alleles between the two groups ($p > 0.05$).

Association of *CYP2C19* and *PON1* Q192R gene polymorphisms and clopidogrel responsiveness

The results of a simple logistic regression model demonstrated that having one copy of *CYP2C19**3 was significantly associated with a 5.71 fold higher risk of clopidogrel resistance (95% CI, 1.72–18.93; p = 0.004) as compared with wild type *CYP2C19* (*1/*1). Although one copy of *CYP2C19**2 was not significantly associated with clopidogrel resistance (p = 0.053), two copy of CYP2C19 (*2/*2) was associated with 12.59 times higher risk of clopidogrel resistance (95%CI, 3.31–47.96; p<0.001). The combined effect of *CYP2C19**2 and *3 estimated that both *2/*2 and *2/*3 genotypes significantly increased the risk of clopidogrel resistances with an unadjusted OR of 13.67 (95%CI, 3.56–52.43; p<0.001) and 23.92 (95%CI, 2.80–204.11; p = 0.004), respectively. After adjusting for the co-dominant effects of *2 and *3 alleles, comparing to *1 allele, *2 was associated with 2.63 times higher risk of clopidogrel resistance (95%CI, 1.62–4.27; p<0.001), and *3 was associated with 6.18 times higher risk of clopidogrel resistance (95%CI, 1.80–21.17; p = 0.004). In contrast, the *PON1* Q192R, both genotypes (QQ/QR) and Q allele, did not significantly associate with clopidogrel resistance (p>0.05).

From multivariable logistic regression analysis, assuming a co-dominant allele effect, having one copy of *CYP2C19**2 (*1/*2) was associated with 2.30 times higher risk than *1/*1 (95%CI, 1.14–4.66); p<0.021), after adjusted for age, sex, and all variables that differed between responders and non-responders (from Table 1). Similarly, one copy of *CYP2C19**3 (*1/*3) was associated with 10.59 times higher risk of clopidogrel resistance compared with *1/*1 (95%CI, 2.39–46.85; p = 0.002). Two copy of *CYP2C19**2 (*2/*2) was associated with 13.23 times higher risk of clopidogrel resistance compared with *1/*1 (95%CI, 2.87–60.88; p = 0.001).

The combined effects of *CYP2C19*2* and *3, after controlling for additional covariates, compared with *1/*1, *CYP2C19**2/*3 was associated with 84.06 times higher risk of clopidogrel resistance (95%CI, 6.89–1026.24; p = 0.001); homozygous

Table 4. Estimated risk of clopidogrel resistance in patients with at least one of the following risk factors: CYP2C19*2, CYP2C19*3, smoking, diabetes mellitus, increase in platelet count adjusted for age and sex.

Risk Factors	Adjusted OR*	95% CI	p-value†
*1/*1	1	-	-
*1/*1+Smoking	3.52	1.53–8.09	0.003
*1/*1+DM	3.33	1.62–6.85	0.001
*1/*1+Platelet	1.05	1.00–1.10	0.034
*1/*1+DM+Smoking	7.78	2.68–22.53	<0.001
*1/*1+DM+Platelet	3.26	1.65–6.45	0.001
*1/*1+DM+Smoking+Platelet	8.12	2.82–23.73	<0.001
*1/*2	2.94	1.65–5.26	<0.001
*2/*2	8.78	3.00–25.71	<0.001
*1/*3	11.26	2.47–51.41	0.002
*2/*3	33.15	7.01–156.72	<0.001
*1/*2+Smoking	7.43	2.76–20.05	<0.001
*2/*2+Smoking	22.03	5.44–89.17	<0.001
*1/*3+Smoking	28.06	4.84–162.83	<0.001
*2/*3+Smoking	83.16	12.51–552.97	<0.001
*1/*2+DM	9.19	3.59–23.52	<0.001
*2/*2+DM	27.23	6.90–107.37	<0.001
*1/*3+DM	34.68	6.75–178.06	<0.001
*2/*3+DM	102.77	17.16–615.29	<0.001
*1/*2+Platelet count	3.12	1.82–5.34	<0.001
*2/*2+Platelet count	9.23	3.15–27.03	<0.001
*1/*3+Platelet count	11.76	2.81–49.29	<0.001
*2/*3+Platelet count	34.86	7.30–166.45	<0.001
*1/*2+Smoking+DM	23.05	6.36–83.56	<0.001
*2/*2+Smoking+DM	68.3	12.96–360.05	<0.001
*1/*3+Smoking+DM	86.99	12.30–615.28	<0.001
*2/*3+Smoking+DM	257.79	31.21–2129.62	<0.001
*1/*2+Smoking+DM+Platelet	24.23	6.67–87.95	<0.001
*2/*2+Smoking+DM+Platelet	71.82	13.62–378.77	<0.001
*1/*3+Smoking+DM+Platelet	91.47	12.82–652.52	<0.001
*2/*3+Smoking+DM+Platelet	271.07	32.56–2256.56	<0.001

*Estimated OR for each risk factor category compared to men with no CYP2C19 mutation (wild type), with average age (66.25 year-old), average platelet count (255,900 platelets/mm^3), who do not smoke and do not have diabetes. Platelet variable is calculated per ×1,000 platelet increased. Log odds for clopidogrel resistance were calculated using multivariate logistic regression as a function of CYP2C19*2+CYP2C19*3+Smoking+Diabetic Status+increased Platelet Count.
†Risk is statistically significant when compared to the reference genotype at p-value<0.05.

*CYP2C19*2* (*2/*2) was associated with 13.09 times higher risk of clopidogrel resistance (95%CI, 2.83–60.57; p = 0.001).

For allelic association, after adjusting for the co-dominant effect of *3 allele, *2 allele carrier was associated with 2.94 times higher risk of clopidogrel resistance compared with *1 allele (95%CI, 1.65–5.26; p<0.001). After adjusting for the effects of *2 allele, *3 allele was associated with 11.26 times higher risk of clopidogrel resistance compared with *1 (95%CI, 2.47–51.40; p = 0.002). In contrast, PON1 QR and QQ genotypes and Q allele showed no association with clopidogrel resistance compared with either RR genotype or R allele as references (Table 3).

The estimated effects of *1, *2, and *3 genotypes, combined with smoking, diabetes status, and increase in platelet count using *1/*1 as a reference genotype, markedly increase the risk of clopidogrel resistance in linear trend as summarized in Table 4.

CYP2C19*2, *3 and PON1 Q192R genotypes and platelet aggregation

The ADP-induced platelet aggregation values across *CYP2C19*2* and *3 genotypes were shown in Table 5. For *CYP2C19*2* genotypes, ADP-induced platelet aggregation significantly differed across genotype groups ($p = 2.98 \times 10^{-5}$). In the patients who were carriers of at least one *2 allele (*1/*2 or *2/*2), ADP induced-platelet aggregation was also significantly different when compared with *1/*1 genotype (p = 0.004). For *CYP2C19*3* genotypes, the ADP-induced platelet aggregation did not differ across genotype groups (p = 0.069). However, when combining *CYP2C19*2* and *3, the ADP-induced platelet aggregations across genotypes were significantly different ($p = 1.98 \times 10^{-6}$). For *PON1* Q192R genotypes, the ADP-induced platelet aggregation did not differ across genotype groups (p = 0.359).

Table 5. ADP induced platelet aggregation level by CYP2C19*2, *3 and PON1 Q192R polymorphisms in clopidogrel treated patients with coronary artery disease.

	Genotypes	n	Platelet Aggregation Level
*CYP2C19*2*	GG (*1/*1)	112	39.16±23.28
(rs4244285; 681G>A)	GA (*1/*2)	84	45.20±23.62
	AA (*2/*2)	15	73.07±39.77
	p-value		2.98×10^{-5}
*CYP2C19*3*	GG (*1/*1)	197	43.10±26.36
(rs4986893; 636G>A)	GA (*1/*3)	14	56.29±20.69
	AA (*3/*3)	0	-
	p-value		0.069
*CYP2C19*2*	*1/*1	106	38.90±23.49
*& CYP2C19*3*	*1/*2	76	43.36±23.28
	*1/*3	6	47.67±19.14
	*2/*3	8	62.75±20.54
	*2/*2	15	73.07±39.77
	p-value		1.98×10^{-6}
PON1	GG (RR)	105	42.14±25.43
(rs662; 575A>G)	AG (QR)	84	45.77±27.30
	AA (QQ)	22	45.86±26.08
	p-value		0.359

p-values assuming additive genetic model represent the association between genotype and ADP-induced platelet aggregation (U) at p-value<0.05.

Interaction between *PON1* Q192R polymorphisms and ADP-induced platelet aggregation level after stratification by *CYP2C19*2* and *CYP2C19*3*

Since both CYP2C19 and PON1 involve in activation of clopidogrel prodrug as suggested by Bouman et al. [20], the interaction effects between CYP2C19 (*2, *3) and PON1 (Q192R) on ADP-induced platelet aggregation were investigated. After stratification by CYP2C19*2 (Figure 1A) and *3 genotypes (Figure 1B), the effects of PON1 (Q192R) polymorphism on ADP-induced platelet aggregation were not modified by neither *CYP2C19*2* nor *CYP2C19*3* allele. Cordell's test for epistatic interaction showed no statistically significant interaction between *CYP2C19*2* or *3 with PON1 Q192R polymorphisms ($p_{int}=0.21$ and 0.91, respectively). Similarly, *CYP2C19*3* did not modify the effects of *CYP2C19*2* on ADP-induced platelet aggregation ($p_{int}=0.65$, Figure 1C). To examine the extent of linkage disequilibrium (LD) in these study samples, standardized LD coefficient (D′) and correlation coefficient (r) were calculated for all pairs of polymorphisms. Table 6 shows the LD matrix generated using D′ and r. No evidence of LD was observed among these three polymorphisms (D′ and r<0.5).

Discussion

Bouman et al's study [20] is the first report to identify that *PON1* Q192R is a major determinant of clopidogrel efficacy using in vitro metabolomic profiling techniques. The PON1 activity was significantly reduced in subjects with homozygous wild type allele (*PON1* QQ192) compared with carriers of the mutant allele. In addition, in a group of patients with stent thrombosis and matched controls without stent thrombosis, *PON1* QQ192 was associated with decreased platelet inhibition by clopidogrel and decreased plasma active thiol metabolite after given a 600 mg clopidogrel loading dose. In addition, *PON1* QQ192 was also associated with an OR of 3.3 for the occurrence of stent thrombosis as compared with QR192 or RR192 genotypes. Later, however, other studies could not document the influence of *PON1* Q192R genotype on clopidogrel antiplatelet aggregation since the publication of the study by Bouman et al [21–23]. In this study, we evaluated the effects of *CYP2C19* and *PON1* genetic polymorphisms on clopidogrel antiplatelet function in Thai population. Similar to the findings from other investigators in African-American and Caucasian populations [21,22], our results have shown that only *CYP2C19*2* and *3 genotypes, but not the *PON1* Q192R genotypes, modified the effect of clopidogrel. The mean aggregation values increased by a strong genetic effect across *CYP2C19* genotype groups in individuals treated with clopidogrel. Also, only *CYP2C19*2* and *3 genotypes but not the *PON1* Q192R genotypes were found to be associated with a higher risk of clopidogrel resistance in CAD patients during treatment with clopidogrel.

The present study was strengthened by testing the influence of these SNPs on platelet aggregation in parallel as measured by MEA assay. Only *CYP2C19*2 and *3 polymorphisms have been demonstrated to be a strong determinant of reduced active clopidogrel metabolite formation corresponding to the studies in Caucasians [14,17,42–52]. Nevertheless, the influence of PON1 on the level of platelet aggregation had a trend towards higher values in QR192 and QQ192 patients (Table 5). This suggested that *PON1* polymorphism may be associated with small differences in platelet inhibition as suggested by the finding of Bouman et al [20]. The small effects of *PON1* Q192R could explain why several reports were unable to confirm this association between *PON1* polymorphism and platelet aggregation in patients who were treated with clopidogrel [21–23,53–57]. Concerning the clinical outcome of patients treated with clopidogrel, our results

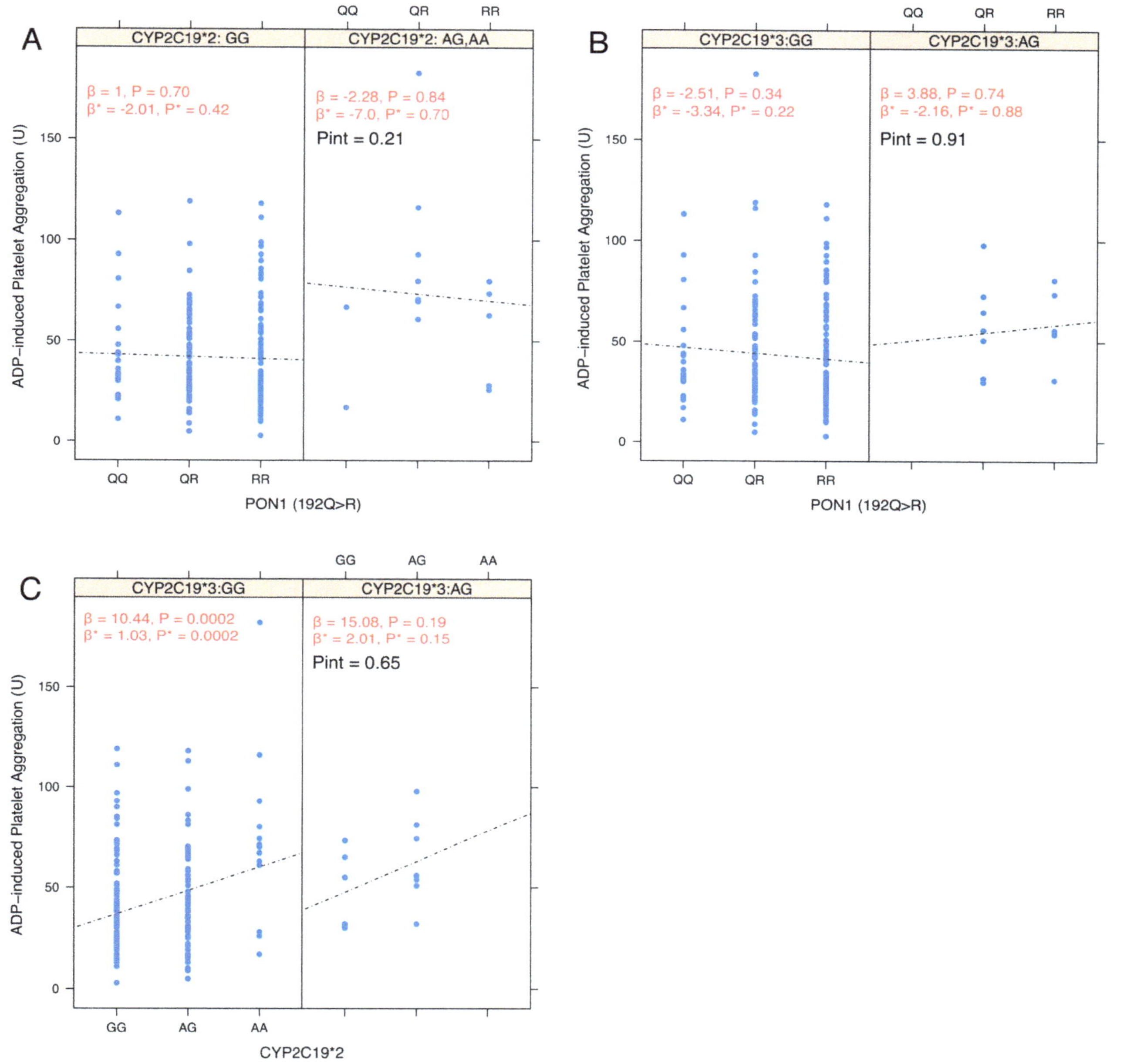

Figure 1. Interaction among polymorphisms in CYP2C19*2, *3 and PON1 Q192R and the effects on ADP-induced platelet aggregation. A) Effects of PON1 Q192R polymorphism on platelet aggregation stratified by *CYP2C19*2* genotype; B) Effects of *PON1* Q192R polymorphism on platelet aggregation stratified by *CYP2C19*3* genotype; C) Effects of *CYP2C19*2* on platelet aggregation stratified by *CYP2C19*3* genotype

Table 6. Standardized linkage disequilibrium coefficient (D′) and correlation coefficient (r) among three polymorphisms in CYP2C19 and PON1.

D′ r	*PON1* Q192R	*CYP2C19*3*	*CYP2C19*2*
PON1 Q192R	-	−0.0276	0.0089
*CYP2C19*3*	0.2258	-	0.0223
*CYP2C19*2*	0.0097	0.0731	-

D′ values are shown in the lower triangle, and *r* values are shown in the upper triangle.

reported here are in agreement with a number of prior studies and confirm the pivotal role of *CYP2C19*2* and *3 as genetic markers for platelet aggregation and clopidogrel response. This present study also demonstrated no association and linkage disequilibrium between *CYP2C19* and *PON1* polymorphisms, which supports the evidence that *CYP2C19* locus, located on chromosome 10, was the only locus which was significantly associated with clopidogrel treatment efficacy in a genome-wide association study (GWAS) [42]. The GWAS did not find evidence for association between SNPs located on or near the *PON1* gene on chromosome 7 and variation in platelet inhibition by clopidogrel [42]. In addition, in a meta-analysis investigating the effect of *CYP2C19* alleles on recurrent stenosis in patients receiving clopidogrel after coronary stenting, the presence of one reduced-function allele was associated with a HR of 2.67, and the presence of two reduced-function alleles was associated with a HR of 3.97 for the recurrence of thrombosis [46]. This study also confirms that the presence of one reduced-function allele of *CYP2C19* was associated with adjusted ORs of 2.94 and 11.26 for *2 and *3, respectively. The presence of two reduced-function alleles was associated with adjusted ORs of 13.09 and 84.06 for *2/*2 and *2/*3, respectively. These findings support the clinical importance of the reduced-function *CYP2C19* polymorphism and clopidogrel resistance on recurrent ischemic events and restenosis after coronary stenting.

In this study, smoking status, diabetes mellitus, and increase in platelet count were shown to be the three major contributing factors that could promote the development of platelet aggregation in CAD patients (Table 4). These conditions have been known to be associated with high oxidative stress, suggesting a possible link between high oxidative stress and response to clopidogrel treatment. This study suggested that not only genetic polymorphisms but also oxidative stress can enhance platelet aggregation to clopidogrel responsiveness in CAD patients.

Limitations of the study include a relatively small sample size, which might contribute to the inability to detect weaker effects of PON1 on clopidogrel response, as compared with the stronger effects of CYP2C19. Although plasma levels of the active metabolite of clopidogrel and PON1 enzyme activity were not measured to confirm the lower level of enzyme activity associated with Q allele, these parameters could be used to indirectly assess the platelet function test as measured by ADP-induced platelet aggregation. Finally, platelet function testing was done with only one single device (Multiplate anslyser), using ADP-induced platelet aggregation, therefore, we could not exclude the possibility that other mechanisms might also explain the clopidogrel resistance as measured by the Multiplate analyser.

Conclusions

This study confirms the impact of *CYP2C19**2 and *3 polymorphisms on antiplatelet effects of clopidogrel in Thai population similar to the results found in Caucasian populations with different genetic background. *PON1* Q192R appeared to have a little modification of efficacy and safety of clopidogrel in CAD patients. A larger study may be needed to confirm the association of the *PON1* Q192 allele with adverse ischemic events in patients receiving clopidogrel treatment. Our results are only relevant to clopidogrel-treated patients; however, knowing the genotypes of *CYP2C19* should aid in selection of antiplatelet therapy. In the future, pharmacogenetic studies may be needed to introduce newer antiplatelet drugs that do not require *CYP2C19* activation and may reduce the overall impact of clopidogrel resistance in patients with CAD.

Acknowledgments

The authors would like to thank Dr. William M. Honsa for English language editorial support. Some parts of this work have been presented in a local meeting at the 39th Congress on Science and Technology of Thailand.

Author Contributions

Conceived and designed the experiments: DT AL BS. Performed the experiments: RK SP AL DT. Analyzed the data: BS SH RK AL. Contributed reagents/materials/analysis tools: DT AL BS. Wrote the paper: AL DT BS SH RK SP BT.

References

1. Moleerergpoom W, Kanjanavanit R, Jintapakorn W, Sritara P (2007) Costs of payment in Thai acute coronary syndrome patients. J Med Assoc Thai 90 Suppl 1: 21–31.
2. Syed FA, Bett J, Walters DL (2011) Anti-platelet therapy for Acute Coronary Syndrome: A review of currently available agents and what the future holds. Cardiovasc Hematol Disord Drug Targets.
3. Smith SC, Jr., Feldman TE, Hirshfeld JW Jr, Jacobs AK, Kern MJ, et al. (2006) ACC/AHA/SCAI 2005 Guideline Update for Percutaneous Coronary Intervention-Summary Article: A Report of the American College of Cardiology/American Heart Association Task Force on Practice Guidelines (ACC/AHA/SCAI Writing Committee to Update the 2001 Guidelines for Percutaneous Coronary Intervention). J Am Coll Cardiol 47: 216–235.
4. Gurbel PA, Tantry US (2006) Drug insight: Clopidogrel nonresponsiveness. Nat Clin Pract Cardiovasc Med 3: 387–395.
5. Gurbel PA, Bliden KP, Hiatt BL, O'Connor CM (2003) Clopidogrel for coronary stenting: response variability, drug resistance, and the effect of pretreatment platelet reactivity. Circulation 107: 2908–2913.
6. Angiolillo DJ, Fernandez-Ortiz A, Bernardo E, Alfonso F, Macaya C, et al. (2007) Variability in individual responsiveness to clopidogrel: clinical implications, management, and future perspectives. J Am Coll Cardiol 49: 1505–1516.
7. Jaremo P, Lindahl TL, Fransson SG, Richter A (2002) Individual variations of platelet inhibition after loading doses of clopidogrel. J Intern Med 252: 233–238.
8. Angiolillo DJ, Fernandez-Ortiz A, Bernardo E, Ramirez C, Sabate M, et al. (2005) Platelet function profiles in patients with type 2 diabetes and coronary artery disease on combined aspirin and clopidogrel treatment. Diabetes 54: 2430–2435.
9. Muller I, Besta F, Schulz C, Massberg S, Schonig A, et al. (2003) Prevalence of clopidogrel non-responders among patients with stable angina pectoris scheduled for elective coronary stent placement. Thromb Haemost 89: 783–787.
10. Mobley JE, Bresee SJ, Wortham DC, Craft RM, Snider CC, et al. (2004) Frequency of nonresponse antiplatelet activity of clopidogrel during pretreatment for cardiac catheterization. Am J Cardiol 93: 456–458.
11. Matetzky S, Shenkman B, Guetta V, Shechter M, Beinart R, et al. (2004) Clopidogrel resistance is associated with increased risk of recurrent atherothrombotic events in patients with acute myocardial infarction. Circulation 109: 3171–3175.
12. Angiolillo DJ, Fernandez-Ortiz A, Bernardo E, Ramirez C, Barrera-Ramirez C, et al. (2005) Identification of low responders to a 300-mg clopidogrel loading dose in patients undergoing coronary stenting. Thromb Res 115: 101–108.
13. Kazui M, Nishiya Y, Ishizuka T, Hagihara K, Farid NA, et al. (2010) Identification of the human cytochrome P450 enzymes involved in the two oxidative steps in the bioactivation of clopidogrel to its pharmacologically active metabolite. Drug Metab Dispos 38: 92–99.
14. Hulot JS, Bura A, Villard E, Azizi M, Remones V, et al. (2006) Cytochrome P450 2C19 loss-of-function polymorphism is a major determinant of clopidogrel responsiveness in healthy subjects. Blood 108: 2244–2247.
15. Brandt JT, Close SL, Iturria SJ, Payne CD, Farid NA, et al. (2007) Common polymorphisms of CYP2C19 and CYP2C9 affect the pharmacokinetic and pharmacodynamic response to clopidogrel but not prasugrel. J Thromb Haemost 5: 2429–2436.
16. Umemura K, Furuta T, Kondo K (2008) The common gene variants of CYP2C19 affect pharmacokinetics and pharmacodynamics in an active metabolite of clopidogrel in healthy subjects. J Thromb Haemost 6: 1439–1441.
17. Simon T, Verstuyft C, Mary-Krause M, Quteineh L, Drouet E, et al. (2009) Genetic determinants of response to clopidogrel and cardiovascular events. N Engl J Med 360: 363–375.

18. Sibbing D, Braun S, Morath T, Mehilli J, Vogt W, et al. (2009) Platelet reactivity after clopidogrel treatment assessed with point-of-care analysis and early drug-eluting stent thrombosis. J Am Coll Cardiol 53: 849–856.
19. Bonello L, Tantry US, Marcucci R, Blindt R, Angiolillo DJ, et al. (2010) Consensus and future directions on the definition of high on-treatment platelet reactivity to adenosine diphosphate. J Am Coll Cardiol 56: 919–933.
20. Bouman HJ, Schomig E, van Werkum JW, Velder J, Hackeng CM, et al. (2011) Paraoxonase-1 is a major determinant of clopidogrel efficacy. Nat Med 17: 110–116.
21. Kreutz RP, Nystrom P, Kreutz Y, Miao J, Desta Z, et al. (2012) Influence of paraoxonase-1 Q192R and cytochrome P450 2C19 polymorphisms on clopidogrel response. Clin Pharmacol 4: 13–20.
22. Sibbing D, Koch W, Massberg S, Byrne RA, Mehilli J, et al. (2011) No association of paraoxonase-1 Q192R genotypes with platelet response to clopidogrel and risk of stent thrombosis after coronary stenting. Eur Heart J 32: 1605–1613.
23. Pare G, Ross S, Mehta SR, Yusuf S, Anand SS, et al. (2012) Effect of PON1 Q192R genetic polymorphism on clopidogrel efficacy and cardiovascular events in the Clopidogrel in the Unstable Angina to Prevent Recurrent Events trial and the Atrial Fibrillation Clopidogrel Trial with Irbesartan for Prevention of Vascular Events. Circ Cardiovasc Genet 5: 250–256.
24. Marsillach J, Aragones G, Beltran R, Caballeria J, Pedro-Botet J, et al. (2009) The measurement of the lactonase activity of paraoxonase-1 in the clinical evaluation of patients with chronic liver impairment. Clin Biochem 42: 91–98.
25. Bhattacharyya T, Nicholls SJ, Topol EJ, Zhang R, Yang X, et al. (2008) Relationship of paraoxonase 1 (PON1) gene polymorphisms and functional activity with systemic oxidative stress and cardiovascular risk. JAMA 299: 1265–1276.
26. Mackness MI, Arrol S, Mackness B, Durrington PN (1997) Alloenzymes of paraoxonase and effectiveness of high-density lipoproteins in protecting low-density lipoprotein against lipid peroxidation. Lancet 349: 851–852.
27. Lawlor DA, Day IN, Gaunt TR, Hinks LJ, Briggs PJ, et al. (2004) The association of the PON1 Q192R polymorphism with coronary heart disease: findings from the British Women's Heart and Health cohort study and a meta-analysis. BMC Genet 5: 17.
28. Regieli JJ, Jukema JW, Doevendans PA, Zwinderman AH, Kastelein JJ, et al. (2009) Paraoxonase variants relate to 10-year risk in coronary artery disease: impact of a high-density lipoprotein-bound antioxidant in secondary prevention. J Am Coll Cardiol 54: 1238–1245.
29. Likidlilid A, Akrawinthawong K, Poldee S, Sriratanasathavorn C (2010) Paraoxonase 1 polymorphisms as the risk factor of coronary heart disease in a Thai population. Acta Cardiol 65: 681–691.
30. Ko YL, Ko YS, Wang SM, Hsu LA, Chang CJ, et al. (1998) The Gln-Arg 191 polymorphism of the human paraoxonase gene is not associated with the risk of coronary artery disease among Chinese in Taiwan. Atherosclerosis 141: 259–264.
31. Imai Y, Morita H, Kurihara H, Sugiyama T, Kato N, et al. (2000) Evidence for association between paraoxonase gene polymorphisms and atherosclerotic diseases. Atherosclerosis 149: 435–442.
32. Ferre N, Tous M, Paul A, Zamora A, Vendrell JJ, et al. (2002) Paraoxonase Gln-Arg(192) and Leu-Met(55) gene polymorphisms and enzyme activity in a population with a low rate of coronary heart disease. Clin Biochem 35: 197–203.
33. Goldstein JA (2001) Clinical relevance of genetic polymorphisms in the human CYP2C subfamily. Br J Clin Pharmacol 52: 349–355.
34. Sibbing D, Braun S, Jawansky S, Vogt W, Mehilli J, et al. (2008) Assessment of ADP-induced platelet aggregation with light transmission aggregometry and multiple electrode platelet aggregometry before and after clopidogrel treatment. Thromb Haemost 99: 121–126.
35. Gerotziafas GT, Zarifis J, Bandi A, Mossialos L, Galea V, et al. (2012) Description of response to aspirin and clopidogrel in outpatients with coronary artery disease using multiple electrode impedance aggregometry. Clin Appl Thromb Hemost 18: 356–363.
36. de Morais SM, Wilkinson GR, Blaisdell J, Nakamura K, Meyer UA, et al. (1994) The major genetic defect responsible for the polymorphism of S-mephenytoin metabolism in humans. J Biol Chem 269: 15419–15422.
37. De Morais SM, Wilkinson GR, Blaisdell J, Meyer UA, Nakamura K, et al. (1994) Identification of a new genetic defect responsible for the polymorphism of (S)-mephenytoin metabolism in Japanese. Mol Pharmacol 46: 594–598.
38. Campo S, Sardo MA, Trimarchi G, Bonaiuto M, Fontana L, et al. (2004) Association between serum paraoxonase (PON1) gene promoter T(-107)C polymorphism, PON1 activity and HDL levels in healthy Sicilian octogenarians. Exp Gerontol 39: 1089–1094.
39. Cordell HJ (2002) Epistasis: what it means, what it doesn't mean, and statistical methods to detect it in humans. Hum Mol Genet 11: 2463–2468.
40. Schwender H, Fritsch A (2013) scrime: Analysis of High-Dimensional Categorical Data such as SNP Data. Available: http://CRAN.R-project.org/package=scrime.
41. R Core Team (2013) R: A language and environment for statistical computing. Vienna, Austria: R Foundation for Statistical Computing. Available: http://www.R-project.org.
42. Shuldiner AR, O'Connell JR, Bliden KP, Gandhi A, Ryan K, et al. (2009) Association of cytochrome P450 2C19 genotype with the antiplatelet effect and clinical efficacy of clopidogrel therapy. JAMA 302: 849–857.
43. Sibbing D, Gebhard D, Koch W, Braun S, Stegherr J, et al. (2010) Isolated and interactive impact of common CYP2C19 genetic variants on the antiplatelet effect of chronic clopidogrel therapy. J Thromb Haemost 8: 1685–1693.
44. Mega JL, Close SL, Wiviott SD, Shen L, Hockett RD, et al. (2009) Cytochrome P450 genetic polymorphisms and the response to prasugrel: relationship to pharmacokinetic, pharmacodynamic, and clinical outcomes. Circulation 119: 2553–2560.
45. Mega JL, Close SL, Wiviott SD, Shen L, Walker JR, et al. (2010) Genetic variants in ABCB1 and CYP2C19 and cardiovascular outcomes after treatment with clopidogrel and prasugrel in the TRITON-TIMI 38 trial: a pharmacogenetic analysis. Lancet 376: 1312–1319.
46. Mega JL, Simon T, Collet JP, Anderson JL, Antman EM, et al. (2010) Reduced-function CYP2C19 genotype and risk of adverse clinical outcomes among patients treated with clopidogrel predominantly for PCI: a meta-analysis. JAMA 304: 1821–1830.
47. Hochholzer W, Trenk D, Fromm MF, Valina CM, Stratz C, et al. (2010) Impact of cytochrome P450 2C19 loss-of-function polymorphism and of major demographic characteristics on residual platelet function after loading and maintenance treatment with clopidogrel in patients undergoing elective coronary stent placement. J Am Coll Cardiol 55: 2427–2434.
48. Trenk D, Hochholzer W, Fromm MF, Chialda LE, Pahl A, et al. (2008) Cytochrome P450 2C19 681G>A polymorphism and high on-clopidogrel platelet reactivity associated with adverse 1-year clinical outcome of elective percutaneous coronary intervention with drug-eluting or bare-metal stents. J Am Coll Cardiol 51: 1925–1934.
49. Sibbing D, Stegherr J, Latz W, Koch W, Mehilli J, et al. (2009) Cytochrome P450 2C19 loss-of-function polymorphism and stent thrombosis following percutaneous coronary intervention. Eur Heart J 30: 916–922.
50. Collet JP, Hulot JS, Pena A, Villard E, Esteve JB, et al. (2009) Cytochrome P450 2C19 polymorphism in young patients treated with clopidogrel after myocardial infarction: a cohort study. Lancet 373: 309–317.
51. Mega JL, Close SL, Wiviott SD, Shen L, Hockett RD, et al. (2009) Cytochrome p-450 polymorphisms and response to clopidogrel. N Engl J Med 360: 354–362.
52. Harmsze AM, van Werkum JW, Ten Berg JM, Zwart B, Bouman HJ, et al. (2010) CYP2C19*2 and CYP2C9*3 alleles are associated with stent thrombosis: a case-control study. Eur Heart J 31: 3046–3053.
53. Simon T, Steg PG, Becquemont L, Verstuyft C, Kotti S, et al. (2011) Effect of paraoxonase-1 polymorphism on clinical outcomes in patients treated with clopidogrel after an acute myocardial infarction. Clin Pharmacol Ther 90: 561–567.
54. Trenk D, Hochholzer W, Fromm MF, Zolk O, Valina CM, et al. (2011) Paraoxonase-1 Q192R polymorphism and antiplatelet effects of clopidogrel in patients undergoing elective coronary stent placement. Circ Cardiovasc Genet 4: 429–436.
55. Fontana P, James R, Barazer I, Berdague P, Schved JF, et al. (2011) Relationship between paraoxonase-1 activity, its Q192R genetic variant and clopidogrel responsiveness in the ADRIE study. J Thromb Haemost 9: 1664–1666.
56. Rideg O, Komocsi A, Magyarlaki T, Tokes-Fuzesi M, Miseta A, et al. (2011) Impact of genetic variants on post-clopidogrel platelet reactivity in patients after elective percutaneous coronary intervention. Pharmacogenomics 12: 1269–1280.
57. Lewis JP, Fisch AS, Ryan K, O'Connell JR, Gibson Q, et al. (2011) Paraoxonase 1 (PON1) gene variants are not associated with clopidogrel response. Clin Pharmacol Ther 90: 568–574.

Association of Endothelial Nitric Oxide Synthase Gene Polymorphisms with Coronary Artery Disease

Himanshu Rai[1*❥], Farah Parveen[2], Sudeep Kumar[1*❥], Aditya Kapoor[1], Nakul Sinha[3]

1 Department of Cardiology, Sanjay Gandhi Post Graduate Institute of Medical Sciences, Lucknow, Uttar Pradesh, India, **2** Department of Medical Genetics, Sanjay Gandhi Post Graduate Institute of Medical Sciences, Lucknow, Uttar Pradesh, India, **3** Department of Cardiology, Sahara India Medical Institute, Gomti Nagar, Lucknow, Uttar Pradesh, India

Abstract

Several association studies of endothelial nitric oxide synthase (*NOS3*) gene polymorphisms with respect to coronary artery disease (CAD) have been published in the past two decades. However, their association with the disease, especially among different ethnic subgroups, still remains controversial. This prompted us to conduct a systematic review and an updated structured meta-analysis, which is the largest so far (89 articles, 132 separate studies, and a sample size of 69,235), examining association of three polymorphic forms of the *NOS3* gene (i.e. Glu298Asp, T786-C and 27bp VNTR b/a) with CAD. In a subgroup analysis, we tested their association separately among published studies originating predominantly from European, Middle Eastern, Asian, Asian-Indian and African ancestries. The pooled analysis confirmed the association of all the three selected SNP with CAD in three different genetic models transcending all ancestries worldwide. The Glu298Asp polymorphism showed strongest association (OR range = 1.28–1.52, and $P<0.00001$ for all comparisons), followed by T786-C (OR range = 1.34–1.42, and $P<0.00001$ for all comparisons) and 4b/a, (OR range = 1.19–1.41, and $P\leq0.002$ for all comparisons) in our pooled analysis. Subgroup analysis revealed that Glu298Asp (OR range = 1.54–1.87, and $P<0.004$ for all comparisons) and 4b/a (OR range = 1.71–3.02, and $P<0.00001$ for all comparisons) have highest degree of association amongst the Middle Easterners. On the other hand, T786-C and its minor allele seem to carry a highest risk for CAD among subjects of Asian ancestry (OR range = 1.61–1.90, and $P\leq0.01$ for all comparisons).

Editor: Jinglu Ai, St Michael's Hospital, University of Toronto, Canada

Funding: The authors have no funding or support to report.

Competing Interests: The authors have declared that no competing interests exist.

* Email: himanshurai1981@gmail.com (HR); sudeepkum@yahoo.com (SK)

❥ These authors contributed equally to this work.

Introduction

Endothelial-derived nitric oxide (NO) has been known to be a major contributor in vascular regulation and has been amply implicated with coronary artery disease (CAD). NO is an important relaxing factor in the human body and is involved in a variety of different important physiological functions. It is synthesized in the human body from L-arginine by at least three isoforms of NO synthase (NOS), viz. inducible NOS, constitutive neuronal NOS and constitutive endothelial NOS (eNOS). [1] NO causes vascular relaxation, it suppresses platelet and leucocyte adhesion to the vascular endothelium [2–4] and reduces smooth muscle cell proliferation and migration [5]. It also scavenges superoxide radicals [2] and limits the oxidation of atherogenic low density lipoproteins [3] resulting in an overall vasoprotective effect. Intracellular NO has thus been considered as an inhibitor of several key processes leading to atherosclerotic plaque formation. [4] Inhibition or reduction of NO on the other hand, may accelerate this process. NO production has been known to be influenced by several polymorphisms of the *NOS3* gene. The *NOS3* gene is located on chromosome 7q35-36, consists of 26 exons with a total size of 21 kb and it encodes for intracellular NO production [6]. This gene is expressionally and functionally regulated through multiple regulatory steps, and entails several polymorphisms [3], some of which have functional consequences.

NOS3 polymorphisms, their role in NO production and their vascular end effects

Hingorani et al., [7] first described a point mutation of guanine (G) to thymine (T) at nucleotide 1917 in exon 7 of the *NOS3* gene, resulting in the replacement of glutamic acid by aspartic acid at codon 298 (Glu298Asp, also known as G894-T, rs1799983). This variant has been shown to be associated with coronary spasm, [8] essential hypertension [9] and the risk of acute myocardial infarction (AMI) [3,10,11]. Controversial results have been obtained over the years when this single nucleotide polymorphism (SNP) was evaluated with respect to its effect on intracellular NO production. Some studies have demonstrated lower concentrations of intracellular NO in genotypes carrying Asp alleles [12], while others have reported lack of association of this SNP with NO production [13]. Apparently, apart from possibly having lower NO concentrations in the human body, genotypes carrying Asp alleles have also been shown to have greater red blood cell (RBC) aggregability [14]. This makes them more prone to suffer from acute coronary events, especially from those of thrombotic origin. Befittingly, over the years this SNP has been shown to be associated to myocardial infarction (MI) [10,11,15], coronary artery spasm [10] and CAD. [2–4,13,16,17] However, association of this SNP with CAD has been a matter of dispute as some studies have also reported its lack of association with the disease. [18–23] Geo-ethnic differences and the role of environmental factors in various populations could have been the prime reason behind these contradictory results.

Another common variant of this gene results by a cytosine replacing a thymine at nucleotide −786 (T786-C, rs2070744) at the 5′-flanking region of the *NOS3* gene. [24] The resulting T786-C variant has been shown to reduce the *NOS3* promoter activity approximately by 50% and has been associated with an increased risk for coronary artery spasm among subjects of Japanese ethnicity. [24] Recently, this polymorphism has also been shown to influence the plasma NO concentrations in hypertensive and type 2 diabetes mellitus patients. [25] It has also has been implicated as a risk factor for developing hypertension. [25] Several published reports strongly suggest that this functional variant in the *NOS3* promoter region (T786-C) is associated with reduction in the promoter efficiency and the level of expressed enzyme, leading to increased CAD risk. [26–28] Apart from hypertension [25,29] and coronary artery spasm, [24] T786-C has also been investigated by several researchers for its association with the presence and severity of CAD, [3,30] and MI. [31] However, some studies have also reported no association with CAD. [32]

There are also several variable number of tandem repeats (VNTRs) with functional significance within *NOS3* gene. Among them polymorphic repeats close to the 5′ end of the gene, the 27-base pair (bp) repeat in intron 4 is one of the most studied. The resulting rare 4-repeat allele has been shown to be associated with CAD among subjects belonging to European ancestry. [33] This 4a/b mutation of *NOS3* gene was found to be associated with MI, among subjects of Turkish descent. [34] Significant association of the 4a/b polymorphism with CAD and MI has been amply reported in several ethnic populations even after adjustment of traditional risk factors. [22,33,35,36] On the other hand, a few groups have also reported lack of association of this SNP with CAD. [37–39]

The only meta-analysis to assess the role of all three *NOS3* SNPs with respect to CAD reported association only in recessive genetic model of Glu298Asp, while dominant and allelic comparisons came out to be non-associated in the pooled analysis (all ethnicities combined). [40] On the other hand, lack of association with CAD was seen for all three genetic models of T786-C and 4b/a. [40] Since the publication of the aforementioned study, [40] a few more recent meta-analyses focusing on either one of the selected SNPs were published reporting varied results of either association or lack of association among different employed genetic models. [41–44] None of them had strict criteria for inclusion of studies, which may have led to inaccurate results. Some of these published meta-analyses also included studies where genotype frequencies among controls deviated from Hardy-Weinberg equilibrium. Such deviation may hint a non-random inclusion of controls among the studies in question, which could have led to inaccurate results. Studies with several surrogate endpoints, such as "coronary artery spasm" and "heart failure", were also included in these previously published meta-analyses. These endpoints may or may not correspond to the disease profile and pathology of CAD in general therefore such studies should have been ideally excluded. On the top of that, ethnic classifications in subgroup analyses were not appropriate in these meta-analyses and the studies were broadly and wrongly classified. We hypothesize that all these described factors may have resulted in biased effect sizes reported in all pooled as well as ethnic subgroups in these previously published meta-analyses. [40–44] It is also noteworthy that no genome wide association study (GWAS) published till date has identified either of these selected SNPs as risk factors for CAD. Thus, a structured meta-analysis of published association studies for *NOS3* polymorphisms, which would aid to improve the existing understanding of these polymorphic forms of this gene in relation to CAD was warranted. Taking this as an objective, we conducted a systematic review and updated meta-analysis to ascertain the role of the three most common *NOS3* gene polymorphisms in CAD. We also tested their association separately among published studies originating predominantly from European, Middle Eastern, Asian, Asian-Indian and African ancestries.

Materials and Methods

Literature Search

The databases of the US National Institutes of Health (PubMed), EMBASE and a MEDLINE Scopus and Web of Knowledge were systematically searched for relevant articles published online by March 2014. Both medical search headings and open text fields were used to identify articles. We systematically searched various databases and the reference lists of the relevant publications using the combination of terms like 'NOS3' OR 'eNOS' OR 'constitutive endothelial NOS' OR 'ecNOS' OR 'endothelial nitric oxide synthase' OR 'endothelial NO synthase' paired with 'atherosclerotic heart disease' OR 'coronary artery disease' OR 'CAD' OR 'MI' OR 'Myocardial Infarction' OR 'AMI' OR Acute Myocardial Infarction OR 'ACS' OR 'Acute Coronary Syndrome' AND 'polymorphism' OR 'mutation' OR 'gene polymorphism' Or 'SNP' OR 'Single Nucleotide Polymorphism'. The search in these databases was restricted to articles relating to humans, covering all relevant English language publications published up to March 2014. All references cited in the resulting studies and in previously published reviews on this topic were examined to identify additional work not indexed in internet databases. Papers without sufficient information were identified and their corresponding authors were contacted via at least three emails (spaced one week apart) requesting needed information. Publications whose corresponding authors did not respond were thenceforth not included. Since data from unpublished studies is unlikely to be trustworthy, we chose not to include it into this present meta-analysis. The decision to include studies was hierarchical; initially study titles, then abstracts and finally the full body of the text were assessed. The following information was recorded from the retrieved studies: author's names, publication year, country where the study was conducted, study design, inclusion criteria for CAD patients and normal controls, methods used for genotyping and the distribution of polymorphic genotypes and alleles in each group.

To be included in the meta-analysis, articles had to assess the association between CAD or MI patients and CAD free controls. Our selection criteria included studies that met all of the following criteria: (1) published in a peer-reviewed journal and independent studies using original data; (2) unrelated case-control or cohort studies; (3) providing complete data with genotype and allele frequencies to calculate the odds ratio (OR) with confidence interval (CI) and p values; (4) CAD patient diagnosis based on coronary angiography/clinical assessment and controls not being CAD patients; (5) all studies included had to be published in English language; and (6) all included studies had to have their genotype distribution among controls consistent with Hardy Weinberg approximations. We excluded the case reports, case studies and the studies not providing adequate information on selection criteria and the actual distribution of genotypes in each group. We also purposefully excluded studies with a surrogate endpoint such as "coronary artery spasm" or "heart failure". Strict adherence to the Preferred Reporting Items for Systematic Reviews and Meta-Analyses-PRISMA statement [45] and the specific recommendations for genetic meta-analysis in the HuGE Review Handbook, version 1.0 was ensured.

Data collection and Statistical Analysis

All required data along with genotypic distribution among cases and controls were recorded from publications (in duplicate) on a paper proforma. Later allele frequency was calculated manually and all the data was then transcribed on to a Microsoft Excel program on a computer. We checked departure from Hardy-Weinberg equilibrium (HWE) among control population for each included study using Michael H. Court's (2005–2008) online calculator (http://www.tufts.edu/~mcourt01/Documents/Court%20lab%20-%20HW%20calculator.xls). Studies with genotype frequency among controls yielding a p value of <0.05, did not conform to HWE approximations and were thus excluded.

All calculations in this meta-analysis were carried out using Review Manager (*RevMan*) [Computer program]. Version 5.3. Copenhagen: The Nordic Cochrane Centre, The Cochrane Collaboration, 2012. The extracted data from all publications were tested using previously described three genetic models i.e. dominant, recessive, and allelic model. [46] Bivariate and random or fixed effect models were used for calculating effect size (i.e. Odds ratios: ORs). For each study, individual and summary ORs and its 95% confidence intervals (CIs) were calculated (for all three genetic models), using either random (DerSimonian-Laird method) [47] or fixed effects model (Mantel-Haenszel method). [48] The pooled odds ratio (OR) with a corresponding 95% confidence interval (CI) was used to assess the degree of association. Based on the individual ORs, the pooled OR was estimated, the significance of which was determined by *Z* test (P<0.05 was considered statistically significant). Summary P value and Z value was also calculated (as listed) for each study group, for each genetic model to express the significance and degree of association. Existence of heterogeneity was tested using a Q test. It was performed using Higgins I^2 statistics (I^2) and Cochran's Q statistics (P_Q) for each group of studies. Those resulting with I^2>50% and P_Q<0.01 were identified as a heterogeneous group. Low, moderate and high heterogeneity was defined according to previously published estimates [49] using cut off points of I^2 values as 25%, 50% and 75%. Using this calculation, I^2 value of <50% and P_Q>0.01 was considered the criterion for selecting fixed effects for analysis. On the other hand, random effects were used for analyses for groups having I^2 values of >50%. In order to define the sources of heterogeneity, subgroup analysis was performed. The subgroups were classified according to predominant ancestry among which the study was conducted. Publication bias was identified by examining Begg's funnel plots [50] and by estimates from the Egger's test. [51] Sensitivity analysis was also performed in each ancestral group in every studied genetic model.

Adjustment of environmental factors is an important aspect in conducting meta-analysis of genetic association studies. However, since genetic variation among individuals is assigned at the time of birth, environmental factors like diet and lifestyle which an individual experiences thenceforth have no role in changing that attribute. [52] These factors, though can have a huge impact over the phenotype, cannot confound to the association between the genotype and the resultant phenotype. It is almost impossible to adjust environmental factors in meta-analyses of this nature. The full data is not available for every included manuscript and we have to work with only the published information. Although in an attempt to adjust the environmental factors, we stratified the studies according to predominant ethnicity among which it was conducted, which was the most we could have done.

Results

The preliminary web search identified a total of 452 potential publications, of which 336 were immediately excluded because of obvious irrelevance after studying their titles and/or abstracts. A total of 116 articles were selected to be reviewed in full text, among which 27 articles were excluded as they met our previously described exclusion criteria. We finally selected 89 articles, which reported 132 separate studies, involving a total sample size of 69,235 to be used in the present meta-analysis. This process is explained in the form of a flowchart in **Figure 1**. The included studies were further broadly classified according to the predominant ancestry among which they were conducted. Accordingly the studies were included in one of the five ancestral groups, viz. European, Middle Eastern, Asian, Asian-Indian or African. The general characteristics of studies classified in each ancestral group, reporting association studies involving any of the three SNPs, along with an estimate of total sample tested are depicted in **Table 1**. Among these included studies, cases were generally recruited in referral centres with documented CAD or MI or ACS, and the controls were without any direct evidence of overt disease. The number of cases among all selected studies varied from 22 to 2,085, while the numbers of controls varied from 21 to 3,918.

Meta-analysis for *NOS3* Glu298Asp polymorphism

Pooled analysis. A total of 60 case control studies [2,3,5,10,11,13–16,18,20–23,28,32,37–39,53–90] investigating the association between Glu298Asp polymorphism and CAD, with a total of 15,957 CAD patients and 14,075 normal controls were included in the pooled analysis (All ancestries combined). (**Tables 1 and 2**) This analysis, using three different genetic models showed moderate to high heterogeneity (I^2 range = 58–72% and P_Q< 0.00001 for all comparisons). (**Table 2**) All three genetic models for Glu298Asp also showed significant association with CAD (OR range = 1.28–1.52, Z value range = 5.14–6.33 and P<0.00001 for all comparisons). (**Table 3 and Figures 2, S1 and S2**)

Subgroup analysis. Among subgroups for Glu298Asp, 17 studies belonged to the European, [2,3,5,15,18,20,21,28,32,37–39,53–65] 14 to the Middle Eastern, [14,16,23,66–76] 10 to the Asian, [10,11,22,77–83] 8 to the Asian-Indian [13,84–90] and 1 to the African [57] group. (**Tables 1 and 2**) The Asian-Indian subgroup in all its genetic models showed low heterogeneity (I^2 range = 18–23% and P_Q range = 0.26–0.28). All other ancestral groups (apart from African which had only 1 study) showed moderate to high heterogeneity (I^2 range = 33–78% and P_Q range = 0.16 to <0.00001). (**Table 2**) Appropriate effects were thus used for further analysis. Four out of 5 ancestral groups (except Africans) showed significant association with CAD in all three genetic models. The Middle Eastern group showed highest levels of association amongst the studied groups (Z value range = 2.92–3.94 and P≤0.004 for all comparisons), followed by European group (Z value range = 2.10–3.37 and P≤0.04 for all comparisons). (**Table 3 and Figures 2, S1 and S2**)

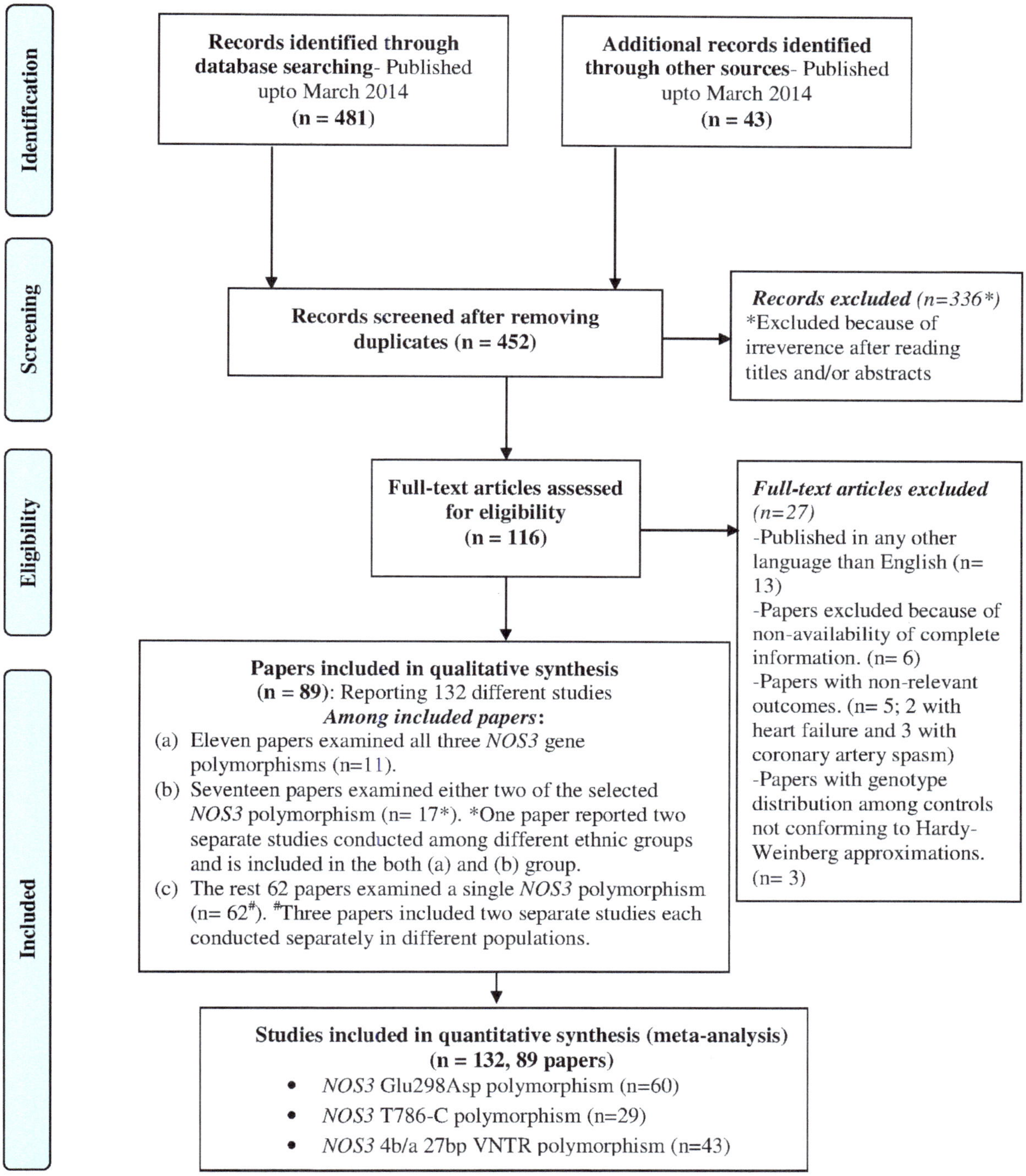

Figure 1. Selection of studies for inclusion.

Meta-analysis for *NOS3* T786-C polymorphism

Pooled analysis. Twenty nine case-control studies [5,17,22,23,27,28,31,32,37,39,54,55,57,58,62,64,65,76,79,82,89–97] with 7,043 CAD patients and 10,409 controls, investigating the association between T786-C polymorphism and CAD were included in the pooled analysis.(**Tables 1 and 2**) Moderate heterogeneity was seen across all genetic models (I^2 range = 35–69%, P_Q range = 0.03 to <0.00001). (**Table 2**) All genetic models also showed significantly associated with CAD showing ORs in the range of 1.34–1.42, Z value ranging from 4.97–5.32 and P values of <0.00001 (for all comparisons). (**Table 3 and Figures 3, S3 and S4**)

Subgroup analysis. Among the ancestral subgroups, 15 studies constituted the European group, [5,27,28,32,37,39,54,55,58,62,64,65,91–93] while 5,6,2 and 1 study respectively constituted Middle Eastern, [17,23,76,94,95] Asian, [22,31,79,82,96,97] Asian-Indian [89,90] and African [57] group. (**Tables 1 and 2**) Moderate to high degree of heterogeneity was seen in almost all ancestral groups

Table 1. Published association studies included in the present meta-analysis.

Study	Year	Country	SNPs studied	MAF (Cases/Controls)			Total sample size (for each SNP)	Outcome
				Glu298Asp	4b/a	T786-C		
EUROPEAN ANCESTRY GROUP								
Wang et al. [33]	1996	Australia	4b/a	-	0.14/0.17	-	702	CAD
Cai et al. [18]	1999	Australia	Glu298Asp	0.32/0.36	-	-	763	CAD
Hingorani et al.(CHAOS) [3]	1999	UK	Glu298Asp	0.48/0.31	-	-	436	CAD
Hingorani et al.(CHAOS-2) [3]	1999	UK	Glu298Asp	0.40/0.31	-	-	432	MI
Poirier et al.(1) [38]	1999	Ireland	Glu298Asp	0.43/0.39	-	-	318	MI
Poirier et al.(2) [38]	1999	France	Glu298Asp	0.34/0.39	-	-	789	MI
Fowkes et al. [99]	2000	UK	4b/a	-	0.16/0.12	-	437	CAD
Pulkkinen et al. [100]	2000	Finland	Glu298Asp, 4b/a	0.32/0.30	0.20/0.16	-	669 for each	CAD
Sigusch et al. [101]	2000	Germany	4b/a	-	0.15/0.17	-	1043	CAD
Alvarez et al. [27]	2001	Spain	4b/a, T786-C	-	0.12/0.14	0.46/0.37	470 for each	PCAD
Granath et al. [37]	2001	Australia	Glu298Asp, 4b/a, T786-C	0.33/0.34	0.14/0.15	0.38/0.38	1194, 1187 and 1196 respectively	PCAD
Gardemann et al. [2]	2002	Germany	Glu298Asp, 4b/a	0.33/0.31	0.14/0.16	-	3250 and 3215 respectively for each	CAD
Colombo et al. [5]	2003	Italy	Glu298Asp, T786-C	0.38/0.31	-	0.51/0.40	415 and 374 respectively for each	CAD
Schmoelzer et al. [20]	2003	Austria	Glu298Asp	0.34/0.31	-	-	488	CAD
Agema et al. [54]	2004	Netherlands	Glu298Asp, 4b/a, T786-C	0.32/0.39	0.15/0.10	0.38/0.36	1329, 1218 and 1096 respectively for each	CAD
Fatini et al. [55]	2004	Italy	Glu298Asp, 4b/a, T786-C	0.39/0/33	0.19/0.15	0.48/0.39	1014 for each	ACS
Letonja et al. [102]	2004	Slovenia	4b/a	-	0.17/0.19	-	260	PCAD
Antoniades et al. [56]	2005	Greece	Glu298Asp	0.36/0.30	-	-	747	MI
Milutinovic et al. [103]	2005	Slovenia	4b/a	-	0.19/0.21	-	403	PCAD
Rao et al.(1) [104]	2005	USA	4b/a	-	0.15/0.14	-	151	CAD
Rios et al. [28]	2005	Brazil	Glu298Asp, T786-C	0.37/0.32	-	0.44/0.34	497 for each	CAD
Dosenko et al. [91]	2006	Ukraine	4b/a, T786-C	-	0.20/0.21	0.34/0.29	304 for each	ACS
Jaramillo et.al. [21]	2006	Chile	Glu298Asp	0.21/0.15	-	-	184	CAD
Rios et al.(1) [57]	2007	Brazil	Glu298Asp, 4b/a	0.29/0.26	0.18/0.23	-	447 for each	CAD
Sampaio et al. [58]	2007	Brazil	Glu298Asp, 4b/a, T786-C	0.31/0.28	0.16/0.19	0.25/0.37	219 for each	PMI
Andrikopoulos et al. [59]	2008	Greece	Glu298Asp	0.33/0.31	-	-	2329	AMI
Jaramillo et al. [92]	2008	Chile	T786-C	-	-	0.24/0.22	221	CAD
Szperl et al. [60]	2008	Poland	Glu298Asp	0.32/0.27	-	-	418	CAD
Vasilakou et al. [61]	2008	Greece	Glu298Asp, 4b/a	0.27/0.30	0.19/0.15	-	370 for each	CAD
Gluba et al. [62]	2009	Poland	Glu298Asp, T786-C	0.50/0.54	-	0.36/0.38	412 for each	PCAD

Table 1. Cont.

Study	Year	Country	SNPs studied	MAF (Cases/Controls)			Total sample size (for each SNP)	Outcome
				Glu298Asp	4b/a	T786-C		
Kincl et al. [105]	2009	Czech republic	4b/a	-	0.18/0.18	-	1161	CAD
Meluzin et al. [93]	2009	Czech republic	4b/a, T786-C	-	0.18/0.15	0.38/0.32	419 for each	CAD
Dafni et al. [15]	2010	Greece	Glu298Asp	0.36/0.29	-	-	422	MI
Isordia-Salas et al. [63]	2010	Mexico	Glu298Asp	0.25/0.14	-	-	360	PMI
Jaramillo et al. [39]	2010	Chile	Glu298Asp, 4b/a, T786-C	0.21/0.18	0.08/0.08	0.24/0.22	224 for each	CAD
Ragia et al. [32]	2010	Greece	Glu298Asp, T786-C	0.31/0.32	-	0.44/0.47	309	CAD
da Costa Escobar Piccoli et al. [64]	2012	Brazil	Glu298Asp, 4b/a, T786-C	0.34/0.26	0.22/0.21	0.36/0.33	241, 240 and 246 respectively for each	ACS
Zigra et al. [65]	2013	Greece	Glu298Asp, T786-C	0.32/0.31	-	0.39/0.19	210	PMI
MIDDLE EASTERN ANCESTRY GROUP								
Aras et al. [66]	2002	Turkey	Glu298Asp	0.33/0.28	-	-	398	CAD
Cine et al. [34]	2002	Turkey	4b/a	-	0.18/0.10	-	513	MI
Afrasyap et al. [67]	2004	Turkey	Glu298Asp	0.34/0.30	-	-	400	CAD
Berdeli et al. [68]	2005	Turkey	Glu298Asp	0.46/0.17	-	-	198	PCAD
Cam et al. [69]	2005	Turkey	Glu298Asp	0.46/0.17	-	-	198	PCAD
Matyar et al. [106]	2005	Turkey	4b/a	-	0.21/0.14	-	266	CAD
Agirbasli et al. [107]	2006	Turkey	4b/a	-	0.14/0.10	-	204	PCAD
Kerkeni et al. [70]	2006	Tunisia	Glu298Asp	0.33/0.22	-	-	220	CAD
Salimi et al. [109]	2006	Iran	4b/a	-	0.17/0.10	-	299	CAD
Tangurek et al. [94]	2006	Turkey	T786-C	-	-	0.37/0.26	211	CAD
Jemaa et al. [110]	2007	Tunisia	4b/a	-	0.22/0.14	-	560	MI
Ciftci et al. [95]	2008	Turkey	T786-C	-	-	0.33/0.19	61	CAD
Alp et al. [23]	2009	Turkey	Glu298Asp, T786-C	0.28/0.25	-	0.29/0.29	268 for each	CAD
Alkharfy et al. [71]	2010	Saudi Arabia	Glu298Asp	0.31/0.19	-	-	287	CAD
Bor-Kucukatay et al. [14]	2010	Turkey	Glu298Asp	0.25/0.18	-	-	157	CAD
Salimi et al. [16]	2010	Iran	Glu298Asp	0.32/0.23	-	-	502	CAD
Agirbasli et al. [108]	2011	Turkey	4b/a	-	0.13/0.15	-	180	PCAD
Motawi et al. [72]	2011	Egypt	Glu298Asp	0.37/0.34	-	-	150	CAD
Gad et al. [73]	2012	Egypt	Glu298Asp	0.27/0.25	-	-	205	AMI
Rahimi et al. [74]	2012	Iran	Glu298Asp	0.26/0.26	-	-	309	CAD
Salimi et al. [17]	2012	Iran	T786-C	-	-	0.33/0.20	502	CAD
Abdel Aziz et al. [75]	2013	Egypt	Glu298Asp	0.39/0.26	-	-	235	PCAD
Ekmekci et al. [111]	2013	Turkey	4b/a	-	0.20/0.09	-	120	PCAD
Kallel et al. [76]	2013	Tunisia	Glu298Asp, 4b/a, T786-C	0.26/0.26	0.22/0.14	0.37/0.35	528 for each	MI

Table 1. Cont.

Study	Year	Country	SNPs studied	MAF (Cases/Controls)			Total sample size (for each SNP)	Outcome
				Glu298Asp	4b/a	T786-C		
ASIAN ANCESTRY GROUP								
Hibi et al. [11]	1998	Japan	Glu298Asp, 4b/a	0.09/0.09	0.12/0.11	-	583 for each	AMI
Ichihara et al. [35]	1998	Japan	4b/a	-	0.14/0.10	-	1005	MI
Odawara et al. [112]	1998	Japan	4b/a	-	013/0.08	-	164	CAD
Shimasaki et al. [10]	1998	Japan	Glu298Asp	0.11/0.07	-	-	892	MI
Nakagami et al. [113]	1999	Japan	4b/a	-	0.25/0.16	-	74	CAD
Nakayama et al. [31]	2000	Japan	T786-C	-	-	0.12/0.04	554	MI
Park et al. [36]	2000	Korea	4b/a	-	0.14/0.12	-	327	AMI
Yoon et al. [77]	2000	Korea	Glu298Asp	0.08/0.07	-	-	238	CAD
Lee et al. [114]	2001	Korea	4b/a	-	0.10/0.12	-	520	CAD
Takagi et al. [96]	2001	Japan	T786-C	-	-	0.12/0.11	4372	MI
Wang et al. [78]	2001	China	Glu298Asp	0.10/0.10	-	-	436	CAD
Hwang et al. [115]	2002	Taiwan	4b/a	-	0.11/0.10	-	219	CAD
Jo et al. [79]	2006	Korea	Glu298Asp, T786-C	0.10/0.09	-	0.16/0.11	932 for each	MI
Kim et al. [22]	2007	Korea	Glu298Asp, 4b/a, T786-C	0.09/0.09	0.13/0.09	0.13/0.09	366, 358 and 367 respectively for each	CAD
Lin et al. [80]	2008	Taiwan	Glu298Asp, 4b/a	0.42/0.22	0.14/0.11	-	198	CVD
Tamemoto et al. [81]	2008	Japan	Glu298Asp	0.18/0.06	-	-	337	CAD
Bae et al. [82]	2010	Korea	Glu298Asp, 4b/a, T786-C	0.09/0.08	0.12/0.09	0.12/0.08	388 for each	CAD
Han et al. [97]	2010	China	T786-C	-	-	0.23/0.15	622	CAD
Min et al. [83]	2010	Korea	Glu298Asp	0.11/0.04	-	-	438	CAD
ASIAN-INDIAN ANCESTRY GROUP								
Mathew et al. [84]	2008	India	Glu298Asp	0.15/0.12	-	-	200	CAD
Angeline et al. [13]	2010	India	Glu298Asp	0.29/0.17	-	-	200	AMI
Bhanushali et al. [85]	2010	India	Glu298Asp	0.18/0.17	-	-	200	CAD
Gururajan et al. [116]	2010	India	4b/a	-	0.28/0.14	-	206	ACS
Saini et al. [86]	2011	India	Glu298Asp	0.12/0.06	-	-	110	CAD
Rai et al. [87]	2012	India	Glu298Asp	0.21/0.17	-	-	427	CAD
Saini et al. [88]	2012	India	Glu298Asp	0.10/0.06	-	-	110	CAD
Arun Kumar et al. [89]	2013	India	Glu298Asp, T786-C	0.15/0.15	-	0.23/0.20	887 for each	MI
Narne et al. [90]	2013	India	Glu298Asp, 4b/a, T786-C	0.21/0.16	0.19/0.19	0.29/0.18	281 for each	CAD
AFRICAN ANCESTRY GROUP								
Hooper et al. [98]	1999	USA	4b/a	-	0.36/0.26	-	295	MI
Rao et al.(2) [104]	2005	USA	4b/a	-	0.36/0.26	-	43	CAD

Table 1. Cont.

Study	Year	Country	SNPs studied	MAF (Cases/Controls)			Total sample size (for each SNP)	Outcome
				Glu298Asp	4b/a	T786-C		
Rios et al.(2) [57]	2007	Brazil	Glu298Asp, 4b/a, T786-C	0.27/0.22	0.21/0.20	0.32/0.22	268 for each	CAD

The studies were grouped according to predominant ancestry among which they were conducted.
Abbreviations used- CAD: Coronary Artery Disease; MI: Myocardial Infarction; AMI: Acute Myocardial Infarction; ACS: Acute Coronary Syndrome; PCAD: Premature CAD; PMI: Premature MI; CVD: Cardiovascular Disease

(except Africans, which had only 1 study), and in amongst almost all comparisons, barring the recessive model amongst the Asians which was rather homogenous (I^2 range = 50–72%, P_Q range = 0.16 to < 0.00001). (**Table 2**) All ancestral subgroups showed significant association in dominant genetic model, similarly all (except Asian-Indians) showed significant association in the allelic model. On the other hand, only Europeans and Asians showed significant association in recessive model. If we disregard the Africans which had only 1 study in its subgroup, Asians showed the highest degree of association consistently in all three models (OR range = 1.61–1.90, Z value range = 2.50–3.56 and P value range = 0.01–0.0004), followed by the Europeans (OR range = 1.21–1.32, Z value range = 2.19–3.96 and P value range = 0.03 to <0.0001). (**Table 3 and Figures 3 S3 and S4**)

Meta-analysis *4b/a (27bp VNTR)* polymorphism

Pooled analysis. Forty three case-control studies, [2,11,22,27,33–37,39,54,55,57,58,61,64,76,80,82,90,91,93,98–116] with 12,477 CAD patients and 9,274 controls analysing the association of 27bp b/a VNTR polymorphism and CAD were included in the pooled analysis. (**Table 2**) Low to moderate heterogeneity was seen among the three genetic models (I^2 = 17–61%, P_Q = 0.17 to <0.00001). (**Table 2**) However, all three genetic models consistently showed significant association with CAD (OR range = 1.19–1.41, Z value range = 3.11–3.99, P≤0.002 for all comparisons). (**Table 3 and Figures 4, S5 and S6**)

Subgroup analysis. A total of 20 studies from European, [2,27,33,37,39,54,55,57,58,61,64,91,93,99–105] 8 from Middle Eastern, [34,76,106–111] 10 from Asian, [11,22,35,36,80,82,112–115] 2 from Asian-Indian [90,116] and 3 from African [57,98,104] group were included for subgroup analysis. (**Table 2**) Middle Eastern, Asian and African groups showed considerably low heterogeneity among the three genetic models (I^2 *range* = 0–33%; P_Q range = 0.18–0.83), while European and Asian-Indian groups showed very low to very high heterogeneity (I^2 *range* = 0–87%; P_Q range = 0.72–0.005). (**Table 2**) The Middle Eastern and Asian groups showed significant association in all three models. It is however noteworthy that the Middle Eastern subgroup showed stronger association (OR range = 1.71–3.02, Z value range = 4.65–7.09, P<0.0001 for all comparisons) than the Asian subgroup (OR range = 1.22–2.48, Z value range = 2.45–3.06, P≤0.01 for all comparisons) consistently in all three models. African group showed moderate association limited only to recessive and allelic models (OR range = 1.37–2.02, Z value range = 2.07–2.34, P≤ 0.02), whereas Asian-Indian group showed marginal association in only the recessive genetic model (OR = 2.63, Z value = 1.99, P value = 0.05). The European group however showed no association in any of the three genetic models (P>0.05). (**Table 3 and Figures 4, S5 and S6**)

Source of heterogeneity

Higher degree of heterogeneity was seen amongst almost all ancestral groups (except Asian-Indians) in all comparisons for Glu298Asp polymorphism. All groups were fairly heterogeneous in all comparisons for T786-C polymorphism. Fairly low heterogeneity was seen amongst Middle Eastern and Asian groups in all comparisons for 4b/a polymorphism. (**Table 2**) Environmental factors like diet, exercise etc. could be the probable reasons behind seen heterogeneity among the groups. We did all we could by classifying studies into five broad subgroups, based on predominant ancestry, in order to determine sources of heterogeneity. Further classification would have only made the samples in each subgroup smaller and their results impotent. (**Table 2**)

Table 2. Basic characteristics of the studied groups classified according to predominant ancestries.

	Heterogeneity (I^2; P_Q)			Number of Studies	Cases (n)/Controls (n)	Total sample
	*Dominant genetic model**	*Recessive genetic model***	*Allelic genetic model****			
Glu298Asp polymorphism						
All ancestries combined	65%; <0.00001	58%; <0.00001	72%; <0.00001	60	15,957/14,075	30,032
European ancestry group	52%; 0.0008	63%; <0.00001	69%; <0.00001	27	10,738/7,748	18,486
Middle Eastern ancestry group	64%; 0.0005	65%; 0.0005	77%; <0.00001	14	2,303/1,752	4,055
Asian ancestry group	78%; <0.00001	33%; 0.16	68%; 0.0008	10	1,649/3,159	4,808
Asian-Indian ancestry group	18%; 0.28	23%; 0.26	21%; 0.27	8	1,120/1,295	2,415
African ancestry group	-	-	-	1	147/121	268
T786-C polymorphism						
All ancestries combined	66%; <0.00001	35%; 0.03	69%; <0.00001	29	7,043/10,409	17,452
European ancestry group	71%; <0.00001	38%; 0.07	72%; <0.00001	15	3,977/3,234	7,211
Middle Eastern ancestry group	50%; 0.09	68%; 0.01	70%; 0.009	5	879/691	1,570
Asian ancestry group	67%; 0.009	0%; 0.69	68%; 0.009	6	1,593/5,642	7,235
Asian-Indian ancestry group	50%; 0.16	70%; 0.07	69%; 0.07	2	447/721	1,168
African ancestry group	-	-	-	1	147/121	268
4b/a polymorphism						
All ancestries combined	60%; <0.00001	17%; 0.17	61%; <0.00001	43	12,477/9,274	21,751
European ancestry group	51%; 0.005	0%; 0.72	47%; 0.01	20	8,779/5,373	14,152
Middle Eastern ancestry group	0%; 0.83	0%; 0.66	0%; 0.80	8	1,356/1,314	2,670
Asian ancestry group	28%; 0.18	0%; 0.72	0%; 0.50	10	1,797/2,039	3,836
Asian-Indian ancestry group	87%; 0.005	0%; 0.65	87%; 0.005	2	266/221	487
African ancestry group	33%; 0.22	0%; 0.58	0%; 0.37	3	279/327	606

Abbreviations: P_Q: Cochran's Q statistics; I^2: Higgin's I^2 statistics.
*Dominant genetic model for Glu298Asp: *TT+GT vs. GG;* for T786-C: *CC+CT vs. TT;* for 4b/a: *4a4a+4a4b vs. 4b4b.*
**Recessive genetic model for Glu298Asp: *TT vs. GG+GT;* for T786-C: *CC vs. TT+CT;* for 4b/a: *4a4a vs. 4a4b+4b4b.*
***Allelic genetic model for Glu298Asp: *Allele T vs. G;* for T786-C: *Allele C vs. T;* for 4b/a: *Allele 4a vs. 4b.*
Notes: Heterogeneity was tested among groups of studies using Higgin's I^2 statistics and Cochran's Q statistics (P_Q). Group showing I^2>50% and P_Q<0.01 were considered heterogeneous, others were considered homogenous.

Potential publication Bias

Potential publication bias among groups of studies for each SNP was assessed by two different statistical tests, viz. Egger's plots [51] and Begg's funnel plots. [50] The recessive genetic model showed least heterogeneity for all three SNPs among all ethnic groups (as seen in **Table 2**), its data was thus selected to generate Egger's plots. No asymmetry in plots was seen for Glu298Asp or 4b/a for the pooled group or any of its ancestral subgroups. Egger's P values for Glu298Asp were 0.56, 0.11, 0.08, 0.42 and 0.56 respectively for pooled and European, Middle Eastern, Asian and Asian Indian subgroups. Similarly Egger's P values for 4b/a were 0.79, 0.15, 0.85, 0.92, 0.88 for pooled and European, Middle Eastern, Asian and African subgroups. Owing to less number of studies (n<3), no P value from Egger's test was generated in African subgroup of Glu298Asp and Asian-Indian subgroup of 4/a polymorphism. In case of T786-C, Egger's plot asymmetry was however seen for pooled (P = 0.002) and European (P = 0.004) subgroup. Rest of the two subgroups showed either symmetry in their plots (P = 0.71 and 0.91 for Middle Eastern and Asian groups respectively) or were their p values was incalculable (i.e. for Asian-Indian and African groups).

Begg's funnel plots, [50] were also generated to assess potential publication bias for each SNP in their three genetic models. Funnel plots are provided for pooled analysis obtained in allelic comparisons for all three studied polymorphisms. (**Figure 5-A, B, C**) Plots for dominant and recessive models for all three SNPs are also provided as (**Figures S7-A, B; S8-A, B; S9-A, B**). Each point in the figure represents OR of a study plotted against standard error (SE) of OR of that particular study. Different indicators of the studies belonging to each ancestry are used in these plots where they are seen to be generally contained within the inverted cone, indicating no significant publication bias, at least in the pooled analyses.

Sensitivity Analysis

Sensitivity analysis was performed in each study group in every genetic model, where we excluded studies one after another and conducted the analysis after each omission. The results in none of the groups and studied genetic models altered substantially to change the results from no association to significant association or the other way around (in groups of ≥5 studies). This indicates that the present meta-analysis is robust in nature.

Discussion

The present meta-analysis and structured systematic review is the most comprehensive till date and comprises of published studies which investigated the association of three most common

Study or Subgroup	Cases Events	Cases Total	Controls Events	Controls Total	Weight	Odds Ratio M-H, Random, 95% CI	Year
3.1.1 European ancestry group							
Cai et al.	389	1210	114	316	2.1%	0.84 [0.65, 1.09]	1999
Poirier et al.(1)	140	326	122	310	1.9%	1.16 [0.85, 1.59]	1999
Hingorani et al.(CHAOS)	285	596	86	276	1.9%	2.02 [1.50, 2.74]	1999
Hingorani et al.(CHAOS-2)	197	498	113	366	2.0%	1.47 [1.10, 1.95]	1999
Poirier et al.(2)	254	736	327	842	2.3%	0.83 [0.68, 1.02]	1999
Pulkkinen et al.	355	1118	67	220	1.9%	1.06 [0.78, 1.45]	2000
Granath et al.	374	1142	419	1246	2.4%	0.96 [0.81, 1.14]	2001
Gardemann et al.	1395	4170	719	2330	2.5%	1.13 [1.01, 1.26]	2002
Colombo et al.	202	536	92	294	1.9%	1.33 [0.98, 1.80]	2003
Schmoelzer et al.	164	480	152	496	2.0%	1.17 [0.90, 1.54]	2003
Agema et al.	491	1510	446	1148	2.4%	0.76 [0.65, 0.89]	2004
Fatini et al.	371	954	359	1074	2.3%	1.27 [1.06, 1.52]	2004
Antoniades et al.	163	456	311	1038	2.2%	1.30 [1.03, 1.64]	2005
Rios et al.	162	438	178	556	2.1%	1.25 [0.96, 1.62]	2005
Jaramillo et al.(1)	47	224	22	144	1.2%	1.47 [0.84, 2.57]	2006
Rios et al.(1)	173	602	76	292	1.9%	1.15 [0.84, 1.57]	2007
Sampaio et al.	72	230	59	208	1.6%	1.15 [0.76, 1.74]	2007
Vasilakou et al.	115	418	96	322	1.9%	0.89 [0.65, 1.23]	2008
Andrikopoulos et al.	1059	3204	453	1454	2.5%	1.09 [0.95, 1.25]	2008
Szperl et al.	97	302	144	534	1.9%	1.28 [0.94, 1.74]	2008
Gluba et al.	158	556	83	268	1.9%	0.88 [0.64, 1.22]	2009
Jaramillo et al.(2)	47	224	40	224	1.4%	1.22 [0.76, 1.95]	2010
Dafni et al.	148	408	125	436	2.0%	1.42 [1.06, 1.89]	2010
Isordia-Salas et al.	90	360	50	360	1.7%	2.07 [1.41, 3.03]	2010
Ragia et al.	97	308	100	310	1.8%	0.97 [0.69, 1.35]	2010
da Costa Escobar Piccoli et al.	88	256	58	226	1.6%	1.52 [1.02, 2.25]	2012
Zigra et al.	68	214	64	206	1.6%	1.03 [0.68, 1.56]	2013
Subtotal (95% CI)		**21476**		**15496**	**52.6%**	**1.15 [1.05, 1.26]**	
Total events	7201		4875				
Heterogeneity: Tau² = 0.03; Chi² = 83.64, df = 26 (P < 0.00001); I² = 69%							
Test for overall effect: Z = 3.08 (P = 0.002)							
3.1.2 Middle Eastern ancestry group							
Aras et al.	183	562	66	234	1.8%	1.23 [0.88, 1.72]	2002
Afrasyap et al.	169	500	90	300	1.9%	1.19 [0.87, 1.62]	2004
Berdeli et al.	105	230	28	166	1.3%	4.14 [2.56, 6.70]	2005
Cam et al.	105	230	28	166	1.3%	4.14 [2.56, 6.70]	2005
Kerkeni et al.	66	200	53	240	1.5%	1.74 [1.14, 2.66]	2006
Alp et al.	81	292	62	244	1.6%	1.13 [0.77, 1.66]	2009
Salimi et al.	155	482	118	522	2.0%	1.62 [1.23, 2.15]	2010
Bor-Kucukatay et al.	42	166	27	148	1.2%	1.52 [0.88, 2.62]	2010
Alkharfy et al.	87	284	54	290	1.6%	1.93 [1.31, 2.85]	2010
Motawi et al.	74	200	34	100	1.3%	1.14 [0.69, 1.89]	2011
Rahimi et al.	108	414	53	204	1.7%	1.01 [0.69, 1.47]	2012
Gad et al.	57	208	50	202	1.5%	1.15 [0.74, 1.78]	2012
Kallel et al.	158	606	116	450	2.0%	1.02 [0.77, 1.34]	2013
Abdel-Aziz et al.	90	232	63	238	1.6%	1.76 [1.19, 2.60]	2013
Subtotal (95% CI)		**4606**		**3504**	**22.4%**	**1.54 [1.24, 1.91]**	
Total events	1480		842				
Heterogeneity: Tau² = 0.13; Chi² = 56.72, df = 13 (P < 0.00001); I² = 77%							
Test for overall effect: Z = 3.94 (P < 0.0001)							
3.1.3 Asian ancestry group							
Hibi et al.	42	452	62	714	1.6%	1.08 [0.71, 1.62]	1998
Shimasaki et al.	61	570	82	1214	1.8%	1.65 [1.17, 2.34]	1998
Yoon et al.	17	220	18	256	0.9%	1.11 [0.56, 2.20]	2000
Wang et al.	42	436	44	436	1.5%	0.95 [0.61, 1.48]	2001
Jo et al.	27	258	141	1606	1.5%	1.21 [0.79, 1.88]	2006
Kim et al.	28	294	38	438	1.3%	1.11 [0.66, 1.85]	2007
Tamemoto et al.	19	108	36	566	1.1%	3.14 [1.73, 5.72]	2008
Lin et al.	101	240	35	156	1.4%	2.51 [1.59, 3.96]	2008
Min et al.	36	336	20	540	1.1%	3.12 [1.77, 5.49]	2010
Bae et al.	36	384	33	392	1.3%	1.13 [0.69, 1.85]	2010
Subtotal (95% CI)		**3298**		**6318**	**13.4%**	**1.51 [1.15, 1.98]**	
Total events	409		509				
Heterogeneity: Tau² = 0.13; Chi² = 28.34, df = 9 (P = 0.0008); I² = 68%							
Test for overall effect: Z = 3.00 (P = 0.003)							
3.1.4 Asian-Indian ancestry group							
Mathew et al.	30	200	24	200	1.1%	1.29 [0.73, 2.30]	2008
Bhanushali et al.	37	200	35	200	1.3%	1.07 [0.64, 1.78]	2010
Angeline et al.	58	200	35	200	1.4%	1.93 [1.20, 3.10]	2010
Saini et al.(1)	15	120	6	100	0.5%	2.24 [0.83, 6.00]	2011
Rai et al.	104	506	60	348	1.8%	1.24 [0.87, 1.77]	2012
Saini et al.(2)	12	120	6	100	0.5%	1.74 [0.63, 4.82]	2012
Narne et al.	66	320	39	242	1.5%	1.35 [0.87, 2.09]	2013
Arun Kumar et al.	86	574	186	1200	2.0%	0.96 [0.73, 1.27]	2013
Subtotal (95% CI)		**2240**		**2590**	**10.0%**	**1.26 [1.05, 1.53]**	
Total events	408		391				
Heterogeneity: Tau² = 0.01; Chi² = 8.82, df = 7 (P = 0.27); I² = 21%							
Test for overall effect: Z = 2.44 (P = 0.01)							
3.1.5 African ancestry group							
Rios et al.(2)	81	294	54	242	1.6%	1.32 [0.89, 1.97]	2007
Subtotal (95% CI)		**294**		**242**	**1.6%**	**1.32 [0.89, 1.97]**	
Total events	81		54				
Heterogeneity: Not applicable							
Test for overall effect: Z = 1.39 (P = 0.17)							
Total (95% CI)		**31914**		**28150**	**100.0%**	**1.29 [1.19, 1.40]**	
Total events	9579		6671				
Heterogeneity: Tau² = 0.06; Chi² = 211.48, df = 59 (P < 0.00001); I² = 72%							
Test for overall effect: Z = 6.33 (P < 0.00001)							
Test for subgroup differences: Chi² = 8.84, df = 4 (P = 0.07), I² = 54.8%							

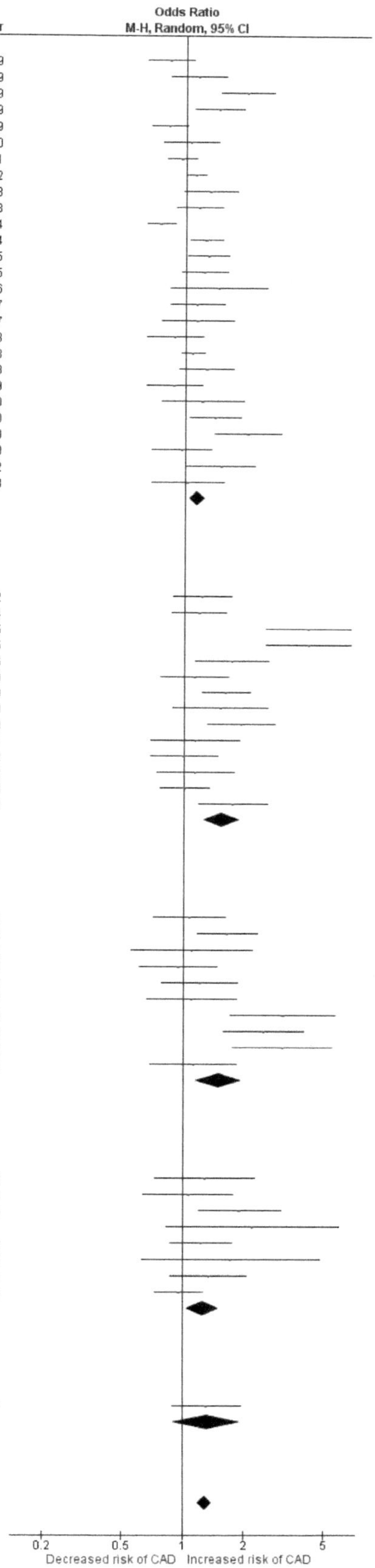

Figure 2. Forest plot depicting results after analyses for the allelic model *(Allele T vs. G)* of *NOS3* Glu298Asp polymorphism. Effect size estimates for all ancestral groups in this plot were obtained using random effects for analysis. Effect size using fixed effects was recalculated for Asian-Indian group which showed homogenous distribution among its included studies. Recalculated effect size estimate for Asian-Indians was, OR, 95%CI = 1.23, 1.05–1.44; Z = 2.59; P = 0.01.

NOS3 gene polymorphisms, (i.e. Glu298Asp, 4b/a and T786-C) with CAD.

All comparisons in the pooled analysis for all three SNPs indicated significant association with CAD. The pooled results of Glu298Asp suggested that the presence of even a single T allele in a genotype effects in an increased risk of CAD. The risk of CAD is even higher if the genotype contains more than 1, T allele. This association is evident by the obtained pooled OR in allelic comparison (OR = 1.29, Z value = 6.33 and $p<0.00001$). (**Table 3 and Figure 2**) The same pattern of association is seen for almost all the ancestral groups (except Africans), where generally higher ORs are seen in recessive models as compared to their dominant models. (**Table 3 and Figures S1 and S2**) Consistent to the seen pattern, the T allele also showed a significant association with CAD in almost all ancestral groups, barring the Africans which had only 1 study. (**Table 3 and Figure 2**) In the case of T786-C polymorphism, our pooled as well as subgroup results also suggested an increased risk in genotypes carrying the minor (C) allele. All three genetic models showed significant association in the pooled analysis. Significant association was also seen in all ancestral subgroups in at least two out of three genetic models. As in the case of Glu298Asp, the risk increased in genotypes of T786-C, which were homozygous to the C allele. However, contrary to the trends seen in case of Glu298Asp and 4b/a, we observed that for T786-C, Asians followed by Europeans showed highest degree of associations across all three genetic models. (**Table 3 and Figure 3**) The presence of 4a allele of 4b/a polymorphism resulted in an increased risk for CAD in the pooled analysis (OR = 1.20) and specifically among two ancestral groups viz. Middle Eastern (OR = 1.71) and Asian (OR = 1.25). (**Table 3 and Figure 4**) Here too, genotypes carrying >1, 4a alleles showed notably higher risk in pooled analysis as well as in the Middle Eastern and Asian subgroups. The pooled as well as the Middle Eastern and Asian subgroups also showed significant association in the allelic model. As far as the 4b/a polymorphism is concerned, Africans showed significant association in recessive and allelic model, while Asian-Indians showed a hint of association in the recessive model. (**Table 3 and Figures 4, S5 and S6**)

Our pooled analysis showed significant associations of all three selected SNPs with CAD in every employed genetic model. Our results are in contrast to the previously published meta-analysis (for all three selected SNPs), [40] which was not able to deduce any significant associations for T786-C and 4b/a and only showed significant association for Glu298Asp under dominant genetic model. One reason for the difference in the results of the present study and the study by Li et al., [40] can be the sheer number of studies included. Since the year 2010 when the study by Li et al. [40] was published, a number of studies came out in the public domain among which several of them reported statistically significant associations. This previous meta-analysis [40] included a much lesser number of studies, thus making the present study a more comprehensive one (56 vs. 132 studies in previous vs. present study respectively). Several other recent meta-analyses which assessed either one of the three *NOS3* SNPs are also now into public domain. [41–44] The pooled analysis for Glu298Asp in the meta-analysis by Tian et al., [43] reported significant associations in dominant (OR = 1.17), recessive (OR = 1.59) and allelic (OR = 1.26) models which are somewhat comparable to those deduced in our study. In the meta-analysis by Tian et al. [43], the Asian subgroup for Glu298Asp showed significant association to CHD in all employed genetic models, the effect sizes of which are similar to those deduced for the Asian subgroup in the present study. There is also a meta-analysis by Zhang et al., [41] who reported significant association (with OR = 1.52), in allelic comparisons of Glu298Asp among Asians, the effect size of which is similar to that deduced in our study (OR = 1.51). We also obtained similar results for Asian subgroup with another previously published meta-analysis for T786-C [42]. In fact our study can be considered as an improvement on all the previously published meta-analyses on polymorphic forms of *NOS3* gene and CAD, [40–44] not only in the terms of higher number of studies included but also in terms of better classification of ancestral groups and assessment of their individual risk. This allowed us to unravel the degree of associations among several other important ancestral groups such as Middle Easterners and Asian-Indians apart from Europeans and Asians which were already amply investigated by several previously published meta-analyses.

There are basically two major merits of the present study which makes it superior to all previously published meta-analyses on this subject. [40–44] Firstly, our study is the most comprehensive till date and we ended up including most number of individual studies which transcribed into the largest sample size ever studied for each of the three *NOS3* SNPs. Secondly, our study had strict inclusion/exclusion criteria, and we excluded studies with surrogate endpoints, and omitted studies in which controls did not conform to HWE proportions (most of which were included in previously published meta-analyses). This methodology ensured that we eliminated studies with potentially biased/inaccurate results, thus possibly presenting a real picture.

The biochemical basis of the association of CAD with various *NOS3* gene polymorphisms has been studied in detail by several researchers. Most schools of thought suggest that all these SNPs of *NOS3* gene viz. Glu298Asp, T786-C and 4b/a 27bp VNTR via various mechanisms affect the serum nitrite/nitrate (NO_x) concentrations in the human body. Over a period of time this imbalance in NO_x concentrations results in "endothelial dysfunction" which finally blooms into an overt form of CAD. It is plausible that this degree of association with CAD and the resulting NO_x concentrations are affected by gene-gene, gene-environment interactions. Compensatory mechanism of the human body against CAD may also increase NO secretion from the vascular endothelium during sudden reperfusion after acute coronary syndromes. [117,118] Therefore it remains unclear whether the increase in NO levels is a "cause" or an "effect" of acute coronary syndromes. Clearly the association between these SNPs and CAD, probably also has different biochemical basis rather than solely brought about by variations in NO_x concentrations.

Positive association of Glu298Asp with CAD/MI has been reported over the years in several published studies. We found that along with a significant association for all three genetic models in our pooled analysis, this SNP seen to be associated with CAD separately among all ancestral groups, with the highest degree of association seen amongst the Middle Easterners.(**Table 3 and Figures 2, S1 and S2**) The reason of this differential risk of CAD seen among different ancestral groups carrying this

Table 3. Meta-analysis results for *NOS3* gene polymorphisms.

	*Dominant genetic model**		*Recessive genetic model***		*Allelic genetic model****	
	OR, 95% CI	**Z; P value**	**OR, 95% CI**	**Z; P value**	**OR, 95% CI**	**Z; P value**
Glu298Asp polymorphism						
All ancestries combined	1.28, 1.17-1.40	5.34; <0.00001	1.52, 1.30-1.79	5.14; <0.00001	1.29, 1.19-1.40	6.33; <0.00001
European ancestry group	1.11, 1.01–1.22	2.10; 0.04	1.36, 1.14–1.63	3.37; 0.0007	1.15, 1.05–1.26	3.08; 0.002
Middle Eastern ancestry group	1.55, 1.25–1.93	3.94; <0.0001	1.87, 1.23–2.85	2.92; 0.004	1.54, 1.24–1.91	3.94; <0.0001
Asian ancestry group	1.60, 1.12–2.29	2.56; 0.01	2.22, 1.21–4.08[F]	2.57; 0.01[F]	1.51, 1.15–1.98	3.00; 0.003
Asian-Indian ancestry group	1.21, 1.01–1.45[F]	2.07; 0.04[F]	1.85, 1.12–3.04[F]	2.42; 0.02[F]	1.23, 1.05–1.44[F]	2.59; 0.01[F]
African ancestry group	1.22, 0.75–1.99	0.81; 0.42	2.84, 0.90–8.94	1.78; 0.07	1.32, 0.89–1.97	1.39; 0.17
T786-C polymorphism						
All ancestries combined	1.42, 1.25–1.62	5.24; <0.00001	1.36, 1.20–1.53[F]	4.97; <0.00001[F]	1.34, 1.20–1.49	5.32; <0.00001
European ancestry group	1.25, 1.02–1.52	2.19; 0.03	1.32, 1.15–1.52[F]	3.96; <0.0001[F]	1.21, 1.05–1.40	2.56; 0.01
Middle Eastern ancestry group	1.59, 1.16–2.18	2.91; 0.004	1.35, 0.69–2.65	0.87; 0.38	1.43, 1.04–1.97	2.20; 0.03
Asian ancestry group	1.67, 1.26–2.23	3.51; 0.0004	1.90, 1.15–3.14[F]	2.50; 0.01[F]	1.61, 1.24–2.10	3.56; 0.0004
Asian-Indian ancestry group	1.53, 1.04–2.26	2.16; 0.03	1.73, 0.38–7.95	0.71; 0.48	1.44, 0.95–2.18	1.71; 0.09
African ancestry group	1.91, 1.17–3.12	2.58; 0.010	1.85, 0.77–4.44	1.37; 0.17	1.70, 1.15–2.52	2.67; 0.008
4b/a polymorphism						
All ancestries combined	1.19, 1.07–1.32	3.11; 0.002	1.41, 1.19–1.67[F]	3.99; <0.0001[F]	1.20, 1.09–1.32	3.77; 0.0002
European ancestry group	1.00, 0.89–1.13	0.06; 0.95	1.03, 0.83–1.26[F]	0.24; 0.81[F]	0.99, 0.93–1.06[F]	0.19; 0.85[F]
Middle Eastern ancestry group	1.73, 1.46–2.05[F]	6.28; <0.00001[F]	3.02, 1.90–4.81[F]	4.65; <0.00001[F]	1.71, 1.47–1.98[F]	7.09; <0.00001[F]
Asian ancestry group	1.22, 1.04–1.42[F]	2.45; 0.01[F]	2.48, 1.38–4.47[F]	3.03; 0.002[F]	1.25, 1.08–1.44[F]	3.06; 0.002[F]
Asian-Indian ancestry group	1.57, 0.53–4.64	0.82; 0.41	2.63, 1.02–6.82[F]	1.99; 0.05[F]	1.56, 0.62–3.94	0.94; 0.35
African ancestry group	1.37, 0.99–1.90[F]	1.87; 0.06[F]	2.02, 1.04–3.91[F]	2.07; 0.04[F]	1.37, 1.05–1.78[F]	2.34; 0.02[F]

Abbreviations: OR, 95% CI: Odds Ratio with its 95% Confidence Interval; [F]: Results derived using Fixed effects for analysis. Random effects were used for all other calculations.
*Dominant genetic model for Glu298Asp: *TT+GT vs. GG;* for T786-C: *CC+CT vs. TT;* for 4b/a: *4a4a+4a4b vs. 4b4b.*
**Recessive genetic model for Glu298Asp: *TT vs. GG+GT;* for T786-C: *CC vs. TT+CT;* for 4b/a: *4a4a vs. 4a4b+4b4b.*
***Allelic genetic model for Glu298Asp: *Allele T vs. G;* for T786-C: *Allele C vs. T;* for 4b/a: *Allele 4a vs. 4b.*

polymorphism is unknown and should be investigated upon. We presume that this difference could had been brought about by the variance in Asp allele frequency (range = 0.04-0.39), as well as several known and unknown gene-gene and gene-environment interactions. The biochemical basis of the association of CAD with Asp allele carriers has although been extensively studied upon however a clear consensus is still lacking. Some studies have reported an association of this SNP with intracellular NO concentration. [12] The mechanism by which the Asp allele possibly reduces NO bioavailability in the human body has also been hypothesized. It has been suggested that the Asp298 is subjected to selective proteolytic cleavage in the endothelial cells and vascular tissues. [119,120] The resultant cleaved fragments especially among the homozygous mutants of this SNP are expected to lack NO synthase activity [13] thus reducing bioavailability of NO in the body. [119,120] Contrary to this notion several studies [13,14,67] have reported lack of association of plasma NO_x concentrations with any of the genotypes or alleles for this SNP. Also, since these associations are often masked, as it is affected by several physiological and pathological conditions, the real effect of *NOS3* gene on plasma NO_x levels is hard to determine. [14] As already discussed genotypes carrying Asp alleles impart greater RBC aggregability. [14] Genotypes having Asp alleles have also been shown to have (i) a reduced blood pressure fall after exercise training, [121] (ii) an enhanced systemic presser response to phenylephrine [12] (iii) lower basal blood flow and reduced vasodilation to adenosine in coronary arteries [122] and (iv) a reduced flow-mediated dilatation of the brachial artery, [123] making them more prone to suffer from coronary events. It is possible that these effects coupled with possible modulation in bioavailability of NO in presence of interactions with other genes and environmental factors may accelerate the process of endothelial dysfunction and subsequent emergence of overt CAD among Asp variants of the *NOS3* gene.

The T786-C gene variant of *NOS3* has also been implicated over the years with CAD occurrence by several investigators. Along with a significant association among all three genetic models in our pooled analysis, Asians seemed to have strongest association with CAD than other ancestral groups. (**Table 3, Figure 3, S3 and S4**) The reason behind this dissimilar degree of association among these ancestral groups is unknown. More in depth studies are warranted to answer this pertinent question. In vitro reporter gene assays performed by Nakayama et al., [24] somewhat explained the possible functional effect of this SNP. They demonstrated that T786-C mutation reduces the promoter activity by as high as 50%, suggesting that in several C allele carriers the L-arginine/NO pathway does not function properly, reducing NO concentrations and causing endothelial dysfunction. [24] Other studies have also shown lower *NOS3* mRNA and serum NO_x levels in genotypes with ≥1, 786C alleles, [26] although contradictory results have also been published. [124] Apart from lower NOx concentrations [26], synergistic effect of *NOS3* Glu298Asp and T786-C polymorphism has also been reported

Study or Subgroup	Cases Events	Cases Total	Controls Events	Controls Total	Weight	Odds Ratio M-H, Random, 95% CI	Year
3.1.1 European ancestry group							
Granath et al.	439	1146	471	1246	4.9%	1.02 [0.87, 1.21]	2001
Alvarez et al.	155	340	223	600	4.1%	1.42 [1.08, 1.86]	2001
Colombo et al.	240	472	111	276	3.8%	1.54 [1.14, 2.08]	2003
Agema et al.	539	1418	280	774	4.8%	1.08 [0.90, 1.30]	2004
Fatini et al.	461	954	416	1074	4.8%	1.48 [1.24, 1.76]	2004
Rios et al.	194	438	187	556	4.2%	1.57 [1.21, 2.03]	2005
Dosenko et al.	152	442	48	166	3.2%	1.29 [0.87, 1.90]	2006
Sampaio et al.	57	230	77	208	3.1%	0.56 [0.37, 0.85]	2007
Jaramillo et al.(1)	54	224	49	218	2.9%	1.10 [0.70, 1.70]	2008
Meluzin et al.	274	724	36	114	3.0%	1.32 [0.86, 2.01]	2009
Gluba et al.	116	556	58	268	3.4%	0.95 [0.67, 1.36]	2009
Jaramillo et al.(2)	54	224	50	224	2.9%	1.11 [0.71, 1.71]	2010
Ragia et al.	137	308	147	310	3.7%	0.89 [0.65, 1.22]	2010
da Costa Escobar Piccoli et al.	95	264	76	228	3.3%	1.12 [0.77, 1.63]	2012
Zigra et al.	83	214	39	206	2.8%	2.71 [1.74, 4.23]	2013
Subtotal (95% CI)		**7954**		**6468**	**54.8%**	**1.21 [1.05, 1.40]**	
Total events	3050		2268				
Heterogeneity: Tau² = 0.05; Chi² = 50.41, df = 14 (P < 0.00001); I² = 72%							
Test for overall effect: Z = 2.56 (P = 0.01)							
3.1.2 Middle Eastern ancestry group							
Tangurek et al.	119	318	27	104	2.5%	1.71 [1.04, 2.79]	2006
Ciftci et al.	20	60	12	62	1.3%	2.08 [0.91, 4.77]	2008
Alp et al.	84	292	70	244	3.3%	1.00 [0.69, 1.46]	2009
Salimi et al.	158	482	104	522	4.0%	1.96 [1.47, 2.61]	2012
Kallel et al.	222	606	156	450	4.2%	1.09 [0.84, 1.41]	2013
Subtotal (95% CI)		**1758**		**1382**	**15.3%**	**1.43 [1.04, 1.97]**	
Total events	603		369				
Heterogeneity: Tau² = 0.09; Chi² = 13.46, df = 4 (P = 0.009); I² = 70%							
Test for overall effect: Z = 2.20 (P = 0.03)							
3.1.3 Asian ancestry group							
Nakayama et al.	87	718	16	390	2.3%	3.22 [1.86, 5.58]	2000
Tagaki et al.	107	908	834	7836	4.5%	1.12 [0.91, 1.39]	2001
Jo et al.	40	258	170	1606	3.3%	1.55 [1.07, 2.25]	2006
Kim et al.	39	294	38	440	2.7%	1.62 [1.01, 2.60]	2007
Han et al.	144	624	92	620	3.9%	1.72 [1.29, 2.30]	2010
Bae et al.	45	384	32	392	2.6%	1.49 [0.93, 2.41]	2010
Subtotal (95% CI)		**3186**		**11284**	**19.3%**	**1.61 [1.24, 2.10]**	
Total events	462		1182				
Heterogeneity: Tau² = 0.07; Chi² = 15.44, df = 5 (P = 0.009); I² = 68%							
Test for overall effect: Z = 3.56 (P = 0.0004)							
3.1.4 Asian-Indian ancestry group							
Arun Kumar et al.	134	574	243	1200	4.3%	1.20 [0.94, 1.52]	2013
Narne et al.	93	320	44	242	3.1%	1.84 [1.23, 2.77]	2013
Subtotal (95% CI)		**894**		**1442**	**7.4%**	**1.44 [0.95, 2.18]**	
Total events	227		287				
Heterogeneity: Tau² = 0.06; Chi² = 3.20, df = 1 (P = 0.07); I² = 69%							
Test for overall effect: Z = 1.71 (P = 0.09)							
3.1.5 African ancestry group							
Rios et al.(2)	95	294	53	242	3.2%	1.70 [1.15, 2.52]	2007
Subtotal (95% CI)		**294**		**242**	**3.2%**	**1.70 [1.15, 2.52]**	
Total events	95		53				
Heterogeneity: Not applicable							
Test for overall effect: Z = 2.67 (P = 0.008)							
Total (95% CI)		**14086**		**20818**	**100.0%**	**1.34 [1.20, 1.49]**	
Total events	4437		4159				
Heterogeneity: Tau² = 0.05; Chi² = 91.44, df = 28 (P < 0.00001); I² = 69%							
Test for overall effect: Z = 5.32 (P < 0.00001)							
Test for subgroup differences: Chi² = 5.59, df = 4 (P = 0.23), I² = 28.4%							

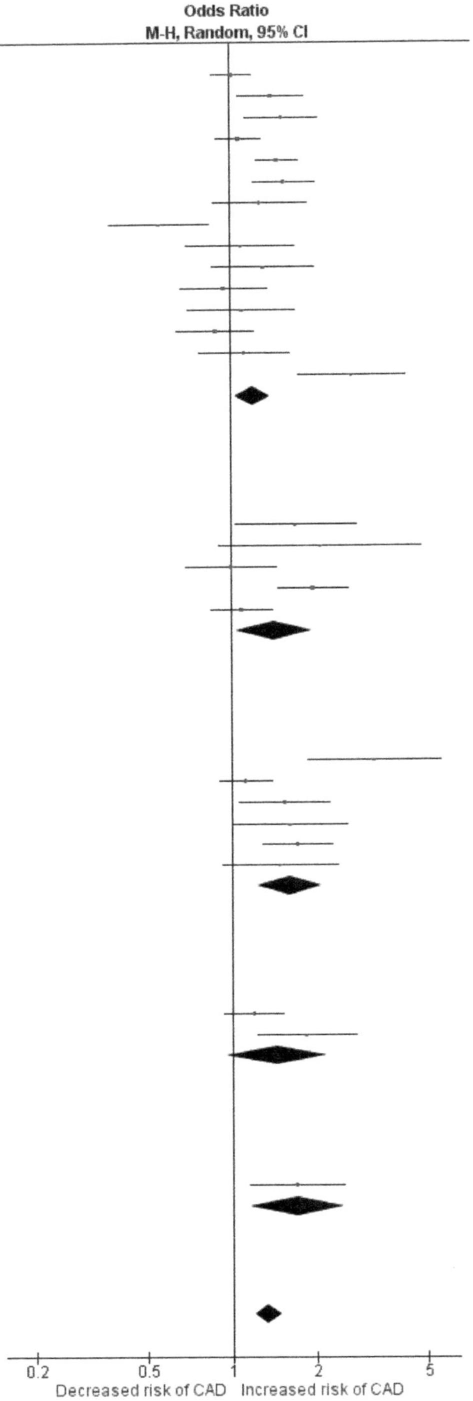

Figure 3. Forest plot depicting results after analyses for the allelic model *(Allele C vs. T)* of *NOS3* T786-C polymorphism. Effect size estimates for all ancestral groups in this plot were obtained using random effects for analysis.

to be the cause of increased CAD risk among carriers of this SNP. [5]

Clear scientific evidence is lacking which can explain the seen association of *NOS3* 4b/a VNTR polymorphism with CAD. In contrast to the previous studies, [40,44] the pooled results of our study yielded significant association amongst all three genetic models. Highest degree of association among the Middle Eastern group was seen in all three genetic models. (**Table 2 and Figures 4, S5 and S6**) The precise reason of this heightened risk amongst subjects of Middle Eastern ancestry is unknown and can only be speculated upon. Here again the influence of environmental factors such as diet and exercise may well be associated

Study or Subgroup	Cases Events	Cases Total	Controls Events	Controls Total	Weight	Odds Ratio M-H, Random, 95% CI	Year
3.1.1 European ancestry group							
Wang et al.	158	1098	52	306	2.8%	0.82 [0.58, 1.16]	1996
Sigusch et al.	183	1260	140	826	3.4%	0.83 [0.65, 1.06]	2000
Pulkkinen et al.	221	1118	36	220	2.5%	1.26 [0.86, 1.85]	2000
Fowkes et al.	45	274	74	600	2.5%	1.40 [0.93, 2.09]	2000
Granath et al.	160	1134	186	1240	3.5%	0.93 [0.74, 1.17]	2001
Alvarez et al.	41	340	84	600	2.5%	0.84 [0.56, 1.26]	2001
Gardemann et al.	589	4118	378	2312	4.0%	0.85 [0.74, 0.98]	2002
Letonja et al.	53	302	42	218	2.2%	0.89 [0.57, 1.40]	2004
Fatini et al.	186	954	166	1074	3.5%	1.32 [1.05, 1.67]	2004
Agema et al.	219	1504	93	932	3.3%	1.54 [1.19, 1.99]	2004
Rao et al.(1)	36	244	8	58	1.0%	1.08 [0.47, 2.47]	2005
Milutinovic et al.	82	430	78	376	2.8%	0.90 [0.64, 1.27]	2005
Dosenko et al.	87	442	35	166	2.3%	0.92 [0.59, 1.42]	2006
Rios et al.(1)	111	602	66	292	2.8%	0.77 [0.55, 1.09]	2007
Sampaio et al.	37	230	40	206	2.0%	0.80 [0.49, 1.30]	2007
Vasilakou et al.	78	418	49	322	2.5%	1.28 [0.86, 1.89]	2008
Meluzin et al.	132	724	17	114	1.8%	1.27 [0.73, 2.20]	2009
Kincl et al.	342	1878	81	444	3.2%	1.00 [0.76, 1.30]	2009
Jaramillo et al.	18	224	18	224	1.4%	1.00 [0.51, 1.98]	2010
da Costa Escobar Piccoli et al.	59	264	46	216	2.3%	1.06 [0.69, 1.64]	2012
Subtotal (95% CI)		**17558**		**10746**	**52.2%**	**1.01 [0.91, 1.12]**	
Total events	2837		1689				
Heterogeneity: Tau² = 0.02; Chi² = 35.91, df = 19 (P = 0.01); I² = 47%							
Test for overall effect: Z = 0.20 (P = 0.84)							
3.1.2 Middle Eastern ancestry group							
Cine et al.	73	414	59	612	2.6%	2.01 [1.39, 2.90]	2002
Matyar et al.	57	266	37	266	2.2%	1.69 [1.07, 2.66]	2005
Salimi et al.	47	282	31	316	2.1%	1.84 [1.13, 2.99]	2006
Agirbasli et al.	29	204	21	204	1.6%	1.44 [0.79, 2.63]	2006
Jemaa et al.	135	620	69	500	2.9%	1.74 [1.27, 2.39]	2007
Agirbasli et al.(1)	82	180	71	180	2.4%	1.28 [0.85, 1.95]	2011
Kallel et al.	131	606	64	450	2.9%	1.66 [1.20, 2.31]	2013
Ekmekci et al.	28	140	9	100	1.1%	2.53 [1.14, 5.63]	2013
Subtotal (95% CI)		**2712**		**2628**	**17.8%**	**1.70 [1.47, 1.98]**	
Total events	582		361				
Heterogeneity: Tau² = 0.00; Chi² = 3.86, df = 7 (P = 0.80); I² = 0%							
Test for overall effect: Z = 7.06 (P < 0.00001)							
3.1.3 Asian ancestry group							
Odawara et al.	11	84	19	244	1.1%	1.78 [0.81, 3.92]	1998
Ichihara et al.	125	910	111	1100	3.2%	1.42 [1.08, 1.86]	1998
Hibi et al.	56	452	78	714	2.7%	1.15 [0.80, 1.66]	1998
Nakagami et al.	20	80	11	68	1.0%	1.73 [0.76, 3.92]	1999
Park et al.	33	242	51	412	2.1%	1.12 [0.70, 1.79]	2000
Lee et al.	59	610	51	430	2.5%	0.80 [0.54, 1.18]	2001
Hwang et al.	34	298	14	140	1.4%	1.16 [0.60, 2.24]	2002
Kim et al.	39	294	40	422	2.1%	1.46 [0.91, 2.33]	2007
Lin et al.	34	240	17	156	1.5%	1.35 [0.73, 2.51]	2008
Bae et al.	46	384	35	392	2.1%	1.39 [0.87, 2.21]	2010
Subtotal (95% CI)		**3594**		**4078**	**19.8%**	**1.25 [1.08, 1.44]**	
Total events	457		427				
Heterogeneity: Tau² = 0.00; Chi² = 8.32, df = 9 (P = 0.50); I² = 0%							
Test for overall effect: Z = 3.06 (P = 0.002)							
3.1.4 Asian-Indian ancestry group							
Gururajan et al.	60	212	27	200	2.0%	2.53 [1.53, 4.19]	2010
Narne et al	60	320	46	242	2.3%	0.98 [0.64, 1.51]	2013
Subtotal (95% CI)		**532**		**442**	**4.3%**	**1.56 [0.62, 3.94]**	
Total events	120		73				
Heterogeneity: Tau² = 0.39; Chi² = 7.88, df = 1 (P = 0.005); I² = 87%							
Test for overall effect: Z = 0.94 (P = 0.35)							
3.1.5 African ancestry group							
Hooper et al.	80	220	98	370	2.7%	1.59 [1.11, 2.27]	1999
Rao et al.(2)	16	44	11	42	0.9%	1.61 [0.64, 4.05]	2005
Rios et al.(2)	62	294	48	242	2.4%	1.08 [0.71, 1.65]	2007
Subtotal (95% CI)		**558**		**654**	**5.9%**	**1.37 [1.05, 1.78]**	
Total events	158		157				
Heterogeneity: Tau² = 0.00; Chi² = 1.98, df = 2 (P = 0.37); I² = 0%							
Test for overall effect: Z = 2.35 (P = 0.02)							
Total (95% CI)		**24954**		**18548**	**100.0%**	**1.20 [1.09, 1.32]**	
Total events	4154		2707				
Heterogeneity: Tau² = 0.05; Chi² = 108.15, df = 42 (P < 0.00001); I² = 61%							
Test for overall effect: Z = 3.77 (P = 0.0002)							
Test for subgroup differences: Chi² = 33.36, df = 4 (P < 0.00001), I² = 88.0%							

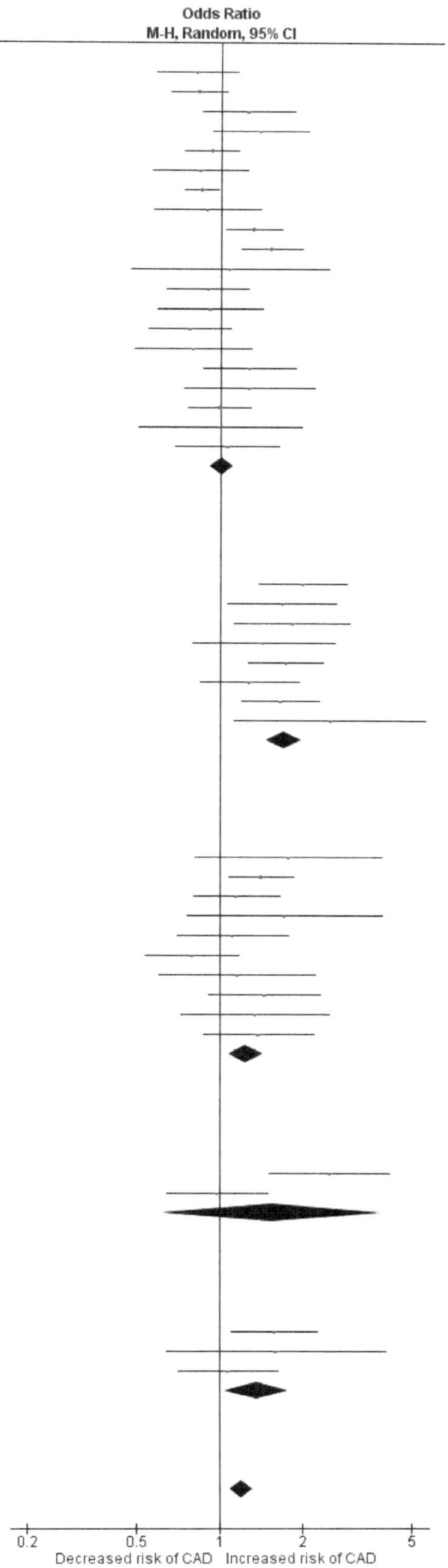

Figure 4. Forest plot depicting results after analyses for the allelic model *(Allele 4a vs. 4b)* of *NOS3* 4b/a VNTR polymorphism. Effect size estimates for all ancestral groups in this plot were obtained using random effects for analysis. Effect sizes using fixed effects were recalculated for European, Middle Eastern, Asian and African groups which showed homogenous distribution among its included studies. Recalculated effect size estimates were, OR, 95%CI = 0.99, 0.93–1.06; Z = 0.19; P = 0.85 for Europeans; OR, 95%CI = 1.71, 1.47–1.98; Z = 7.09; P<0.00001 for Middle Easterners; OR, 95%CI = 1.25, 1.08–1.44; Z = 3.06; P = 0.002 for Asians and OR, 95%CI = 1.37, 1.05–1.78; Z = 2.34; P = 0.02 for Africans.

with the increased risk. Conflicting reports between the intron-4 variant and NO pathway activity are there in the public domain. Genotypes carrying ≥1 mutant alleles have been shown to have lower plasma NO levels and reduced protein expression, [125,126] although some studies have demonstrated otherwise. [77,124,127] As this polymorphism is located in the intron region of the gene, even if it is not functional it might act as a risk factor and act in linkage disequilibrium with other regulatory regions and functional gene variants of the *NOS3* gene. [124]

We believe that the present study has successfully answered the research question that it aimed at the outset and is statistically powered enough to the stand by the results it obtained. Although, there is a scope for limitations in every meta-analysis of genetic association studies and ours was no exception either. Firstly, we believe that there was under representation of the South-Asian region, and we found no published data on the subject from several South-Asian countries like Bangladesh, Sri Lanka and Pakistan etc., which have a sizable population inflicted with CAD. Secondly possibility of errors in genotyping, presence of selection bias and risk of inadequate sample size among different studies cannot be ruled out. It is also noteworthy that in case of polygenic diseases like CAD, an association study cannot test causality, it can merely measure statistical associations. Also, during meta-analysis of association studies we cannot ensure interference of linkage disequilibrium of the selected SNP with another closely linked site and its extent of effect on the overall association. Even after using two statistical tools, we could not detect any hint of publication bias amongst our study groups, at least for Glu298Asp and 4b/a polymorphisms. However, Egger's plot asymmetry was observed, with significant p values for pooled and European subgroup of T786-C polymorphism. Since the accuracy of Egger's test is debatable, and this asymmetry in the aforementioned plots could have possibly been due to factors like inter-study variations or small study effects among European subgroup for T786-C. Even then, the role of existing publication bias cannot be completely ruled out. This also qualifies to be listed as another small limitation in the present study.

Conclusions

In conclusion, since the criteria for inclusion and exclusion of studies are critical parts of a meta-analysis and can substantially affect results, we find that the present study is the most comprehensive till date and is systematically planned to funnel out erroneous studies. We thus feel that our study projects the real picture, and confirms the association of the three common *NOS3* gene polymorphisms i.e. Glu298Asp, T786-C and 4a/b VNTR with CAD transcending all ancestries worldwide. Results amongst different ancestral subgroups were rather illuminating. Amongst the studied *NOS3* SNPs, both Glu298Asp and 4b/a showed strongest association among the Middle Eastern subgroup. On the other hand, T786-C and its minor allele seem to carry the highest risk for CAD among subjects of Asian ancestry. Our study significantly improves the understanding of the relation between this gene and CAD and its association amongst subjects of all major ancestries. These findings should thenceforth be assessed clinically for its implications in prevention and treatment strategies of CAD.

Supporting Information

Figure S1 Forest plot depicting results of meta-analysis of studies reporting *NOS3* Glu298Asp polymorphism assessed under dominant *(TT+GT vs. GG)* genetic model. Effect size estimates for all ancestral groups in this plot were obtained using random effects for analysis. Effect sizes using fixed effects were recalculated for Asian-Indian group which showed homogenous distribution among its included studies. Recalculated effect size estimate for Asian-Indians was, OR, 95%CI = 1.21, 1.01–1.45; Z = 2.07; P = 0.04.

Figure S2 Forest plot depicting results of meta-analysis of studies reporting *NOS3* Glu298Asp polymorphism assessed under recessive *(TT vs. GG+GT)* genetic model. Effect size estimates for all ancestral groups in this plot were obtained using random effects for analysis. Effect sizes using fixed effects were recalculated for Asian and Asian-Indian groups which

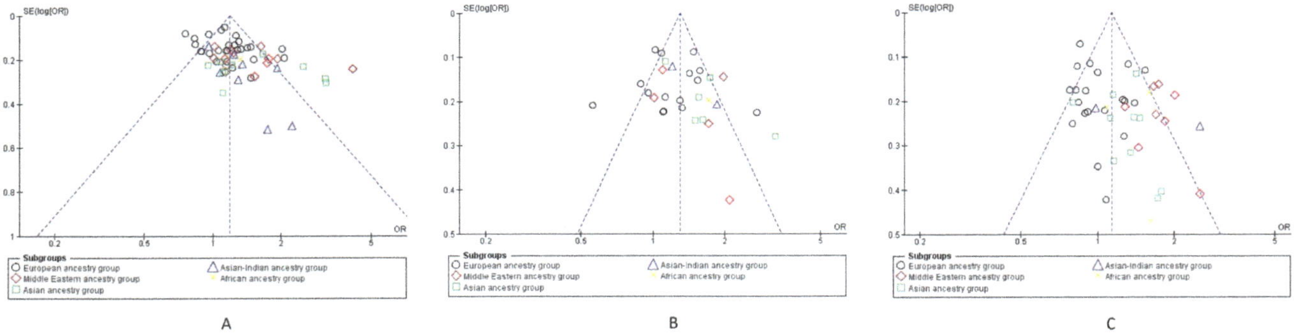

Figure 5. Begg's funnel plots for testing publication bias in Allelic comparisons. Each point in each figure represents OR of a study plotted against the standard error (SE) its OR. Different indicators of the studies belonging to each ancestral group are used in these plots. **Figure 5A**: *Allele T vs. G* for Glu298Asp; **Figure 5B**: *Allele C vs. T* for T786-C; **Figure 5C**: *Allele 4a vs. 4b* for 4b/a.

showed homogenous distribution among its included studies. Recalculated effect size estimates were, OR, 95%CI = 2.22, 1.21–4.08; Z = 2.57; P = 0.01 and OR, 95%CI = 1.85, 1.12–3.04; Z = 2.42; P = 0.02 for Asians and Asian-Indians respectively.

Figure S3 Forest plot depicting results of meta-analysis of studies reporting *NOS3* T786-C polymorphism assessed under dominant *(CC+CT vs. TT)* genetic model. Effect size estimates for all ancestral groups in this plot were obtained using random effects for analysis.

Figure S4 Forest plot depicting results of meta-analysis of studies reporting *NOS3* T786-C polymorphism assessed under recessive *(CC vs. TT+CT)* genetic model. Effect size estimates for all ancestral groups in this plot were obtained using fixed effects for analysis. Effect sizes using random effects were recalculated for three ancestral subgroups viz. Middle Eastern, Asian-Indian and African, which showed homogenous distribution among its included studies. Recalculated effect size estimates were, OR, 95%CI = 1.35, 0.69-2.65; Z = 0.87; P = 0.38 for Middle Easterners; OR, 95%CI = 1.73, 0.38–7.95; Z = 0.71; P = 0.48 for Asian-Indians and OR, 95%CI = 1.85, 0.77–4.44; Z = 1.37; P = 0.17 for Africans.

Figure S5 Forest plot depicting results of meta-analysis of studies reporting *NOS3* 4b/a VNTR polymorphism assessed under dominant *(4a4a+4a4b vs. 4b4b)* genetic model. Effect size estimates for all ancestral groups in this plot were obtained using random effects for analysis. Effect sizes using fixed effects were recalculated for Middle Eastern and Asian groups which showed homogenous distribution among its included studies. Recalculated effect size estimates were, OR, 95%CI = 1.73, 1.46–2.05; Z = 6.28; P = <0.00001 and OR, 95%CI = 1.22, 1.04–1.42; Z = 2.45; P = 0.01 for Middle Easterners and Asians respectively.

Figure S6 Forest plots depicting results of meta-analysis of studies reporting *NOS3* 4b/a VNTR polymorphism assessed under recessive *(4a4a vs. 4a4b+4b4b)* genetic model. Since all the ancestral groups showed homogenous distribution among its included studies, effect size estimates for all groups in this plot were obtained using fixed effects for analysis.

Figure S7 Begg's funnel plots for testing publication bias in comparisons under different genetic models for *NOS3* Glu298Asp polymorphism. Each point in each figure represents OR of a study plotted against the standard error (SE) its OR. Different indicators of the studies belonging to each ancestral group are used in these plots. **Figure S7A**: Begg's Plot for comparisons under dominant genetic model *(TT+GT vs. GG)*; **Figure S7B**: Begg's Plot for comparisons under recessive genetic model *(TT vs. GG+GT)*.

Figure S8 Begg's funnel plots for testing publication bias in comparisons under different genetic models for *NOS3* T786-C polymorphism. Each point in each figure represents OR of a study plotted against the standard error (SE) its OR. Different indicators of the studies belonging to each ancestral group are used in these plots. **Figure S8A**: Begg's Plot for comparisons under dominant genetic model *(CC+CT vs. TT)*; **Figure S8B**: Begg's Plot for comparisons under recessive genetic model *(CC vs. TT+CT)*.

Figure S9 Begg's funnel plots for testing publication bias in comparisons under different genetic models for *NOS3* 4b/a VNTR gene polymorphism. Each point in each figure represents OR of a study plotted against the standard error (SE) its OR. Different indicators of the studies belonging to each ancestral group are used in these plots. **Figure S9A**: Begg's Plot for comparisons under dominant genetic model *(4a4a+4a4b vs. 4b4b)*; **Figure S9B**: Begg's Plot for comparisons under recessive genetic model *(4a4a vs. 4a4b+4b4b)*.

Data S1 The raw data collected from all the published association studies included in the present meta-analysis.

Checklist S1 PRISMA Checklist.

Author Contributions

Conceived and designed the experiments: HR SK. Analyzed the data: HR FP SK. Contributed reagents/materials/analysis tools: HR FP SK. Wrote the paper: HR FP SK AK NS.

References

1. Moncada S, Higgs A (1993) The L-arginine-nitric oxide pathway. N Engl J Med 329(27): 2002–2012.
2. Gardemann A, Lohre J, Cayci S, Katz N, Tillmanns H, et al. (2002) The T allele of the missense Glu(298)Asp endothelial nitric oxide synthase gene polymorphism is associated with coronary heart disease in younger individuals with high atherosclerotic risk profile. Atherosclerosis 160(1): 167–175.
3. Hingorani AD, Liang CF, Fatibene J, Lyon A, Monteith S, et al. (1999) A common variant of the endothelial nitric oxide synthase (Glu298—>Asp) is a major risk factor for coronary artery disease in the UK. Circulation 100(14): 1515–1520.
4. Colombo MG, Andreassi MG, Paradossi U, Botto N, Manfredi S, et al. (2002) Evidence for association of a common variant of the endothelial nitric oxide synthase gene (Glu298—>Asp polymorphism) to the presence, extent, and severity of coronary artery disease. Heart 87(6): 525–528.
5. Colombo MG, Paradossi U, Andreassi MG, Botto N, Manfredi S, et al. (2003) Endothelial nitric oxide synthase gene polymorphisms and risk of coronary artery disease. Clin Chem 49(3): 389–395.
6. Marsden PA, Heng HH, Scherer SW, Stewart RJ, Hall AV, et al. (1993) Structure and chromosomal localization of the human constitutive endothelial nitric oxide synthase gene. J Biol Chem 268(23): 17478–17488.
7. Hingorani A, Jia H, Stevens P, Monteith M, Brown M (1995) A Common Variant in Exon 7 of the Endothelial Constitutive Nitric Oxide Synthase Gene: Identification by Single Strand Conformation Polymorphism Analysis. Clinical Science 88(Pt s32): 21P-21P. (Abstract).
8. Yoshimura M, Yasue H, Nakayama M, Shimasaki Y, Sumida H, et al. (1998) A missense Glu298Asp variant in the endothelial nitric oxide synthase gene is associated with coronary spasm in the Japanese. Hum Genet 103(1): 65–69.
9. Miyamoto Y, Saito Y, Kajiyama N, Yoshimura M, Shimasaki Y, et al. (1998) Endothelial nitric oxide synthase gene is positively associated with essential hypertension. Hypertension 32(1): 3–8.
10. Shimasaki Y, Yasue H, Yoshimura M, Nakayama M, Kugiyama K, et al. (1998) Association of the missense Glu298Asp variant of the endothelial nitric oxide synthase gene with myocardial infarction. J Am Coll Cardiol 31(7): 1506–1510.
11. Hibi K, Ishigami T, Tamura K, Mizushima S, Nyui N, et al. (1998) Endothelial nitric oxide synthase gene polymorphism and acute myocardial infarction. Hypertension 32(3): 521–526.
12. Philip I, Plantefeve G, Vuillaumier-Barrot S, Vicaut E, LeMarie C, et al. (1999) G894T polymorphism in the endothelial nitric oxide synthase gene is associated with an enhanced vascular responsiveness to phenylephrine. Circulation 99(24): 3096–3098.
13. Angeline T, Isabel W, Tsongalis GJ (2010) Endothelial nitric oxide gene polymorphisms, nitric oxide production and coronary artery disease risk in a South Indian population. Exp Mol Pathol 89(3): 205–208.

14. Bor-Kucukatay M, Demir S, Akbay R, Dursunoglu D, Akdag B, et al. (2010) Relationship between hemorheology and Glu(298)Asp polymorphism of endothelial nitric oxide synthase gene in patients with coronary artery disease. Mol Biol Rep 37(1): 171–178.
15. Dafni C, Drakoulis N, Landt O, Panidis D, Reczko M, et al. (2010) Association of the eNOS E298D polymorphism and the risk of myocardial infarction in the Greek population. BMC Med Genet 11: 133.
16. Salimi S, Firoozrai M, Zand H, Nakhaee A, Shafiee SM, et al. (2010) Endothelial nitric oxide synthase gene Glu298Asp polymorphism in patients with coronary artery disease. Ann Saudi Med 30(1): 33–37.
17. Salimi S, Naghavi A, Firoozrai M, Zand H, Tavilani H, et al. (2012) Association of plasma nitric oxide concentration and endothelial nitric oxide synthase T-786C gene polymorphism in coronary artery disease. Pathophysiology 19(3): 157–162.
18. Cai H, Wilcken DE, Wang XL (1999) The Glu-298—>Asp (894G—>T) mutation at exon 7 of the endothelial nitric oxide synthase gene and coronary artery disease. J Mol Med (Berl) 77(6): 511–514.
19. Nassar BA, Bevin LD, Johnstone DE, O'Neill B J, Bata IR, et al. (2001) Relationship of the Glu298Asp polymorphism of the endothelial nitric oxide synthase gene and early-onset coronary artery disease. Am Heart J 142(4): 586–589.
20. Schmoelzer I, Renner W, Paulweber B, Malaimare L, Iglseder B, et al. (2003) Lack of association of the Glu298Asp polymorphism of endothelial nitric oxide synthase with manifest coronary artery disease, carotid atherosclerosis and forearm vascular reactivity in two Austrian populations. Eur J Clin Invest 33(3): 191–198.
21. Jaramillo PC, Munoz MA, Lanas MC, Lanas ZF, Salazar LA (2006) Endothelial nitric oxide synthase G894T gene polymorphism in Chilean subjects with coronary artery disease and controls. Clin Chim Acta 371(1-2): 102–106.
22. Kim IJ, Bae J, Lim SW, Cha DH, Cho HJ, et al. (2007) Influence of endothelial nitric oxide synthase gene polymorphisms (-786T>C, 4a4b, 894G>T) in Korean patients with coronary artery disease. Thromb Res 119(5): 579–585.
23. Alp E, Menevse S, Tulmac M, Kan D, Yalcin R, et al. (2009) Lack of association between matrix metalloproteinase-9 and endothelial nitric oxide synthase gene polymorphisms and coronary artery disease in Turkish population. DNA Cell Biol 28(7): 343–350.
24. Nakayama M, Yasue H, Yoshimura M, Shimasaki Y, Kugiyama K, et al. (1999) T-786—>C mutation in the 5'-flanking region of the endothelial nitric oxide synthase gene is associated with coronary spasm. Circulation 99(22): 2864–2870.
25. Sandrim VC, de Syllos RW, Lisboa HR, Tres GS, Tanus-Santos JE (2006) Endothelial nitric oxide synthase haplotypes affect the susceptibility to hypertension in patients with type 2 diabetes mellitus. Atherosclerosis 189(1): 241–246.
26. Miyamoto Y, Saito Y, Nakayama M, Shimasaki Y, Yoshimura T, et al. (2000) Replication protein A1 reduces transcription of the endothelial nitric oxide synthase gene containing a -786T—>C mutation associated with coronary spastic angina. Hum Mol Genet 9(18): 2629–2637.
27. Alvarez R, Gonzalez P, Batalla A, Reguero JR, Iglesias-Cubero G, et al. (2001) Association between the NOS3 (-786 T/C) and the ACE (I/D) DNA genotypes and early coronary artery disease. Nitric Oxide 5(4): 343–348.
28. Rios DL, Callegari-Jacques SM, Hutz MH (2005) Endothelial nitric oxide synthase and fractalkine chemokine receptor polymorphisms on angiographically assessed coronary atherosclerosis. Clin Chim Acta 362(1-2): 138–146.
29. Hyndman ME, Parsons HG, Verma S, Bridge PJ, Edworthy S, et al. (2002) The T-786—>C mutation in endothelial nitric oxide synthase is associated with hypertension. Hypertension 39(4): 919–922.
30. Rossi GP, Cesari M, Zanchetta M, Colonna S, Maiolino G, et al. (2003) The T-786C endothelial nitric oxide synthase genotype is a novel risk factor for coronary artery disease in Caucasian patients of the GENICA study. J Am Coll Cardiol 41(6): 930–937.
31. Nakayama M, Yasue H, Yoshimura M, Shimasaki Y, Ogawa H, et al. (2000) T(-786)—> C mutation in the 5'-flanking region of the endothelial nitric oxide synthase gene is associated with myocardial infarction, especially without coronary organic stenosis. Am J Cardiol 86(6): 628–634.
32. Ragia G, Nikolaidis E, Tavridou A, Arvanitidis KI, Kanoni S, et al. (2010) Endothelial nitric oxide synthase gene polymorphisms -786T> C and 894G> T in coronary artery bypass graft surgery patients. Hum Genomics 4(6): 375–383.
33. Wang XL, Sim AS, Badenhop RF, McCredie RM, Wilcken DE (1996) A smoking-dependent risk of coronary artery disease associated with a polymorphism of the endothelial nitric oxide synthase gene. Nat Med 2(1): 41–45.
34. Cine N, Hatemi AC, Erginel-Unaltuna N (2002) Association of a polymorphism of the ecNOS gene with myocardial infarction in a subgroup of Turkish MI patients. Clin Genet 61(1): 66–70.
35. Ichihara S, Yamada Y, Fujimura T, Nakashima N, Yokota M (1998) Association of a polymorphism of the endothelial constitutive nitric oxide synthase gene with myocardial infarction in the Japanese population. Am J Cardiol 81(1): 83–86.
36. Park JE, Lee WH, Hwang TH, Chu JA, Kim S, et al. (2000) Aging affects the association between endothelial nitric oxide synthase gene polymorphism and acute myocardial infarction in the Korean male population. Korean J Intern Med 15(1): 65–70.
37. Granath B, Taylor RR, van Bockxmeer FM, Mamotte CD (2001) Lack of evidence for association between endothelial nitric oxide synthase gene polymorphisms and coronary artery disease in the Australian Caucasian population. J Cardiovasc Risk 8(4): 235–241.
38. Poirier O, Mao C, Mallet C, Nicaud V, Herrmann SM, et al. (1999) Polymorphisms of the endothelial nitric oxide synthase gene - no consistent association with myocardial infarction in the ECTIM study. Eur J Clin Invest 29(4): 284–290.
39. Jaramillo PC, Lanas C, Lanas F, Salazar LA (2010) Polymorphisms of the NOS3 gene in Southern Chilean subjects with coronary artery disease and controls. Clin Chim Acta 411(3-4): 258–262.
40. Li J, Wu X, Li X, Feng G, He L, et al. (2010) The endothelial nitric oxide synthase gene is associated with coronary artery disease: a meta-analysis. Cardiology 116(4): 271–278.
41. Zhang K, Bai P, Shi S, Zhou B, Wang Y, et al. (2012) The G894T polymorphism on endothelial nitric oxide synthase gene is associated with increased coronary heart disease among Asia population: evidence from a Meta analysis. Thromb Res 130(2): 192–197.
42. Liu D, Jiang Z, Dai L, Zhang X, Yan C, et al. (2013) Association between the -786T>C 1polymorphism in the promoter region of endothelial nitric oxide synthase (eNOS) and risk of coronary artery disease: A systematic review and meta-analysis. Gene pii: S0378-1119(13)01333-4.
43. Tian GX, Zeng XT, Wang XB, Zhang L, Zhang W, et al. (2013) Association between the endothelial nitric oxide synthase gene Glu298Asp polymorphism and coronary heart disease: a metaanalysis of 39 casecontrol studies. Mol Med Rep 7(4): 1310–1318.
44. Yang Y, Du K, Liu Z, Lu X (2014). Endothelial nitric oxide synthase (eNOS) 4b/a gene polymorphisms and coronary artery disease: evidence from a meta-analysis. Int J Mol Sci 15(5): 7987–8003.
45. Panic N, Leoncini E, de Belvis G, Ricciardi W, Boccia S (2013) Evaluation of the endorsement of the preferred reporting items for systematic reviews and meta-analysis (PRISMA) statement on the quality of published systematic review and meta-analyses. PLoS One 8(12): e83138.
46. Lewis CM (2002) Genetic association studies: design, analysis and interpretation. Brief Bioinform 3(2): 146–153.
47. DerSimonian R, Laird N (1986) Meta-analysis in clinical trials. Control Clin Trials 7(3): 177–188.
48. Mantel N, Haenszel W (1959) Statistical aspects of the analysis of data from retrospective studies of disease. J Natl Cancer Inst 22(4): 719–748.
49. Higgins JP, Thompson SG, Deeks JJ, Altman DG (2003) Measuring inconsistency in meta-analyses. Bmj 327(7414): 557–560.
50. Begg CB, Mazumdar M (1994) Operating characteristics of a rank correlation test for publication bias. Biometrics 50(4): 1088–1101.
51. Egger M, Davey Smith G, Schneider M, Minder C (1997) Bias in meta-analysis detected by a simple, graphical test. Bmj 315(7109): 629–634.
52. Clayton D, McKeigue PM (2001) Epidemiological methods for studying genes and environmental factors in complex diseases. The Lancet 358(9290): 1356–1360.
53. Pulkkinen A, Viitanen L, Kareinen A, Lehto S, Vauhkonen I, et al. (2000) Intron 4 polymorphism of the endothelial nitric oxide synthase gene is associated with elevated blood pressure in type 2 diabetic patients with coronary heart disease. J Mol Med (Berl) 78(7): 372–379.
54. Agema WR, de Maat MP, Zwinderman AH, Kastelein JJ, Rabelink TJ, et al. (2004) An integrated evaluation of endothelial constitutive nitric oxide synthase polymorphisms and coronary artery disease in men. Clin Sci (Lond) 107(3): 255–261.
55. Fatini C, Sofi F, Sticchi E, Gensini F, Gori AM, et al. (2004) Influence of endothelial nitric oxide synthase gene polymorphisms (G894T, 4a4b, T-786C) and hyperhomocysteinemia on the predisposition to acute coronary syndromes. Am Heart J.147(3): 516–521.
56. Antoniades C, Tousoulis D, Vasiliadou C, Pitsavos C, Chrysochoou C, et al. (2005) Genetic polymorphism on endothelial nitric oxide synthase affects endothelial activation and inflammatory response during the acute phase of myocardial infarction. J Am Coll Cardiol.46(6): 1101–1109.
57. Rios DL, D'Onofrio LO, Souza JK, Queiroz AM, Raduy-Maron L, et al. (2007) Smoking-dependent and haplotype-specific effects of endothelial nitric oxide synthase gene polymorphisms on angiographically assessed coronary artery disease in Caucasian- and African-Brazilians. Atherosclerosis 193(1): 135–41.
58. Sampaio MF, Hirata MH, Hirata RD, Santos FC, Picciotti R. et al. (2007) AMI is associated with polymorphisms in the NOS3 and FGB but not in PAI-1 genes in young adults. Clin Chim Acta 377(1-2): 154–162.
59. Andrikopoulos GK, Grammatopoulos DK, Tzeis SE, Zervou SI, Richter DJ, et al. (2008) Association of the 894G>T polymorphism in the endothelial nitric oxide synthase gene with risk of acute myocardial infarction. BMC Med Genet 9: 43.
60. Szperl M, Dzielinska Z, Roszczynko M, Malek LA, Makowiecka-Ciesla M, et al. (2008) Genetic variants in hypertensive patients with coronary artery disease and coexisting atheromatous renal artery stenosis. Med Sci Monit 14(12): Cr611–616.
61. Vasilakou M, Votteas V, Kasparian C, Pantazopoulos N, Dedoussis G, et al. (2008) Lack of association between endothelial nitric oxide synthase gene

polymorphisms and risk of premature coronary artery disease in the Greek population. Acta Cardiol 63(5): 609–614.

62. Gluba A, Banach M, Rysz J, Piotrowski G, Fendler W, et al. (2009) Is polymorphism within eNOS gene associated with the late onset of myocardial infarction? A pilot study. Angiology 60(5): 588–595.
63. Isordia-Salas I, Leanos-Miranda A, Borrayo-Sanchez G (2010) The Glu298Asp polymorphism of the endothelial nitric oxide synthase gene is associated with premature ST elevation myocardial infarction in Mexican population. Clin Chim Acta 411(7-8): 553–557.
64. da Costa Escobar Piccoli J, Manfredini V, Hamester FI, Bandinelli JB, Turkienicz IM, et al. (2012) Interaction between endothelial nitric oxide synthase gene polymorphisms (-786T>C, 894G>T and intron 4 a/b) and cardiovascular risk factors in acute coronary syndromes. Arch Med Res 43(3): 205–11.
65. Zigra AM, Rallidis LS, Anastasiou G, Merkouri E, Gialeraki A (2013) eNOS gene variants and the risk of premature myocardial infarction. Dis Markers 34(6): 431–436.
66. Aras O, Hanson NQ, Bakanay SM, Tsai MY, Gulec S (2002) Endothelial nitric oxide gene polymorphism (Glu298Asp) is not associated with coronary artery disease in Turkish population. Thromb Haemost;87(2): 347–349.
67. Afrasyap L, Ozturk G (2004) NO level and endothelial NO synthase gene polymorphism (Glu298Asp) in the patients with coronary artery disease from the Turkish population. Acta Biochim Biophys Sin (Shanghai) 36(10): 661–666.
68. Berdeli A, Sekuri C, Sirri Cam F, Ercan E, Sagcan A., et al. (2005) Association between the eNOS (Glu298Asp) and the RAS genes polymorphisms and premature coronary artery disease in a Turkish population. Clin Chim Acta 351(1-2): 87–94.
69. Cam SF, Sekuri C, Tengiz I, Ercan E, Sagcan A., et al. (2005) The G894T polymorphism on endothelial nitric oxide synthase gene is associated with premature coronary artery disease in a Turkish population. Thromb Res 116(4): 287–292.
70. Kerkeni M, Addad F, Chauffert M, Myara A, Ben Farhat M, et al. (2006) Hyperhomocysteinemia, endothelial nitric oxide synthase polymorphism, and risk of coronary artery disease. Clin Chem 52(1): 53–58.
71. Alkharfy KM, Al-Daghri NM, Al-Attas OS, Alokail MS, Draz HM, et al. (2010) Endothelial nitric oxide synthase gene polymorphisms (894G> T and -786T> C) and risk of coronary artery disease in a Saudi population. Arch Med Res 41(2): 134–141.
72. Motawi T, Shaker O, Taha M, Sedrak H, Nabil M (2011) Endothelial nitric oxide synthase and angiotensinogen gene polymorphism in coronary artery diseases in Egypt. Angiology 62(2):191–7.
73. Gad MZ, Abdel Rahman MF, Hashad IM, Abdel-Maksoud SM, Farag NM, et al. (2012) Endothelial nitric oxide synthase (G894T) gene polymorphism in a random sample of the Egyptian population: comparison with myocardial infarction patients. Genet Test Mol Biomarkers 16(7): 695–700.
74. Rahimi Z, Nourozi-Rad R (2012) Association of endothelial nitric oxide synthase gene variant (G894T) with coronary artery disease in Western Iran. Angiology 63(2): 131–137.
75. Abdel-Aziz TA, Mohamed RH (2013) Association of endothelial nitric oxide synthase gene polymorphisms with classical risk factors in development of premature coronary artery disease. Mol Biol Rep 40(4): 3065–3071.
76. Kallel A, Sbai MH, Sediri Y, Abdessalem S, Mourali MS, et al. (2013) Polymorphisms of the NOS3 gene and risk of myocardial infarction in the Tunisian population. Cytokine 64(3): 646–651.
77. Yoon Y, Song J, Hong SH, Kim JQ (2000) Plasma nitric oxide concentrations and nitric oxide synthase gene polymorphisms in coronary artery disease. Clin Chem 46(10): 1626–1630.
78. Wang CL, Hsu LA, Ko YS, Ko YL, Lee YH (2001) Lack of association between the Glu298Asp variant of the endothelial nitric oxide synthase gene and the risk of coronary artery disease among Taiwanese. J Formos Med Assoc 100(11): 736–740.
79. Jo I, Moon J, Yoon S, Kim HT, Kim E, et al. (2006) Interaction between -786TC polymorphism in the endothelial nitric oxide synthase gene and smoking for myocardial infarction in Korean population. Clin Chim Acta 365(1-2):86–92.
80. Lin NT, Lee MJ, Lee RP, Hong AI, Chen HI (2008) Analysis of endothelial nitric oxide synthase gene polymorphisms with cardiovascular diseases in eastern Taiwan. Chin J Physiol 51(1): 42–47.
81. Tamemoto H, Ishikawa SE, Kawakami M (2008) Association of the Glu298Asp polymorphism of the eNOS Gene with ischemic heart disease in Japanese diabetic subjects. Diabetes Res Clin Pract 80(2): 275–279.
82. Bae J, Kim IJ, Hong SH, Sung JH, Lim SW, et al. (2010) Association of endothelial nitric oxide synthase polymorphisms with coronary artery disease in Korean individuals with or without diabetes mellitus. Exp Ther Med 1(4): 719–724.
83. Min BW, Na JY, Juhng SW, Park MS, Park JT, et al. (2010) A polymorphism (G894T) in eNOS increases the risk of coronary atherosclerosis rather than intracranial atherosclerosis in Koreans. Acta Neurol Belg 110(3): 255–262.
84. Mathew J, Narayanan P, Sundaram R, Jayaraman B, Dutta TK, et al. (2008) Lack of association between Glu(298) asp polymorphism of endothelial nitric oxide synthase (eNOS) gene and coronary artery disease in Tamilian population. Indian Heart J 60(3): 223–227.
85. Bhanushali AA, Das BR (2010) Genetic variants at the APOE, lipoprotein lipase (LpL), cholesteryl ester transfer protein (CETP), and endothelial nitric oxide (eNOS) genes and coronary artery disease (CAD): CETP Taq1 B2B2 associates with lower risk of CAD in Asian Indians. J Community Genet 1(2): 55–62.
86. Saini V, Bhatnagar MK, Bhattacharjee J (2011) Association of endothelial dysfunction with endothelin, nitric oxide and eNOS Glu298Asp gene polymorphism in coronary artery disease. Dis Markers 31(4): 215–22.
87. Rai H, Fitt J, Sharma AK, Sinha N, Kumar S, et al. (2012) Lack of association between Glu298Asp polymorphism and coronary artery disease in North Indians. Mol Biol Rep 39(5): 5995–6000.
88. Saini V, Bhatnagar MK, Bhattacharjee J (2012) Endothelial nitric oxide synthase Glu298Asp (G894T) gene polymorphism in coronary artery disease patients with type 2 diabetes mellitus. Diabetes Metab Syndr 6(2): 106–9.
89. Arun Kumar AS, Umamaheswaran G, Padmapriya R, Balachandar J, Adithan C (2013) Endothelial nitric oxide synthase gene polymorphisms and the risk of acute myocardial infarction in a South Indian population. Mol Biol Rep 40(2): 1275–81.
90. Narne P, Ponnaluri KC, Singh S, Siraj M, Ishaq M (2013) Association of the genetic variants of endothelial nitric oxide synthase gene with angiographically defined coronary artery disease and myocardial infarction in South Indian patients with type 2 diabetes mellitus. J Diabetes Complications 27(3): 255–261.
91. Dosenko VE, Zagoriy VY, Lutay YM, Parkhomenko AN, Moibenko AA (2006) Allelic polymorphism in the promoter (T—>C), but not in exon 7 (G—>T) or the variable number tandem repeat in intron 4, of the endothelial nitric oxide synthase gene is positively associated with acute coronary syndrome in the Ukrainian population. Exp Clin Cardiol 11(1): 11–13.
92. Jaramillo PC, Lanas C, Lanas F, Salazar LA (2008) -786T>C polymorphism of the endothelial nitric oxide synthase gene in Chilean subjects with coronary artery disease and controls. Clin Chim Acta 387(1-2): 105–108.
93. Meluzin J, Vasku A, Kincl V, Panovsky R, Sramkova T (2009) Association of coronary artery disease, erectile dysfunction, and endothelial nitric oxide synthase polymorphisms. Heart Vessels 24(3): 157–163.
94. Tangurek B, Ozer N, Sayar N, Terzi S, Yilmaz H, et al. (2006) The relationship between endothelial nitric oxide synthase gene polymorphism (T-786 C) and coronary artery disease in the Turkish population. Heart Vessels 21(5): 285–290.
95. Ciftci C, Melil S, Cebi Y, Ersoz M, Cagatay P, et al. (2008) Association of endothelial nitric oxide synthase promoter region (T-786C) gene polymorphism with acute coronary syndrome and coronary heart disease. Lipids Health Dis 7: 5.
96. Takagi S, Goto Y, Nonogi H, Baba S, Iwai N (2001) Genetic polymorphisms of angiotensin converting enzyme (I/D) and endothelial nitric oxide synthase (T(-788)C) genes in Japanese patients with myocardial infarction. Thromb Haemost Germany p. 1339–40.
97. Han Y, Xu W, Zhang W, Liu N, Ji Y (2010) T-786C polymorphism in the endothelial nitric oxide synthase gene is associated with increased risk of coronary artery disease in a Chinese population. Pharmacology 85(4): 211–216.
98. Hooper WC, Lally C, Austin H, Benson J, Dilley A, et al. (1999) The relationship between polymorphisms in the endothelial cell nitric oxide synthase gene and the platelet GPIIIa gene with myocardial infarction and venous thromboembolism in African Americans. Chest 116(4): 880–6.
99. Fowkes FG, Lee AJ, Hau CM, Cooke A, Connor JM, et al. (2000) Methylene tetrahydrofolate reductase (MTHFR) and nitric oxide synthase (ecNOS) genes and risks of peripheral arterial disease and coronary heart disease: Edinburgh Artery Study. Atherosclerosis 150(1): 179–185.
100. Pulkkinen A, Viitanen L, Kareinen A, Lehto S, Vauhkonen I, et al. (2000) Intron 4 polymorphism of the endothelial nitric oxide synthase gene is associated with elevated blood pressure in type 2 diabetic patients with coronary heart disease. J Mol Med (Berl) 78(7): 372–379.
101. Sigusch HH, Surber R, Lehmann MH, Surber S, Weber J, et al. (2000) Lack of association between 27-bp repeat polymorphism in intron 4 of the endothelial nitric oxide synthase gene and the risk of coronary artery disease. Scand J Clin Lab Invest 60(3): 229–235.
102. Letonja M (2004) The eNOS gene polymorphism does not have a major impact on lipid parameters and premature coronary artery disease in Caucasian women. Acta Cardiol 59(6): 618–622.
103. Milutinovic A, Hruskovicova H (2005) The eNOS gene polymorphism does not have a major impact on lipid parameters and premature coronary artery disease in Slovene men (Caucasians). Folia Biol (Praha) 51(2): 47–49.
104. Rao S, Austin H, Davidoff MN, Zafari AM (2005) Endothelial nitric oxide synthase intron 4 polymorphism is a marker for coronary artery disease in African-American and Caucasian men. Ethn Dis 15(2): 191–7.
105. Kincl V, Vasku A, Meluzin J, Panovsky R, Semenka J, et al. (2009) Association of the eNOS 4a/b and -786T/C polymormphisms with coronary artery disease, obesity and diabetes mellitus. Folia Biol (Praha) 55(5): 187–191.
106. Matyar S, Attila G, Acarturk E, Akpinar O, Inal T (2005) eNOS gene intron 4 a/b VNTR polymorphism is a risk factor for coronary artery disease in Southern Turkey. Clin Chim Acta 354(1-2): 153–158.
107. Agirbasli D, Agirbasli M, Williams SM, Phillips JA 3rd (2006) Interaction among 5,10 methylenetetrahydrofolate reductase, plasminogen activator inhibitor and endothelial nitric oxide synthase gene polymorphisms predicts the severity of coronary artery disease in Turkish patients. Coron Artery Dis 17(5): 413–417.

108. Agirbasli M, Guney AI, Ozturhan HS, Agirbasli D, Ulucan K., et al. (2011) Multifactor dimensionality reduction analysis of MTHFR, PAI-1, ACE, PON1, and eNOS gene polymorphisms in patients with early onset coronary artery disease. Eur J Cardiovasc Prev Rehabil 18(6): 803–809.
109. Salimi S, Firoozrai M, Nourmohammadi I, Shabani M, Mohebbi A (2006) Endothelial nitric oxide synthase gene intron4 VNTR polymorphism in patients with coronary artery disease in Iran. Indian J Med Res 124(6): 683–688.
110. Jemaa R, Kallel A, Ben Ali S, Omar S, Chabrak S, et al. (2007) Association of a 27-bp repeat polymorphism in intron 4 of endothelial constitutive nitric oxide synthase gene with myocardial infarction in Tunisian patients. Clin Chem Lab Med 45(11): 1476–80.
111. Ekmekci A, Ozcan KS, Gungor B, Abaci N, Osmonov D., et al. (2013) The relationship between endothelial nitric oxide synthase 4a/4b gene polymorphism and premature coronary artery disease. Acta Cardiol 68(5): 464–468.
112. Odawara M, Sasaki K, Tachi Y, Yamashita K (1998) Endothelial nitric oxide synthase gene polymorphism and coronary heart disease in Japanese NIDDM. Diabetologia 41(3): 365–366.
113. Nakagami H, Ikeda U, Maeda Y, Yamamoto K, Hojo Y, et al. (1999) Coronary artery disease and endothelial nitric oxide synthase and angiotensin-converting enzyme gene polymorphisms. J Thromb Thrombolysis 8(3): 191–5.
114. Lee WH, Hwang TH, Oh GT, Kwon SU, Choi YH, et al. (2001) Genetic factors associated with endothelial dysfunction affect the early onset of coronary artery disease in Korean males. Vasc Med 6(2): 103–108.
115. Hwang JJ, Tsai CT, Yeh HM, Chiang FT, Hsu KL, et al. (2002) The 27-bp tandem repeat polymorphism in intron 4 of the endothelial nitric oxide synthase gene is not associated with coronary artery disease in a hospital-based Taiwanese population. Cardiology 97(2): 67–72.
116. Gururajan P, Gurumurthy P, Victor D, Srinivasa Nageswara Rao G, Sai Babu R, et al. (2011) Plasma total nitric oxide and endothelial constitutive nitric oxide synthase (ecNOS) gene polymorphism: a study in a South Indian population. Biochem Genet 49(1-2): 96–103.
117. Salom MG, Arregui B, Carbonell LF, Ruiz F, Gonzalez-Mora JL, et al. (2005) Renal ischemia induces an increase in nitric oxide levels from tissue stores. Am J Physiol Regul Integr Comp Physiol 289(5): R1459–1466.
118. Kelm M, Feelisch M, Deussen A, Strauer BE, Schrader J (1991) Release of endothelium derived nitric oxide in relation to pressure and flow. Cardiovasc Res 25(10): 831–836.
119. Tesauro M, Thompson WC, Rogliani P, Qi L, Chaudhary PP, et al. (2000) Intracellular processing of endothelial nitric oxide synthase isoforms associated with differences in severity of cardiopulmonary diseases: cleavage of proteins with aspartate vs. glutamate at position 298. Proc Natl Acad Sci U S A 97(6): 2832–2835.
120. Persu A, Stoenoiu MS, Messiaen T, Davila S, Robino C, et al. (2002) Modifier effect of ENOS in autosomal dominant polycystic kidney disease. Hum Mol Genet. 11(3): 229–241.
121. Rankinen T, Rice T, Perusse L, Chagnon YC, Gagnon J, et al. (2000) NOS3 Glu298Asp genotype and blood pressure response to endurance training: the HERITAGE family study. Hypertension 36(5): 885–889.
122. Naber CK, Baumgart D, Altmann C, Siffert W, Erbel R, et al. (2001) eNOS 894T allele and coronary blood flow at rest and during adenosine-induced hyperemia. Am J Physiol Heart Circ Physiol 281(5): H1908–1912.
123. Savvidou MD, Vallance PJ, Nicolaides KH, Hingorani AD (2001) Endothelial nitric oxide synthase gene polymorphism and maternal vascular adaptation to pregnancy. Hypertension 38(6): 1289–1293.
124. Jeerooburkhan N, Jones LC, Bujac S, Cooper JA, Miller GJ, et al. (2001) Genetic and environmental determinants of plasma nitrogen oxides and risk of ischemic heart disease. Hypertension 38(5): 1054–1061.
125. Tsukada T, Yokoyama K, Arai T, Takemoto F, Hara S, et al. (1998) Evidence of association of the ecNOS gene polymorphism with plasma NO metabolite levels in humans. Biochem Biophys Res Commun 245(1): 190–193.
126. Wang XL, Sim AS, Wang MX, Murrell GA, Trudinger B, et al. (2000) Genotype dependent and cigarette specific effects on endothelial nitric oxide synthase gene expression and enzyme activity. FEBS Lett 471(1): 45–50.
127. Wang XL, Mahaney MC, Sim AS, Wang J, Wang J., et al. (1997) Genetic contribution of the endothelial constitutive nitric oxide synthase gene to plasma nitric oxide levels. Arterioscler Thromb Vasc Biol 17(11): 3147–3153.

24

Association of Aminoacyl-tRNA Synthetases Gene Polymorphisms with the Risk of Congenital Heart Disease in the Chinese Han Population

Min Da[1], Yu Feng[1], Jing Xu[2], Yuanli Hu[1], Yuan Lin[3], Bixian Ni[3], Bo Qian[1], Zhibin Hu[3], Xuming Mo[1]*

1 Department of Cardiothoracic Surgery, The Affiliated Nanjing Children's Hospital of Nanjing Medical University, Nanjing, Jiangsu, P.R. China, 2 Department of Thoracic and Cardiovascular Surgery, The First Affiliated Hospital of Nanjing Medical University, Nanjing, Jiangsu, P.R. China, 3 Department of Epidemiology and Biostatistics, State Key Laboratory of Reproductive Medicine, Nanjing Medical University, Nanjing, Jiangsu, P.R. China

Abstract

Aminoacyl-tRNA synthetases (ARSs) are in charge of cellular protein synthesis and have additional domains that function in a versatile manner beyond translation. Eight core ARSs (*EPRS, MRS, QRS, RRS, IRS, LRS, KRS, DRS*) combined with three nonenzymatic components form a complex known as multisynthetase complex (MSC).We hypothesize that the single-nucleotide polymorphisms (SNPs) of the eight core ARS coding genes might influence the susceptibility of sporadic congenital heart disease (CHD). Thus, we conducted a case-control study of 984 CHD cases and 2953 non-CHD controls in the Chinese Han population to evaluate the associations of 16 potentially functional SNPs within the eight ARS coding genes with the risk of CHD. We observed significant associations with the risk of CHD for rs1061248 [G/A; odds ratio (OR) = 0.90, 95% confidence interval (CI) = 0.81–0.99; $P = 3.81\times10^{-2}$], rs2230301 [A/C; OR = 0.73, 95%CI = 0.60–0.90, $P = 3.81\times10^{-2}$], rs1061160 [G/A; OR = 1.18, 95%CI = 1.06–1.31; $P = 3.53\times10^{-3}$] and rs5030754 [G/A; OR = 1.39, 95%CI = 1.11–1.75; $P = 4.47\times10^{-3}$] of *EPRS* gene. After multiple comparisons, rs1061248 conferred no predisposition to CHD. Additionally, a combined analysis showed a significant dosage-response effect of CHD risk among individuals carrying the different number of risk alleles ($P_{trend} = 5.00\times10^{-4}$). Compared with individuals with "0–2" risk allele, those carrying "3", "4" or "5 or more" risk alleles had a 0.97-, 1.25- or 1.38-fold increased risk of CHD, respectively. These findings indicate that genetic variants of the *EPRS* gene may influence the individual susceptibility to CHD in the Chinese Han population.

Editor: Yong-Gang Yao, Kunming Institute of Zoology, Chinese Academy of Sciences, China

Funding: This work was supported in part by National Natural Science Foundation of China (grant numbers 81370277 and 81300128); Jiangsu Provincial Special Program of Medical Science (grant number BL2013013); Ph.D. Programs Foundation of Ministry of Education of China (grant number 20123234120015); and Jiangsu Natural Science Foundation (grant number BK20131025). The funders had no role in study design, data collection and analysis, decision to publish, or preparation of the manuscript.

Competing Interests: The authors have declared that no competing interests exist.

* Email: mohsuming15@sina.com

These authors contributed equally to this work.

Introduction

Congenital heart disease(CHD) is the most common human birth defect and the leading cause of perinatal mortality, with an incidence of approximately 6–8 per 1000 live births or even higher [1,2,3]. With the advances in surgical techniques, the prognosis of children with complicated and uncomplicated CHDs continues to improve, but the reported incidence remains unchanged [4]. The etiology of CHD is complex and possibly includes the interaction of inherited factors and environmental exposures [5,6,7]. A multitude of research studies have identified both chromosomal abnormality and gene mutations as causation for the syndromic heart malfunction [8]. However, the origin of non-syndromic CHD, which accounts for most of all congenital cardiac abnormalities, is waiting to be uncovered further.

Over the past decades, plenty of genes have been identified as candidates to be responsible for CHD [9,10,11]. However, aminoacyl-tRNA synthetases (ARSs) that seemed to be in charge of only cellular protein synthesis were overlooked. ARSs catalyze the attachment of amino acids to their cognate tRNAs with high fidelity [12,13]. Recent research has shown that eukaryote ARSs, distinguished from their prokaryotic counterparts, have additional domains and motifs such as glutathione S-transferase (GST), WHEP domains, leucine zipper domains, and α-helicalappendices that function beyond translation [14] and may link with a variety of human diseases, such as cancer, neuronal pathologies, autoimmune disorders, and disrupted metabolic conditions [13,15]. Recently, the nontranslational functions of vertebrate ARSs have been associated with cytoplasmic forms and nuclear and secreted extracellular forms that impact cardiovascular development pathways [16].

Eight core aminoacyl-tRNA synthetases (ARSs), bifunctional glutamyl-prolyl-tRNA synthetase (*EPRS*), isoleucyl-tRNA synthetase (*IRS*), leucyl-tRNA synthetase (*LRS*), methionyl-tRNA synthetase (*MRS*), glutaminyl-tRNA synthetase (*QRS*), lysyl-tRNA synthetase (*KRS*), aspartyl-tRNA synthetase (*DRS*), and arginyl-tRNA synthetase (*RRS*), form a macromolecular protein complex with three auxiliary factors, designated ARS-interacting multi-functional protein 1 (AIMP1), AIMP2 and AIMP3. This complex is known as the multisynthetase complex (MSC). The MSC may act as a depot for ARSs, which could be subsequently released from the macromolecular complexes to participate in auxiliary tasks beyond translation [17], generate a channel for the delivery of tRNAs [18,19] and help the proofreading of newly synthesized nuclear tRNAs in the nucleus [20].

According to the expressed sequence tags (EST) profile in the public database UniGene (http://www.ncbi.nlm.nih.gov/UniGene), all eight of the core ARS coding genes were expressed in human heart tissues, with transcripts ranging from 44 to 502 per million (**Figure S1**). Thus, it is plausible that changes in the core ARSs may affect heart development and are related to the occurrence of CHD. However, to date, no research has reported a relation between the genetic variants of the core ARS genes and CHD susceptibility.

To determine the effect of genetic variants in the core ARS genes on CHD development, we conducted a case-control study by investigating the genotype frequency distribution of the 16 potential functional polymorphisms in the eight members of the MSC.

Materials and Methods

Ethics Statement

This study was approved by the institutional review board of Nanjing Medical University and adhered to the tenets of the Declaration of Helsinki. The design and performance of the current study involving human subjects were clearly described in a research protocol. All participants and/or their parents were voluntary and completed the informed consent in writing before taking part in this research.

Study populations

The case-control analysis included 984 affected children with sporadic CHD and 2953 unrelated non-CHD controls. All subjects were genetically unrelated ethnic Han Chinese. Subjects for the study were consecutively recruited from the Affiliated Nanjing Children's Hospital of Nanjing Medical University and the First Affiliated Hospital of Nanjing Medical University, Nanjing, China, from March 2009 to December 2011. All CHD patients were diagnosed based on echocardiography, with some diagnoses further confirmed by cardiac catheterization and/or surgery. Potential study subjects were initially surveyed with a brief questionnaire at clinics to determine whether they were willing to participate in a research study; we then conducted a face-to-face interview to obtain demographic information. Cases that had clinical features of developmental syndromes, multiple major developmental anomalies or known chromosomal abnormalities were excluded. The exclusion criteria also included a positive family history of CHD in a first-degree relative (parents, siblings and children), maternal diabetes mellitus, phenylketonuria, maternal teratogen exposure (e.g., pesticides and organic solvents), and maternal therapeutic drug exposure during the intrauterine period. Controls were non-CHD outpatients from the same geographic areas. They were recruited from the hospitals listed above during the same time period. Controls with congenital anomalies or cardiac disease were excluded. For each participant, approximately 2 ml of whole blood was obtained to extract genomic DNA for genotyping analysis.

SNP selection and genotyping

Eight ARSs (*EPRS, MRS, QRS, RRS, IRS, LRS, KRS, DRS*) that formed MSC were selected. For each ARS-coding gene, we first used the public HapMap single nucleotide polymorphism (SNP) database (phase II+ III Feb 09, on NCBI B36 assembly and dbSNP b126) to search for SNPs that localized within gene regions, with MAF≥0.05, in the Chinese Han population. Then, a web-based analysis tool was used to predict the function of these SNPs (http://snpinfo.niehs.nih.gov/snpinfo/snpfunc.htm). Finally, a total of 27 potentially functional SNPs were selected in 8 ARS-coding genes. We next conducted linkage disequilibrium (LD) analysis by the Haploview 4.2 software, and only one SNP was selected in the case of multiple SNPs in the same haplotype block (r^2>0.8). Eighteen (rs1061160, rs1061248, rs2230301 and rs5030754 in *EPRS*; rs508904 in *MRS*; rs193466, rs2305737 and rs244903 in *RRS*; rs1058751, rs10820966 and rs556155 in *IRS*; rs10988 in *LRS*; rs2233805 and rs3784929 in *KRS*; rs2164331, rs309142, rs309143 and rs6738266 in *DRS*) of 27 SNPs remained. Two SNPs (rs6738266 and rs2164331) were excluded due to primer design failure.

Genomic DNA was isolated from leukocyte pellets of venous blood by proteinase K digestion, followed by phenol-chloroform extraction and ethanol precipitation. Nanodrop and DNA electrophoresis were used to check the quality and quantity of DNA samples before genotyping. The genotyping was performed by Illumina Infinium BeadChip (Illumina, Inc.). All SNPs were successfully genotyped with call rates >95% (**Table 1**).

Statistical analyses

The differences between the CHD patients and control subjects were evaluated in the distributions of demographic characteristics, selected variables, and frequencies of genotypes of the 16 polymorphisms using Student's t-test (for continuous variables) or the χ^2 test (for categorical variables). The χ^2 test determined the Hardy-Weinberg equilibrium of the genotype distribution of polymorphisms in the control group. LD between SNPs was evaluated using Haploview 4.2.Odds ratios (ORs) and 95% confidence intervals (CIs) were estimated by logistic regression analyses in the additive model to estimate the associations between the variants genotypes and risk of CHD. Chi-square-based Q-test was applied to test the heterogeneity of associations between subgroups, and the heterogeneity was considered significant when $P<0.05$. All statistical analyses were performed using the Statistical Analysis System software (v.9.1.3; SAS Institute, Cary, NC, USA). All tests were two-sided, and $P<0.05$ was considered significant.

Results

An overview of the study design using a flowchart was performed as shown in **Figure 1**. We systematically investigated the association of potentially functional SNPs with CHD susceptibility in 984 cases and 2953 controls in a Chinese population. There were no statistically significant differences for the distributions of age and gender between cases and controls ($P=0.261$ and $P=0.832$, respectively). Among the 984 CHD patients, 312 had atrial septal defect (ASD), 585 were diagnosed with ventricular septal defect (VSD), and 87 were diagnosed with ASD combined with VSD.

The genotype distributions of the 16 SNPs and the associations with CHD risk are summarized in **Table 2**. The observed genotype frequencies of these SNPs were in agreement with Hardy-Weinberg equilibrium in the controls (P value from 0.16 to 1.00) except rs10988 ($P=0.04$). Among the 16 SNPs, significant

Table 1. Primary information for 16 functional SNPs in ARS-coding genes.

Gene	ARS	Chr. (cytoband)	SNP	Position (bp)[a]	Location	Predicted function[b]	MAF[c]	Allele[c]	HWE[d]	Genotyping call rate (%)
EPRS	Glutamyl-prolyl-tRNA synthetase	1q41	**rs1061248**	219968681	3'UTR	miRNA[e]	0.378	G/A	0.63	99.5
			rs1061160	219981426	exon	Splice sites[f]	0.366	G/A	0.76	99.8
			rs5030754	219983387	exon	Splice sites	0.012	G/A	0.82	99.9
			rs2230301	220024283	exon	Splice sites, nsSNP[g]	0.073	A/C	0.90	99.9
DRS	Aspartyl-tRNA synthetase	2q21.3	rs309143	135956608	intron	TFBS[h]	0.207	A/G	0.40	99.8
			rs309142	1395957754	intron	TFBS	0.488	A/G	0.29	99.8
LRS	Leucyl-tRNA synthetase	5q32	rs10988	146120433	exon	nsSNP	0.280	G/A	0.04	99.9
RRS	Arginyl-tRNA synthetase	5q34	rs244903	168486505	exon	Splice sites, nsSNP	0.146	A/G	0.35	99.7
			rs193466	1684865598	intron	TFBS	0.305	A/G	0.58	99.7
			rs2305737	168519256	3'UTR	Splice sites, miRNA	0.146	C/A	0.71	99.8
IRS	Isoleucyl-tRNA synthetase	9q22.31	rs1058751	92210634	3'UTR	miRNA	0.122	A/T	0.22	99.5
			rs556155	92223355	exon	nsSNP	0.195	A/G	0.25	99.9
			rs10820966	92293147	intron	TFBS	0.078	A/T	0.16	99.9
MRS	Methionyl-tRNA synthetase	12q13.3	rs508904	57488311	intron	TFBS	0.289	A/G	0.70	99.8
KRS	Lysyl-tRNA synthetase	16q23.1	rs3784929	75643129	intron	TFBS	0.159	G/A	0.66	99.8
			rs2233805	75647244	intron	TFBS	0.049	A/G	1.00	99.9

[a]Derived from the UCSC Genome Browser on Human Feb. 2009 (GRCh37/hg19) Assembly (http://genome.ucsc.edu/);
[b]Derived from an online tool-SNPinfo (http://snpinfo.niehs.nih.gov/snpfunc.htm);
[c]Major/minor allele;
[d]Hardy-Weinberg equilibrium test among controls;
[e]miRNA: microRNA
[f]Splice sites: Exonic splicing enhancer (ESE) or exonic splicing silencer (ESS) binding sites;
[g]nsSNP: non-synonymous polymorphisms.
[h]TFBS: Transcription factor binding sites;

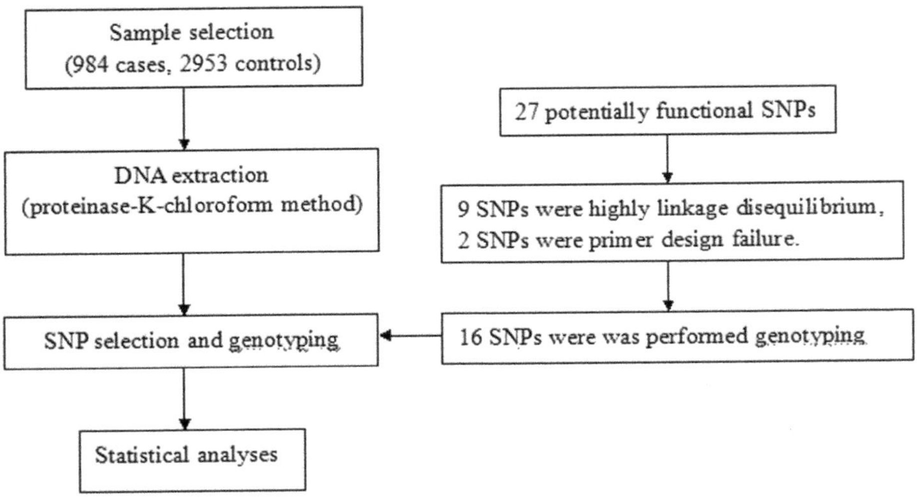

Figure 1. Study design procedures for association of ARSs gene polymorphisms with the risk of congenital heart disease in the Chinese Han population.

associations were observed between 4 SNPs (rs1061248, rs1061160, rs5030754 and rs2230301) and CHD risk following a logistic regression analysis in the additive model. All four SNPs were in the *ERPS* gene. The G allele of rs1061248 and the A allele of rs2230301 were associated with a decreased risk of CHD [additive model: odds ratio (OR) = 0.90, 95% confidence interval (CI) = 0.81–0.99, $P = 3.81 \times 10^{-2}$; and OR = 0.73, 95%CI = 0.60–0.90, $P = 3.53 \times 10^{-3}$, respectively]; however, the G allele of rs1061160 and the G allele of rs5030754 were associated with an increased risk of CHD (OR = 1.18, 95%CI = 1.06–1.31, $P = 1.28 \times 10^{-3}$; and OR = 1.39, 95%CI = 1.11–1.75, $P = 4.47 \times 10^{-3}$, respectively). We further calculated P values for the false discovery rate to perform multiple comparisons. After comparisons, we found that rs2230301, rs5030754 and rs1061160 correlated with CHD risk, whereas rs1061248 lost its significant association with the risk of CHD. In contrast, no obvious evidence of a significant association between the other 12 SNPs and CHD risk was found.

We have listed the results of the genotypic association analysis in **Table 3**. In dominant genetic model, for rs1061160 and rs5030754 polymorphisms, AG+AA and AG+GG genotypes were associated with an increased risk of CHD compared with the GG genotype, respectively(OR = 1.25, 95%CI = 1.07–1.46; OR = 1.44, 95%CI = 1.14–1.82). For rs2230301 polymorphism, AC+CC genotypes were associated with a decreased risk of CHD compared with the AA genotype(OR = 0.73, 95% CI = 0.59–0.91).

Additionally, we performed haplotype analysis (**Table 4**). As shown, the haplotype "GAAA" (combination of risk alleles of the four SNPs) was associated with an increased risk of CHD, whereas the protective allele combination "AGGC" was associated with a decreased risk of CHD. In the stratification analysis, we further evaluated the associations of the four SNPs in *EPRS* with CHD risk in subgroups stratified by gender and specific CHD phenotypes. As shown in **Table 5**, similar effects were observed among the subgroups.

We also conducted a combined analysis of the four promising SNPs to test their joint effects on CHD risk. There was a significant dosage-response effect among individuals carrying the different number of risk alleles and CHD risk ($P_{trend} = 5.00 \times 10^{-4}$). Compared with individuals with "0–2" risk allele, those carrying "3", "4" or "5 or more" risk alleles had a 0.97- (95% CI = 0.69–1.37), 1.25- (95% CI = 1.05–1.50) or 1.38-fold (95% CI = 1.14–1.68) increased risk of CHD, respectively (**Table 6**).

Discussion

In this study, we systematically investigated the association of potentially functional SNPs in ARS-coding genes of the MSC with CHD susceptibility in 984 cases and 2953 controls in a Chinese population. We observed significant association of four SNPs (rs1061248, rs1061160, rs5030754 and rs2230301) in the *EPRS* gene with the risk of CHD, and the risk remarkably accelerated in the individuals who carried more risk alleles. Although ASD and VSD represent the most common congenital heart malfunctions, the accurate pathogenesis is poorly understood. Based on previous research, the ARS-coding genes of MSC take part in diverse functional activities, and some of them have been proven to be crucial for heart development and proper functioning. Few studies have linked the variants of MSC genes to congenital heart disease. To our knowledge, we provide the first evidence that SNPs in *EPRS*, one of the core coding genes in MSC, may modulate the process of CHD.

Some ARSs in MSC have been demonstrated to have a close correlation with cardiovascular development. Glutamyl-prolyl-tRNA synthetase (*EPRS*) is a bifunctional enzyme that could translationally suppress vascular endothelial growth factor-A (VEGF-A) to regulate angiogenesis [21] and seems to act as a key gatekeeper of inflammatory gene translation [22]. Lysyl-tRNA synthetase (*KRS*) is secreted to trigger pro-inflammatory response [23] and plays a key role via Ap4A as an important signaling molecule in the transcriptional activity of microphthalmia transcription factor(MITF) [24], which has been demonstrated to be necessary in heart growth [25]. Glutaminyl-tRNA synthetase (*QRS*) can bind and inhibit the apoptotic activity of apoptosis signal-regulating kinase 1 (ASK1) [26], which has been demonstrated to be a new intracellular regulator of p38 MAPK activation in cardiac myogenic differentiation [27]. Han and colleagues [28] reported that Leucyl-tRNA synthetase (*LRS*) acts as a vital

Table 2. Summary of associations between 16 SNPs of MSC genes with congenital heart disease.

Chr. (cytoband)	Gene	SNP	Allele[a]	Case[b] (N = 984)	Control[b] (N = 2953)	MAF[c] Cases	MAF[c] Controls	HWE[d]	Additive model OR(95%CI)	Additive model P	P_{FDR}[e]
1q41	*EPRS*	**rs1061248**	G/A	217/486/271	741/1459/744	0.47	0.50	0.63	**0.90 (0.81–0.99)**	**3.81×10^{-2}**	**0.152**
		rs1061160	G/A	184/486/311	465/1402/1083	0.44	0.40	0.76	**1.18 (1.06–1.31)**	**1.82×10^{-3}**	**0.029**
		rs5030754	G/A	1/113/869	6/241/2704	0.06	0.04	0.82	**1.39 (1.11–1.75)**	**4.47×10^{-3}**	**0.023**
		rs2230301	A/C	3/114/865	20/440/2490	0.06	0.08	0.90	**0.73 (0.60–0.90)**	**3.53×10^{-3}**	**0.028**
2q21.3	*DRS*	rs309143	A/G	38/308/634	100/927/1921	0.20	0.19	0.40	1.03 (0.91–1.17)	6.40×10^{-1}	1.024
		rs309142	A/G	172/499/310	526/1472/949	0.43	0.43	0.29	1.01 (0.91–1.12)	9.11×10^{-1}	0.911
5q32	*LRS*	rs10988	G/A	47/340/596	120/1041/1789	0.22	0.22	0.04	1.02 (0.90–1.16)	7.32×10^{-1}	0.901
5q34	*RRS*	rs244903	A/G	15/213/754	50/622/2270	0.12	0.12	0.35	1.01 (0.87–1.18)	9.06×10^{-1}	0.966
		rs193466	A/G	74/399/509	229/1162/1553	0.28	0.28	0.58	1.02 (0.91–1.14)	7.72×10^{-1}	0.505
		rs2305737	C/A	20/270/691	60/744/2145	0.16	0.15	0.71	1.10 (0.95–1.26)	2.12×10^{-1}	0.565
9q22.31	*IRS*	rs1058751	A/T	0/150/828	11/412/2516	0.08	0.07	0.22	1.04 (0.86–1.27)	6.71×10^{-1}	0.976
		rs556155	A/G	16/206/760	34/627/2291	0.12	0.12	0.25	1.03 (0.88–1.21)	6.79×10^{-1}	0.905
		rs10820966	A/T	10/213/760	40/681/2230	0.12	0.13	0.16	0.91 (0.77–1.06)	2.21×10^{-1}	0.505
12q13.3	*MRS*	rs508904	A/G	105/442/433	301/1268/1380	0.33	0.32	0.70	1.07 (0.96–1.20)	2.01×10^{-1}	0.643
16q23.1	*KRS*	rs3784929	G/A	33/302/644	95/849/2005	0.19	0.18	0.66	1.08 (0.95–1.23)	2.40×10^{-1}	0.480
		rs2233805	A/G	0/31/951	1/106/2844	0.02	0.02	1.00	0.86 (0.57–1.29)	4.63×10^{-1}	0.823

[a]Major/minor allele;
[b]Variant homozygote/Heterozygote/Wild type homozygote;
[c]Minor allele frequency among cases/controls;
[d]Hardy-Weinberg equilibrium test among controls.
[e]Multiple comparisons P values for false discovery rate.

Table 3. Summary of genotypic association analysis of four SNPs of the *EPRS gene* with congenital heart disease.

SNP	Genotype	Cases	Controls	OR (95%CI)	*P*
rs1061248	GG	271	744	1.00	-
	AG	486	1459	0.91 (0.77–1.09)	3.11×10^{-1}
	AA	217	741	**0.80 (0.65–0.99)**	$\mathbf{3.74\times10^{-2}}$
	AG+AA	703	2200	0.88 (0.75–1.03)	1.15×10^{-1}
rs1061160	GG	311	1083	1.00	-
	AG	486	1402	**1.21 (1.03–1.42)**	$\mathbf{2.35\times10^{-2}}$
	AA	164	465	**1.38 (1.11–1.70)**	$\mathbf{3.07\times10^{-3}}$
	AG+AA	650	1867	**1.25 (1.07–1.46)**	$\mathbf{4.54\times10^{-3}}$
rs5030754	GG	869	2704	1.00	-
	AG	113	241	**1.46 (1.15–1.85)**	$\mathbf{1.72\times10^{-3}}$
	AA	1	6	0.52 (0.06–4.31)	5.44×10^{-1}
	AG+GG	114	247	**1.44 (1.14–1.82)**	$\mathbf{2.51\times10^{-3}}$
rs2230301	AA	865	2490	1.00	-
	AC	114	440	**0.75 (0.60–0.93)**	$\mathbf{8.99\times10^{-3}}$
	CC	3	20	0.43 (0.13–1.46)	1.76×10^{-1}
	AC+CC	117	460	**0.73 (0.59–0.91)**	$\mathbf{4.90\times10^{-3}}$

mediator for amino acid signaling to mTORC1, and the latter has been found to be related to the normal development of cardiovascular tissue [29].

Human *EPRS*, the largest polypeptide from the complex, is a bifunctional enzyme in which the two domains exhibiting each catalytic activity are linked by three tandem WHEP motifs [30]. *EPRS* contains 29 exons and 28 introns. In response to interferon-γ (IFNγ), *EPRS* is phosphorylated and released from its residence in the MSC. MSC then forms another multi-component complex, known as IFN-γ–activated inhibitor of translation (GAIT), with other regulatory proteins at a 3′UTR region that is involved in the translational silencing of target transcripts, such as VEGF-A [31,32,33]. As documented in many studies, VEGF-A shares a close relationship with CHD, and both the increased and decreased expression of VEGF-A during heart development can result in various CHD [34,35,36]. The SNP rs2230301, a missense SNP located at the 23rd exon of the *EPRS* gene, may act as a part of the exonic splicing enhancer based on the online tool SNPinfo [37]. The missense mutation would change the sequence of *EPRS* and may lead to protein misfolding and malfunction. We used a web-based analysis tool to predict the potential function of the SNPs, and rs2230301 was predicted to be a missense variant that may result in an amino acid alteration from aspartic acid (Asp) to glutamic acid (Glu) (http://snpinfo.niehs.nih.gov/snpinfo/snpfunc.htm). The NCBI database confirmed the results (http://www.ncbi.nlm.nih.gov/). However, the predicted results differed from the *in-silico* analysis. To further validate the function of this variant, some functional studies should be performed in some follow-up studies. The SNP rs1061248 is located at the 3′ regulatory region of the *EPRS* gene with a predicted function as a MicroRNA-binding site. Considering its potentially functional role, it is likely that this polymorphism might alter miRNA binding, thereby modulating the biological function of *EPRS*. The two synonymous SNPs rs1061160 and rs5030754 were localized on the seventh exon and the eleventh exon, respectively. Recently, a synonymous SNP was reported to alter the function of the protein in certain circumstances [38].

Several limitations of the present study need to be addressed. First, we did not replicate the results in additional individuals; this may contribute to potential false positive errors. The present analysis was restricted to individuals of Chinese Han descent, and therefore, the findings may not hold true for individuals of other

Table 4. The haplotypic association of the four SNPs of the *EPRS* gene with congenital heart disease.

Haplotype[a]	case (%)	control (%)	OR (95%CI)	*P*
AGGA	905 (45.99)	2835 (48.0)	1.00 (referent)	
GAGA	740 (37.60)	2075 (35.13)	1.12 (0.99–1.25)	5.34×10^{-2}
GGGC	100 (5.08)	370 (6.26)	0.85 (0.67–1.07)	1.62×10^{-1}
GGGA	84 (4.27)	259 (4.39)	1.02 (0.79–1.31)	9.04×10^{-1}
GAAA	113 (5.74)	253 (4.28)	**1.40 (1.11–1.77)**	$\mathbf{4.91\times10^{-3}}$
AGGC	20 (1.02)	107 (1.81)	**0.59 (0.36–0.95)**	$\mathbf{3.00\times10^{-2}}$
Others	6 (0.30)	7 (0.12)	2.69 (0.90–8.01)	7.65×10^{-2}

[a]SNP order: rs1061248, rs1061160, rs5030754 and rs2230301.

Table 5. Stratified analysis on the associations between four SNPs in *EPRS* with congenital heart disease.

Characteristics	rs1061248					rs1061160				
	Case [a]	Control [a]	OR (95%CI) [b]	P^b	P^c	Case [a]	Control [a]	OR (95%CI) [b]	P^b	P^c
Gender										
male	105/241/138	472/856/464	0.87 (0.76–1.00)	4.90×10^{-2}	0.527	91/237/160	286/844/667	1.16 (1.00–1.33)	4.79×10^{-2}	0.751
female	112/245/133	269/603/280	0.93 (0.80–1.09)	3.74×10^{-1}		93/249/151	179/558/416	1.20 (1.03–1.40)	1.83×10^{-2}	
Diagnostic groups										
ASD	71/139/98	741/1459/744	0.84 (0.71–0.99)	4.27×10^{-2}	0.483	68/146/98	465/1402/1083	1.26 (1.07–1.49)	6.44×10^{-3}	0.489
VSD	126/299/154	741/1459/744	0.91 (0.80–1.03)	1.41×10^{-1}		104/294/184	465/1402/1083	1.16 (1.02–1.32)	2.21×10^{-2}	
ASD/VSD	20/48/19	741/1459/744	1.03 (0.76–1.39)	8.71×10^{-1}		12/46/29	465/1402/1083	1.03 (0.76–1.40)	8.52×10^{-1}	
Characteristics	**rs5030754**					**rs2230301**				
	Case [a]	Control [a]	OR(95%CI) [b]	P^b	P^c	Case [a]	Control [a]	OR(95%CI) [b]	P^b	P^c
Gender										
male	1/58/429	4/135/1659	1.58 (1.16–2.15)	3.90×10^{-3}	0.211	3/64/421	13/280/1504	0.83 (0.63–1.09)	1.77×10^{-1}	0.260
female	0/55/440	2/106/1045	1.18 (0.84–1.65)	3.37×10^{-1}		0/50/444	7/160/986	0.65 (0.47–0.90)	9.74×10^{-3}	
Diagnostic groups										
ASD	0/42/270	6/241/2704	1.62 (1.15–2.27)	5.54×10^{-3}	0.119	0/31/280	20/440/2490	0.59 (0.41–0.86)	5.93×10^{-3}	0.281
VSD	1/67/516	6/241/2704	1.40 (1.07–1.85)	1.56×10^{-2}		2/76/506	20/440/2490	0.83 (0.65–1.06)	1.37×10^{-1}	
ASD/VSD	0/4/83	6/241/2704	0.53 (0.19–1.43)	2.08×10^{-1}		1/7/79	20/440/2490	0.62 (0.31–1.21)	1.62×10^{-1}	

[a]Major/minor allele;
[b]Calculated by additive model;
[c]*P* for heterogeneity.

Table 6. Combined effects of rs1061248, rs1061160, rs1061160, and rs2230301 on CHD.

Number of risk alleles[a]	Case (%)	Control (%)	OR (95% CI)[b]	P^b
0–2	262 (26.95)	939 (31.96)	1.00	
3	50 (5.14)	184 (6.26)	0.97 (0.69–1.37)	8.79×10^{-1}
4	384 (39.51)	1098 (37.37)	1.25 (1.05–1.50)	1.37×10^{-2}
≥5	276 (28.40)	717 (24.40)	1.38 (1.14–1.68)	1.20×10^{-3}
Trend				5.00×10^{-4}

[a]rs1061248 G, rs1061160 A, rs5030754 A, and rs2230301 A were assumed as risk alleles;
[b]Calculated by additive model.

races and ethnicities. Additionally, the limited sample size may contribute to the failed validation in the stratified analysis concerning the association between the SNPs and CHD. We performed the statistic power analysis of the significant SNPs in the studied population. The powers of three SNPs (rs1061248, rs5030754, and rs2230301) are lower than 0.6 because the sample size of our study is relatively small (984 CHD cases and 2953 non-CHD controls) and the effects of our target common SNPs are weak. Further replication of the association signal in an independent cohort for the four SNPs would support the conclusions. Therefore, the results are required to be further replicated by well-designed studies in additional large-scale Chinese Han populations.

In conclusion, we conducted a case-control study to investigate the role of genetic variants in ARS-coding genes of MSC in the development of CHD in a Chinese population. We observed that four SNPs (rs1061248, rs1061160, rs5030754, and rs2230301) in the *EPRS* gene may confer susceptibility to sporadic CHD and that the risk significantly increased with the number of risk alleles. However, further studies with functional evaluations are warranted to elucidate the potentially biological mechanisms of these polymorphisms in the development of CHD.

Supporting Information

Figure S1 Expressed sequence tags (EST) profile of the 8 core ARSs coding genes.

Author Contributions

Conceived and designed the experiments: XM. Performed the experiments: MD YF JX. Analyzed the data: YH YL BN BQ. Contributed reagents/materials/analysis tools: ZH. Contributed to the writing of the manuscript: MD YF JX XM.

References

1. Hoffman JI, Kaplan S (2002) The incidence of congenital heart disease. J Am Coll Cardiol 39: 1890–1900.
2. Botto LD, Correa A, Erickson JD (2001) Racial and temporal variations in the prevalence of heart defects. Pediatrics 107: E32.
3. Rosamond W, Flegal K, Friday G, Furie K, Go A, et al. (2007) Heart disease and stroke statistics–2007 update: a report from the American Heart Association Statistics Committee and Stroke Statistics Subcommittee. Circulation 115: e69–171.
4. Gatzoulis MA (2004) Adult congenital heart disease: a cardiovascular area of growth in urgent need of additional resource allocation. Int J Cardiol 97 Suppl 1: 1–2.
5. van der Bom T, Zomer AC, Zwinderman AH, Meijboom FJ, Bouma BJ, et al. (2011) The changing epidemiology of congenital heart disease. Nat Rev Cardiol 8: 50–60.
6. Jenkins KJ, Correa A, Feinstein JA, Botto L, Britt AE, et al. (2007) Noninherited risk factors and congenital cardiovascular defects: current knowledge: a scientific statement from the American Heart Association Council on Cardiovascular Disease in the Young: endorsed by the American Academy of Pediatrics. Circulation 115: 2995–3014.
7. Huhta J, Linask KK (2013) Environmental origins of congenital heart disease: the heart-placenta connection. Semin Fetal Neonatal Med 18: 245–250.
8. Pierpont ME, Basson CT, Benson DW Jr, Gelb BD, Giglia TM, et al. (2007) Genetic basis for congenital heart defects: current knowledge: a scientific statement from the American Heart Association Congenital Cardiac Defects Committee, Council on Cardiovascular Disease in the Young: endorsed by the American Academy of Pediatrics. Circulation 115: 3015–3038.
9. Wessels MW, Willems PJ (2010) Genetic factors in non-syndromic congenital heart malformations. Clin Genet 78: 103–123.
10. Wolf M, Basson CT (2010) The molecular genetics of congenital heart disease: a review of recent developments. Curr Opin Cardiol 25: 192–197.
11. Garg V (2006) Insights into the genetic basis of congenital heart disease. Cell Mol Life Sci 63: 1141–1148.
12. Schimmel P (1987) Aminoacyl tRNA synthetases: general scheme of structure-function relationships in the polypeptides and recognition of transfer RNAs. Annu Rev Biochem 56: 125–158.
13. Park SG, Ewalt KL, Kim S (2005) Functional expansion of aminoacyl-tRNA synthetases and their interacting factors: new perspectives on housekeepers. Trends Biochem Sci 30: 569–574.
14. Guo M, Yang XL, Schimmel P (2010) New functions of aminoacyl-tRNA synthetases beyond translation. Nat Rev Mol Cell Biol 11: 668–674.
15. Park SG, Schimmel P, Kim S (2008) Aminoacyl tRNA synthetases and their connections to disease. Proc Natl Acad Sci U S A 105: 11043–11049.
16. Guo M, Schimmel P (2013) Essential nontranslational functions of tRNA synthetases. Nat Chem Biol 9: 145–153.
17. Ray PS, Arif A, Fox PL (2007) Macromolecular complexes as depots for releasable regulatory proteins. Trends Biochem Sci 32: 158–164.
18. Simos G, Grosshans H, Hurt E (2002) Nuclear export of tRNA. Results Probl Cell Differ 35: 115–131.
19. Hopper AK, Phizicky EM (2003) tRNA transfers to the limelight. Genes Dev 17: 162–180.
20. Nathanson L, Deutscher MP (2000) Active aminoacyl-tRNA synthetases are present in nuclei as a high molecular weight multienzyme complex. J Biol Chem 275: 31559–31562.
21. Ray PS, Fox PL (2007) A post-transcriptional pathway represses monocyte VEGF-A expression and angiogenic activity. EMBO J 26: 3360–3372.
22. Mukhopadhyay R, Jia J, Arif A, Ray PS, Fox PL (2009) The GAIT system: a gatekeeper of inflammatory gene expression. Trends Biochem Sci 34: 324–331.
23. Park SG, Kim HJ, Min YH, Choi EC, Shin YK, et al. (2005) Human lysyl-tRNA synthetase is secreted to trigger proinflammatory response. Proc Natl Acad Sci U S A 102: 6356–6361.
24. Lee YN, Nechushtan H, Figov N, Razin E (2004) The function of lysyl-tRNA synthetase and Ap4A as signaling regulators of MITF activity in FcepsilonRI-activated mast cells. Immunity 20: 145–151.
25. Tshori S, Gilon D, Beeri R, Nechushtan H, Kaluzhny D, et al. (2006) Transcription factor MITF regulates cardiac growth and hypertrophy. J Clin Invest 116: 2673–2681.
26. Aizenshtat LI, Rozenblyum YZ (1975) The OPD-1 trial frame for children. Biomed Eng (NY) 8: 177–178.
27. Choi TG, Lee J, Ha J, Kim SS (2011) Apoptosis signal-regulating kinase 1 is an intracellular inducer of p38 MAPK-mediated myogenic signalling in cardiac myoblasts. Biochim Biophys Acta 1813: 1412–1421.
28. Han JM, Jeong SJ, Park MC, Kim G, Kwon NH, et al. (2012) Leucyl-tRNA synthetase is an intracellular leucine sensor for the mTORC1-signaling pathway. Cell 149: 410–424.
29. Malhowski AJ, Hira H, Bashiruddin S, Warburton R, Goto J, et al. (2011) Smooth muscle protein-22-mediated deletion of Tsc1 results in cardiac

hypertrophy that is mTORC1-mediated and reversed by rapamycin. Hum Mol Genet 20: 1290–1305.

30. Rho SB, Lee JS, Jeong EJ, Kim KS, Kim YG, et al. (1998) A multifunctional repeated motif is present in human bifunctional tRNA synthetase. J Biol Chem 273: 11267–11273.
31. Arif A, Jia J, Moodt RA, DiCorleto PE, Fox PL (2011) Phosphorylation of glutamyl-prolyl tRNA synthetase by cyclin-dependent kinase 5 dictates transcript-selective translational control. Proc Natl Acad Sci U S A 108: 1415–1420.
32. Sampath P, Mazumder B, Seshadri V, Gerber CA, Chavatte L, et al. (2004) Noncanonical function of glutamyl-prolyl-tRNA synthetase: gene-specific silencing of translation. Cell 119: 195–208.
33. Ray PS, Jia J, Yao P, Majumder M, Hatzoglou M, et al. (2009) A stress-responsive RNA switch regulates VEGFA expression. Nature 457: 915–919.
34. Zhao W, Wang J, Shen J, Sun K, Zhu J, et al. (2010) Mutations in VEGFA are associated with congenital left ventricular outflow tract obstruction. Biochem Biophys Res Commun 396: 483–488.
35. Ackerman C, Locke AE, Feingold E, Reshey B, Espana K, et al. (2012) An excess of deleterious variants in VEGF-A pathway genes in Down-syndrome-associated atrioventricular septal defects. Am J Hum Genet 91: 646–659.
36. Vannay A, Vasarhelyi B, Kornyei M, Treszl A, Kozma G, et al. (2006) Single-nucleotide polymorphisms of VEGF gene are associated with risk of congenital valvuloseptal heart defects. Am Heart J 151: 878–881.
37. Xu Z, Taylor JA (2009) SNPinfo: integrating GWAS and candidate gene information into functional SNP selection for genetic association studies. Nucleic Acids Res 37: W600–605.
38. Kimchi-Sarfaty C, Oh JM, Kim IW, Sauna ZE, Calcagno AM, et al. (2007) A "silent" polymorphism in the MDR1 gene changes substrate specificity. Science 315: 525–528.

Permissions

All chapters in this book were first published in PLOS ONE, by The Public Library of Science; hereby published with permission under the Creative Commons Attribution License or equivalent. Every chapter published in this book has been scrutinized by our experts. Their significance has been extensively debated. The topics covered herein carry significant findings which will fuel the growth of the discipline. They may even be implemented as practical applications or may be referred to as a beginning point for another development.

The contributors of this book come from diverse backgrounds, making this book a truly international effort. This book will bring forth new frontiers with its revolutionizing research information and detailed analysis of the nascent developments around the world.

We would like to thank all the contributing authors for lending their expertise to make the book truly unique. They have played a crucial role in the development of this book. Without their invaluable contributions this book wouldn't have been possible. They have made vital efforts to compile up to date information on the varied aspects of this subject to make this book a valuable addition to the collection of many professionals and students.

This book was conceptualized with the vision of imparting up-to-date information and advanced data in this field. To ensure the same, a matchless editorial board was set up. Every individual on the board went through rigorous rounds of assessment to prove their worth. After which they invested a large part of their time researching and compiling the most relevant data for our readers.

The editorial board has been involved in producing this book since its inception. They have spent rigorous hours researching and exploring the diverse topics which have resulted in the successful publishing of this book. They have passed on their knowledge of decades through this book. To expedite this challenging task, the publisher supported the team at every step. A small team of assistant editors was also appointed to further simplify the editing procedure and attain best results for the readers.

Apart from the editorial board, the designing team has also invested a significant amount of their time in understanding the subject and creating the most relevant covers. They scrutinized every image to scout for the most suitable representation of the subject and create an appropriate cover for the book.

The publishing team has been an ardent support to the editorial, designing and production team. Their endless efforts to recruit the best for this project, has resulted in the accomplishment of this book. They are a veteran in the field of academics and their pool of knowledge is as vast as their experience in printing. Their expertise and guidance has proved useful at every step. Their uncompromising quality standards have made this book an exceptional effort. Their encouragement from time to time has been an inspiration for everyone.

The publisher and the editorial board hope that this book will prove to be a valuable piece of knowledge for researchers, students, practitioners and scholars across the globe.

List of Contributors

Truls Råmunddal, Christian Dworeck, Oskar Angerås, Jacob Odenstedt, Dan Ioanes, Göran Matejka, Per Albertsson and Elmir Omerovic
Department of Cardiology, Sahlgrenska University Hospital, Gothenburg, Sweden

Loes Hoebers and Jose P. S. Henriques
Department of Cardiology, Academic Medical Center, Amsterdam, The Netherlands

Göran Olivecrona and Jan Harnek
Department of Coronary Heart Disease, Skåne University Hospital, Scania, Sweden

Ulf Jensen, Mikael Aasa and Risto Jussila
Department of Cardiology, Stockholm South General Hospital, Stockholm, Sweden

Stefan James and Bo Lagerqvist
Department of Medical Sciences, Uppsala University, Uppsala, Sweden

Fabien A. Picard and Jean-Michel Juliard
Cardiology Department, Assistance Publique-Hôpitaux de Paris, Hôpital Bichat, Université Paris-Diderot, Sorbonne-Paris Cité, Paris, France

Pascal Gueret and Stéphane Champagne
Cardiology Department, Assistance Publique-Hôpitaux de Paris, Hôpital Henri Mondor, Université Paris-Est-Cré teil, Cré teil, France

Jean-Pierre Laissy
Radiology Department, Assistance Publique-Hô pitaux de Paris, Hô pital Bichat, Université Paris-Diderot, Sorbonne-Paris Cité, Paris, France
Dé partement Hospitalo-Universitaire FIRE, INSERM U-1148, Assistance Publique-Hô pitaux de Paris, Hô pital Bichat, Université Paris-Diderot, Sorbonne-Paris Cité, Paris, France

Florence Leclercq
Cardiology Department, Centre Hospitalier Universitaire Arnaud de Villeneuve Montpellier, France

Didier Carrié
Cardiology Department, Centre Hospitalier Universitaire de Rangueil, Toulouse, France

Patrick Henry
Cardiology Department, Assistance Publique-Hôpitaux de Paris, Hôpital Lariboisière, Université Paris-Diderot, Sorbonne-Paris Cité, Paris, France

Ralph Niarra
Epidemiology and Clinical Research Unit, Assistance Publique-Hôpitaux de Paris, Hôpital Europé en Georges-Pompidou, Paris, France
Unité INSERM Centre D'investigation Épidé miologique 4, Paris, France

Gilles Chatellier
Epidemiology and Clinical Research Unit, Assistance Publique-Hôpitaux de Paris, Hôpital Europé en Georges-Pompidou, Paris, France
Unité INSERM Centre D'investigation Épidé miologique 4, Paris, France
Université Paris Descartes, Sorbonne Paris Cité , Faculté de Mé decine, Paris, France
NHLI Imperial College, ICMS Royal Brompton Hospital, London, United Kingdom

Philippe Gabriel Steg
Cardiology Department, Assistance Publique-Hôpitaux de Paris, Hôpital Bichat, Université Paris-Diderot, Sorbonne-Paris Cité , Paris, France
Département Hospitalo-Universitaire FIRE, INSERM U-1148, Assistance Publique-Hô pitaux de Paris, Hôpital Bichat, Université Paris-Diderot, Sorbonne-Paris Cité, Paris, France
NHLI Imperial College, ICMS Royal Brompton Hospital, London, United Kingdom

Jing-Fang Hsu and Fang-Yu Chen
L5 Research Center, China Medical University Hospital, Taichung, Taiwan

Tzu-Chieh Chou
Department of Public Health, China Medical University, Taichung, Taiwan
Department of Health Risk Management, China Medical University, Taichung, Taiwan

Jonathan Lu and Shu-Hua Chen
Vascular and Medicinal Research, Texas Heart Institute, Houston, Texas, United States of America

Ching-Chu Chen
Department of Internal Medicine, China Medical University Hospital, Taichung, Taiwan

Jeffrey L. Chen
Physical Medicine & Rehabilitation, Department of Orthopedic Surgery, University of California San Diego, San Diego, California, United States of America

MacArthur Elayda
Biostatistics and Epidemiology, Texas Heart Institute, Houston, Texas, United States of America

Christie M. Ballantyne
Department of Medicine, Baylor College of Medicine, Houston, Texas, United States of America

Steven Shayani
Mount Sinai Medical Center, New York, New York, United States of America
New York Heart Research Foundation, New York, New York, United States of America

Chu- Huang Chen
L5 Research Center, China Medical University Hospital, Taichung, Taiwan
Vascular and Medicinal Research, Texas Heart Institute, Houston, Texas, United States of America
Department of Medicine, Baylor College of Medicine, Houston, Texas, United States of America
Department of Medicine, Kaohsiung Medical University, Kaohsiung, Taiwan

Stephen Burgess, Daniel F. Freitag, Hassan Khan, Donal N. Gorman and Simon G. Thompson
Cardiovascular Epidemiology Unit, Department of Public Health and Primary Care, University of Cambridge, Cambridge, Cambridgeshire, United Kingdom

Chun-Tai Mao, Ming- Jui Hung and Chao-Hung Wang
Heart Failure Center, Division of Cardiology, Department of Internal Medicine, Chang Gung Memorial Hospital, Keelung, Taiwan
College of Medicine, Chang Gung University, Taoyuan, Taiwan

Ming-Lung Tsai, Chao-Yung Wang, Ming-Shien Wen and I-Chang Hsieh and Chun-Chi Chen
Division of Cardiology, Department of Internal Medicine, Chang Gung Memorial Hospital, Taipei, Taiwan
College of Medicine, Chang Gung University, Taoyuan, Taiwan

Tien-Hsing Chen
Division of Cardiology, Department of Internal Medicine, Chang Gung Memorial Hospital, Taipei, Taiwan
Department of cardiology, Chang Gung Memorial Hospital, Xiamen, China
College of Medicine, Chang Gung University, Taoyuan, Taiwan

Milan Gautam., Atsushi Izawa, Yuji Shiba, Hirohiko Motoki, Takahiro Takeuchi, Ayako Okada, Takeshi Tomita, Yusuke Miyashita, Jun Koyama and Uichi Ikeda
Department of Cardiovascular Medicine, Shinshu University School of Medicine, Matsumoto, Nagano, Japan

Kosuke Minai, Takayuki Ogawa, Makoto Kawai, Kimiaki Komukai, Toshikazu Tanaka, Kazuo Ogawa, Tomohisa Nagoshi, Satoshi Arase, Satoshi Morimoto, Yasunori Inoue, Hiroshi Sekiyama, Akihiro Urabe, Seiichiro Matsuo, Kenichi Hongo and Michihiro Yoshimura
Division of Cardiology, Department of Internal Medicine, The Jikei University School of Medicine, Tokyo, Japan

Gelin Xu, Zhizhong Zhang, Qiushi Lv, Yun Li, Ruidong Ye, Yunyun Xiong, Yongjun Jiang and Xinfeng Liu
Department of Neurology, Jinling Hospital, Nanjing University School of Medicine, Nanjing, Jiangsu Province, China

Bernhard Haring
Department of Internal Medicine I, Comprehensive Heart Failure Center, University of Würzburg, Würzburg, Bavaria, Germany

Noelle Gronroos and Alvaro Alonso
Division of Epidemiology and Community Health, University of Minnesota, Minneapolis, Minnesota, United States of America

Jennifer A. Nettleton
Division of Epidemiology, Human Genetics and Environmental Sciences, School of Public Health, University of Texas Health Science Center at Houston, Houston, Texas, United States of America

Moritz C. Wyler von Ballmoos
Department of Surgery & Division of Cardiothoracic Surgery, Froedtert Memorial Hospital & Medical College of Wisconsin, Milwaukee, Wisconsin, United States of America

Elizabeth Selvin
Department of Epidemiology and the Welch Center for Prevention, Epidemiology and Clinical Research, Johns Hopkins Bloomberg School of Public Health, Baltimore, Maryland, United States of America

Bijun Zhao and Shiqiang Yu
Department of Cardiovascular Surgery, Xijing Hospital, The Fourth Military Medical University, Xi'an, China

Yuan Lin, Kai Zhang and Hongbing Shen
State Key Laboratory of Reproductive Medicine, Nanjing Medical University, Nanjing, China
Department of Epidemiology and Biostatistics and Key Laboratory of Modern Toxicology of Ministry of Education, School of Public Health, Nanjing Medical University, Nanjing, China

Bixian Ni and Hongxia Ma
Department of Epidemiology and Biostatistics and Key Laboratory of Modern Toxicology of Ministry of Education, School of Public Health, Nanjing Medical University, Nanjing, China

Jing Xu, Xiaowei Wang and Yijiang Chen
Department of Thoracic and Cardiovascular Surgery, The First Affiliated Hospital of Nanjing Medical University, Nanjing, China

Yuanli Hu, Min Da and Xuming Mo
Department of Cardiothoracic Surgery, Nanjing Children's Hospital, Nanjing Medical University, Nanjing, China

Chenyue Ding
Center of Clinical Reproductive Medicine, First Affiliated Hospital, Nanjing Medical University, Nanjing, China

Jiayin Liu
State Key Laboratory of Reproductive Medicine, Nanjing Medical University, Nanjing, China
Center of Clinical Reproductive Medicine, First Affiliated Hospital, Nanjing Medical University, Nanjing, China

Shiwei Yang
Department of Cardiology, Nanjing Children's Hospital, Nanjing Medical University, Nanjing, China

Jiahao Sha
State Key Laboratory of Reproductive Medicine, Nanjing Medical University, Nanjing, China
Department of Histology and Embryology, Nanjing Medical University, Nanjing, China

Ragnar O. Vilmundarson
Ruddy Canadian Cardiovascular Genetics Centre, University of Ottawa Heart Institute, Ottawa, Ontario, Canada,
Department of Biochemistry, Microbiology andImmunology, University of Ottawa, Ottawa, Ontario, Canada

Naif A. M. Almontashiri
Ruddy Canadian Cardiovascular Genetics Centre, University of Ottawa Heart Institute, Ottawa, Ontario, Canada
Department of Biochemistry, Microbiology andImmunology, University of Ottawa, Ottawa, Ontario, Canada
Center for Genetics and Inherited Diseases, Taibah University, Almadina, Saudi Arabia

Nima Ghasemzadeh
Department of Medicine, Emory University, Atlanta, Georgia, United States of America

Sonny Dandona and Arshed A. Quyyumi
Department of Medicine, McGill University, Montreal, Canada

Alexandre F. R. Stewart
Ruddy Canadian Cardiovascular Genetics Centre, University of Ottawa Heart Institute, Ottawa, Ontario, Canada
Department of Biochemistry, Microbiology andImmunology, University of Ottawa, Ottawa, Ontario, Canada
Department of Medicine, University of Ottawa, Ottawa, Ontario, Canada

Robert Roberts
Ruddy Canadian Cardiovascular Genetics Centre, University of Ottawa Heart Institute, Ottawa, Ontario, Canada
Department of Medicine, University of Ottawa, Ottawa, Ontario, Canada

Hsiao-Huei Chen
Department of Medicine, University of Ottawa, Ottawa, Ontario, Canada
Ottawa Hospital Research Institute, Ottawa, Ontario, Canada

Gang Xu
Department of Preventive Medicine, School of Basic Medicine, Jiangxi University of Traditional Chinese Medicine, Nanchang, Jiangxi, China

Xuemei Sui and Steven N. Blair
Department of Exercise Science, Arnold School of Public Health, University of South Carolina, Columbia, South Carolina, United States of America

Shiwei Liu and Yichong Li
National Center for Chronic and Noncommunicable Disease Control and Prevention, Chinese Center for Disease Control and Prevention, Beijing, China

Jie Liu
Division of Chronic Disease Control and Prevention, Jiangxi Province Center for Disease Control and Prevention, Nanchang, Jiangxi, China

Junxiu Liu
Department of Epidemiology and Biostatisitcs, Arnold School of Public Health, University of South Carolina, Columbia, South Carolina, United States of America

Shouqing Huang
The Second People's Hospital Affiliated to Fujian University of Traditional Chinese Medicine, Fuzhou, Fujian, China

Zhengzhen Wang
Division of Exercise Rehabilitation, Beijing Sport University Sport Rehabilitation College, Beijing, China

Ingerid Arbo
K.G. Jebsen Center of Exercise in Medicine, Department of Circulation and Medical Imaging, Faculty of Medicine, Norwegian University of Science and Technology, Trondheim, Norway

Erik Madssen
K.G. Jebsen Center of Exercise in Medicine, Department of Circulation and Medical Imaging, Faculty of Medicine, Norwegian University of Science and Technology, Trondheim, Norway
Department of Pulmonary Medicine, St. Olavs Hospital, Trondheim, Norway

Ingrid Granøien and Liv Walderhaug
Ålesund Hospital, Ålesund, Norway

Trine Moholdt
K.G. Jebsen Center of Exercise in Medicine, Department of Circulation and Medical Imaging, Faculty of Medicine, Norwegian University of Science and Technology, Trondheim, Norway
Women's Clinic, St. Olavs Hospital, Trondheim, Norway

Chi Zhang
Department of Neurosurgery, Shanghai Seventh People's Hospital, Shanghai, China

Zhi-Yong Wang
Department of Information, Changhai Hospital, Second Military Medical University Shanghai, China

Ying-Yi Qin and Fei-Fei Yu
Department of Health Statistics, Second Military Medical University, Shanghai, China

Yu-Hao Zhou
Department of Rehabilitation Institute, Shanghai Seventh People's Hospital, Shanghai, China

Manuel Muñoz-Torres and Beatriz García-Fontana
Bone Metabolic Unit (RETICEF), Endocrinology Division, Hospital Universitario San Cecilio, Instituto de Investigación Biosanitaria de Granada, Granada, Spain

Antonia Garcia-Martín
Bone Metabolic Unit (RETICEF), Endocrinology Division, Hospital Universitario San Cecilio, Instituto de Investigación Biosanitaria de Granada, Granada, Spain
Endocrinology, Hospital Comarcal del Noroeste, Caravaca de la Cruz, Murcia, Spain

Rebeca Reyes-Garcia
Bone Metabolic Unit (RETICEF), Endocrinology Division, Hospital Universitario San Cecilio, Instituto de Investigación Biosanitaria de Granada, Granada, Spain
Endocrinology Unit, Hospital General Universitario Rafael Mendez, Lorca, Murcia Spain

Sonia Morales-Santana
Bone Metabolic Unit (RETICEF), Endocrinology Division, Hospital Universitario San Cecilio, Instituto de Investigación Biosanitaria de Granada, Granada, Spain
Proteomic Research Service, Fundación para la Investigación Biosanitaria de Andalucía Oriental -Alejandro Otero- (FIBAO), Granada, Spain

Ana Coto-Montes
Department of Morphology and Cellular Biology (RETICEF), Faculty of Medicine, University of Oviedo, Oviedo, Spain

Manuel Muñoz-Garach
Critical Care and Emergencies Unit, Hospital Universitario San Cecilio, Granada, Spain

Pedro Rozas-Moreno
Endocrinology Division, Hospital General de Ciudad Real, Ciudad Real, Spain

Jørgen Jeppesen
Department of Internal Medicine, Glostrup Hospital, University of Copenhagen, Glostrup, Denmark

Julie K. K. Vishram
Department of Internal Medicine, Glostrup Hospital, University of Copenhagen, Glostrup, Denmark, Research Centre for Prevention and Health, Glostrup Hospital, University of Copenhagen, Glostrup, Denmark

Anders Borglykke, Anne H. Andreasen and Torben Jørgensen
Research Centre for Prevention and Health, Glostrup Hospital, University of Copenhagen, Glostrup, Denmark

Hans Ibsen
Division of Cardiology, Holbæk University Hospital, Holbæk, Denmark

Luigi Palmieri, Simona Giampaoli and Chiara Donfrancesco
Cerebro and Cardiovascular Epidemiology Unit, National Centre of Epidemiology Surveillance and Health Promotion, National Institute of Health, Rome, Italy

Frank Kee
UKCRC Centre of Excellence for Public Health Research (NI), The Queen's University of Belfast, Belfast, Northern Ireland

Giuseppe Mancia
Clinica Medica e Istituto Auxologico Italiano, Monza, Milano, Italy

Giancarlo Cesana
Research Centre on Public Health, University of Milano Bicocca, Monza, Italy

Kari Kuulasmaa and Veikko Salomaa
National Institute for Health and Welfare (THL), Helsinki, Finland

Susana Sans
Department of Health, Barcelona, Spain

Jean Ferrieres
Department of Cardiology, Toulouse University School of Medicine, Rangueil Hospital, Toulouse, France

Jean Dallongeville
Institut Pasteur de Lille, Lille, France

Stefan Söderberg
Department of Public Health and Clinical Medicine, Cardiology and Heart Centre, Umeå University, Umeå, Sweden

Dominique Arveiler and Aline Wagner
Department of Epidemiology and Public Health, University of Strasbourg, Faculty of Medicine, Strasbourg, France

Hugh Tunstall-Pedoe
Cardiovascular Epidemiology Unit, University of Dundee, Ninewells Hospital and Medical School, Dundee, United Kingdom

Wojciech Drygas
Department of Epidemiology, CVD Prevention and Health Promotion, National Institute of Cardiology, Warsaw, Poland

Michael H. Olsen
Department of Endocrinology, Center of Individualized Medicine in Arterial Diseases (CIMA), Odense University Hospital, Odense, Denmark, and Hypertension in Africa Research Team (HART), North-West University, Potchefstroom, South Africa

Eisuke Amiya, Masafumi Watanabe, Munenori Takata, Atsuko Ozeki, Aya Watanabe, Shuichi Kawarasaki, Tomoko Nakao, Yumiko Hosoya and Issei Komuro
Department of Cardiovascular Medicine, Graduate School of Medicine, The University of Tokyo, Tokyo, Japan

Shogo Watanabe
Department of Cardiovascular Medicine, Graduate School of Medicine, The University of Tokyo, Tokyo, Japan
Department of Pathophysiological Laboratory Sciences, Nagoya University Graduate School of Medicine, Aichi, Japan

Kohzo Nagata
Department of Pathophysiological Laboratory Sciences, Nagoya University Graduate School of Medicine, Aichi, Japan

Ryozo Nagai
Jichi Medical School, Tochigi, Japan

Walter Noordzij, Andor W. Glaudemans, Riemer H. Slart and Rudi A. Dierckx
Department of Nuclear Medicine and Molecular Imaging, University of Groningen, University Medical Center Groningen, Groningen, The Netherlands

André P. van Beek and Anouk N. van der Horst-Schrivers
Department of Endocrinology, University of Groningen, University Medical Center Groningen, Groningen, The Netherlands

René A. Tio
Department of Cardiology, University of Groningen, University Medical Center Groningen, Groningen, The Netherlands

Elisabeth G. de Vries and Annemiek M. Walenkamp
Department of Medical Oncology, University of Groningen, University Medical Center Groningen, Groningen, The Netherlands

Bram van Ginkel
Faculty of Medicine, University of Groningen, University Medical Center Groningen, Groningen, The Netherlands

Chang-Hoon Lee
Department of Internal Medicine, Seoul National University College of Medicine, Seoul, Republic of Korea

Bo Kyung Koo
Department of Internal Medicine, Seoul National University College of Medicine, Seoul, Republic of Korea
Department of Internal Medicine, Boramae Medical Center, Seoul, Republic of Korea

Bo Ram Yang
Division of Clinical Epidemiology, Medical Research Collaborating Center, Seoul National University College of Medicine, Seoul, Republic of Korea
Department of Preventive Medicine, Seoul National University College of Medicine, Seoul, Republic of Korea

Seung-sik Hwang
Department of Social and Preventive Medicine, Inha University School of Medicine, Incheon, Republic of Korea

Nam-Kyong Choi
Division of Clinical Epidemiology, Medical Research Collaborating Center, Seoul National University College of Medicine, Seoul, Republic of Korea
Institute of Environmental Medicine, Seoul National University Medical Research Center, Seoul, Republic of Korea

Josef Yayan
Department of Internal Medicine, Division of Pulmonary, Allergy, and Sleep Medicine, Saarland University Medical Center, Homburg/Saar, Germany

Hui-Chen Cheng and Shui-Mei Lee
Department of Ophthalmology, School of Medicine, National Yang-Ming University, Taipei, Taiwan
Department of Ophthalmology, Taipei Veterans General Hospital, Taipei, Taiwan

Jorn-Hon Liu
Department of Ophthalmology, School of Medicine, National Yang-Ming University, Taipei, Taiwan
Department of Ophthalmology, Taipei Veterans General Hospital, Taipei, Taiwan
Department of Ophthalmology, Cheng Hsin Rehabilitation Medical Center, Taipei, Taiwan

Po-Kang Lin
Department of Ophthalmology, School of Medicine, National Yang-Ming University, Taipei, Taiwan
Department of Ophthalmology, Taipei Veterans General Hospital, Taipei, Taiwan
Graduate Institute of Biomedical Electronics and Bioinformatics, National Taiwan University, Taipei, Taiwan
Biomedical Electronics Translational Research Center, National Chiao Tung University, Hsinchu, Taiwa

Damrus Tresukosol
Division of Cardiology, Department of Internal Medicine, Faculty of Medicine, Siriraj Hospital, Mahidol University, Siriraj, Bangkoknoi, Bangkok, Thailand

Ruttakarn Kamkaew, Saiphon Poldee and Atip Likidlilid
Department of Biochemistry, Faculty of Medicine, Siriraj Hospital, Mahidol University, Siriraj, Bangkoknoi, Bangkok, Thailand

Bhoom Suktitipat
Department of Biochemistry, Faculty of Medicine, Siriraj Hospital, Mahidol University, Siriraj, Bangkoknoi, Bangkok, Thailand
Integrative Computation BioScience Center (ICBS), Mahidol University, Salaya, Nakhon Prathom, Thailand

Saowalak Hunnangkul and Boonrat Tassaneetrithep
Department of Health Research and Development, Faculty of Medicine, Siriraj Hospital, Mahidol University, Siriraj, Bangkoknoi, Bangkok, Thailand

Himanshu Rai, Aditya Kapoor and Sudeep Kumar
Department of Cardiology, Sanjay Gandhi Post Graduate Institute of Medical Sciences, Lucknow, Uttar Pradesh, India

Farah Parveen
Department of Medical Genetics, Sanjay Gandhi Post Graduate Institute of Medical Sciences, Lucknow, Uttar Pradesh, India

Nakul Sinha
Department of Cardiology, Sahara India Medical Institute, Gomti Nagar, Lucknow, Uttar Pradesh, India

Min Da, Yu Feng, Yuanli Hu, Bo Qian and Xuming Mo
Department of Cardiothoracic Surgery, The Affiliated Nanjing Children's Hospital of Nanjing Medical University, Nanjing, Jiangsu, P.R. China

Jing Xu
Department of Thoracic and Cardiovascular Surgery, The First Affiliated Hospital of Nanjing Medical University, Nanjing, Jiangsu, P.R. China

Yuan Lin, Bixian Ni and Zhibin Hu
Department of Epidemiology and Biostatistics, State Key Laboratory of Reproductive Medicine, Nanjing Medical University, Nanjing, Jiangsu, P.R. China

Index